AI in Clinical Medicine

AI in Clinical Medicine

A Practical Guide for Healthcare Professionals

Lead Editor

Michael F. Byrne

Co-editors

Nasim Parsa, Alexandra T. Greenhill, Daljeet Chahal, Omer Ahmad, Ulas Bagci

Editorial Manager

Chrystal Palatý

WILEY Blackwell

Library of Congress Cataloging-in-Publication Data
Names: Byrne, Michael F., editor.
Title: AI in clinical medicine : a practical guide for healthcare
   professionals / lead editor, Michael F. Byrne ; co-editors, Nasim Parsa, Alexandra T. Greenhill, Daljeet Chahal,
   Omer Ahmad, and Ulas Bagci.
Description: Hoboken, NJ : Wiley-Blackwell, 2023. | Includes
   bibliographical references and index.
Identifiers: LCCN 2022045648 | ISBN 9781119790648 (hardback) | ISBN
   9781119790624 (ePDF) | ISBN 9781119790679 (epub) | ISBN 9781119790686
   (oBook)
Subjects: MESH: Artificial Intelligence | Clinical Medicine | Medical
   Informatics
Classification: LCC R859.7.A78 | NLM W 26.55.A7 | DDC
   610.285/63–dc23/eng/20221209
LC record available at https://lccn.loc.gov/2022045648

Cover Design: Wiley
Cover Image: used with the permission of Aidan Meller of the Ai-Da Robot project – www.ai-darobot.com

Set in 11.5/13.5pt STIXTwoText by Straive, Pondicherry, India

Printed in Singapore
M115502_170223

Dedication

I dedicate this book to my beloved parents, Tom and Philomena, who truly nurtured and encouraged me, and genuinely made countless sacrifices to give me the wonderful opportunities in life that I have; to my brother and best friend, Sean, always there for support and laughs; and, of course, to my truly wonderful, patient, supportive, loving, and beautiful wife, Vivian. I hope this book goes some small way to show my gratitude to all of them.

—Michael F. Byrne, Lead Editor

Contents

List of Contributors

Editor Biographies

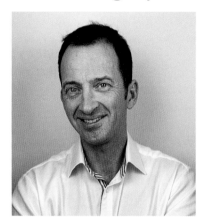

Lead Editor,
Dr Michael F. Byrne

Dr Michael F. Byrne is a Clinical Professor of Medicine in the Division of Gastroenterology, and Director of the Interventional Endoscopy Fellowship programme at Vancouver General Hospital/University of British Columbia.

He is also CEO of Satisfai Health (and founder of ai4gi), a company aiming to deliver precision endoscopy to gastroenterology using artificial intelligence and allied technologies.

Dr Byrne is a graduate of both Cambridge and Liverpool Universities, and trained in advanced endoscopy at Duke University. He holds a doctorate degree from Cambridge University for his molecular science bench research work on *Helicobacter pylori* and Cyclooxygenase.

He is widely regarded as one of the leading physician experts in artificial intelligence as applied to gastroenterology. He is in huge demand as a medical AI reviewer for all the top medical journals, and is frequently described as one of *the* pioneers in bringing AI to gastroenterology and endoscopy.

He has presented at many international conferences, particularly in relation to artificial intelligence and gastroenterology.

He has published over 150 papers in peer-reviewed journals, and over 200 abstracts.

Dr Byrne is a clinical innovator and physician entrepreneur with more than 25 years' experience as a practising physician.

Editorial Team

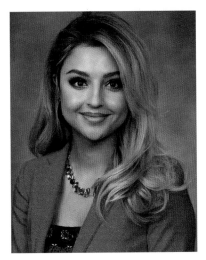

Dr Nasim Parsa

Dr Nasim Parsa is a board-certified gastroenterologist and clinical researcher. She attended Tehran University of Medical Sciences, completed her gastroenterology fellowships at the University of Missouri, and pursued an additional year of training in advanced oesophageal disorders at the Mayo Clinic. She is also the Vice President of Medical Affairs at Satisfai Health Inc., a leading medical solution provider specializing in AI applications in gastroenterology.

Through her work as a clinician and researcher, she has published extensively, with over 30 peer-reviewed publications and over 40 abstract presentations at national and international meetings. She has been an invited reviewer for several prestigious journals, including *Gastroenterology* and *Gastrointestinal Endoscopy*. She is committed to serving her profession, and is currently serving on several GI Society committees, including the Educational Affair Committee for the American College of Gastroenterology (ACG), the Education Committee of the International Society for the Disease of the Esophagus, and the Quality Leadership Council of the American Gastroenterological Association (AGA).

Dr Parsa is passionate about improving patient outcomes through cutting-edge technology and the meaningful implementation of AI in clinical practice. She is the youngest member of the *AI in Clinical Medicine* editorial team, and has made significant editorial contributions to this book.

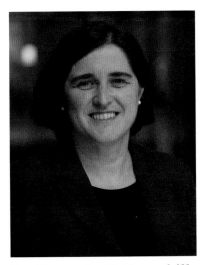

Dr Alexandra T. Greenhill

Dr Alexandra T. Greenhill is one of the leading physicians in health innovation, and the CEO/Chief Medical Officer of Careteam Technologies. After a more than 15-year career in director and C-level leadership roles, she has spent the last few years leading and advising some of the most innovative healthtech companies. She is a TEDx and keynote speaker, has been recognized as one of the Top 40 under 40, Most Influential Women in STEM, and WXN Most Powerful Woman, and has received the Queen Elizabeth II Medal of Service.

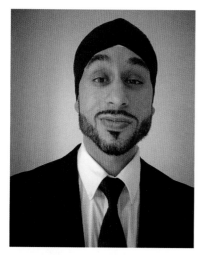

Dr Daljeet Chahal

Dr Daljeet Chahal completed his bachelor's degree at the University of Northern British Columbia, followed by his master's and medical degrees through the University of British Columbia. He completed his internal medicine and gastroenterology training in Vancouver. Dr Chahal is currently completing advanced hepatology training at the Mount Sinai Hospital in New York. He has an interest in applying machine learning technologies to various aspects of clinical medicine, and hopes to incorporate such technologies into his future clinical practice and research endeavors.

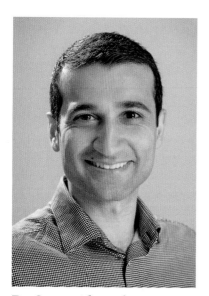

Dr Omer Ahmad

Dr Omer Ahmad is a gastroenterologist and senior clinical research scientist at University College London, with a specialist interest in interventional endoscopy, advanced imaging techniques, and computer vision.

His academic work focused on the clinical translation of artificial intelligence in endoscopy, providing experience across the entire translational pipeline for AI software as a medical device. His pioneering interdisciplinary research at UCL led to the development of AI software for real-time use during colonoscopy, which is currently being used in clinical practice. He was awarded the young clinical and translational scientist of the year by the British Society of Gastroenterology. His specific research interests include identifying barriers to the implementation of artificial intelligence in healthcare. He has published numerous international initiatives related to the effective validation and implementation of AI solutions. He also serves as an expert member on AI working groups for international endoscopy societies and is developing educational programmes to improve foundational knowledge of AI for clinicians.

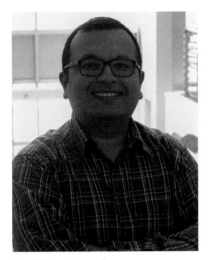

Dr Ulas Bagci

Dr Ulas Bagci is an Associate Professor at Northwestern University's Radiology, ECE, and Biomedical Engineering Departments in Chicago, and Courtesy Professor at the Center for Research in Computer Vision, Department of Computer Science, at the University of Central Florida. His research interests include artificial intelligence, machine learning, and their applications in biomedical and clinical imaging. Dr Bagci has more than 250 peer-reviewed articles in these areas. Previously, he was a staff scientist and lab co-manager at the National Institutes of Health's Radiology and Imaging Sciences Department, and Center for Infectious Diseases Imaging. Dr Bagci holds two NIH R01 grants (as Principal Investigator), and serves as a Steering Committee member of AIR (artificial intelligence resource) at the NIH. He has also served as an area chair for MICCAI for several years, and is an Associate Editor of top-tier journals in his fields such as *IEEE Transactions on Medical Imaging*, *Medical Physics*, and *Medical Image Analysis*. Dr Bagci teaches machine learning, advanced deep learning methods, computer and robot vision, and medical imaging courses. He has several international and national recognitions, including best paper and reviewer awards.

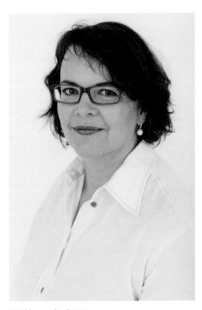

**Editorial Manager –
Dr Chrystal Palatý**

Dr Chrystal Palatý has provided project management and medical writing services to her clients in the medical and health research sectors since founding her company, Metaphase Health Research Consulting Inc. (www.metaphase-consulting.com), in 2007. She earned her PhD in Experimental Medicine from the University of British Columbia, then continued her research with a postdoctoral position in cell cycle control at the University of Toronto, and molecular mechanisms of DNA repair at Toronto's Hospital for Sick Children Research Institute.

AI in Clinical Medicine: A Practical Guide for Healthcare Professionals was her most challenging project to date and also one of the most rewarding. She especially enjoyed working with all the editors and authors.

Alphabetical List of Authors

Aazad Abbas, MD(c)
Temerty Faculty of Medicine,
University of Toronto, Toronto, Canada

Yasmin Abedin, BSc, MBBS, MSc
Computer Science, University College
London, London, UK

Aakanksha Agarwal,
MBBS, MD, DNB
Fellow in Musculoskeletal Radiology,
Department of Radiology, University of
British Columbia, Vancouver,
BC, Canada

Omer F. Ahmad, BSc, MBBS, MRCP
Wellcome EPSRC Centre for
Interventional and Surgical Sciences
(WEISS), University College London,
London, UK

Sharib Ali, MSc, PhD
Lecturer, School of Computing, Faculty
of Engineering and Physical Sciences,
University of Leeds, Leeds, UK

Syed Muhammad Anwar, PhD
University of Engineering and
Technology, Taxila, Pakistan
Sheikh Zayed Institute for Pediatric
Surgical Innovation, Children's National
Hospital, Washington, DC, USA

Charles E. Aunger, MSc, FBCS
Managing Director, Health2047,
Menlo Park, CA, USA

Ulas Bagci
Machine and Hybrid Intelligence Lab,
Department of Radiology, Department
of Biomedical Engineering,
Department of Electrical and
Computer Engineering, Northwestern
University, Chicago, IL, USA

Junaid Bajwa, BSc, MBBS, MRCGP,
MRCS, FRCP, MSc, MBA
Chief Medical Scientist, Microsoft
Research (Global)
Physician, NHS, UK

Judy L. Barkal
Health2047, Menlo Park, CA, USA

Tyler M. Berzin, MD, MS, FASGE
Center for Advanced Endoscopy,
Division of Gastroenterology,
Beth Israel Deaconess Medical Center
and Harvard Medical School,
Boston, MA, USA

Ramin E. Beygui, MD, MSc, FACS
Professor of Surgery, UCSF School of
Medicine, University of California, San
Francisco, CA, USA
Medical Director, Washington
Hospital Healthcare System,
Fremont, CA, USA

Abhishek Bhattarcharya, BA, BS
School of Medicine, University of
Michigan, MI, USA

David Burns MD, PhD
Division of Orthopaedic Surgery,
Department of Surgery, University
of Toronto, Toronto, Canada

Michael F. Byrne, BA, MA, MD
(Cantab), MB, ChB
Clinical Professor of Medicine,
Division of Gastroenterology,
Vancouver General Hospital, The
University of British Columbia,
Vancouver, Canada
CEO and Founder, Satisfai Health,
Vancouver, Canada

Leo Anthony Celi
Institute for Medical Engineering and
Science, Massachusetts Institute
of Technology, Cambridge, MA, USA
Department of Medicine, Beth Israel
Deaconess Medical Center,
Boston, MA, USA
Department of Biostatistics, Harvard
T.H. Chan School of Public Health,
Boston, MA, USA

Dipayan Chaudhuri, MD, FRCPC
Division of Critical Care, Department
of Medicine, McMaster University,
Hamilton, ON, Canada
Department of Health Research
Methods, Evidence and Impact,
McMaster University, Hamilton,
ON, Canada

Jennifer Y. Chen, BA
Department of Dermatology,
University of California,
San Francisco, CA, USA
Dermatology Service, San Francisco
VA Health Care System,
San Francisco, CA, USA

Nolan Chen, BSc
Computer Science and Engineering,
Biology, University of California,
Berkeley, CA, USA

Leonid L. Chepelev, MD,
PhD, FRCPC
Assistant Professor, University of
Toronto, ON, Canada

Lawrence K. Cohen, PhD
Health2047, Menlo Park, CA, USA

Henri Colt, MD, FCCP, FAWM
Emeritus Professor, University
of California, Irvine, CA USA
Certified Affiliate, APPA

Kevin Deasy, BSc, MB, BCh, MRCPI
Clinical Associate, Respiratory
Medicine, Cork University Hospital,
Cork, Ireland

Ugur Demir
Machine and Hybrid Intelligence Lab,
Department of Radiology and
Department of Electrical and Computer
Engineering, Northwestern University,
Chicago, IL, USA

Alastair K. Denniston
College of Medical and Dental
Sciences, University of Birmingham,
Birmingham, UK
Centre for Regulatory Science and
Innovation, Birmingham Health
Partners, University of Birmingham,
Birmingham, UK
National Institute of Health
Research Biomedical Research Centre
for Ophthalmology, Moorfields
Hospital London NHS Foundation
Trust and University College
London, Institute of Ophthalmology,
London, UK
University Hospitals Birmingham
NHS Foundation Trust,
Birmingham, UK

Lakshmi Deshpande
Design Lead at XR Labs, Tata
Consultancy Services, Mumbai, India

Girish Dwivedi, MD, PhD,
FCSANZ, FRACP
Department of Cardiology, Fiona
Stanley Hospital, Murdoch,
WA, Australia
Harry Perkins Institute of Medical
Research, Murdoch, WA, Australia
Medical School, University of
Western Australia, Crawley,
WA, Australia

Alanna Ebigbo
Internal Medicine III, Department of
Gastroenterology and Infectious
Diseases, University Hospital
Augsburg, Augsburg, Germany

Jesse M. Ehrenfeld, MD, MPH,
FAMIA, FASA
Medical College of Wisconsin,
Milwaukee, WI, USA

Rehman Faryal, MBBS
Department of Haematology, Mater
Misericordiae University Hospital,
Dublin, Ireland

Darren Gates, MBChB(Hons),
MRCPCH, DTM&H
Paediatric Intensive Care Consultant
and AI Clinical Lead, Alder Hey
Children's Hospital, Liverpool, UK

Sara Gerke
Assistant Professor of Law, Penn State
Dickinson Law, Carlisle, PA, USA

Nima John Ghadiri, MA, MB, BChir,
MClinEd, MRCP, FHEA
Consultant Medical Ophthalmologist,
University of Liverpool, Liverpool
University Hospitals NHS Foundation
Trust, Liverpool, UK

Adrian Goudie, MBBS, FACEM
Emergency Department, Fiona Stanley
Hospital, Murdoch, Australia

Alexandra T. Greenhill, MD, CCFP
Associate Clinical Professor,
Department of Family Medicine,
University of British Columbia,
Vancouver, Canada
CEO and Chief Medical Officer,
Careteam Technologies,
Vancouver, Canada

Lin Gu, PhD
Researcher Scientist, RIKEN AIP,
Tokyo, Japan
Special Researcher, University of
Tokyo, Tokyo, Japan

Dexter Hadley, MD, PhD
Founding Chief, Division of
Artificial Intelligence
Assistant Professor of Pathology
Departments of Clinical and
Computer Sciences, University of
Central Florida, College of Medicine,
Orlando, FL, USA

Diana Han
College of Medical and Dental
Sciences, University of Birmingham,
Birmingham, UK
Centre for Regulatory Science and
Innovation, Birmingham Health
Partners, University of Birmingham,
Birmingham, UK

Michael Hardisty, PhD
Division of Orthopaedic Surgery,
Department of Surgery, University
of Toronto, Toronto, Canada
Holland Bone and Joint Program,
Sunnybrook Research Institute,
Toronto, Canada

Stephanie Harmon, PhD
Staff Scientist, National Cancer
Institute, National Institutes of Health,
Bethesda, MD, USA

Iain Hennessey, MBChB(Hons),
BSc(Hons), MMIS, FRCS(Paed
Surg), FRSA
Consultant Paediatric Surgeon
and Clinical Director of Innovation,
Alder Hey Children's Hospital,
Liverpool, UK

Dora Huang
Department of Gastroenterology &
Hepatology, Beth Israel Deaconess
Medical Center, Boston, MA, USA

Ismail Irmakci
Machine and Hybrid Intelligence Lab,
Department of Radiology,
Northwestern University,
Chicago, IL, USA

Sabeena Jalal, MBBS, MSc, Msc,
Research Fellow, Vancouver General
Hospital, Vancouver, BC, Canada

Vesna Janic, BSc
Satisfai Health, Vancouver, BC, Canada

Junaid Kalia MD, BCMAS
Vice President, VeeMed Inc,
Roseville, CA, USA
Founder, AINeuroCare.com,
Prosper, TX, USA
Neurocritical Care, Stroke and Epilepsy
Specialist

Isaak Kavasidis
Department of Electrical, Electronic
and Computer Engineering, University
of Catania, Catania, Italy

Pearse A. Keane
National Institute of Health Research
Biomedical Research Centre for
Ophthalmology, Moorfields Hospital
London NHS Foundation Trust and
University College London, Institute
of Ophthalmology, London, UK

Elif Keles
Machine and Hybrid Intelligence Lab,
Department of Radiology, Northwestern
University, Chicago, IL, USA

Marcus Kennedy, MD FRCPI FCCP
Interventional Pulmonologist, Cork
University Hospital, Cork, Ireland

Barry Kevane, MB, PhD,
MRCPI, FRCPath
ConwaySPHERE, Conway Institute,
University College Dublin,
Dublin, Ireland
Department of Haematology, Mater
Misericordiae University Hospital,
Dublin, Ireland
School of Medicine, University College
Dublin, Dublin, Ireland

Taimoor Khan, BEng
StarFish Medical, Toronto, ON, Canada

Colm Kirby, MB, BCh BAO, MRCPI
Department of Rheumatology, Tallaght
University Hospital, Dublin, Ireland

Sandeep S. Kohli, MD, FRCPC
Division of Critical Care, Department of
Medicine, Oakville Trafalgar Memorial
Hospital, Oakville, ON, Canada
Assistant Clinical Professor (adjunct),
Department of Medicine, McMaster
University, Hamilton, ON, Canada

Vesela Kovacheva, MD, PHD
Attending Anesthesiologist and
Director of Translational and Clinical
Research, Division of Obstetric
Anesthesia, Department of
Anesthesiology, Perioperative and Pain
Medicine, Brigham and Women's
Hospital, Boston, MA, USA
Assistant Professor of Anesthesia,
Harvard Medical School,
Boston, MA, USA

Xiaoxuan Liu
College of Medical and Dental
Sciences, University of Birmingham,
Birmingham, UK
Centre for Regulatory Science and
Innovation, Birmingham Health
Partners, University of Birmingham,
Birmingham, UK

University Hospitals Birmingham NHS
Foundation Trust, Birmingham, UK

Juan Lu, MPE
Harry Perkins Institute of Medical
Research, Murdoch, WA, Australia
Medical School, University of Western
Australia, Crawley, WA, Australia

Kevin Ma, PhD
Postdoctoral Fellow, National Cancer
Institute, National Institutes of Health,
Bethesda, MD, USA

Brian Mac Namee, PhD, BA (Mod)
School of Computer Science, University
College Dublin, Dublin, Ireland

Lucy Mackillop
Consultant Obstetric Physician, Oxford
University Hospitals NHS Foundation
Trust, Oxford, UK
Chief Medical Officer – Data and
Research, EMIS Group plc, Leeds, UK
Honorary Senior Clinical Lecturer,
Nuffield Department of Women's and
Reproductive Health, University of
Oxford, Oxford, UK

Patricia B. Maguire, PhD, BSc
ConwaySPHERE Research Group,
Conway Institute, University College
Dublin, Dublin, Ireland
School of Biomolecular & Biomedical
Science, University College Dublin,
Dublin, Ireland
UCD Institute for Discovery, University
College Dublin, Dublin, Ireland
AI Healthcare Hub, Institute for
Discovery, University College Dublin,
Dublin, Ireland

Amarpreet Mahil, BSc
Department of Radiology, Vancouver
General Hospital, Vancouver,
BC, Canada

Sam Mathewlynn
Senior Registrar in Obstetrics and
Gynaecology, Oxford University
Hospitals NHS Foundation Trust,
Oxford, UK
Digital Fellow, National Centre for
Maternity Improvement, London, UK

Sherif Mehralivand, MD
Molecular Imaging Branch,
National Institutes of Health,
Bethesda, MD, USA

Helmut Messmann
Internal Medicine III, Department
of Gastroenterology and Infectious
Diseases, University Hospital
Augsburg, Augsburg, Germany

Prasun J. Mishra, PhD
President and Chair, American
Association for Precision Medicine
(AAPM), Belmont, CA, USA
Founder, Agility Pharmaceuticals and
Precision BioPharma Inc.,
Belmont, CA, USA

Mohammed F. Mohammed, MBBS
SB-RAD CIIP, ER/Trauma
Abdominal Imaging and Nonvascular
Intervention Radiologist, Department
of Radiology, King Faisal Specialist
Hospital & Research Center, Riyadh,
Saudi Arabia

Grainne Murphy, MB, BCh BAO,
PhD, MRCPI
Department of Rheumatology, Cork
University Hospital, Cork, Ireland

Lisa Murphy BSc, MBChB, MSc
Senior Policy Manager, NHS England
Centre for Improving Data
Collaboration, London, UK

Timothy É. Murray, MB, MCh, MBA, MRCS, FFR, FRCPC, EBIR
Diagnostic and Interventional Radiologist, Department of Radiology, St. Paul's Hospital, Vancouver, BC, Canada
Clinical Assistant Professor, Department of Radiology, University of British Columbia, Vancouver, BC, Canada

Fionnuala Ní Áinle, MB, PhD, MRCPI, FRCPath
ConwaySPHERE, Conway Institute, University College Dublin, Dublin, Ireland
School of Medicine, University College Dublin, Dublin, Ireland
Department of Haematology, Mater Misericordiae University Hospital and Rotunda Hospital, Dublin, Ireland

Dr Savvas Nicolaou, MD, FRCPC
Professor, University of British Columbia, Vancouver, BC, Canada
Department of Radiology, Vancouver General Hospital, Vancouver, BC, Canada

Zachary O'Brien
Australian and New Zealand Intensive Care Research Centre, Department of Epidemiology and Preventive Medicine, Monash University, Melbourne, VIC, Australia
Department of Critical Care, University of Melbourne, Melbourne, VIC, Australia

Jesutofunmi A. Omiye, MD
Stanford University School of Medicine, Stanford, CA, USA

Simone Palazzo
Department of Electrical, Electronic and Computer Engineering, University of Catania, Catania, Italy

Christoph Palm, Dipl.-Inform.
Regensburg Medical Image Computing (ReMIC), Ostbayerische Technische Hochschule Regensburg (OTH Regensburg), Regensburg, Germany

Maryam Panahiazar, PhD, MSc
Bioinformatics, Computer Science and Engineering, University of California, San Francisco, CA, USA

L. Eric Pulver, DDS, FRCD(C), Dip
Oral & Maxillofacial Surgery
Chief Dental Officer, Denti.AI Technology Inc., Toronto, ON, Canada
Adjunct clinical faculty, Indiana University Dental School, Indianapolis, IN, USA

Sarah Quidwai, MB, BCh BAO, MRCPI
Department of Rheumatology, Tallaght University Hospital, Dublin, Ireland

Krishan Ramdoo
Tympa Health Technologies Ltd, London, UK
Division of Surgery and Interventional Sciences, University College London, London, UK
Royal Free Hospital, London, UK

Harish RaviPrakash
AstraZeneca, Waltham, MA, USA

Jesús Rogel-Salazar
Tympa Health Technologies Ltd, London, UK
Blackett Laboratory, Department of Physics, Imperial College London, London, UK
Department of Physics, Astronomy and Mathematics, School of Physics, Engineering and Computer Science, University of Hertfordshire, Hatfield, UK

Elsie G. Ross, MD, MSc
Division of Vascular Surgery, Stanford
University School of Medicine,
Stanford, CA, USA

Gagandeep Sachdeva
College of Medical and Dental
Sciences, University of Birmingham,
Birmingham, UK

Federica Proietto Salanitri
Department of Electrical, Electronic
and Computer Engineering, University
of Catania, Catania, Italy

Matt Schwartz
Chief Executive Officer, Virgo Surgical
Video Solutions, Inc.,
Carlsbad, CA, USA

Mark A. Shapiro, MA, MBA
Chief Operating Officer, xCures, Inc.,
Oakland, CA, USA

Adnan Sheikh, MD FRCPC
Professor, University of British
Columbia, Vancouver, BC, Canada

Helen Simons, MEng
StarFish Medical, Victoria, BC, Canada

Concetto Spampinato
Department of Electrical, Electronic
and Computer Engineering, University
of Catania, Catania, Italy

Jonathon Stewart, MBBS,
MMed(CritCare)
Emergency Department, Fiona Stanley
Hospital, Murdoch, WA, Australia
Harry Perkins Institute of Medical
Research, Murdoch, WA, Australia
Medical School, University of Western
Australia, Crawley, WA, Australia

Jack W. Stockert, MD, MBA
Health2047, Menlo Park, CA, USA

Ian Strug
Chief Customer Officer, Virgo Surgical
Video Solutions, Inc.,
Carlsbad, CA, USA

Siddharthan Surveswaran, PhD
Department of Life Sciences, CHRIST
(Deemed to be University),
Bangalore, India

Akshay Swaminathan, BA
Stanford University School of
Medicine, Stanford, CA, USA

Paulina B. Szklanna, PhD, BSc
ConwaySPHERE, Conway Institute,
University College Dublin,
Dublin, Ireland
School of Biomolecular & Biomedical
Science, University College Dublin,
Dublin, Ireland
AI Healthcare Hub, Institute for
Discovery, University College Dublin,
Dublin, Ireland

Marty Tenenbaum, PhD, FAAAI
Chairman, Cancer Commons,
Mountain View, CA, USA

Jay Toor MD, MBA
Division of Orthopaedic Surgery,
Department of Surgery, University of
Toronto, Toronto, Canada

Baris Turkbey, MD
Molecular Imaging Branch, National
Institutes of Health, Bethesda,
Maryland, USA

Dmitry Tuzoff
Founder and CEO, Denti.AI
Technology Inc., Toronto,
ON, Canada
PhD researcher, Steklov Institute of
Mathematics, St Petersburg, Russia

Lyudmila Tuzova
Co-founder and lead researcher,
Denti.AI Technology Inc., Toronto,
ON, Canada
MSc student, Georgia Institute of
Technology, Atlanta, GA, USA

Niels van Berkel, PhD
Department of Computer Science,
Aalborg University, Aalborg, Denmark

Trent Walradt, MD
Department of Internal Medicine, Beth
Israel Deaconess Medical Center,
Harvard Medical School,
Boston, MA, USA

Maria L. Wei, MD, PhD
Professor, Department of Dermatology,
University of California, San
Francisco, CA, USA
Dermatology Service, San Francisco VA
Health Care System, San
Francisco, CA, USA

Luisa Weiss, PhD, MSc, BSc
ConwaySPHERE, Conway Institute,
University College Dublin,
Dublin, Ireland
School of Biomolecular & Biomedical
Science, University College Dublin,
Dublin, Ireland

Jason Yao, MD
McMaster University, Hamilton,
ON, Canada

Albert T. Young, MD, MAS
Department of Dermatology, Henry
Ford Hospital, Detroit, MI, USA

Shu Min Yu, BSc
Department of Radiology, Vancouver
General Hospital, Vancouver,
BC, Canada

Foreword

Ten years ago, the technology world was fascinated with *SMAC*. The perfect storm of social networks, mobile computing, analytics, and cloud computing seemed to be happening all at once. Facebook would soon go public. The iPad and iPhone had captured the world's imagination, a wonderful, keyboard-free device with more power than the supercomputers of the 1990s. Cloud computing had just begun, scoffed at by many, but growing fast. Companies everywhere were beginning to apply analytics at scale, reimagining themselves as digital natives. SMAC. Social, Mobile, Analytics, and Cloud. What could *possibly* be next?

That summer two papers were released, in seemingly different domains.

- Geoffrey Hinton et al. published 'ImageNet classification with deep convolutional neural networks', a breakthrough in AI that demonstrated how computers could actually *see*. His software combined the power of video game consoles (graphics processing units or GPUs) with recent advances in analytics and cloud computing, creating the first AI that could correctly identify over 1000 different items from millions of images. Hinton and his peers ignited a Cambrian explosion of computer systems that could perceive.
- Jennifer Doudna et al. published 'A programmable dual-RNA–guided DNA endonuclease in adaptive bacterial immunity', which to me demonstrated the human ability to modify the programming of biological cells. Jennifer and her team could not only read the source code of life, their biological apparatus could now *change* it. A universe of possibilities opened up, forever changing genomics, medicine, and biology.

As I write this Foreword today, kids in elementary school are dancing to TikTok videos, where video 'filters' change their appearance in hilarious ways. These filters implement a far more sophisticated version of Hinton's algorithm, now running on mobile phones. The Pinocchio of my youth now appears as realistic long noses in videos of their parents at a family dining table, with kids giggling in delight.

Biology students are regularly reading the DNA of strawberries, using hand-held sequencers with the same power of the larger machines Doudna had in her lab. Astronauts are sequencing their blood on the space station, a prelude to precision medicine and the world's best care for adventurers that take an eight-month trip to Mars on SpaceX rockets.

These powerful technologies amplify who we are as humans, and portend a truly exciting future. We can now build computers that see, hear, taste, and feel, then describe what they perceive in human terms. We're beginning to understand the source code of life, and from that detect cancers and wellness transitions, far earlier and in less invasive ways than today's biopsies and mammograms.

That's both exciting – but also unnerving. Humans must make assumptions about the world to function properly. Our *reticular focus* subconsciously filters signals that bombard our everyday senses, allowing us to focus on what *we think* matters. That inherent and often hidden bias is crucial for proper use of our neocortex.

We've all experienced this phenomenon. Having a baby? Suddenly, you see babies, baby carriages, and pregnant women seemingly everywhere. Looking to buy a new car? Your favourite car seems to appear at all your favorite spots.

These activities, of course, were always there. We just weren't paying attention.

That brings me to this wonderful book, either a heavy, thick tome in your hands at home, or perhaps on a mobile phone that you're reading at 30,000 feet on a flight.

Michael F. Byrne, lead editor of this book, has an incredible skill for finding humans from all walks of life, brilliant and accomplished in their own way, and inspiring them to contribute for the collective good. He found me speaking at a conference on AI and gastroenterology in San Diego, one foggy afternoon in May of 2022. I've been in AI for over 30 years – starting when it 'didn't work' back at MIT to today, where I've been leading a team at Google of Applied AI in precision medicine and science. If you've met Michael, you'll know he's hard to turn down!

In this book you'll dive into such fun topics as the history of AI, the use of machine vision to detect polyps, or machines that can interpret and process clinical notes. My brother hopes all this work can lead to the elimination of keyboards in medical offices, 'zero clicks', using technology to give everyone more valuable time with patients.

Hold on to this book. Meet the authors, reach out to them on LinkedIn, seek them at conferences or in your daily work. You all form a community collective. Realize that we all have a reticular focus. Only together can we perceive the proverbial elephant in the room. AI is truly a team sport, where diversity of thought, perception, and background is *required* by human biology and science.

Michael's collection of brilliant, accomplished authors are the seed of a broader community that will redefine clinical practice in medicine, powered by AI and the source code of life. As a reader, you too can contribute, and I strongly encourage you to reach out.

How do we ensure that AI is treated in an ethical way? What sort of projects are meaningful and worthy of our time, and which should we avoid? How do humans and AI effectively collaborate for better patient outcomes? Working together, we all see what's truly out there, the bigger picture, the classic three blind humans perceiving the elephant. We need to. By overlapping our assumptions and rooting out unfair bias, we can build truly wonderful systems and science.

To the authors of this book, the editors, and especially to Michael, thank you for diving in, taking the time to think carefully about AI and how it can change the field of medicine. I'm excited to see what this community will achieve together in the next decade. Your diversity of thought is paramount to advancing the state of the art, protecting and ensuring healthy lives for millions of patients, now and for centuries to come.

Read on. Your journey has just begun.

Scott Penberthy
Director of Applied AI, Google

Preface

Michael F. Byrne

Why This Book, Why Now?

When I was approached by the publisher, Wiley, at a large gastroenterology conference in San Diego over two years ago, it was not immediately clear to me that this would quickly morph from a commitment to lead a book on AI in my field of gastroenterology to a significantly bigger undertaking – namely, leading a book for AI in the entire field of clinical medicine! After the initial consternation about this decision, my excitement grew week by week as my support team came together and the writing started in earnest.

With the book beginning to take some initial shape, my enthusiasm sky-rocketed as it was abundantly clear to me that now, more than at any time in the history of AI in medicine, we truly needed a practical guide in this field. The speed of development and adoption of AI in clinical medicine has increased so much since I took on this project that I became totally convinced that we were doing something very necessary and timely. I sincerely hope that this book does not disappoint.

The Promise of AI in Clinical Medicine

Artificial intelligence is an overarching term used to describe the use of machine learning algorithms and software. In healthcare applications, AI mimics human cognition in the analysis, presentation, and comprehension of complex data, such as in medical imaging.

AI is a rapidly growing technology, involving much of what we do day to day, from the smart devices on our wrists to the virtual library we access online. We are, rightly, seeing AI applications and advancement in clinical medicine. In the last few years, deep learning techniques and data availability have resulted in an explosion of applications/potential applications of AI to the whole of clinical medicine. We are moving ahead in our applications for radiology, pathology, dermatology, endoscopy, surgery, robotics, drug discovery, and more. It's not a matter of when anymore: we are already living in the AI age, and we can expect and celebrate that AI is increasingly being applied for medical purposes to address some of our biggest clinical challenges.

For this reason, physicians across the entire healthcare spectrum and at all stages of their careers need to have at least a basic appreciation of the AI tools that are already in use in clinical medicine, and a knowledge base to grasp those that come down the pike. We wrote this book for inquisitive pre-med or medical students, graduate-level students, practising physicians, academics, and nursing and allied health professionals – basically, everyone involved in healthcare. The content includes information that is understandable for the clinician who wants to integrate and apply this knowledge to improve patient care. This book is also valuable for those already in the medical AI space, including entrepreneurs and those who are developing clinical tools, as well as regulatory/policy/political personnel involved in digital health.

Our goal was that *AI in Clinical Medicine: A Practical Guide for Healthcare Professionals* would become the definitive reference book for the emerging and exciting use of AI throughout clinical medicine. This book:

- Describes where AI is currently being used to change practice in specific medical domains.
- Discusses the applicability of AI, and provides successful cases of AI approaches in the setting of specific specialties.
- Addresses some of the unique challenges associated with AI in clinical medicine.
- Includes bulleted lists of
  - Learning objectives.
  - Key insights.
  - Clinical vignettes (where appropriate).
  - Brief examples of where AI is successfully deployed.
  - Brief examples of potential problematic uses of AI, and possible risks or issues.

The background artwork on the front cover was created by Ai-da, the world's first ultra-realistic artist robot. I was keen to bring some art to this book, as the practice of medicine is an art as well as a science. In my opinion, this will not and should not change as we incorporate some of the AI solutions described in this book to our clinical practice. I will quote Aidan Meller, creative director and project manager for the Ai-da robot project, as his words say much better what I am trying to say!

> *Today, a dominant opinion is that art is created by the human, for other humans. This has not always been the case. The ancient Greeks felt art and creativity came from the Gods. Inspiration was divine inspiration. Today, a dominant mind-set is that of humanism, where art is an entirely human affair, stemming from human agency. However, current thinking suggests we are edging away from humanism, into a time where machines and algorithms influence our behaviour to a point where our 'agency' isn't just our own. It is starting to get outsourced to the decisions and suggestions of algorithms, and complete human autonomy starts to look less robust. Ai-Da creates art, because art no longer has to be restrained by the requirement of human agency alone. (Aidan Meller,*
> www.aidanmeller.com)

We know that we have some readers who are fearful and apprehensive about the advent of AI in clinical medicine. Our hope is that this book reassures them about the future role of AI and the interplay with clinicians. Other readers are excitedly anticipating that, once implemented, AI will take over all aspects of their jobs. The messages in our book may disappoint them. This book, for the most part, presents a realistic vision of where AI is used now, and where it is most likely to go.

What We Didn't Cover in This Edition

This book will not present exhaustive detail of the history, development, or technical foundations of AI, nor delve into really niche areas of AI in clinical practice. As there are already many other general AI resources available, the book will not explore in great detail the different AI models, the different types and details of neural networks, AI in statistical learning, AI for general clinical data analysis, AI for genomics, or AI for drug discovery.

We were simply unable to cover every aspect of clinical medicine to which AI applies or can apply. We can only direct our readers to online publications in these areas, and we hope to include these topics in future editions of this book.

How This Book Is Organized

The book contains four sections. The idea is that you can dip in and out of each section as you need to.

- *Section 1*. This short section gives readers the basic vocabulary that they require and a framework for thinking about AI, and highlights the importance of robust AI training for physicians.
- *Section 2*. AI Foundations covers foundational ideas and concepts. This includes the history of AI, and chapters on the basics and a deeper dive into some of the definitions used in AI.
- *Section 3*. Applications to different clinical areas provide a discipline-specific deep dive into how AI is applied in that given area. Specialties overlap to a certain degree, so most readers will be interested in at least two or three of those chapters. Readers can select the chapters they want without having to read everything in this section. The chapters are not hyper-specialized, but do represent a 101 level that will equip readers with what they need to be able to explore further by reading more specialized books and published medical articles in that domain.
- *Section 4*. On emerging trends and applications of AI in medicine in the future, this section addresses some of the wider issues, challenges, and solutions with regard to AI. This includes issues related to the evolution of AI regulation, data privacy legislation, and AI-enabled consumer-facing health technology. The section discusses challenges with bias, consent, and ethical

use of data, as well as the design, validation, and testing of algorithms, and implementation issues. It includes applications and insights in relation to AI in medicine in the future, those that are undecided, awaiting approval, being developed, or being envisaged. This is a section for content that builds on the first three, and is meant for more advanced consideration of how AI is and will be used in medicine, how to prepare for all the possibilities, and how to get involved in shaping the directions and decisions for the evolution of AI.

In addition to recommendations for further reading, many of our authors have included longer lists of references. These are available online at www.wiley.com/go/byrne/aiinclinicalmedicine.

Acknowledgements

Covid-19 changed the way that we work and live. We wish to first acknowledge the large team of influential, international experts ranging from AI developers to globally leading medical specialists who diligently wrote this book during a challenging time for humanity. Our authors represent countries from all over the planet – too many countries to mention individually! They come from many different backgrounds and different environments, and they have generously shared their abundant and insightful perspectives on AI in clinical medicine. They prioritized our book at a time when healthcare personnel and resources were already spread thinly, and when they were overstretched during multiple waves of the pandemic. We sincerely thank all of our authors.

The support and hard work of our editorial team were essential on this long road. I want to personally thank Nasim Parsa for her exceptional edits to many of the chapters; Alexandra Greenhill for her inspirational guidance and her senior leadership; Dal Chahal for quick responses, total dedication, and for being the nicest guy ever; Omer Ahmad for insightful comments, quirky humour, and for bringing his influential network; and, last but not least, Ulas Bagci for being at my side right from the beginning of this project, and playing a significant role in getting this book off the ground.

I wish to thank my friends and collaborators, Mike Galvin and Brian Isaac, at Bammai. They supplied a lot of the fuel for this project by way of endless enthusiasm, and invaluable contacts. They also provided the Handzin collaboration platform, which was essential during the early days of this project, and allowed us all to connect even when other social media platforms went down.

I also want to express my gratitude to my physician colleagues in my Gastroenterology group at Vancouver General Hospital and the University of British Columbia for understanding why I was often unavailable for other academic endeavours during this book editing.

Thank you to my colleagues at my medical AI start-up, Satisfai Health, who recognized the importance of this project to me and to the field in general. They gave me time and resources to pursue this book. I hope that this contribution to the area reflects well on them.

A solid thank you to Chrystal Palatý, PhD, our managing editor, and her team of English language editing experts. Chrystal managed to juggle 105 authors, 46 chapters, and 6 editors and delivered an occasional reprimand or two to keep us all in order! Thank you to Jenny Boon from Capricorn Communications and Jenn Currie from JC Consulting, for their hard work as lay-readers and copy-editors, and for their gentle advice on how to make these chapters more reader friendly for our audience. Thank you to Dr. Shirley Jiang and Aishwi Roshan for their work as medical lay-readers, helping to further improve some of the chapters.

As you may have noticed, I have dedicated this book to my family, which of course includes my wife, Vivian. Over the duration of this project, Vivian and I dated, fell in love, and got married. Throughout this time, she has been my biggest supporter, and her endless patience and sense of humour have allowed me to work on this venture with a smile on my face, at least sometimes!

To our valued partners at Wiley – James Watson, Kerry Powell, Ella Elliot, and all others who helped us finalize this book – a very big thank-you.

While this book is global in scope, I would like to gratefully acknowledge that I personally live and work in Vancouver, BC, Canada, on the traditional, ancestral, and unceded territory of the Coast Salish peoples – Sḵwx̱wú7mesh (Squamish), Stó:lō and Səl̓ílwətaʔ/Selilwitulh (Tsleil-Waututh), and xʷməθkʷəy̓əm (Musqueam) Nations. I also was fortunate enough to spend a fair bit of time in beautiful Whistler working on this book. Whistler is located on the unceded territories of the Lil'wat Nation and Squamish Nation who have lived on those lands since time immemorial.

Cover Acknowledgement

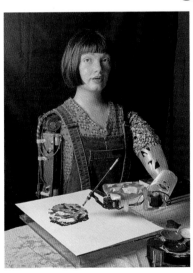

Ai-Da is the world's first ultra-realistic artist robot. Created in February 2019, she had her first solo show at the University of Oxford, called *Unsecured Futures*. She has since travelled and exhibited work internationally, and shown at many major museums. She continues to create art that challenges our notions of living in a post-humanist era. More information at www.ai-darobot.com.

Relevant AI Terms

Activation function: A mathematical function that defines if a neuron is activated or not, contributing to the output of that neuron.

Active learning: A training strategy where algorithms can proactively select and prioritize unlabelled data for learning, thereby maximizing model performance.

Adaptive vs locked algorithms: Locked algorithms provide the same output each time the same input is received. Adaptive algorithms, for example continuous learning algorithms, change behaviour using a defined learning process.

AI winters: Overwhelming AI promises that have resulted in disappointments time and again.

Artificial general intelligence: Artificial intelligence that can understand or learn any task that a human can.

Artificial narrow intelligence: Artificial intelligence that is designed to perform a limited or specific task.

Artificial neural networks: A computational system that is loosely inspired by neurons in the biological brain.

Augmentation bias: A situation whereby humans over-rely on automation, blindly accepting automated decisions and disregarding contradictory information.

Backpropagation: A method for training neural network algorithms where the input is fed into the model, an initial prediction is made and compared against the desired output decision, and the difference (error) is then propagated back through the neural network to update the weights of the model in order to reduce the error.

Batch normalization: A technique to train deeper neural networks faster, and to provide a more stable learning process. Mini-batches of a full dataset are used, for which re-centering and re-scaling processes are conducted.

Classifier: An algorithm that predicts a categorical variable, e.g. a type of cancer.

Closed-loop system: A system in which AI-determined interventions would be implemented autonomously.

Clustering analysis: A statistical technique where observations are grouped based on the similarity observed in several variables of interest. It is very useful in exploratory data analysis.

Continual learning: This technique allows neural network models to continuously learn and evolve based on the input from the increasing amounts of data dynamically while retaining previously learnt features.

Convolutional neural network (CNN): A type of neural network that is often used with images and time-series data. It is composed of a layer structure. One type of layer used in these networks is the convolutional layer. The convolutional layers contain trainable filters that filter input data, creating feature map outputs that, when combined with other structures, can be used to perform many tasks (detection, segmentation, classification).

Cross-validation: A technique used to repeatedly split samples into training and validation sets during the model training. In this way, the model sees all data. This technique is generally used when limited data samples are present. The process creates 'folds' or 'partitions' of data samples.

Data augmentation: A technique to increase the number of training data samples by adding slightly modified copies, for example by adding different colours or rotating images in the case of imaging data samples.

Data dimensionality: The number of variables (columns) in a dataset. The higher the dimensionality, the more samples (rows) are needed to train the algorithm.

Data normalization: Rescaling of data within a common range (for example, 0–1). This is an essential step in the learning process and can be considered part of data preparation.

Data preparation: A major step that includes data collection, cleaning (removing noisy data), structuring, and enriching raw data into a desired output for model training.

Deep learning: Multi-layer artificial neural networks with input and output layers, and hidden layers composed of linear and non-linear modules.

Domain adaptation: Training a model on a source data distribution (also known as the 'source domain') that has labels, such that it tackles the domain shift problem by leveraging partially labelled or unlabelled target data samples (different distribution, or 'target domain'). For example, using the trained model on computed tomography data with some magnetic resonance images (MRI) to enable disease diagnosis on unlabelled MRI data.

Domain generalization: Incorporating knowledge from multiple source data distributions (also known as the 'source domain') into a single model that can then generalize on unseen samples coming from a different distribution, or 'target domain'.

Dropout layers: Randomly selecting and switching off some neurons (i.e. set input to 0). This helps to prevent overfitting on training samples. It is not applied during validation or testing stages.

Edge-case scenarios: Rare occurrences that an AI algorithm has not encountered in training data.

Edge computing: Computation that is performed locally or near the data source.

Ensemble technique: Combining several model predictions to produce an optimal prediction. For example, using three different neural network models and taking the output that is repeated in two of the models (i.e. highest voting, referred to as a *max-voting* approach).

Epoch: Training a neural network with all training samples makes an epoch. An epoch can have one or more mini-batches.

Expert-in-the-loop system: A system where clinicians retain control of final decisions regarding patient care.

Explainable artificial intelligence (XAI) or interpretable deep learning: Methods that allow humans to understand and interpret predictions made by AI models.

Federated learning: A method used to train AI models, using data from multiple locations, without the data being transferred outside of the original location.

Fine tuning: Utilizing the trained model weights as initialization for the model training on new data samples. This is a good practice as it speeds up the training process, and overcomes the problem of a small dataset.

Forward pass: Calculation and storage of intermediate weights in an order between the input layer and the output layer.

Frequency domain: An analysis of signals or mathematical functions, in reference to frequency instead of time.

Fully connected networks: Neural networks that are composed of a series of layers with neurons (nodes) in each layer that are connected to every neuron in the adjacent layers.

Generalization: The ability of a trained model to make predictions on new unseen data.

Ground truth: A reference standard.

Hidden layer: A layer in between the input and output layers of a neural network, where a weighted set of inputs is taken to produce an output through an activation function.

High-dimensional data: A dataset in which the number of features, p, is larger than the number of observations, N, often written as $p >> N$. For example, high-dimensional data is common in healthcare datasets where the number of features for a given individual can be massive (blood pressure, resting heart rate, immune system status, surgical history, height, weight, existing conditions, etc.). In these datasets, it is common for the number of features to be larger than the number of observations (https://www.statology.org/high-dimensional-data).

Hyperparameters: Parameters that control the learning process and can affect the learnt outcome (for example, learning rate, number of neurons, number of epochs). Often hyperparameters need to be tuned in order to obtain optimal results.

ImageNet: A large dataset of annotated images that are used for computer vision research.

Iteration: One complete forward pass and backward pass (backpropagation).

Learning rate: A rate that needs to be optimized, usually in an incremental step-wise fashion, via trial and error.

Logistic regression: A statistical model to determine the probability of a discrete outcome given an input variable.

Loss function: A mathematical function that compares the output generated by neural networks with the expected outcome. Generally, the loss function needs to be minimized.

Natural language processing: The area of study concerned with processing and analysing human language; this includes speech recognition, language understanding, and generating language.

Neuron: Similar to a biological neuron, in that it computes a weighted average of its inputs and passes this along to other neurons.

Non-neural algorithm: Machine learning algorithms other than artificial neural networks (e.g. logistic regression, random forest, etc.). Also referred to as classical algorithms.

Open imaging datasets: Repositories of imaging data that are accessible to the public and researchers.

Optimization: Adjusting a set of weights to effectively minimize a loss function during training.

Out-of-distribution (OOD) detection: A machine learning classifier's ability to identify instances where a new class (one not in the training set) is encountered.

Output layer: The last layer of a neural network that produces the result.

Overfitting: When the model learns the training set data distribution exhaustively, and cannot generalize.

Performance metrics: Values that tell you how well your model has learnt to give a desirable output (for example, accuracy) on held-out data samples.

Recurrent neural network: An artificial neural network that works for time-series data or data involving sequences.

Reinforcement learning: A type of learning in AI that allows an agent to learn in an interactive environment by trial and error using feedback from its own actions.

Sample and label: Supervised learning requires raw data and ground truth (a label assigned by an expert). In the example of a cancer lesion observed in a colonoscopy, validated from biopsy results, the sample refers to the image and the label refers to the biopsy finding assigned to the image.

Self-supervised learning: A technique that uses self-made simple tasks without requiring labels as pretext (for example, finding self-made rotation angles, or solving a puzzle by shuffling the input sample). This allows models to learn rich feature representations that can then be used for task-specific training (for example, classifying tumours) with fewer data, or even improve the performance of a model in a supervised setting.

Stopping criteria: A defined threshold for when to discontinue model training to avoid overfitting.

Testing dataset: An independent data sample that has a similar probability distribution to the training dataset but is *not used during the training process*. The objective is to allow the model to generalize using these previously unseen data samples.

Time-series data: Collection of data points or observations that is amassed over an interval of time.

Training dataset: Data samples used to train a machine learning model for outcome prediction.

Transfer learning: A process where a model that has already been pre-trained on a dataset is used again as a starting point for a model on a different task. This is a good practice as it speeds up the training process and overcomes the problem of small datasets.

Transformers: A type of neural network that utilizes self-attention mechanisms, weighting the significance of different parts of the input data.

Underfitting: A model not capable of learning the distribution of the data.

Validation dataset: Data samples used to understand the learning process during training. The validation dataset permits tuning of hyperparameters, and helps to determine if the training process should be stopped. Validation datasets generally use 10–20% of samples.

About the Companion Website

This book is accompanied by a companion website.

www.wiley.com/go/byrne/aiinclinicalmedicine

This website includes:

- Figures from the book for downloading
- Additional chapter end further readings
- Additional chapter end references

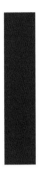

Overview of Medical AI: The What, the Why, and the How

1

An Introduction to AI for Non-Experts

Sharib Ali[1] and Michael F. Byrne[2,3]

[1] *School of Computing, Faculty of Engineering and Physical Sciences, University of Leeds, Leeds, UK*

[2] *Division of Gastroenterology, Vancouver General Hospital, The University of British Columbia, Vancouver, Canada*

[3] *Satisfai Health, Vancouver, Canada*

Learning Objectives

- Introduce the terms 'AI' and 'machine learning'.
- Understand key ideas and concepts of machine learning, including widely used machine learning strategies.
- Describe how to get started in AI and learn about the pitfalls to avoid while training your first machine learning model.

1.1 Introduction

Artificial intelligence was conceptualized in the first half of the twentieth century, with the term 'AI' coined at Dartmouth College in 1956. Due to high costs and technical limitations such as limited computer memory, AI research during this period was difficult. However, from 1957 to 1974, AI research began to flourish due to improving computational capabilities, such as increased storage and faster processing speeds. Advances in data storage and processing technologies have continued over time and contribute largely to the progress of AI research that we are currently witnessing in the twenty-first century.

In simple terms, AI refers to the ability of computers to perform tasks that usually require human intelligence – for example, the ability to examine an X-ray image to identify areas consistent with pathology, such as a fracture. AI is an umbrella term that comprises any system or methodologies that demonstrate such ability. AI includes explicitly programmed mathematical models (for example, automated car parking based on line identification and alignment) and data-driven models (for example, learning from data to predict weather without strictly programmed conditions).

Machine learning is a subset of AI that uses statistical learning algorithms to interpret and learn from data to predict future events. Examples of machine learning in our daily lives include Netflix recommendations based on what we watch, or a Google search engine that prioritizes search results based on the keywords provided.

AI in Clinical Medicine: A Practical Guide for Healthcare Professionals, First Edition. Edited by Michael F. Byrne, Nasim Parsa, Alexandra T. Greenhill, Daljeet Chahal, Omer Ahmad, and Ulas Bagci.
© 2023 John Wiley & Sons Ltd. Published 2023 by John Wiley & Sons Ltd.
Companion website: www.wiley.com/go/byrne/aiinclinicalmedicine

In this chapter we will focus on understanding key ideas and concepts of machine learning, strategies that are widely used, key ingredients of neural networks, how to get started, and some pitfalls that are important to avoid while training your first successful machine learning model.

1.2 Machine Learning

Machine learning uses algorithms to analyse and interpret data, and to make intelligent decisions based on the learnt understanding of the features present in provided data. While traditional machine learning requires pre-defined features of interest (for example, shape of tumour, size of tumour, heterogeneity etc., derived by some mathematical or statistical function) to understand the data and infer a decision, modern machine learning techniques, also known as neural networks (NN), can automatically determine which features are important. Multiple decision nodes, commonly referred to as neurons, can be stacked in the same mathematical layer or in multiple layers, with each neuron having some non-linear activation functions (simple maths functions that can switch a neuron 'on' or 'off') that help it learn complex features representative of the provided data samples (for example, patterns in data samples that mathematical models cannot define; see Figure 1.1). Traditional machine learning algorithms can be trained using fewer data samples, as compared to NNs that require large data samples for training. Machine learning algorithms are first developed using a 'training' dataset, and their validity is then usually confirmed by evaluating the algorithms using a separate dataset, also known as the 'testing' dataset. The goal is to ensure that the algorithm is generalizable and applicable to various data.

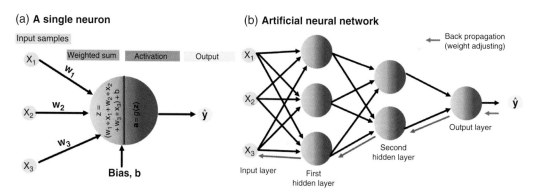

Figure 1.1: One layered neural network, and an artificial neural network. (a) A single neuron process is illustrated. Input samples are multiplied with learnable weights and summed. A constant value (bias, b, usually set to zero) is added. An activation function is then used to add non-linearity that allows the network to learn complex features. (b) Artificial neural network with multiple neurons in each layer and concatenated to other layers between the input and the output. Backpropagation for the learning process is shown by red arrows pointing backwards, while forward black arrows represent a forward pass (i.e. weights are added and stored at each layer). Figure created by Dr Sharib Ali.

1.3 Strategies to Train Algorithms

Four strategies are widely used in training machine learning solutions that vary by the amount and type of supervision involved, as shown in Figure 1.2:

- *Supervised learning.* The training data consist of samples and associated desired outputs, known as 'labels'. For example, data with X-ray images with labels 'pneumonia' (say, class 1) and 'no pneumonia' (say, class 0) are provided for training a model, which is then used to classify a new X-ray image as either 0 or 1.
- *Semi-supervised learning.* Only some of the samples in the training data have labels, while many samples are unlabelled.
- *Unsupervised learning.* The training data do not have labels, so the machine learning model tries to learn without explicit instruction, looking only at learnt features. Some examples are clustering approaches (for example, widely used k-means), principal component analysis (PCA), and t-distributed stochastic neighbour embedding (t-SNE).
- *Reinforcement learning.* There is a reward and penalty scheme that makes the system (agent) learn. The greatest reward is given if the agent learns on its own (for example, DeepMind's AlphaGo program).

1.4 Underfitting and Overfitting

It is essential to understand whether a machine learning model is training effectively or not, as that will directly affect the model generalization on unseen data (test data; see Figure 1.3). If the model is too simple to learn the underlying structures in the provided data, it will fail to fit optimally on both training samples and new samples (test data). Failure is quite easy to detect as it will be reflected in the training performance. In contrast, overfitting is hard to detect if the model does very well on

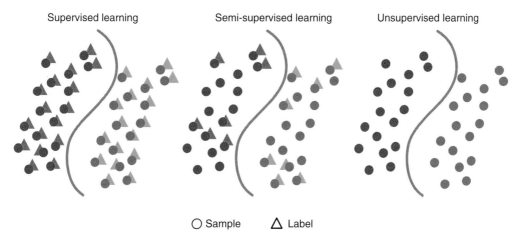

Supervised learning   Semi-supervised learning   Unsupervised learning

○ Sample   △ Label

Figure 1.2: Machine learning strategies. Circles represent data samples while triangles denote labels. A paired circle and triangle means a sample with its corresponding label. The grey line defines the decision boundary between the two classes. Figure created by Dr Sharib Ali.

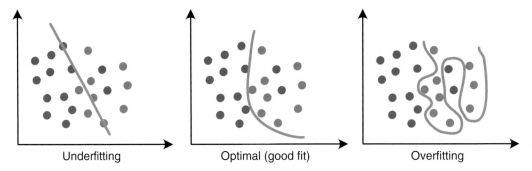

Figure 1.3: Illustration of performance judgement that affects model generalization on unseen data. Different sample colours represent two sample categories, and the grey line denotes the decision boundary. Here, we want to accurately classify the two sample categories (magenta and purple) into distinct classes. Figure created by Dr Sharib Ali.

the training data but fails to generalize on the test data. The goal when training a machine learning algorithm is to ensure that the algorithm 'learns' appropriate features that ensure an excellent fit on test data, while minimizing overfitting on training data.

1.5 Data Preparation and Its Importance

Data preparation is a fundamental part of any machine learning algorithm. After a problem (also referred to as a task) is identified, the data that would allow computers to understand this specific task need to be collected, including samples and labels (where required). Here, the term 'label' refers to a ground truth value provided from an expert annotation or by linking an accurate outcome (for example, a biopsy finding). As part of data preparation, data normalization is crucial to ensure that the algorithm learns effectively. The process includes rescaling raw input data within a definite range, usually between 0 and 1.

The dataset (a collection of samples and labels) need to be divided into the following categories (see Figure 1.4):

- *Training data*: data with features that are associated with an intended outcome for an AI/machine learning model.
- *Validation data*: held-out samples (separate from the training data) that are used during training to understand how well the model is doing and tune the associated parameters.
- *Test data*: independent data not used during training, and used only after the model has learnt (for example, using a trained machine learning model on a data cohort from an outpatient clinic for predicting breast cancer on new patients in that clinic).

It is important that data are well prepared, including the normalization step, as poorly prepared data can affect the learning process (for example, models can give unexpected results, or take infinite time to learn due to data ambiguity, etc.). If there are some outliers it may be better to discard or fix them manually rather than not addressing them at all. Always remember a now familiar adage in AI: 'garbage in, garbage out'. The validation dataset is key to understanding how well the machine

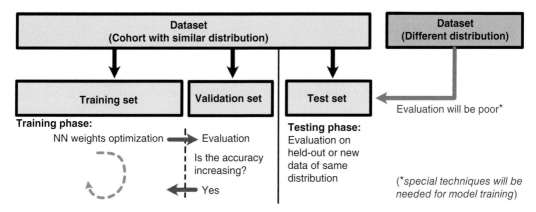

Figure 1.4: Training, validation and testing phases in machine learning model development. NN, neural network. Figure created by Dr Sharib Ali.

learning model performs, and whether the training is promoting overfitting or underfitting (Figure 1.3). Other key elements and other essential steps for training a machine learning model are shown in Table 1.1.

Table 1.1: Navigating Through The Key Steps of Machine Learning

Key	Description
Data preparation	A major step that includes data collection, cleaning (*removing noisy data*), structuring, and enriching raw data into a desired output for model training
Data normalization	Rescaling of data within a common range (for example, 0–1). This is an essential step in the learning process and can be considered part of data preparation
Sample and label	Supervised learning requires raw data and ground truth (a label assigned by an expert). In the example of a cancer lesion observed in a colonoscopy, validated from biopsy results, the sample refers to the image and the label refers to the biopsy finding assigned to the image
Training dataset	Data samples used to train a machine learning model for outcome prediction
Validation dataset	Data samples used to understand the learning process during training. The validation dataset permits tuning of hyperparameters, and helps to determine if the training process should be stopped. Validation datasets generally use 10–20% of samples. Hyperparameters are parameters whose values control the learning process and determine the values of model parameters.
Testing dataset	An independent data sample that has a similar probability distribution as the training dataset but is **not used during the training process**. The objective is to allow the model to generalize using these previously unseen data samples
Cross-validation	A technique used to repeatedly split samples into training and validation sets during the model training. In this way, the model sees all data. This technique is generally used when limited data samples are present. The process creates 'folds' or 'partitions' of data samples
Performance metrics	Values that indicate how well the model has learnt to provide a desirable output (for example, accuracy) on held-out data samples

1.6 Artificial Neural Network

Artificial neural networks (ANNs) are biologically inspired computational networks consisting of neurons. Historically, this could consist of a single neuron, as depicted in Figure 1.1a, or be in a complex and non-linear form, constructed as input, hidden, and output layers, as shown in Figure 1.1b. Here, the network weights are computed through learning and training methods. During this process, an error function (often referred to as a 'loss function') is minimized by comparing the predicted sample $\hat{y}$ and the known label, say y (in supervised learning). The gradients are then computed backwards (shown by red arrows in Figure 1.1b) for the estimated error, and the weights are adjusted in each layer right up to the first layer. This complete process is called one iteration, and the process with all data samples is called an epoch. Typically, this is done using an optimizer, often available in computational library packages. The weights usually are adjusted only in small-step sizes, provided heuristically (trial and error), and at a learning rate usually set to a small value, e.g. from 0.1 to 0.0001. Validation data are often used to understand the optimal learning rate for given data. Models with larger intermediate layers (hidden layers) are typically called deep neural networks. The network depth, or number of hidden layers, depends on, and is proportional to, the size of the dataset and the complexity of the task. Some of the key components of a NN are briefly described in Table 1.2.

NNs are used to solve various real-world problems such as pattern recognition, control and manipulation, and prediction. They have been applied in diverse fields, including medical, financial, entertainment, banking, and automotive.

Table 1.2: Neural Network Components

Key	Description
Neuron	Similar to a biological neuron, in that it computes a weighted average of its inputs and passes this along to other neurons
Activation function	A mathematical function that defines if a neuron is activated or not, contributing to the output of that neuron
Hidden layers	A layer in between the input and output layers of a neural network, where a weighted set of inputs is taken to produce an output through an activation function
Output layers	The last layer of a neural network that produces the result
Dropout layers	Randomly selecting and switching off some neurons (i.e. set input to 0). This helps to prevent overfitting on training samples. It is not applied during the validation or testing stages
Batch normalization	A technique to train deeper neural networks faster, and to provide a more stable learning process. Mini-batches of a full dataset are used, for which recentring and rescaling processes are conducted

Table 1.2: (Continued)

Key	Description
Learning rate	A rate that needs to be optimized, usually in an incremental step-wise fashion, via trial and error
Loss function	A mathematical function that compares the output generated by neural networks with the expected outcome. Generally, the loss function needs to be minimized
Optimization	Adjusting a set of weights to effectively minimize a loss function during training
Forward pass	Calculation and storage of intermediate weights in an order between the input layer and the output layer
Backpropagation	A method for training neural network algorithms where the input is fed into the model, an initial prediction is made and compared against the desired output decision, and the difference (error) is then propagated back through the neural network to update the weights of the model in order to reduce the error
Iteration	One complete forward pass and backward pass (back propagation)
Epoch	Training a neural network with all training samples makes an epoch. An epoch can have one or more mini-batches
Stopping criteria (early stopping)	A defined threshold for when to discontinue model training to avoid overfitting
Hyperparameters	Parameters that control the learning process and can affect the learnt outcome (for example, learning rate, number of neurons, number of epochs). Often hyperparameters need to be tuned in order to obtain optimal results
Convolutional neural network	A type of neural network that is often used with images and time-series data. It has a layered structure. One type of layer used in these networks is the convolutional layer. This contains trainable filters that filter input data, creating feature map outputs that, when combined with other structures, can be used to perform many tasks (detection, segmentation, classification)

1.7 Training a Neural Network: All You Need to Know

Thus far, we have illustrated how to prepare the data and the key ingredients of an NN. In this section, we will learn how to interpret the behaviour of an NN during training so that it provides similar performance on unseen test samples. Note that the validation set used during the training process does not provide the accuracy that will be reported for network performance. The objective here, rather, is to find out how well the model generalizes to the test samples (unseen data samples).

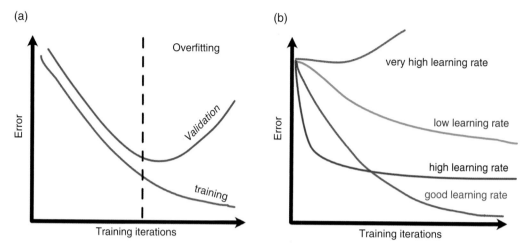

Figure 1.5: Error (also known as loss) minimization during training iterations. (a) The dotted vertical line shows where to stop training and overfitting on held-out data. (b) The influence of learning rate on error minimization over training iterations. Figure created by Dr Sharib Ali.

We make the following suggestions:

- *Keep track of your training.* It is essential to split the use of training data and validation data during training. The validation dataset will help you to understand when the network is starting to overfit or underfit. Figure 1.5a shows how the error in the validation data starts to increase after training iterations. This is the point at which training should be discontinued.
- *Tune your learning rate.* A good learning rate will better generalize the model to test data. Plotting errors for different learning rates can help elucidate where the training is heading. Figure 1.5b demonstrates how a good learning rate results in a progressive decrease in the error.
- *Size of data.* If the dataset size is small and the NN is complex, the error function will saturate quickly, giving zero gradients (vanishing gradients). This does not mean that the network has learnt all features, but rather that the features learnt are tiny and eventually become zero. An optimally sized network, according to the data size, is needed.
- *Regularization.* This is an ideal way of dealing with overfitting problems in NNs. We would advise using some prior understanding of data, and rescuing a model from the pitfall of overfitting (see cross-validation in Table 1.1; dropout layers in Table 1.2; data augmentation in Table 1.3).

1.8 Advanced Techniques

A summary of advanced techniques widely applied in machine learning is given in Table 1.3.

Transfer learning is a successful technique from which machine learning models can benefit. Transfer learning is when the previously learnt weights from one domain are applied as initialization for another domain. There are different ways of

Table 1.3: Advanced Techniques In Machine Learning

Key	Description
Data augmentation	A technique to increase the number of training data samples by adding slightly modified copies. For example, adding different colours, or rotating images in the case of imaging data samples
Transfer learning	A process where a model that has already been pre-trained on a dataset is used again as a starting point for a model on a different task. This is a good practice, as it speeds up the training process and overcomes the problem of small datasets
Ensemble technique	Combining several model predictions to produce an optimal prediction. For example, using three different neural network models and taking the output that is repeated in two of the models (i.e. highest voting, referred to as the *max-voting* approach)
Active learning	A training strategy where algorithms can proactively select and prioritise unlabelled data for learning, thereby maximizing model performance
Domain generalization	Incorporating knowledge from multiple source data distributions (also known as the 'source domain') into a single model that can then generalize on unseen samples coming from a different distribution, or 'target domain'
Domain adaptation	Training a model on source data distribution (also known as the 'source domain') that has labels, such that it tackles the domain shift problem by leveraging partially labelled or unlabelled target data samples (different distribution, or 'target domain'). For example, using the trained model on computed tomography (CT) data with some magnetic resonance imaging (MRI) images to enable disease diagnosis on unlabelled MRI data
Self-supervised learning	A technique that uses self-made simple tasks without requiring labels as pretext (for example, finding self-made rotation angles, or solving a puzzle by shuffling the input sample). This allows models to learn rich feature representations that can then be used for task-specific training (for example, classifying tumours) with fewer data, or even improving the performance of a model in a supervised setting
Continual learning	This technique allows neural network models to continuously learn and evolve based on the input from the increasing amounts of data dynamically while retaining previously learnt features

performing transfer learning, such as fine-tuning on all the layers, which means retraining the entire network parameters with new data or fine-tuning some layers only (i.e. freezing some layers). Ensemble techniques are also quite successful. They can strengthen the prediction performance by averaging the prediction labels of several networks or taking those predictions given by two out of three networks (also known as max-voting). However, due to increased network complexity, these models can be limited by the test time. Limited labels are a big problem for training supervised NN models as these models are very data hungry. Active learning is a technique that overcomes this problem: users are permitted to interact with the system and provide labels for a few 'query' samples in order to boost training accuracy.

What if the data come from a different distribution than described in the chapter thus far? In this context, researchers are designing NN models that can generalize to an unseen distribution (also known as domain generalization), or use some such data as a part of algorithm development to help networks learn to understand or map to the new distribution (also known as domain adaptation). Recently, self-supervised learning methods are gaining popularity as they do not require any labels in order to learn better feature representations, something that is however required for any supervised model to achieve a task. These techniques apply a pseudo-task (also known as a pretext) to strengthen the model's ability to understand discriminative and important features. These models are then used for a defined task, for example classification of pneumonia in X-ray images, with only a few samples. Continual learning is another new and important technique that is used to learn from dynamic data flow, while retaining previously learnt information. For example, if more training samples are collected and added to the training set, the entire network will generally need to be retrained. Continual learning, however, allows the addition of new samples without the need to retrain the network.

KEY INSIGHTS

- AI, in particular NNs, are being widely used in various fields to automate data analysis and interpretation, and to provide a prediction that otherwise requires human intelligence.
- The key elements in training an NN are problem identification, data preparation, understanding the size of data, network choice, and hyperparameter optimization.
- Data must be split into training, validation, and testing sets. Similarly, understanding when a network overfits or underfits is essential to achieving a desirable model output.
- While NNs provide ample opportunities to obtain the desired outcome, they also have limitations as they are dependent on expert labels. However, NNs undoubtedly provide a way forward in many domains, including medicine, to minimize operator dependence and subjectivity and to serve as a second opinion, at least for now.

For Further Reading please see www.wiley.com/go/byrne/aiinclinicalmedicine.

2

General Framework for Using AI in Clinical Practice

Judy L. Barkal[1], Jack W. Stockert[1], Jesse M. Ehrenfeld[2], Charles E. Aunger[1], and Lawrence K. Cohen[1]

[1] *Health 2047, Menlo Park, CA, USA*

[2] *Medical College of Wisconsin, Milwaukee, WI, USA*

Learning Objectives

- Understand the current scope, potential, limitations, and implications of using AI in clinical practice.
- Learn how to identify and evaluate opportunities to apply AI-powered solutions in practice.
- Become familiar with what questions to ask about AI solution suitability in each context.
- Develop an approach for discussing AI-enabled tools with patients.
- Understand key factors, limitations, and risks when implementing AI solutions.

2.1 Introduction

It is hard to escape the frequent news about emerging AI solutions that make amazing claims of accuracy in performing clinical tasks. Physicians are tasked with evaluating the utility as well as quality of AI solutions developed for use in clinical practice. Does AI improve patient outcomes? Can AI provide helpful assistance with certain tasks, or will AI increase physician workload and cognitive burden? Promises of improvements using other technologies (including electronic health records) have not always been realized in practice, leaving many sceptics to wonder if AI could become another unfulfilled promise. In this chapter, we offer a general framework that enables exploration of AI so that informed decisions can be made about when and where AI might add value in clinical use. Our discussion is not intended to delve into detailed evaluations of any specific AI or clinical specialties and we avoid deep technology discussions. The framework helps physicians explore and evaluate AI from multiple perspectives, and offers guiding questions for contemplating potential impacts of adopting AI in clinical practice as well as discussing AI use with patients.

AI in Clinical Medicine: A Practical Guide for Healthcare Professionals, First Edition. Edited by Michael F. Byrne, Nasim Parsa, Alexandra T. Greenhill, Daljeet Chahal, Omer Ahmad, and Ulas Bagci.
© 2023 John Wiley & Sons Ltd. Published 2023 by John Wiley & Sons Ltd.
Companion website: www.wiley.com/go/byrne/aiinclinicalmedicine

The authors of this chapter favour augmented intelligence as the preferred conceptualization of artificial intelligence that focuses on AI's assistive role, emphasizing that its design enhances human intelligence rather than replaces it. We do not mean to say that some roles and tasks cannot be eliminated or no longer require human oversight and intervention, but rather that all solutions must be taken in the context of their human user in the medical setting (e.g. healthcare profession, individual patient). Additionally, in our opinion augmented intelligence is a more appropriate term, as artificial general intelligence is still a hypothetical concept and all currently available AI solutions are focused/narrow applications. However, in this chapter, and throughout the book, the more common umbrella term of artificial intelligence will be consistently used and abbreviated as AI.

2.2 AI in Clinical Use Framework

The framework we use for our discussion is shown in Figure 2.1. Each component of the framework addresses an important area for inquiry and evaluation of AI in any clinical context. The goal of the framework is to help guide the exploration of AI options while considering how adopting AI may impact clinical practice.

In our discussion, we use the term 'AI makers' to refer to any entity that offers AI solutions for clinical use. Our discussion often makes references to the 'AI user' and 'physician', who may also be a clinician or other healthcare professional who is interacting with AI in clinical use.

Let's get started by discussing the core of our framework: the patient physician trust.

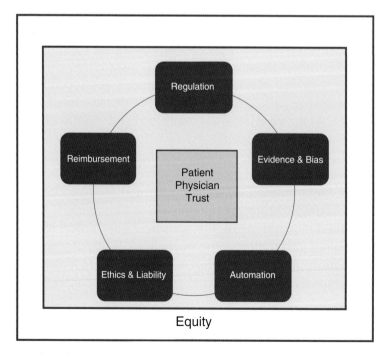

Figure 2.1: AI in clinical use framework.

Source: Barkal, Stockert, Ehrenfeld, Cohen.

2.3 Patient Physician Trust

When exploring AI in clinical use, the potential impact of AI on patient physician trust is a primary consideration. The precious bond of trust between patient and physician must be preserved if AI is to be successfully adopted in clinical use. Recent research into what patients think about AI in clinical use revealed that they trust humans more than AI, mainly because they perceive AI as being standardized and inflexible, unable to deal with their unique characteristics and situation [1]. These studies have further demonstrated that patients prefer humans over AI – even when humans might be more prone to making diagnostic mistakes or errors in a variety of clinical contexts. Earning greater trust of AI is not just a challenge for AI makers, but also a challenge for physicians to inform patients how AI contributes to shared decision-making, explain when AI is or is not an option, and help patients understand choices about their care. As we will discuss later in this chapter, the ability to provide this type of insight to patients about AI tools is just as dependent on the AI makers as it is on physicians using the tool.

Physicians have expressed wariness about whether AI is safe and whether AI can perform tasks at least as well as humans. Physicians regularly use medical devices and technology without really pausing to ask 'Does it work?' or 'Is it safe?' Physicians' trust is based on knowing that the devices have been authorized or approved by regulators prior to market release. Their own experiences and observation of reliable performance in practice also inform their views and trust. Note that this latter part is a continually developed position, with each use informing future use.

The same level of trust does not yet apply to AI. Regulatory guidance is evolving, as are AI solutions with regulatory approval for clinical use, and the transparency of continual learning from use in training and practice is insufficient. It is not surprising that physicians might be sceptical about what AI will do in a real-world clinical situation and ask:

- Does AI work?
- Does AI work for my patients?
- Can AI improve health outcomes?
- Who is liable if AI 'makes a mistake'?

The answers to these basic questions nearly always lead to more complex questions:

- How does AI work and how does it learn?
- Does AI system performance change over time or is it a locked model?
- How are AI claims monitored? How transparent is the continual learning system?
- How will I know what AI is doing?
- What training will I need to use AI?
- How can I explain AI to my patients?
- How do patients and their data interact with the AI? What are the implications for my practice?

Each question seems to spawn new questions that are reasonable and expected from a physician who considers using AI. These questions are similar to those prompted by any new tool/device, therapeutic technique, or medication being considered for clinical use. To address basic questions about whether AI is safe and works, we start with the regulation component of our framework.

2.4 Regulation

When looking at the regulation of AI, we find a growing number of AI tools that have received regulatory approval or authorization. The regulatory guidance of AI continues to evolve through pilot programs with AI makers and partnerships with industry experts. Regulators refer to AI as 'Software as a Medical Device' (SaMD). The regulatory authorities and global standards groups are working together and examining approaches for regulating AI, which differs from traditional medical devices. Table 2.1, from the International Medical Device Regulators Forum (IMDRF), assigns categories to healthcarc SaMD based on intended use and patient risk. (See Chapter 36 for more discussion on this topic.)

Global regulators have provided reference materials that describe regulatory processes for AI approval and the current state of regulatory approvals, often including a searchable database.

The AI user's first inquiry is to understand regulatory approval or authorization:

- Is the AI approved or authorized by regulatory authorities?
- If so, by which ones, what SaMD category, and for what intended clinical use(s)?

If AI has received regulatory approval or authorization, then its assigned risk category can help identify the level of risk, and its label (also approved by the regulator) should specify any significant risks and limitations for the use of AI with patients. The approved intended use can offer a preliminary answer for 'Does the AI work?' and clarifies the intended clinical function that AI performs.

If regulatory approval or authorization does not exist, then experimental use procedures need to be followed as part of an AI evaluation, including the need for

Table 2.1: International Medical Device Regulators Forum Software as a Medical Device (SaMD) Categories.

State of healthcare situation or condition	Significance of information provided by SaMD to healthcare decision		
	Treat or diagnose	Drive clinical management	Inform clinical management
Critical	IV	III	II
Serious	III	II	I
Non-serious	II	I	I

Source: [2] / IMDRF.

patient consent. Medical regulators will require proof that the AI performs its intended use function safely and reliably with patients in a clinical situation. The source, type, volume, and variety of clinically valid data will be examined by medical regulators, along with the accuracy of AI results, as part of quality management processes. Since regulators may not have yet reviewed the AI for clinical validity, key questions to ask are:

- Is the AI based on clinically validated data?
- If so, what is the data source, what quantity of data was used, how were the data validated for quality, and how were AI results validated for accuracy?
- Were clinically qualified AI users involved?

In some cases AI is embedded in a consumer-grade device, such as a wearable or smart phone. Consumer regulators may approve a device as safe to operate, but do not validate the clinical quality of device operation. While these AI solutions can sometimes provide interesting and perhaps helpful advisory information, the sensor data used by consumer-grade AI is typically not clinically validated and is of limited medical use. A consumer-grade AI may prompt a patient to reach out to the physician or seek medical care, but is not a substitute for clinically validated devices that can be used for clinical decisions. It is important to recognize, however, that many consumers will not differentiate between devices that are consumer grade and those that are medical grade and clinically validated [3]. (See Chapter 44 for more discussion on this topic.)

The framework discussion does not address consumer-grade AI further because of its limitations for clinical use. The discussion proceeds with the assumption that AI has regulatory approval or is in the experimental stage prior to regulatory approval. In addition, we assume that the AI is capable of generating accurate results based on clinically validated data (AI 'works').

We should point out that the global regulatory framework for AI in clinical medicine is evolving. As of this writing, in the US the Food and Drug Administration (FDA) through its Center for Devices and Radiological Health (CDRH) is still developing its regulatory pathway. US regulators have indicated that they are considering a total product lifecycle-based regulatory framework for AI-enabled devices that would allow for modifications to be made from real-world learning and adaptation. However, there are still many unanswered questions about requirements for algorithm transparency and labelling.

Let's proceed in our discussion to address the physician's next question: 'Does the AI work for my patients?'

2.5 Evidence and Bias

A technologist might view evidence and bias as a way to describe 'generalizable' AI, or how well AI performs under new conditions with new input data. In medicine, a somewhat analogous situation might be when a newly approved drug first becomes available for treating patients who were not part of the clinical trial. The collection of real-world data (RWD) from patients treated with the new drug is analysed to create real-world evidence (RWE) that helps determine how the new drug performs in populations not previously tested, and may help characterize bias in the clinical trial. (See Chapter 42 for more discussion on this topic.)

When a physician asks 'Does the AI work for my patients?' the underlying questions are about evidence and bias.

- Is there evidence that AI works for patients who are similar to my patients? Similarities may include race, ethnicity, gender, age, health status, genetics, or many other characteristics.
- To what extent has bias been introduced in the AI? Bias may result if AI training data have little to no similarity to the physicians' patients. There could be bias in patient data, or source and type of data, such as one brand of medical equipment or a particular clinical site. Bias can also be introduced at the AI maker from the teams that program, train, and validate AI. Even if the AI maker used a third party to do quality assessments of AI results and performance, or to provide education and training for users of AI, bias may still be present. (See Chapter 39, Biases in Machine Learning and Healthcare, for more discussion on this topic).

   Discussion of AI bias can help physicians understand overall where an AI solution applies or doesn't apply to their patients and current clinical practices. Physicians may tailor questions based on medical specialty or unique clinical practice conditions. For example, a physician who treats patients who speak many different languages may need multilingual AI capabilities for patients and clinical staff.
- Has the AI been used in clinical settings that are similar to mine? Prepare questions that delve into what distinguishes your clinical practice, and inquire about AI training and validation similarities [4].

Our discussion just begins to scratch the surface of evidence and bias inquiries into AI for a given clinical specialty and use. Much more can be learnt by doing hands-on evaluations of AI, with access to AI makers for deeper questions. In the early stages of evaluation, physicians can gather information to learn if the AI maker has built credible evidence that the AI works for their patients, in clinical practices like theirs, and confirm what steps have been taken to avoid unwanted bias in the AI data and results [5]. (See Chapter 41 for more discussion on this topic.)

2.6 Automation

Our framework uses the term 'automation' to describe the role of AI and the human–AI interaction in a clinical workflow. News stories often hype AI as being fully autonomous or artificial general intelligence. As already noted, in reality AI in clinical use is automating some tasks more narrowly to augment the physician's

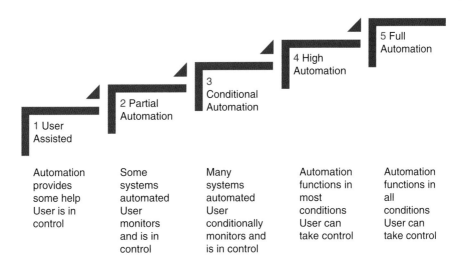

Figure 2.2: Levels of AI automation.

Source: Adapted from [6] / Barkal, Stockert, Ehrenfeld, Cohen.

clinical work. As described in our introduction, we therefore prefer the conceptualization of AI as augmented intelligence that enhances human intelligence.

Uses in other industries, like autopilots in airplanes or self-driving cars, refer to levels of AI automation. The Society of Automotive Engineers established six levels of driving automation, where level 0 means no automation and level 5 means full automation unless the human wants control [6]. AI in clinical practice can also be described as having levels of automation. As in other industries, even the highest level of AI automation keeps physician decision-makers in control. Figure 2.2 describes different levels of AI automation.

The AI user needs to understand the AI automation capabilities (which regulators have approved) and how to interact with AI as part of a clinical workflow:

- What is AI capable of doing automatically, and what am I expected to do?
- What view do I have into what tasks AI is doing?
- How do I take control from AI when needed?
- How is the AI system updating/evolving (e.g. continuously, discretely, at regular intervals)? How can I monitor AI system updates?

Possible automation levels may be discussed or demonstrated by AI makers, but details are learnt through education and training for the specific AI being evaluated for clinical use.

Any level of automation also relies on physicians monitoring the quality of AI results, including the quality of what information AI is using to generate results:

- Will I be able to view AI inputs and the AI results that were generated?
- Will I see what confidence AI assigns to results?
- How immediate are results?

When an AI user does not know what AI is doing, this is often called 'black box' AI. 'Explainable' AI may provide the AI user with more information, but may still not actually explain how AI algorithms work. 'Transparent' AI offers greater insight into how AI algorithms work. The AI user needs to ask AI makers to provide detail about how AI algorithms work, how to monitor AI accuracy, and under what conditions AI is qualified (and regulator approved) to perform a specified level of automation. As the concept of transparency continues to evolve through ongoing regulatory framework discussions, there have been some interesting suggestions about AI labelling that could help further clarify what AI transparency means [7].

In addition, AI makers should address AI operational questions:

- How can I monitor AI automated tasks?
- How do I know when the AI is in an error condition or unreliable state?
- How do I 'disengage' AI and take control?

Answers to these questions can help physicians better understand how AI operates and what actions they may still need to take. In addition, physicians may begin to gauge how AI might offer some opportunities to help reduce physician workload.

A key desirable feature of AI automation is the interface with the AI user. There has been considerable research into human–computer interaction (HCI) that can offer helpful guidance to physicians who are evaluating AI and innovators who want to make AI more usable by physicians [8]. In addition, there are many lessons to be learnt from other industries. Experiences with autopilots and self-driving car technology can offer many valuable lessons, including those from analysing safety-critical situations with similarities to clinical practice [9–11].

AI users often inquire whether the AI user interface alerts when AI has errors, or perhaps when AI accuracy is declining, as might occur when AI is being applied to a novel patient/population. These questions emphasize safety and preventing harm to the patient:

- How will AI alert me to errors?
- Will the AI 'stop operation' to prevent patient harm?
- Will I be warned to 'take over' when AI stops?
- What warnings or alerts will AI provide if accuracy is declining?

The questions about AI automation help the physician know what assistance AI can provide and what limitations may be present in current AI automation. Transparency about what AI is doing, and the quality of AI results, helps physicians compare AI performance with that of humans, and hopefully start to build trust when using AI in clinical practice.

Next in our framework discussion of ethics and liability, we cover physicians' questions about not knowing what AI is doing, and perhaps not being able to recognize AI errors.

2.7 Ethics and Liability

The framework discussion of ethics and liability focuses on risks and assignment of accountability when AI is part of the clinical workflow. We continue to build on previous discussions of AI 'black box' algorithms, and how AI automation fits into the overall clinical workflow. The regulatory category assigned to AI is also important to understand AI's intended function and potential risks to patients.

If a patient is harmed when AI is part of the clinical workflow, then difficult questions will be raised:

- Was the AI at fault?
- Were the physicians at fault?
- Were there multiple faults?
- Is the physician, medical organization, or the AI maker liable for what happened?

Liability for medical errors typically falls under tort law [12]. A tort is a civil claim in which a party requests damages for injuries caused by a harmful, wrongful act of another. A physician may be liable for negligence, a healthcare organization may be assigned 'vicarious liability' due to actions of employees, and manufacturers may have product liability for products that are deemed 'not reasonably safe'.

The application of tort law to clinical use of AI is still being evaluated. We present three suggestions currently being discussed by diverse experts:

- Assign 'personhood' to AI, and require AI to have malpractice-type insurance in cases of negligence assigned to AI.
- Assign 'common enterprise liability' where all parties involved in the implementation and use of AI share the liability and burden of making the harmed patient whole, and no fault is assigned to any single party.
- Assign liability to clinical AI users, with responsibility for evaluating and implementing 'black box' AI algorithms into standard of care, and for validating algorithmic results.

AI in clinical use is still expected to follow the normal clinical practice of having physicians explain the risks to patients, and obtaining patient consent for the use of AI. Whether use of an AI product in the clinical workflow requires separate consent or is covered by a patient's general consent to treatment is currently still an unanswered question.

Another area of potential AI liability is security, patient privacy, and patient confidentiality. AI makers must demonstrate reliable, tested security platforms and tools for preventing tampering or theft of patient and physician data. Start by asking AI makers:

- What security platform, tools, procedures, and services do you use to ensure data is safe and secure, as well as ensure compliance with security regulations?

Data are an integral part of any AI. Patient privacy and confidentiality must be preserved. AI makers rely on patient data to develop algorithms and products. This use of patient data often goes beyond intended use in clinical care, and may constitute a commercial use of patient data. As such, the AI maker may need patients' permission to use their data in AI products and services. Seeking legal counsel is advised, as there are many complex considerations for specific contexts. (See Chapter 37 for more discussion on this topic.)

Here we describe some general questions that AI users may want to ask AI makers:

- Do you obtain patient consent for data use in your AI products and services? And how do you ensure that if patients withdraw consent, their data will no longer be used?
- How do you protect patient data from being identified and ensure regulatory compliance?

Any discussion of liability would not be complete without mention of AI's capability to do 'continuous learning'. When typical AI encounters new data and new conditions, it attempts to improve algorithms and accuracy automatically. Technically, this means AI algorithms could change 'in the field' and become different from what AI makers have built and validated. This naturally raises concerns about liability, and to date regulators do not allow regulatory-approved AI to change in the field. Changes must be done by AI makers, and regulators must approve the modified AI for clinical use. In this way, AI has a compliance and safety model similar to more traditional medical devices. AI makers and regulators, along with AI users, are working on ideas to address the risks and liabilities while taking advantage of AI's capability to improve accuracy with new data and situations. If AI is ever permitted to learn in the field, then regulators and AI makers must agree on how to control AI quality, mitigate risks, and maintain safety and reliability. Regulatory websites and reference materials are a good place to keep abreast of what's happening with AI continuous learning.

Physicians can keep in mind the previous discussions and ask AI makers:

- What evidence serves as the foundation for regulatory approval or authorization and supports that AI 'works'?
- What AI features have not been trained or validated (i.e. are still experimental)?
- How do you develop human–computer interfaces that help physicians easily understand what AI is doing and advising them to do?
- How do you develop training and education that help physicians become highly skilled using AI, including training physicians in AI error scenarios where they must override AI and take control?

As AI advances, questions of ethics and liability will persist, and resolutions of tort law are still needed. Further, regulatory bodies must evolve new constructs around oversight, safety, and security. Physicians can use the AI evaluation phase to learn more about what AI makers provide to help ensure AI does not bring harm to patients. In addition, physicians can develop a better understanding of skills, training, and responsibilities for using AI in clinical practice, and therefore provide valued input into the evolution of our regulatory, ethical, and policy frameworks [13].

2.8 Reimbursement

The focus on reimbursement in our framework is not to provide an exhaustive exploration of the topic, but to help AI users explore whether paths for reimbursement exist for AI in clinical use, and what roles and responsibilities AI users and AI makers may have when seeking reimbursement.

To begin, potential payers or 'who pays' for AI can be difficult to identify without AI makers having RWE of improved patient outcomes. Government insurers and private insurance companies nearly always require RWE before agreeing to cover a new service such as the use of AI. There may be opportunities to work with payers on how much and how diverse RWE needs to be, but the AI maker needs to have plans for RWE in the path for reimbursement.

Some AI makers may cover costs while gathering RWE to submit to regulators for approval and to payers for coverage. Others expect that AI users or even patients will pay to see if improved outcomes are possible. Sometimes, shared cost coverage among multiple parties might be proposed. Some initial questions to ask AI makers are:

- Who pays for AI?
- Who generates the supporting information and documentation for billing?
- Who is responsible for billing the payers?

If no government or private insurance payer has been identified, then some key follow-up questions are:

- Are you collecting RWE to share with regulators? With insurers?
- What is the impact on my patients regarding data requirements?
- What role and responsibilities do you expect me to have? How am I compensated (if at all)?

Some proven paths to reimbursement for AI already exist. There are AI makers using level 1 automation to assist with clinical tasks, such as remote patient monitoring (RPM) for patients with confirmed diagnoses of chronic conditions. These AI can leverage already established RPM reimbursement codes. In this AI use case, the automation saves considerable staff time compared to manual processes, and often allows more patients to be monitored effectively. As in all level 1 automation, AI is assisting the physician with some clinical tasks. The physician is providing the services. The physician may want to ask:

- How will responsibilities for reimbursement processes be shared?
- How will AI create opportunities for improving outcomes and reducing costs (e.g. in value-based care arrangements)?

Documenting current and future reimbursement approaches helps physicians assess the cost and resource burden for them, their staff, and possibly their patients. If the decision is later made to adopt AI, project leaders will also need resource estimates to plan accordingly.

Reimbursement presents challenges for both AI makers and AI users, as well as payers who may be unfamiliar with AI for clinical use. Additional considerations may help guide the evaluation process:

- If the AI maker has no cogent plan for, or experience with, developing RWE, it may be reasonable to consider other options from AI makers who do. Reimbursement is unlikely to be possible without some type of RWE that might include how AI could improve patient outcomes.
- If the AI maker intends for patients to be part of their cost coverage strategy, AI users may want to consider other more equitable options that are accessible to all patients regardless of their ability to pay. In addition, the research on patient preferences discussed earlier found that patients exhibited lower reservation prices for machines (AI), which may also impact reimbursement considerations [14].
- If the AI maker's business model presumes that the AI user will pay for using their AI, what evidence will you need to estimate your return on that investment (e.g. improved patient outcomes, increased value-based payments)? Consider AI options that help you build that evidence.

Physicians want to improve patient outcomes. Evaluating AI takes time and resources. Deploying and maintaining AI is a major undertaking that involves many stakeholders and resources. Developing a sustainable business model for AI is a key step towards the successful adoption of AI in clinical use. (For a discussion of alternate delivery and funding models, refer to Chapter 45).

2.9 Equity

Equity is the framework component that influences and impacts all other components. Our previous discussion of bias addressed physicians' questions about whether AI works for their patients, and whether evidence shows that AI improves health outcomes for their patients. If AI makers do not have or cannot provide RWE that shows improved health outcomes from diverse patient populations, then the AI may have built-in bias and may not be available to all patients. Another consideration is that the AI maker may have introduced inequities during development. For example, AI makers may ignore accessibility for patients who cannot afford to pay if AI is not covered by reimbursement. Another example might be lack of AI accessibility to patients without literacy in English or any language.

It is important to recognize that AI can also contribute to positive impacts by enabling greater access to care for populations that are underserved. For example, millions of patients with diabetes who cannot see an ophthalmologist whose practice is far away might receive screening for diabetic retinopathy in their primary care setting enabled by a regulator-approved AI diagnostic tool [15].

Physicians can ask AI makers about whether AI is equitable:

- Is AI accessible to patients from diverse racial, ethnic, and socioeconomic backgrounds?
- If so, what accessibility features are part of AI?

It is also important to consider the diversity of AI users who will interact with AI. Ask AI makers:

- What education is provided, and what training will AI users need?
- What steps have been taken to ensure that all AI users can safely and reliably understand and use AI in practice? What features enable safe use by diverse populations of AI users?
- During AI adoption, how do you help build trust and confidence for diverse AI users?

AI users can have a leading role in raising equity awareness by expressing concerns and facilitating conversations with AI makers throughout each step of the AI product life cycle, from concept to evaluation, implementation, and surveillance. AI in clinical use needs to be accessible and applicable to diverse patients, and usable by diverse AI users, to achieve improved patient outcomes for all [16]. (For a further discussion on equity, refer to Chapter 40).

It is an exciting time for AI and medicine. AI in clinical use will transform how physicians deliver care, how they interact with patients, and how patients manage their conditions between physician visits. This framework is a start to guide meaningful discussions with AI makers, AI users, healthcare stakeholders, and, most importantly, patients. As AI in clinical use continues to evolve, physicians have a unique opportunity to lead in setting expectations for AI makers and help with shaping the adoption of AI in clinical care to improve patient outcomes.

KEY INSIGHTS

Our discussion of a general framework for identifying and evaluating AI for clinical use poses questions and touches on key areas to explore and help guide AI users. Here we summarize key considerations for each framework component:

- *Regulation*: **Does AI have regulatory approval or authorization, and use clinically validated data?**
- *Evidence and bias*: **Does the AI maker have RWE of improved patient outcomes? Is there bias in AI data or algorithms?**

- *Automation*: What is the level of AI automation? Are AI algorithms transparent? What is the human–AI interface, and how well does it function?
- *Ethics and liability*: What risks might cause patient harm? How is liability assigned? How does the AI maker meet security, patient privacy, and confidentiality regulations?
- *Reimbursement*: Is there an already established or viable path forward for AI coverage and payment? What are my role and responsibility in obtaining coverage and payment?
- *Equity*: Is AI accessible regardless of patient socioeconomic situation? Does AI improve patient outcomes for all?

References

1. Cadario R, Longoni C, Morewedge CK. Understanding, explaining, and utilizing medical artificial intelligence. *Nature Human Behaviour* 2021;5:1636–1642. https://doi.org/101038/s41562-021-01146-0.
2. Software as a Medical Device Working Group. *Software as a Medical Device (SaMD): Clinical Evaluation*. International Medical Device Regulators Forum, September 2017. https://www.imdrf.org/sites/default/files/docs/imdrf/final/technical/imdrf-tech-170921-samd-n41-clinical-evaluation_1.pdf.
3. Bui L. Using AI to help find answers to common skin conditions. *The Keyword*, 18 May 2021. https://blog.google/technology/health/ai-dermatology-preview-io-2021.
4. Crigger E, Reinbold K, Hanson C, Kao A, Blake K, Irons M. Trustworthy augmented intelligence in health care. *Journal of Medical Systems* 2022;46:12.
5. Wong A, Otles E, Donnelly JP et al. External validation of a widely implemented proprietary sepsis prediction model in hospitalized patients. *JAMA Internal Medicine* 2021;181:1065–1070.
6. SAE International. Taxonomy and definitions for terms related to driving automation systems for on-road motor vehicles. *SAE Standards* 2021:J3016(TM)(April):30–32. https://www.sae.org/standards/content/j3016_202104.
7. US Food and Drug Administration. *Virtual Public Workshop – Transparency of Artificial Intelligence/Machine Learning-Enabled Medical Devices*. 14 October 2021. https://www.fda.gov/medical-devices/workshops-conferences-medical-devices/virtual-public-workshop-transparency-artificial-intelligencemachine-learning-enabled-medical-devices

For additional references please see www.wiley.com/go/byrne/aiinclinical medicine.

3

AI and Medical Education

Alexandra T. Greenhill

Department of Family Medicine, University of British Columbia, Vancouver, Canada
Careteam Technologies, Vancouver, Canada

Learning Objectives

▦ Recognize the importance of advancing understanding of AI, and appreciate the current gaps in AI knowledge for physicians in training and in practice (medical school, residency, and fellowship training) and for continuous professional development (CPD)/continued medical education (CME).

▦ Identify core competencies and key topics, challenges, and opportunities for introducing AI into medical education.

▦ Review current applications and future opportunities for using AI to enhance medical education, specifically in learning support and for knowledge testing.

3.1 Introduction

The teaching and practice of medicine remain fundamentally focused on information acquisition and application, but there is an urgent need to change this. Today, the constant increase and change in medical knowledge exceed the capacity of physicians to stay current. Additionally, the emergence of new technologies requires a different approach to practising medicine, where the key skills of physicians will be either to find and judiciously apply the right information to the right situation or to evaluate the suggestion of AI-enabled technology. The incredibly rapid rise of innovative technologies, including AI, applied to clinical medicine has created a huge and growing knowledge gap for physicians in training and in practice.

There is consensus across the medical profession that there is an urgent need to increase the overall level of technology and AI literacy, including basic concepts, current state of the art, and future implications of AI [1–12]. There is also a recognized need for many physicians to go beyond literacy, in order to reach proficiency and performance across the spectrum of creating, using, validating, and regulating AI technologies for all medical domains, and to lead the transformation of healthcare. This very book was intended to help in this effort, and this chapter will focus on how to accomplish the required transformation within medical education.

AI in Clinical Medicine: A Practical Guide for Healthcare Professionals, First Edition. Edited by Michael F. Byrne, Nasim Parsa, Alexandra T. Greenhill, Daljeet Chahal, Omer Ahmad, and Ulas Bagci.
© 2023 John Wiley & Sons Ltd. Published 2023 by John Wiley & Sons Ltd.
Companion website: www.wiley.com/go/byrne/aiinclinicalmedicine

Here we present various perspectives on the necessary upskilling of the medical profession, from those in training to those in practice, as AI impacts curriculum content, delivery, and testing. For the rest of this chapter, unless specifically indicated, the term 'medical education' will be used to encompass a lifelong learning continuum aimed at physicians in training (medical school, residency, and fellowship) and in practice (continuous professional development [CPD], continued medical education [CME], certifications, and advanced degrees). This chapter will also review the best practices and future opportunities to use AI for clinical education itself.

While the chapter will focus on physicians, there is a great opportunity to make all of these changes together with all of the different professions within healthcare, both to combine efforts and to ensure better interprofessional collaboration, as increasingly healthcare is delivered through team-based care.

3.2 Competency in AI: Preparing for the Era of AI in Medicine

While there is general excitement about AI as a new competency for physicians, it is imperative to understand: (i) why there is a need to formally incorporate this domain into medical education; (ii) what the current state is; and (iii) what the core elements of the curriculum are for this domain. These three dimensions mirror what is occurring in other professions beyond healthcare, as all are impacted by what the World Economic Forum has named the 'fourth industrial revolution' – the rapid change in technology, industries, and societal patterns and processes in the twenty-first century due to increasing interconnectivity and smart automation, and fusion of advances in new technologies such as AI, robotics, the Internet of Things (IoT), genetic engineering, and quantum computing [13].

3.2.1 'Upskilling' the Medical Profession in the Field of AI

Medical education has undergone several important transformations in the last two centuries, from the increased use of the scientific method and formal training rather than apprenticeship, to the move to patient-centred bedside clinical training that Dr William Osler, the 'father of modern medicine', initiated at the start of the twentieth century through the Flexner report, to the three massive changes that have gained momentum since the 1990s: (i) problem-based learning (PBL), case-based learning (CBL), and team-based learning (TBL); (ii) evidence-based medicine (EBM) and evidence-informed practice; and (iii) the increased importance of non-clinical competencies, as outlined, for example, in the CanMEDs framework [14].

In the last two decades, beyond the significant advances in diagnosis and treatment options, there has been an incredible acceleration in the use of technology, including AI, across all medical domains – clinical care, administration, policy, education, and research. There is a widely recognized need for physicians to correspondingly also (i) transform what it means to be competent within the new era as defined by rapid innovation cycles and constant change; and (ii) ensure that they are ready to meaningfully contribute to the creation and use of these new technologies in order to move from promise to results.

Medical organizations play a key role, and are stepping up in the last few years by creating policy and raising awareness of the need for action [2–7]. From various initiatives, it is clear that the medical profession's only real question pertains to whether physicians will lead or follow this inevitable transformation. Some physicians are understandably hesitant to commit, given concerns about the possibility of harm to patients or replacement of health professionals [8,15].

It is imperative to learn from the past, as when the first wave of eHealth technologies (primarily electronic medical records [EMRs]) was thrust into the clinical setting, there was a significant lack of involvement from physicians at all steps – from technology design to implementation. EMRs have now been shown to have caused increased workload and burnout of clinicians due to usability and workflow issues, while largely failing to deliver on the promise behind the massive investment and effort – which was to improve quality and safety while reducing costs. This trend has led to heavy scepticism and resistance around the adoption of the many new health technologies that have followed EMRs. In addition, healthcare consistently and significantly lags behind every cycle of technology innovation that transforms society and work, a lag due not only to the resistance of adoption from end users, but also to the delay from the additional requirements to ensure that these new tools meet medical regulations, quality, and safety standards, as well as from issues with funding their development and use.

The Lancet Commission on 'Education of Health Professionals for a New Century: Transforming Education to Strengthen Health Systems in an Interdependent World' The Lancet Commission [1] called for medical education to have three levels of learning: informative, which creates experts; formative, which creates professionals; and transformative, which creates change agents.

To avoid the mistakes of the past, there is a need for greater literacy in AI for all physicians, in order to ensure a greater role for physicians in the creation and roll-out of the 'Health 2.0' wave that is happening right now [8–12].

3.2.2 Current State and Gaps in AI in Medical Education

Medical education is still largely based on traditional curricula that vary by length and emphasis between countries, but the core competencies of these curricula are globally similar, and still focus on memorization and application of knowledge [16]. The availability of technology, data, and AI requires additional capabilities related to competences in effectively integrating and applying information from a growing array of sources, and also in the fundamental understanding of technology, innovation, and AI in medicine [11,12,16]. In addition, we are being asked to consider how to teach care and compassion in the context of technology and AI [11,12,17,18].

Most health professionals, including those in medicine, have no or insufficient AI education, despite calls from physicians to increase competence in this key emerging domain, and their strong interest in learning more [2,11,12,16,19–23]. Medical training accreditation and certification examination organizations have not added expectations about new trainee capabilities related to AI. Such expectations could act as a strong driver of change for a medical programme's curriculum. Most medical schools do not offer any exposure to AI in the undergraduate or postgraduate medical curriculum, and those who do limit it to a few hours or days at most [21,22].

As the speed of the advances in AI is ever increasing, the education gap becomes more and more significant. This gap exists for other domains beyond healthcare, but the additional challenge is that medical education is already one of the most intensive and longest, and it is difficult on a practical level to add this additional competency.

An increasing number of CME/CPD courses and conferences include the mention of AI as applied to a given topic at the discretion of the faculty. This may take the form of presentations and workshops on AI. In addition to medical school and CME/CPD, physicians in training and in practice can choose from an increasing number of emerging AI courses, programmes, certificates, and degrees. Some of these are specific to healthcare and some are not, and there are also combined programmes such as MD/MBA, MD/MPH, and MD/PhD [21].

Most physicians in training and in practice who are interested in AI often resort to self-directed and informal learning. While currently there are limited opportunities to transform these into a recognized certificate, it is possible to contemplate the emergence of certification through an organization that reviews a particular portfolio, similar to the credentialing now available to physicians in leadership positions.

3.2.3 Defining the Curriculum and Core Competencies Related to AI in Medicine

As identified earlier, there is an urgent need to augment the medical education curriculum at all levels, with three core dimensions related to AI in medicine:

- *Competence in the effective integration and use of information* from a growing array of sources that are generated using technology and AI [8,11,12,16,21].
- *Communication, empathy, care, and compassion* in the context of technology and AI [8,11,12,17,18].
- *AI literacy, proficiency, and competency* in order to harness AI tools effectively to improve outcomes and experiences for patients [8,10–12,16,21]. This will be the focus of the rest of this section.

It must be noted first that the curriculum and core competencies for AI in medicine greatly overlap with the curriculum and core competencies for overall technology and innovation in medicine. Therefore, the optimal approach would be not to treat AI as a standalone competency, but rather to increase the overall teaching about technology and innovation in medicine, with an increased emphasis on AI as a significant and unique domain of knowledge, seamlessly integrated across different aspects of the curriculum [16].

The other important trend to recognize is that there is a need to learn from efforts for AI literacy directed at the general public. This includes K-12 education, as well as efforts by all the other non-medical domains impacted by this fourth industrial revolution to enable non-technical professionals to gain AI literacy and competency in their education and at work.

There is relatively little known about effective methods and best practices for AI education for non-technical learners in general, let alone physicians, and current approaches are based on adapting from expert opinion and from lessons learnt in the education of non-technical learners about technology and innovation. There is a significant 'ontological mismatch' that must be overcome as, while computer science and medicine share some overlap, there are significant differences in vocabulary, concepts, and approaches [10].

Finally, it must be emphasized that AI is still a nascent domain of knowledge that is subject to rapid transformation. Therefore, it would be ideal if we could help physicians gain foundational skills that would enable them to continue to learn as the knowledge base expands and refines. In addition, AI learning should focus on principles and processes rather than the ability to use specific platforms, devices, or products.

The Revised Bloom Taxonomy [24] can serve as a model (Figure 3.1) to understand the continuum of skills and abilities in AI from literacy to proficiency to performance. For these latter two, as mentioned previously, there is an increasing number of courses, programmes, certificates, and degrees being offered, both general and specific to healthcare, that have different content depending on the area of focus.

For AI literacy, there are numerous emerging frameworks that are aimed at developing AI literacy-focused curricula for medical education, with AI literacy

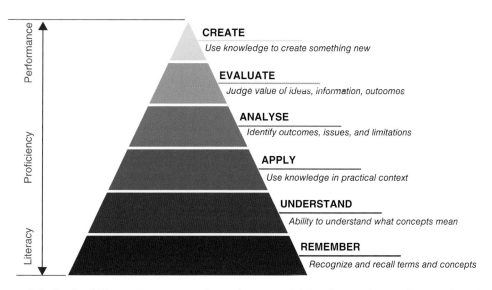

Figure 3.1: Revised Bloom Taxonomy adapted as a model for the continuum for AI education.

defined as a set of competencies that enables individuals to critically evaluate AI technologies, communicate and collaborate effectively with AI, and use AI as a tool [25,26]. At a minimum, physicians should know how to [27]:

- *Use the AI solution.* Identify when it is indicated, what inputs are required to receive meaningful results, and how to correctly apply the solution.
- *Interpret the results obtained.* Understand and assess the results with a reasonable degree of accuracy, including awareness of sources of error and bias.
- *Explain the use of AI and the results obtained.* Be able to communicate the results and the processes to patients and colleagues.

To enable these three core skills and abilities, the following key competency dimensions would help increase AI literacy for physicians in training and in practice [8,10–12,15–16,25,26,28]:

- Understand the definitions, core concepts, and principles of AI and data science in general, and specific to medicine.
- Understand possible applications, opportunities, strengths, and limitations.
- Understand the key dimensions, such as ethics, bias, transparency, data protection, safety and liability, as well as societal, legal, and economic considerations.
- Understand how AI can support and augment medical decision-making.
- Gain knowledge of clinical-grade and consumer-facing applications of AI within the given specialty.
- Identify the appropriate use cases and perform critical appraisal of AI solutions for effective and efficient use for patient care, education, research, or quality improvement.
- Build knowledge of how to explain to the patient, where appropriate, the AI applications used, and if required obtain informed consent.
- Interpret and explain the results and insights from using AI for patient care, education, research, or quality improvement.
- Understand the principles of dissemination and implementation of innovations.
- Consider areas for possible future applications of AI, and the effects of such applications.

3.3 AI Tools to Enhance Medical Education Itself

The use of AI in education in general, and particularly in medicine, shows great potential to transform the effectiveness and experience of the learning process, building on the learnings from the early computer-based education (CBE) efforts. The field of AI in education (AIED) is rapidly developing, and has immediate and significant implications for medical education especially the ability to deliver high-quality adaptive education at scale, and to increase access for remote areas and for developing countries. However, it is important to emphasize the current limits of these technologies, and that AI does not replace existing approaches but rather augments them. There is a recognized need to study and validate how to fulfil the promise of AI in education in general, and in medical education in particular [1,28].

The rest of this section will provide an overview into two main domains where AI is currently being used for medical education: learning support and knowledge testing [29].

3.3.1 AI for Learning Support

Among the many options for how AI can enhance the delivery of learning support, here is a quick overview of solutions currently in early use across different medical education programmes, and showing success in case reports and studies:

- *Curriculum content development and optimization.* AI can collect information about the process and outcomes of learning, and can inform educators about the progress and trajectory of both individual learners and the group in order to guide content development and optimization [12]. AI can also reduce the burden of intensive curriculum tracing, mapping, and reviewing processes by helping make sense of the complex interplay between educational strategies, course content, learning outcomes, educational experiences, and assessments [30].
- *Personalized learning plans and feedback.* AI can assist in the gathering and analysis of information about an individual's learning needs and preferences, conduct knowledge assessments, and recommend a learning plan that is tailored to the individual. This can enable a true strengths-based approach, where learning is focused on what the person needs to improve on and in the learner's preferred style, instead of the cohort-based approach. In addition, this can address one of the big challenges of CME/CPD, because when physicians know a lot of the content, it is harder for them to sustain interest in order to identify and learn new or changed information. The AI systems can also monitor progress, provide personalized feedback, and keep optimizing the learning plan, as well as provide the learners and teachers with insights into the students' learning habits and opportunities to improve them.
- *Adaptive/smart content for learning on demand or embedded in context.* AI enables the delivery of content that is adaptive/smart as it learns from what the learner knows, or is interested in, and presents the right new information in the optimal sequence. AI has also enabled the emergence of micro-learning: namely, the presentation of new knowledge in live time, triggered by a situation where the practitioner may be hesitant on how to proceed, may be potentially making a mistake, or where there is new knowledge available.
- *Intelligent virtual tutoring.* Chatbots, also known as teacherbots, can provide effective personalized 24/7 support for learners that is increasingly preferred by students to the support provided by teaching assistants, because of the

rapidity, convenience, and effectiveness of the virtual tutor [31]. Rules-based AI can also enable the rapid and inexpensive creation of intelligent tutoring systems, based on the AI analysing a few examples of how a human solves a given query with a body of content. The teachers can then rapidly review and correct the AI-produced tutoring outline, saving time and effort.

- *Clinical scenarios and digital virtual patients (DVP).* AI can use anonymized data from EMRs to rapidly generate real-world scenarios for clinical practice. There is promising evidence that DVPs can more effectively improve skills (clinical reasoning, procedural skills, and a mix of procedural and team skills), and at least as effectively improve knowledge as traditional case learning in both high-income and low- and middle-income countries, demonstrating the global applicability of virtual patients DVPs [32].
- *AI-enhanced high-fidelity simulations, extended reality (XR), and interactive learning environments (ILE).* Still in their very early days because they are expensive to create and validate AI-enhanced high-fidelity simulations and XR solutions that often incorporate AI are emerging as the most exciting solutions in medical education. They could increase patient safety, for example, as students can practise as long as they need to, and do not have to learn by starting directly with patients. XR solutions enable learning experiences that either blend physical and virtual elements, known as augmented reality (AR), or provide a totally virtual immersive experience called virtual reality (VR). These ILEs are sophisticated experiences that can be applied to a range of clinical topics, from 3D visualization of anatomy to risk-free practice of procedures, medical equipment training, and communication and social skills learning. They can be integrated with virtual tutoring and adaptive learning to further personalize the learning process [33].

3.3.2 AI for Knowledge Testing

One of the challenges in medical education testing is the availability, cost, reliability, and biases of physicians who create and administer tests and clinical skills assessments. AI has shown promise, and will be increasingly used to augment humans for conducting knowledge testing:

- *Generation of testing questions and cases.* It can be time-consuming and expensive to generate formative and summative test questions and cases. As knowledge rapidly shifts on an increasing basis, there is a challenge in ensuring that testing content is up to date. From a given body of knowledge, AI can be used to easily and quickly generate new, high-quality test items that can then be reviewed and adapted by a human expert. This drives down the cost of assessment, and limits the need to reuse questions.
- *Optimized testing.* In the 1990s, educators started experimenting with computerized adaptive testing (CAT), which used the responses provided to adjust

the level of difficulty of the next questions to match the knowledge and ability of a test taker. CAT scoring is based on both the number of correct answers provided and the difficulty of the items completed. AI is now used as a next-generation tool to create and score smarter tests that assess the learner's knowledge and skills in an optimal amount of time.

- *Automated scoring.* AI has been shown to correctly score student performance on both written and in-person components of clinical skills assessment, using natural language processing to score each student's diagnosis in real time. This provides immediate insight into their performance. In addition, applying AI to video recordings of physician–patient interactions and developing algorithms to analyse these encounters is being evaluated, measuring aspects like non-verbal communication, empathy, and eye contact [34].

3.4 Perspectives and Best Practices in Implementing Changes to the Medical Curriculum

The first recommendation of the Lancet Commission was that there is a need for 'adoption of competency-based curricula that are responsive to rapidly changing needs rather than being dominated by static coursework' [1]. While there was no specific mention of AI, this recognizes the massive importance in moving from ideas to rapid and widespread adoption of new concepts in medical education.

There are a few published studies and reports on how to incorporate AI into the medical curriculum that can be used as a starting point [8]. Incorporating new topics into the already heavily charged medical curriculum is always challenging, including overcoming barriers such as long-standing faculty practices and funding streams, university policies and procedures, and incremental reform by regulatory and accreditation bodies [11,12]. Similarly, the adoption of AI learning technologies is often limited in scale and scope, and frequently fails to transform teaching practices unless key requirements are present, related to the technology itself, the working environment, and the individual charged with the dissemination and implementation of the innovation [35,36].

The three main opportunities to create rapid adoption of AI in medical education are as follows:

- *Support medical educators themselves in understanding and embracing AI*, in order to be able both to teach the curriculum and to leverage AI capabilities for the purpose of education. Medical schools lack the faculty expertise required to teach AI-related content. AI has been the domain of computer science, mathematics, and engineering faculties. In addition, beyond theoretical AI literacy, lack of mentorship and faculty role modelling poses a significant challenge for the application of this knowledge in practice

[8,11,12,19]. A focus on a 'train the trainer' approach would have a significant impact on the speed of dissemination of both the AI in medicine curriculum and the use of AI in medical education.

- *Add accreditation and certification requirements related to AI* for medical training programmes, licensing, and CME/CPD programmes, which often lead to more rapid change in medical education curricula [8].
- *Collaborate to reduce the considerable costs* of developing the AI curriculum in medicine, as well as inherent in the development and validation of AI-based educational tools, especially for a specialized and complex knowledge domain like healthcare. There is an exciting opportunity for transformation of the curriculum through collaborations involving medical educators across the world, and this has the added benefit of helping developing countries create greater access to higher-quality medical education [8].

3.5 Future Directions

Medical educators and AI experts need to work together to successfully diffuse AI knowledge across the lifelong learning continuum for physicians, and also to introduce more education about technology in general. Much can also be learnt and adapted from efforts for AI literacy for the public, K-12 education system, and other professions.

As the medical domain has some of the most stringent requirements for quality, safety, and ethics, there needs to be a massive effort to study and validate the many promises that AI will enhance medical education.

Looking into the future, it is a matter of when, not if, the medical profession will acquire a general level of AI literacy, and incorporate AI as a tool within the many others used for clinical care, administration, policy, education, and research. Medical education around AI will then be simply embedded within the context of the specific topic being taught rather than being a standalone domain of knowledge.

KEY INSIGHTS

- **Despite the rapid increase in use of AI in clinical practice, knowledge about technology in general, and AI in particular, is nearly absent from medical education for physicians in training (medical school, residency, and fellowship) and in practice (CPD and CME certifications and advanced degrees). AI literacy, proficiency, and competency are widely recognized as necessary for the medical profession to thrive in the technology-driven transformation of medicine.**
- **Medical training programmes need to rapidly consider how to incorporate understanding of technology in general, and AI in particular, into the medical education curriculum. In addition, additional**

competencies relevant to practising in an AI-enabled environment, such as management of increased information load and providing care with empathy and compassion, need to be addressed.

- Education about AI for physicians in practice can be done through AI-focused courses, and also by incorporating AI into the clinical subjects covered in the medical training curriculum and in CPD/CME courses.
- AI can be used to enhance medical education itself, especially in the two areas of learning support and knowledge testing.
- Numerous challenges exist to the development and dissemination of AI in medical training for the profession, as well as using AI to enhance medical education. The three key opportunities to accelerate these trends are to help educate the educators, introduce accreditation and certification requirements for medical education programmes, and create adequate funding for the efforts to increase AI in medical education.

Disclosure Statement

Alexandra T. Greenhill is an advisor to a number of technology companies providing healthcare solutions for clinical practice and for consumers, both directly and through accelerators such as New Ventures BC, Founders Institute, FoundersBoost, and The Forum. None of the companies she works with or advises have been mentioned in this chapter.

References

1. Frenk J, Chen L, Bhutta ZA et al. Health professionals for a new century: transforming education to strengthen health systems in an interdependent world. *Lancet* 2010;376(9756):1923–1958. https://doi.org/10.1016/S0140-6736(10)61854-5.
2. American Medical Association. *Digital Health Study: Physicians' Motivations and Requirements for Adopting Digital Clinical Tools.* Chicago, IL: American Medical Association; 2016. https://www.ama-assn.org/media/11681/download.
3. Canadian Medical Association. *Shaping the Future of Health and Medicine.* 2018. https://www.cma.ca/sites/default/files/pdf/Activities/Shaping%20the%20Future%20of%20Health%20and%20Medicine.pdf.
4. Matheny M, Thadaney Israni S, Ahmed M, Whicher D, eds. *Artificial Intelligence in Health Care: The Hope, the Hype, the Promise, the Peril.* NAM Special Publication. Washington, DC: National Academy of Medicine; 2019.
5. Bilimoria K, Harish V, McCoy L et al. *Training for the Future: Preparing Medical Students for the Impact of Artificial Intelligence.* Ontario: Ontario Medical Students Association; 2019. https://omsa.ca/sites/default/files/policy_or_position_paper/115/position_paper_preparing_medical_students_for_artificial_intelligence_2019_feb.pdf.

6. Harish V, Bilimoria K, Mehta N et al. *Preparing Medical Students for the Impact of Artificial Intelligence on Healthcare.* Ottawa: Canadian Federation of Medical Students; 2020. https://www.cfms.org/files/meetings/agm-2020/resolutions/ai_healthcare/ PreparingMedStudentsForAI.pdf.

7. Royal College of Physicians and Surgeons of Canada. *Artificial Intelligence (AI) and Emerging Digital Technologies.* Ottawa: Royal College of Physicians and Surgeons of Canada; 2020. https://www.royalcollege.ca/rcsite/health-policy/initiatives/ ai-task-force-e.

For additional references and Further Reading, please see www.wiley.com/go/byrne/ aiinclinicalmedicine.

AI Foundations

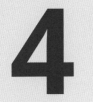

4

History of AI in Clinical Medicine

Isaak Kavasidis, Federica Proietto Salanitri, Simone Palazzo, and Concetto Spampinato

Department of Electrical, Electronic and Computer Engineering, University of Catania, Catania, Italy

---

Learning Objectives

- Understand the evolution of AI in clinical medicine from the 1960s to the present time.
- Review key milestones of AI in clinical medicine, including some of the setbacks resulting in AI winters.
- Become familiar with the language, fundamental tools, and concepts underpinning AI, machine learning, and deep learning in clinical medicine.
- Gain perspective on the differences in explainable artificial intelligence (XAI) methods.
- Briefly discuss future directions for AI in clinical medicine.

4.1 Introduction

In clinical practice, huge volumes of data are routinely produced. These include, but are not limited to, images (magnetic resonance imaging [MRI], computed tomography [CT], sonography, radiography), time series (electroencephalography [EEG], electromyography [EMG], electrocardiography [ECG]), audio (speech, Doppler), and free-text documents (both structured and unstructured reports, comments, and annotations). This, in conjunction with the complete digitalization of medical data, has established a fertile ground for the massive processing and training of AI to ultimately aid in the performance of tasks in clinical practice. Despite the emergence of AI in the 1950s, however, digital medical data have only become ubiquitous during the last two decades.

Between the 1960s and 1980s, lack of adequate data and computing capacity led to the first so-called AI winter. This was provoked by generalized criticism regarding the performance and efficiency of AI that ultimately hampered interest in further research and development. Moreover, the medical community was slow in adopting fundamentally diverse methods to practice; practitioners were reluctant to trust technology to optimize healthcare, and to improve patient well-being.

AI in Clinical Medicine: A Practical Guide for Healthcare Professionals, First Edition. Edited by Michael F. Byrne, Nasim Parsa, Alexandra T. Greenhill, Daljeet Chahal, Omer Ahmad, and Ulas Bagci.
© 2023 John Wiley & Sons Ltd. Published 2023 by John Wiley & Sons Ltd.
Companion website: www.wiley.com/go/byrne/aiinclinicalmedicine

AI has come a long way since then. It now meets the application needs of medicine through the sheer number-crunching capacity that it offers. We can readily find applications of AI, namely deep learning, in clinical medicine. This includes the generation of diagnoses through medical imaging and signal analysis, precise treatment planning through chatbots and simple questionnaires, and surgical assistance through autonomous AI-guided robotic systems.

4.2 The Beginnings of AI in Medicine

The adoption of AI in medicine can be tracked back to the mid-1960s. Initially, AI was based on conditional methods, or 'if-then-else' rules. These statistical methods usually exploited Bayes' theorem to perform simple predictions, such as whether or not a patient will develop coronary heart disease based on health indicators [1]. The utility of conditional methods subsequently evolved into the use of more complex logic paradigms, fuzzy logic [2], for simple medical decisions or classification problems, such as evaluating the health index of patients [3]. Fuzzy logic had the advantage of being simple in its inner workings, which lent itself to easy knowledge translation for its use and subsequent establishment in the medical community. Compared to more recent machine learning approaches, fuzzy logic is still an active research topic in the use of AI in medicine, demonstrating its reliability as an indispensable tool.

Despite AI being in its infancy during this period, there was an urgent and unmet need for expert systems in large-scale computing. Existing computers were programmed to provide answers based on a set of rules. In medicine, examples of such systems were MYCIN, an expert system for treating bacterial blood infections, which led to the evolution of the knowledge-enhanced domain-independent EMYCIN; and PUFF, a specialized tool based on EMYCIN for interpreting pulmonary function data.

4.3 The Development of Artificial Neural Networks

In 1943, McCulloch and Pitts [4] set the mathematical foundations for a tool that attempted to emulate the human brain, namely an artificial neuron. Fifteen years later, Rosenblatt [5] presented the perceptron, a simplified model of the artificial neuron. Technical limitations in execution – that is, training and validation – hindered further research.

Nevertheless, in the 1980s the introduction of the error backpropagation algorithm (i.e. an algorithm where the input is fed into the model, an initial decision is made and compared against the desired output decision, and the difference is then used to update the parameters of the model) rejuvenated interest in artificial neural networks (ANNs) by demonstrating their potential in solving multiple, complex, non-linear problems. The capacity to deal with non-linearities, in conjunction with their simplicity, enabled widespread acceptance of ANNs in medical research.

While other methods, such as non-linear regression, required very detailed mathematical models to compute, ANNs could automatically discover patterns in input data. In other words, the popularity of ANNs grew from the fact that they needed nothing more than input data and the data labels to be trained.

However, it was precisely this freedom in architectural design that led to some practical problems. Training and validating many network architectures (number of hidden layers, number of neurons in each layer, etc.) was cumbersome, given that computing capacity was not as readily available then as it is now. Scientists and engineers often struggled with the bias-variance dilemma. These challenges, which frequently led to overfitting (i.e. the model learns exhaustively the training set data distribution and cannot generalize) and underfitting (i.e. the model is not capable enough to learn the distribution of the data), together with the invention of another, simpler parametric model that could work even better, led to the second, but shorter, AI winter.

4.4 The Era of Support Vector Machines and Feature Descriptors

As the research community shifted its attention away from neural networks, a new tool, the support vector machine (SVM), emerged [6]. SVMs were found to overcome many of the issues that neural networks inherently had by design. First, they required fewer data to train – data storage, transfer, and annotation were not as easy as they are now. They also required much less computing and design time. Moreover, SVMs were able to guarantee convergence to the global minimum (i.e. the function learnt is the one that produces the minimum possible error), something that neural networks cannot always achieve, even today.

The power of SVMs also enabled more generic features to be used. Until then, feature construction and selection were often 'handcrafted', such as angles and textures in images, words or phrases in textual data, and peaks and frequency spectrums in bio-signals. With SVMs, the scientific community concentrated its efforts on *feature engineering,* or the identification of generalizable (feature) descriptors invariant to rotation, scaling, and affine transformations. The premise of feature engineering is the extraction of a numerical representation from the most general or significant components of data for the training of AI models.

A variety of methods for generalizable feature extraction include scale-invariant feature transformation (SIFT) [7], where, as the name suggests, descriptors remained uniform for similar objects but with different sizes or scales, as well as orientation- and rotation-invariant (ORB) approaches [8], where descriptor vectors are uniform for similar objects but with varying orientations and rotations. These features could then be exploited together with matching algorithms to locate anatomical structures, ignoring the normal (and abnormal) variability that comes with human nature and medical devices. In text data, through natural language processing (NLP), such features could be used to decipher the concept of an article or the summary of medical reports. Also, NLP has been successfully applied to knowledge discovery, together with the emergence of Big Data, where many previously unknown associations between physiological processes could be discovered. An example of an SVM-based method is demonstrated by Guyon et al. [9], where an SVM is used to diagnose cancer based on the genomic profile of patients.

4.5 Dominance of Deep Learning

While feature descriptors were dominating the AI scene between the 1990s and 2000s, many of the drawbacks (e.g. computation times and sensitivity to data disturbances worsening the lack of generalization) of existing methods persisted.

As larger datasets became available, variance and model complexities subsequently increased to unprecedented levels, revealing the limitations of the feature engineering methods. Thus, the research focus shifted again to learning feature representation directly from data, but this time the feature selection procedure was completely unsupervised by humans (i.e. the model itself decides which features to extract). Also, the fast progress of gaming hardware (graphics processing units [GPU]) in performing massive matrix multiplications enabled the scientific community to shift towards parallelizable paradigms under which neural networks resurged again. The increased availability of computing resources lent itself to the development of more complex architectures comprising multiple hierarchical processing layers. In other words, the *deep learning* era had begun.

Even though the foundations of deep learning were defined in the late 1980s with the discovery of the backpropagation training algorithm [10], it was not until 2012 when deep learning was readily applied. AlexNet, one of the first convolutional neural network–based deep learning models [11], demonstrated its superiority over not only traditional machine learning but also human capabilities on certain tasks. Since then, deep learning–based methods, including convolutional neural networks and recurrent neural networks, are being integrated into medical applications almost everywhere. U-NETs (the name coming from their shape being like the letter U) [12], one of the most exploited deep learning model architectures in medical applications, and their variants are routinely used for making segmentation masks of individual organs. Such segmentation masks can subsequently be used 'as is' for visualization purposes or as the basis for further processing.

An indicator of the advancement of AI in medicine is best exemplified by the previously widespread adoption of IBM's Watson AI platform in healthcare for managing patient treatment plans, suggesting alternative treatment options and drug discovery, as well as the recent US Food and Drug Administration (FDA)-approved 'Arterys', which aids in medical imaging diagnosis.

Deep learning has undoubtedly revolutionized the analysis and discovery of complex patterns, which has resulted in the simplification of many medical tasks. However, this had led to concerns about how deep learning models make decisions, and whether the criteria for making such decisions reflect actual, real, and objective scientific knowledge.

4.6 Interpretability of Deep Models

The unclear processes underlying deep networks place a limitation on their general interpretability. This, in turn, limits the wider adoption of deep learning in areas of high-stakes decision-making, as in clinical practice. There is an urgent and unmet need to endow deep learning models with explainable mechanisms that would lead to easier comprehension by end-users of decisions made by the models. Explainable AI (XAI) can indeed provide explanations for model decisions (see Figure 4.1). (XAI is also referred to as interpretable deep learning, and the two terms are commonly interchanged.) This is also required by recent regulations, such as the European Union's General Data Protection Regulation (GDPR, Article 15), which supports the rights of patients to receive information about how a medical decision is made.

AI researchers are increasingly employing XAI to shed light on their algorithms' inner workings. XAI methods can be classified according to the following three criteria: model based versus post hoc, model specific versus model agnostic, and global versus local (i.e. the scope of the explanation):

- *Model-based methods* attempt to construct explainable features by enforcing sparsity. However, they cannot be used in models with thousands or millions of parameters, such as deep models.
- *Post-hoc methods* train a neural network and then explain the behaviour of the trained model by inspecting the learnt features. This ultimately provides a visual explanation of the relative importance of input data using saliency maps [13].
- *Model-agnostic explanations* operate only on the relationships between input and output of the models by perturbating the inputs and observing how the outputs change as a consequence. In this case, no knowledge is required about the model and, as such, they are also considered post-hoc methods.
- *Model-specific explanations* are limited only to particular classes of models, and have subsequent reduced applicability to multiple cases.

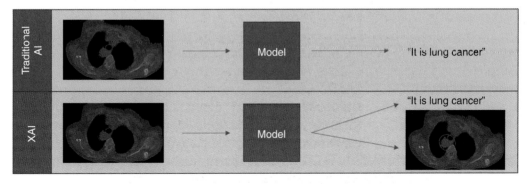

Figure 4.1: Traditional AI (top) versus explainable AI (XAI, bottom). Traditional AI does not provide any means to understand the basis for the model's decision. On the other hand, XAI does what traditional AI does, but additionally offers evidence on the parts of data that aided the model to make that decision (e.g. in the image it highlights the tumour through the use of heatmaps).

XAI methods have been largely applied to medical image analysis by providing either a visual or textual explanation for the decisions made by a model. Among the visual explanation solutions, also called saliency mapping, we can find the popular backpropagation-based approaches, such as GradCAM [13]. GradCAM uses gradient information flowing into the last convolutional layer of a CNN to assign importance values to each neuron for a particular decision of interest. For example, it has been used to highlight the pathological areas of a lymph node biopsy and identify metastatic tissue [14]. It can also identify and explain the parts of a CT scan most associated with genes involved in lung cancer [15]. GradCAM was used too in an integrated platform to locate and differentiate COVID-19 lung lesions on CT scans [16].

Textual explanation of deep models is a form of XAI that basically provides image captioning on visual data. This approach is combined with a visual description to enhance explanation capabilities. For example, Lee et al. proposed image captioning with visual explanation for breast mammograms whereby radiology reports were linked to visual saliency maps [17].

Despite XAI methods having gained momentum, those performing post-hoc explanations are not exempt from criticism. In 2019, Rudin et al. reported several examples of explanations by post-hoc methods that do not provide enough insight for users to be able to understand what it is happening within the 'black box' [18]. This lack of understanding is sufficient for the authors of this chapter to advise the use of model-based rather than post-hoc XAI methods.

4.7 Transformers: Better Performance and Inherent Interpretability through Self-Attention

As already highlighted, CNN-based architectures have played a major role in medical imaging research. However, more recently a novel type of architecture, the transformer, has entered the scene.

Transformers are deep learning models that were initially designed to deal with Seq2Seq (sequence-to-sequence, i.e. an input sequence produces an output sequence) tasks. They consist of two main low-level operation blocks: an attention-based block for modelling inter-element relations (e.g. how a tumour is shown in sequential CT slices), and a multi-layer perceptron (MLP) modelling intra-element relations (e.g. different parts of a tumour in a single CT slice). A pipeline of attention and MLP blocks intertwined with residual connections has been shown to allow for generalization over multiple tasks. Transformers have demonstrated remarkable performance in many fields of artificial intelligence, such as NLP, audio processing, and more recently in computer vision tasks [19].

Transformer-based architectures are very efficient in medical imaging analysis due to several key advantages. They capture long-range dependencies, provide an intrinsic method to explain model decisions, and can achieve similar performance to traditional deep learning.

Vanilla Transformers were designed to model sequential one-dimensional data, but after the pioneering works of Dosovitskiy et al. showing that transformers can be adapted to process bi-dimensional data (Vision Transformers or ViTs), numerous approaches have been presented based on transformers, and are being continuously adapted to medical practice [20]. Many approaches are focused on image segmentation by combining transformer modules with traditional deep learning ones [21,22].

The use of transformers in medical image analysis is growing. However, this trend requires larger datasets. The original ViT was trained with 300 million-labelled images, which is not feasible in today's medical settings because data is not readily available.

The introduction of transformers enables interpretability; their attention mechanism strategy makes them inherently more explainable. The attention scores can be exploited to interpret and visually demonstrate the decisions either by using the last layer [23] or by traversing the whole model starting from the decision back to the input [24]. Transformers thus represent a unified solution, combining effectiveness in solving complex tasks (comparable to that of traditional deep learning counterparts) and providing adequate explanations surrounding decision-making. Most importantly, these two features are obtained without significant tweaking of the model, and they combine the advantages of model-based and post-hoc XAI.

4.8 The (Near) Future

Progress is measured by the day as new inventions are added to the arsenal of available medical tools that aid in the diagnosis and treatment of disease.

Currently the research community is interested in finding more reliable methods for explaining AI. Indeed, knowing why an AI model makes a particular decision in clinical practice is as important as its performance. Transformers, with their self-attention and clear user interpretability, are the logical candidates for this endeavour, although more traditional deep learning architectures can achieve the same interpretability by employing gradient-based methods.

AI performs better when it is trained on large-scale labelled datasets. Despite this, it is the act of labelling that introduces the biggest barrier to AI's current application. Creating large-scale datasets is relatively easy given the thousands or maybe millions of medical data points acquired every day in clinical practice. However, to label this data is rather unfeasible. For this reason, research efforts are also focused on unsupervised learning methods [25–28].

For the near future, safe short-term predictions can be made. Deep learning has already reached a peak in performance, and more dynamic architectures are starting to be considered. For example, dynamic routing between neurons led to the development of Capsule networks [29], and they can be used to model better hierarchical relationships.

Given that the goal of AI research is to reach human-level adaptability and performance in many different and complex tasks, new neuron models have been proposed to better simulate the functionality of biological neurons. Such research has resulted in so-called third-generation neural networks, or spiking neural networks (SNNs), that are able to internally represent the concept of time in the data flow, with the promise of greater efficiency, adaptability, and performance.

KEY INSIGHTS

- ■ **Deep learning in medicine has already reached a peak in performance, and more dynamic architectures are being considered.**
- ■ **Due to the insufficiency of post-hoc explanations, model-based rather than post-hoc XAI methods are recommended.**
- ■ **Knowing why an AI model makes a particular decision in clinical practice is as important as its performance. Transformers, with their self-attention and clear user interpretability, are the ideal candidates to address this need.**

Funding

This work has been partially supported by:

- ▤ The REHASTART project funded by Regione Sicilia (PO FESR 2014/2020 – Azione 1.1.5, N. 08ME6201000222,CUP G79J18000610007).
- ▤ The 'Go for IT' project funded by the Conference of Italian University Rectors (CRUI).

References

1. Warner HR, Toronto AF, Veasy LG. Experience with Baye's theorem for computer diagnosis of congenital heart disease. *Annals of the New York Academy of Sciences* 1964;115(2):558–567.
2. Shortliffe EH, Buchanan BG. A model of inexact reasoning in medicine. *Mathematical Biosciences* 1975;23(3–4):351–379.
3. Fanshel S, Bush JW. A health-status index and its application to health-services outcomes. *Operations Research* 1970;18(6):1021–1066.
4. McCulloch WS, Pitts W. A logical calculus of the ideas immanent in nervous activity. *Bulletin of Mathematical Biophysics* 1943;5(4):115–133.
5. Rosenblatt F. The perceptron: a probabilistic model for information storage and organization in the brain. *Psychological Review* 1958;65(6):386.
6. Boser BE, Guyon, IM, Vapnik VN. A training algorithm for optimal margin classifiers. *Proceedings of the Fifth Annual Workshop on Computational Learning Theory*. New York: Association for Computing Machinery; 1992, 144–152.
7. Lowe DG. Distinctive image features from scale-invariant keypoints. *International Journal of Computer Vision* 2004;60(2):91–110.

For additional references and Further Reading, please see www.wiley.com/go/byrne/aiinclinicalmedicine.

5

History, Core Concepts, and Role of AI in Clinical Medicine

Christoph Palm

Regensburg Medical Image Computing (ReMIC), Ostbayerische Technische Hochschule Regensburg (OTH Regensburg), Regensburg, Germany

---

Learning Objectives

- Gain perspective on the evolution, hype, and reality of AI in general and related to clinical medicine.
- Gain insight into the various AI terms and methods.
- Understand the different roles AI can play in clinical medicine, and how this is expected to change the physician's role.

5.1 Introduction

The term artificial intelligence or AI is broad, and several different terms are used in this context that must be organized and demystified. This chapter will review the key concepts and methods of AI, and will introduce some of the different roles for AI in relation to the physician.

Figure 5.1 presents a timeline of AI in clinical medicine.

Human imagination has envisioned many possible AI scenarios, ranging from servants for the people to a superintelligence that overpowers humanity. However, the timeline demonstrates that the short history of AI is characterized by a continuous cycle of ambitious promises, high – perhaps too high – expectations, and ongoing repeated disappointments that have been called 'AI winters' by some experts. The AI community has contributed to this situation by making several grandiose announcements. The invitation to the Dartmouth workshop in 1955 stated that 'every aspect of learning or any other feature of intelligence can in principle be so precisely described that a machine can be made to simulate it' [2]. IBM advertised that its health AI system with 'Doctor Watson' can take over the doctor's responsibilities [6]. Furthermore, Geoffrey Hinton made the following comments: 'Deep learning is going to be able to do everything' and 'People should stop training radiologists now. It's completely obvious that in five years deep learning is going to

AI in Clinical Medicine: A Practical Guide for Healthcare Professionals, First Edition. Edited by Michael F. Byrne, Nasim Parsa, Alexandra T. Greenhill, Daljeet Chahal, Omer Ahmad, and Ulas Bagci.
© 2023 John Wiley & Sons Ltd. Published 2023 by John Wiley & Sons Ltd.
Companion website: www.wiley.com/go/byrne/aiinclinicalmedicine

do better than radiologists' (https://www.youtube.com/watch?v=2HMPRXstSvQ). Despite making significant progress, AI is still far away from achieving human-level intelligence and, obviously, radiologists and physicians in general are still needed!

5.2 Core Concepts of AI

AI is an intelligent agent that is expected to act reasonably in a complex world to achieve a goal or solve a problem. Different types of AI can be differentiated by their increasing ability to perceive the surrounding environment, and by the consequences of decisions and actions:

- Problem-solving AI agents have knowledge only about possible actions, and can look ahead to define reasonably appropriate action sequences for specific situations.
- AI agents with a representation of the complex world can derive new representations, and are able to deduce what to do to achieve a specific goal.
- In a more realistic scenario, more complex AI agents can deal with uncertainty regarding their state of being and the result after a sequence of actions.
- A learning AI agent builds a model of the world from observational data, which leads to problem-solving [2].

Machine learning focuses on the study of learning AI agents. Programming, in the traditional sense, refers to the implementation of an algorithm that transforms input data into output data. Such a program is stable and does not change without the input of a programmer. Alternatively, programs with a *learning* component are also implemented by a human programmer. However, some parameters of such programs

(a)

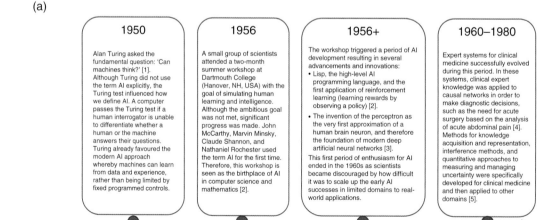

Figure 5.1: (a–d) Timeline of AI in clinical medicine from 1950 to the present.

are not hardcoded but can be changed by a learning process. This learning process can be triggered by:

- The input data and labels.
- Clustering of common input data features.
- Reinforcement based on the processing outcome.

A visual representation of this can be found in Chapter 6. In the context of AI, these three variants of learning are called *supervised, unsupervised,* and *reinforcement* learning, respectively. In simple terms, supervised learning uses labelled input and output data. If the data set is large, from different sources, heterogeneous, and essentially unlabelled, unsupervised methods are applied. In reinforcement learning, the learner interacts with the environment to extract the output or make decisions.

Several learning algorithms already in use include support vector machines and random forests. However, neural networks (NNs) are receiving increasing attention because of their superior performance. An NN consists of layers of neurons, with a specific input and output layer and several hidden layers. Each neuron of a hidden layer essentially has a linear component computing the weighted sum of its input values and a so-called activation function as a non-linear component. AlexNet, mentioned in Chapter 4, consisted of 11 hidden layers in 2012, but current NNs contain more than 100 hidden layers. Since the early NNs had only one layer (or in the case of the perceptron only one neuron), all these larger NNs are called deep neural networks and are subsumed by the term deep learning.

AI is often used as a blanket term for all methods involving a learning process. Because deep learning is part of machine learning, and machine learning is part of AI, AI and machine learning and even AI and deep learning are frequently used synonymously. *However, if we take the term AI seriously, then AI is defined as software that can reason, can adapt to new situations, can find new and hidden relationships,*

(b)

1980s	1990s	2000

...Unfortunately, clinical decision support by expert systems did not make it into daily practice due to the lack of large clinical trials to demonstrate the real-world impact of such systems, problems collecting data from heterogeneous clinical data management systems, the lack of quality measures to support formal evaluations, and the general complexity and amount of uncertainty in the clinical domain.

The back-propagation algorithm was reinvented to allow parameters to be optimized, most frequently using gradient descent approaches [2]. We say 'reinvention' because back-propagation was introduced in the early 1960s, but by the late 1980s was being used by artificial neural networks (NNs) – including computational NNs – which emerged from the perceptron. Back-propagation is one of the key elements of modern AI approaches that provides an efficient way to compute partial derivatives in a high-dimensional feature space.

The shift to a probabilistic model based on Bayes decision rules was an important AI milestone. Introduced in 1763 by Thomas Bayes, the principles of Bayesian learning became more and more important for data-driven machine learning. Bayesian learning predicts the most probable hypothesis based on available data, taking the uncertainty of data and decisions into account [2]. This is a departure from Boolean logic, which allows only binary outcomes of true of false, or 0 or 1. Bayesian learning integrates expert knowledge about the domain into a priori probabilities. Combining several simple and mathematically manageable Gaussian distributions into probabilistic mixture models permits the modelling of very complex situations.

Speech recognition and later machine translation were very successful at integrating these mixture models into hidden Markov models, accommodating the probability of state transitions in the temporal course of phonemes (the smallest units of speech), words, and sentence fragments for the first time. In dark rooms where X-ray images or computed tomography scans are assessed, the translation of the spoken narrative into written text to be stored in the patient record is time-saving for the radiologist. Unfortunately, high-quality recognition at this time required a restricted vocabulary, limiting speech recognition to specific domains.

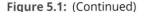

Figure 5.1: (Continued)

can integrate prior knowledge, and is creative and innovative; in short, software that is comparable to human intelligence. It is of note that this does not necessarily mean that AI must mimic the human brain in detail. Although this goal is a driving force for the research community, we are still far away from developing this kind of AI, something known as strong AI or artificial general intelligence.

AI's basic achievement is the creation of software that is capable of learning a very specific task and may be very successful in performing this task. In clinical medicine, this type of AI is increasingly able to outperform humans on certain specific functions because it can be trained with huge volumes of data, including exceptionally rare cases that physicians may never encounter in their careers. However, this type of AI is unable to transfer the learnt knowledge from one domain to the next, and if the task is changed, it has to start from the beginning and learn the new task from new data. This kind of AI is called weak AI or artificial narrow intelligence.

Methods like domain adaptation and transfer learning are being developed to overcome these limitations. These methods extend the boundaries of weak AI, by forcing the AI to use some learnt features or statistical distributions from one task to make learning the next task easier. Whether the weak AI is able to *understand* the initial task and, therefore, now understands the relationship to the second task remains a philosophical question.

The science fiction view of AI suggests that AI should not be limited to artificial general intelligence (at the same level as humans), but could potentially surpass human intelligence. A requirement for AI to make this major next step to artificial superintelligence would be the acquisition of self-awareness. As this kind of AI is not limited to a physical body like human intelligence, it would have much more potential. For example, it could be transferred to other locations in the world and beyond in milliseconds. The only requirements would be a digital transfer connection and a computer to receive the artificial superintelligence at the other end.

(c)

2011

More data and larger storage capabilities led to the development of data-mining approaches to learn from such vast amounts of data. However, the challenge of Big Data is not only the sheer number of data, but the heterogeneity of data sources, unlabelled data, unstructured data, and incomplete data. After IBM Watson won the *Jeopardy* game show in 2011, IBM Watson Health started to build a clinical decision system for oncology. The concept was simple: analyse a vast amount of clinical data to provide the clinician with personalized advice for the treatment of a specific patient. Key concept: 'patient similarity analytics', patients with similar attributes but different treatments and outcomes are compared [6].

...IBM believed that, with this analysis, the best treatment could be derived from the Big Data pool, removing the requirement for elaborate and expensive clinical studies. After huge financial and resource investment, including hundreds of programmers working on the software, the system failed, and the development ceased in 2015. This demonstrates that the complexity of the medical domain cannot be underestimated, and that the quality and completeness of data are perhaps more important than the amount of data.

2011+

The relaunch of NNs after 2011 is attributed to Yoshua Bengio, Geoffrey Hinton, and Yann LeCun (Turing Award winners 2018), as well as Jürgen Schmidhuber. The term 'deep learning' was introduced for this new generation of NNs and refers to multi-layer artificial NNs, with input and output layers and hidden layers composed of linear and non-linear modules [8]. The deep learning approach builds on all methods introduced previously, and is enabled by faster computers, parallelization of basic operations on graphical processing units (GPUs), and larger storage.

...A key advantage of the deep learning approach is that the networks are fed by raw data (e.g. the pixel values in case of images), allowing back-propagation-based optimization to learn the relevant features by itself. The programmer designs the network architecture and data preprocessing, but the network learns from the data.

Figure 5.1: (Continued)

It is beyond this book to deeply speculate on the nature of the relationship between humans and an artificial superintelligence. Will humans have to fear this kind of AI? Or will AI and humans co-exist because humans will simply be unimportant irritants to AI, like mosquitos are to humans? Perhaps humans will prevail, because they developed AI to fulfil human-defined objectives [7]. Only time will tell.

5.3 Roles of AI in Relation to Physicians

As a relatively new partner joining the patient–physician relationship, AI has to prove that it will re-humanize and not de-humanize clinical medicine [13]. The role of AI as a virtual medical assistant should be made clear, where it should serve as augmented intelligence for the clinician while keeping the human in the loop [14]. Some examples are now described.

5.3.1 AI as a Measuring Device

When making a diagnosis, clinicians rely on objective measurements ranging from body temperature to blood pressure to blood counts. However, clinicians also rely on subjective data, including the results of physical examinations as well as imaging results. AI methods are very proficient at medical image analysis, providing objective information like radiomics features, including tumour location and size, tumour border characterization, and higher-order statistics describing grey level or colour variations of the tumour tissue.

5.3.2 AI as a Planning and Simulation Tool

Complicated interventional procedures, for example in neurosurgery, require advanced planning and experienced decision-making about the optimal way to remove tumour tissue. While imaging allows the head to be visualized beforehand,

(d)

2012	2015		2017+	2020
The deep convolutional neural network (CNN) AlexNet won the ImageNet (www.image-net.org) competition, reducing by nearly 50% the error rate of the previous year, when shallow networks were used [9]. The ImageNet dataset, containing thousands of real-world images from cats and dogs, to cars and trees, to children and frogs, is still important because it frequently serves as the basis for NNs' initialization of parameters, something called transfer learning.	Similar to when IBM Watson won *Jeopardy*, the public recognized the new advent of AI when DeepMind's AlphaGo won the game Go, which has long been viewed as the most challenging of classic games for AI [10]. Methodologically, AlphaGo made use of a recurrent NN, where the networks learned from the outcome of the game while one AlphaGo version plays against another. Remarkably, AlphaGo used game moves not previously shown by human players.	…Some might judge this as a creative process, which was one of the early goals of AI: the idea that computers that are able to reason can react to new situations and be creative. However, AlphaGo did not understand the game, and if the playing field was reduced by one row and one column, it would be unable to perform as before. However, AlphaGo could adapt to the new situation by retraining quite quickly.	Deep learning has directly boosted the performance of AI in clinical medicine. In selected application domains, AI can achieve or exceed physician performance, as highlighted by the 2017 *Nature* paper by Andre Esteva et al., which describes dermatologist-level classification of skin cancer by an AI model [11]. This system used only raw images and their respective labels, and did not integrate the clinically relevant ABCD rules for skin cancer diagnosis. This changed the learning paradigm from one requiring handcrafted features that simulate the physicians' perspective to one that used data-learned features. Similar to the challenge faced by expert systems, large clinical trials using deep learning systems are still rare. The next challenge is to translate promising research results into clinical practice.	DeepMind successfully transformed the ideas and the lessons learned from AlphaGo, and applied them to a very complex biomedical problem: protein folding. AlphaFold won the CASP14 challenge by a large margin [12]. This breakthrough will certainly impact clinical medicine, as the accurate prediction of the three-dimensional protein structure based on the amino acid sequence has the potential to revolutionize the understanding of molecular processes and the development of new drugs and therapies.

Figure 5.1: (Continued)

AI can show the optimal access path, can mark high-risk structures, and can simulate the whole procedure in advance. This AI information, combined with haptic feedback, will allow surgeons to practise and perfect a complex, high-risk procedure using a realistic virtual scenario prior to the actual operation.

5.3.3 AI as a Helpmate

AI can serve as a helpmate to clinicians to reduce the burden in their daily practice by completing some of the more routine tasks or by helping to diagnose simple and non-critical cases with high sensitivity and specificity. For example, patients with a long medical history may have an enormous volume of health information in their medical records, including medical reports, imaging results, and prescription records. AI can identify and present the most important information to the clinician to prevent them from missing a relevant detail, especially in more acute situations.

This will allow the physician to concentrate on complicated cases and to follow up with the patient. For now at least, the accurate diagnosis of more challenging cases is only possible for a radiologist rather than AI, as only the radiologist has the appropriate training and ability to address the entire spectrum of possible clinical scenarios. In addition, differentiating non-critical from critical cases is an important skill for radiologists, so this still needs to be included in their training.

5.3.4 AI as a Monitoring Tool

Patients in intensive care units are continuously monitored, whereas in hospital wards this monitoring is selective. Wearable sensors allow AI to monitor and analyse the health condition of patients 24/7, and can alert nurses and clinicians if a change in status occurs. For this application, AI can take a patient's case history, medication, and disease process into consideration.

5.3.5 AI as a Mentor (or Minder)

With AI in the role of a mentor, the physician acts independently. The AI monitors the diagnosis, therapy decisions, or intervention (in the case of surgical robotics). AI can assess potential risks and intervene to provide information when something is missed, or can highlight high-risk structures in the operating field.

5.3.6 AI as an Assistant

Computer-aided diagnosis supports the physician in interpreting medical images by analysing suspicious lesions, calculating probabilities for tumorous tissue, or indicating the location of polyps in colonoscopy. During surgery, augmented reality can be used to support the surgeon by overlaying tissue borders, identifying high-risk structures, and assisting with camera positioning during minimally invasive surgery.

5.3.7 AI as an Independent Second Examiner

Currently, most physicians reach diagnostic decisions without AI support. In many cases, AI can now be used to make a diagnosis without physician input, and as an independent second examiner. In cases where the physician and AI diagnoses agree, no further action is required. If the diagnoses differ, the physician will be prompted to refer to further information to confirm the previous diagnosis or revise the previous decision.

5.4 Concluding Remarks

Undoubtedly, AI will play a major role in nearly all domains of clinical medicine in the future. The examples provided in this chapter, as well as many other examples in this book, demonstrate that the physician can use AI for assistance, error prevention, and timesaving, to substantially improve the practice of clinical medicine.

KEY INSIGHTS

- **Since its origin in the 1950s, AI has consistently made a positive impact on clinical medicine.**
- **The complexity of the medical domain cannot be underestimated, and the quality and completeness of data are perhaps more important than the amount of data.**
- **AI as a new partner supplementing the patient–physician relationship will increasingly support physicians in different roles.**

References

1. Turing AM. I. – Computing machinery and intelligence, *Mind* 1950;LIX(236):433–460.
2. Russel S, Norvig P. *Artificial Intelligence: A Modern Approach*, 4th edn. Harlow: Pearson; 2021.
3. Rosenblatt F. The perceptron: a probabilistic model for information storage and organization in the brain. *Psychological Review* 1958;65(6):386–408.
4. Samarghitean C, Vihinen M. Medical expert systems. *Current Bioinformatics* 2008;3:56–65.
5. Shortliffe EH. The adolescence of AI in medicine: will the field come of age in the ′90s? *Artificial Intelligence in Medicine* 1993;5(2):93–106.
6. Wachter RM. *The Digital Doctor: Hope, Hype, and Harm at the Dawn of Medicine's Computer Age.* New York: McGraw-Hill Education; 2015.
7. Bostrom N. *Superintelligence: Paths, Dangers, Strategies.* Oxford: Oxford University Press; 2014.

For additional references please see www.wiley.com/go/byrne/aiinclinical medicine.

6

Building Blocks of AI

Ulas Bagci, Ismail Irmakci, Ugur Demir, and Elif Keles

Machine and Hybrid Intelligence Lab, Department of Radiology, Northwestern University, Chicago, IL, USA

Learning Objectives

- Define the building blocks of AI: data, algorithms, and optimization.
- Introduce the current application and recent advancements of AI in healthcare.
- Discuss unique challenges of the application of AI in clinical medicine, and potential solutions to these challenges.

6.1 Introduction and AI Definitions

Artificial intelligence (AI) is playing an increasingly important role in modern medicine. Physicians of the future and other healthcare professionals will be expected to work closely with AI tools and therefore must have a clear understanding of AI, or at least the general principles. This chapter will summarize the building blocks of AI algorithms to provide a solid foundation for the rest of the book.

AI is a broad term and is defined as the intelligence demonstrated by machines (see Figure 6.1). However, in current jargon-heavy use, the term AI is typically used nowadays to refer to machine learning, specifically deep learning. Technically speaking, machine learning is a subset of AI. Machine learning encompasses the methods that enable computers (algorithms) to perceive their environment with associated data (parsing and learning from data), and take actions that maximize their chance of achieving goals (prediction about something in the world). Deep learning is a subfield of machine learning. It enables computers to solve the aforementioned prediction problems by using neural networks, a specific method in the machine learning field.

Much of the recent success in AI, particularly in deep learning, has been driven by two important factors:

- Hardware developments that provide more memory and faster, more complex computation.
- Big datasets containing enough examples to represent diverse patterns.

AI in Clinical Medicine: A Practical Guide for Healthcare Professionals, First Edition. Edited by Michael F. Byrne, Nasim Parsa, Alexandra T. Greenhill, Daljeet Chahal, Omer Ahmad, and Ulas Bagci.
© 2023 John Wiley & Sons Ltd. Published 2023 by John Wiley & Sons Ltd.
Companion website: www.wiley.com/go/byrne/aiinclinicalmedicine

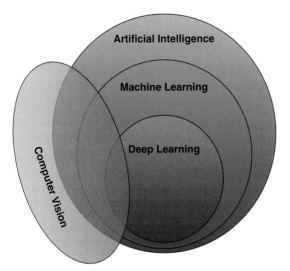

Figure 6.1: Venn diagram of AI nomenclature.

Source: [1] / Walters Kluwer Health.

In addition to these advances, new optimization algorithms have been established for large-scale data processing [2].

Deep learning has been at the centre of almost all recent advances in AI applications for medicine. Deep learning algorithms can learn from data to mimic human actions, and thus solve complex real-world problems. Given enough data, deep learning discovers the rules (patterns) underlying these data. Such patterns can be extracted (learnt) from the data to solve important healthcare problems in many areas of clinical medicine. There are three essential components of successful deep learning algorithms:

- Data collection and labelling.
- Choice of algorithms (learners).
- Model optimization and evaluation.

These are the basic building blocks of AI for pretty much anything, including the medical field (Figure 6.2).

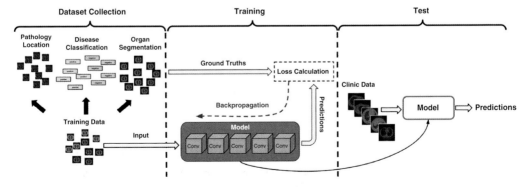

Figure 6.2: A typical framework illustrating deep learning design principles (essential components): data collection and labelling on the left, choice of algorithms and model optimization in the middle, and evaluation/testing on the right.

6.1.1 Data Collection and Labelling

Collecting a large dataset with high sample variation is a key and necessary step for the successful execution of a deep learning algorithm. All deep learning algorithms require large training datasets, which begs the question: how 'intelligent' are systems that rely on large-scale data while humans can infer conclusions even with very few data?

The requirements for data and labelling are best illustrated with a description of supervised learning. In supervised learning, which is the most mature, common, and successful learning method, the training data include labels (i.e. ground truth, or target values) associated with those data. Hence, any supervised medical deep learning application starts with data collection and labelling. The term 'label' refers to the detection or tagging of the data with appropriate content. For example, in a binary classification of tumour images, cancerous images might be labelled as '1' while cystic tumours or normal tissue would be labelled as '0'. Labels can also identify certain locations in the image with bounding boxes. Moreover, labels can be at the pixel level, with each pixel identified as specific tissue. However, this labelling procedure is very costly and tedious because, in most cases, the examples must be evaluated by domain experts (e.g. radiologists, pathologists, and other specialists), and labelled to make them ready to train deep learning models.

As an example, for a supervised learning algorithm to learn how to detect lung cancer from computed tomography (CT) scans, expert clinicians need to draw outlines for lung nodules, delineate them, and even label nearby organs. This procedure is even more challenging and tedious for radiation oncology applications where multiple organs and tumours require pixel-by-pixel labelling. In a different application, such as digital pathology, pixel-by-pixel analysis requires labels (i.e. ground truths) on pathology slides that are much larger than conventional radiology scans, thus requiring even more effort. In general, annotations are often noisy, the inter- and intra-observer variations may change considerably from application to application, and the heterogeneity of data from one centre to another makes data collection and labelling a major burden when developing medical deep learning applications.

Often, more labelled data are needed to improve the effectiveness of the model. The idea behind this is that having more data results in a higher likelihood of having more diverse and unbiased content, something that is necessary for highly accurate deep learning training. Once large-scale reliable data are collected, they are used as input, while the labels are used to guide training of the model. In short, deep learning applications improve with more experience, just like humans. One needs more data to drive the deep learning process, and these data need high-quality labels.

6.1.2 Choice of Algorithms (Learners)

Machine learning methods can be categorized based on how much labelled data they require for their training. The three broad categories are:

- Supervised learning.
- Semi-supervised learning.
- Unsupervised learning.

As already described, in *supervised learning*, all the samples in the dataset have to be labelled. Supervised methods aim to find a correlation between the patterns in the samples and the associated labels to solve a task. Since modern machine learning needs a large number of annotated datasets, supervised learning can be a burden for experts, especially in medicine. However, supervised models have undeniable supremacy in terms of performance.

Semi-supervised learning addresses the problem of labelling burden by requiring only a small number of labelled samples along with a large set of unlabelled examples. The models start to learn to solve the task from the labelled examples, and further improve their performance by incorporating a large set of given examples in an iterative way. In each iteration, originally labelled data are updated with new data that have predicted labels. While semi-supervised learning provides a much cheaper way of creating machine learning models, it can lead to too many classification (prediction) errors as data in the first step may have noisy labels, and there is no guarantee that the predicted labels for unlabelled data are completely true.

Unsupervised learning does not use any labels, and algorithms blindly cluster the data based on the patterns available in the data. This approach can be useful to learn the hidden patterns within the samples in the dataset without requiring expert knowledge. Common patterns and similarities between the data points allow them to be sorted and grouped together. An AI system that requires minimal labelling is of course attractive in AI in general, and more so in clinical AI applications.

Once the clinical AI problem is defined with an appropriate *learner* choice (supervised, semi-supervised, unsupervised), *deep learning architectures* can then be chosen depending on the complexity of the problem.

There are many candidate deep learning algorithms, each with their own unique advantages and disadvantages; these are well described in the literature. Most deep learning models generally use the same underlying type of algorithm – namely, convolutional neural networks (CNNs; Figure 6.3). CNNs consist of hundreds of

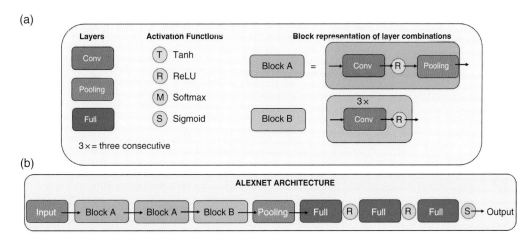

Figure 6.3: Illustration of a convolutional neural network (CNN). (a) How CNN components are organized. (b) The construction of the AlexNet architecture.

layers connected to each other. A layer can be considered as a mathematical function. In each layer there are several *filters* extracting patterns from the data, and these extracted patterns are used as input to the next connected layer(s), like connected biological neurons in the human body. These filters are initially defined with random values, and when training a deep learning algorithm, contents of the filters are 'learnt'. This is the famous 'learning' part of deep learning procedures. Randomly initiated filter contents are iteratively refined during training of the deep learning architectures, and the system converges into stable values once the desired outcome is achieved (see next section for optimization).

Convolution is one of the most commonly used 'filters' in layers of the deep networks that extracts *local patterns* from the input data. A layer with a convolution operation is usually called a 'convolution layer'. The very common term CNN takes its name from this convolution operation with consecutive layers (see Figure 6.3a). A layer may also include simpler mathematical operations such as down-sampling the data (e.g. pooling), or simply thresholding the data. Stacking a set of convolution layers allows the model to discover *global patterns*. The earlier deep network architectures such as AlexNet [3] (example representation in Figure 6.3b), VGG [4], and InceptionNet [5] followed a simple design by combining convolutional layers next to each other (Figure 6.3a). ResNet [6] was one of the earliest models that adapted skip connections, allowing deeper models to be trained. The skip connection strategy allows previous layers to be connected to the later layers in a non-sequential way, with the benefit of avoiding potential loss of information in the patterns when there is a large number of layers.

A significant part of the success in deep learning lies in the careful design of the neural network architecture for the problem at hand. In other words, there is no single deep learning architecture (design) that works for all prediction problems. Depending on the problem complexity, the design of the underlying neural network architecture may need to change. Hence, extensive architectural engineering has resulted in the almost daily emergence of deeper and more advanced deep architectures. In early architectures, such as AlexNet [3], there are eight layers to handle image classification problems (Figure 6.3b). Later, ResNet [6] architectures used 18, 50, and even more than 100 layers as time passed. Technological advances in algorithms and graphic processing units (GPUs) allowed more layers and more complicated connections between layers to be used. More complex problems require deeper networks (i.e. a higher number of layers in the network design) and greater volumes of data with sufficient diversity. Once large-scale data are collected, deep learning architectures can be adjusted according to the problem type (more layers, different connections between earlier and later layers, etc). Table 6.1 summarizes the most commonly used architectural components of deep learning design, which can be changed according to the problem type.

Architecture choices can also be made according to the problem types. There are three problem types in AI in medical imaging: image segmentation, object detection (an object can be a tumour, organ, or any other anatomical or pathological entity), and image classification (e.g. diagnosis). For example, *image segmentation* requires

Table 6.1: Some of the common components of deep learning architectures. AI practitioners use these components to design neural networks by changing their locations, number, and content.

Common components of deep learning architectures	Types	Description
Layers (each layer is a function)	Convolution	The most basic layer. Perform convolution over the input and propagate the output to other layers (often other convolution operations), extracting features from the input via convolution operation
	Densely connected layers	Previous layer outputs are also considered as inputs in a convolution layer. In this way, the relation of inputs–outputs is enriched
	Pooling	Outputs after the convolution operations are high-dimensional. Pooling helps to reduce this dimension while still keeping good information in the feature vectors
	Recurrent	For temporal events, having a circular connection helps extract better and more reliable features
	Normalization	From each layer and activation, features are extracted at different scales. Normalization helps standardize the features within a certain range
Activation function	SoftMax, rectified linear units (RELU – mostly used), hyperbolic tangent (tanh), sigmoid, and others	Feature vectors are extracted after each layer, then they are activated by an activation function to add some non-linearity into the features. Since linear functions turn into non-linear ones with activation functions, more complex relations can be modelled. In this way, activation functions enhance the network performance
Optimization algorithms	SGD (stochastic gradient descent), root mean square propagation (RMSprop), ADAM (mostly used) and others	Optimization algorithms tune the weights of the neural networks. Different optimization functions have different techniques as to how to fine-tune these weights. SGD is the basic one, while ADAM is the adaptive and mostly used optimization algorithm
Loss functions	Mean square error (MSE), cosine distance, cross entropy (mostly used), and others	Loss function is defined as a part of the problem definition (objective). For instance, cross entropy and mean square are used together in segmentation problems, while cosine distance is used in measuring similarity of vectors

every image pixel to have labels, while recognition (classification) of a disease requires only one label per image (cancer vs non-cancer). Similarly, object detection requires some image pixels to have object labels while the rest is considered as background. These are called *classification algorithms*. There are also *survival prediction algorithms*, which can be considered as the fourth type. By simply changing the last layer in the network, the deep learning architecture will operate as a *regression network* (continuous variables will be the output). Table 6.2 shows this stratification in brief.

6.1.3 Model Optimization and Evaluation

▓ *Optimization.* After the preferred deep learning architecture is chosen (or a new architecture is developed based on one of the deep learning architectures in the literature), an optimization algorithm, called *backpropagation*, is run iteratively. The purpose of this step is for the architecture to learn the relationship between the data and the labels. As an example, typical CNN-based architecture is given input data (such as a medical scan) and learns the underlying patterns via a training procedure (Figure 6.2). Each layer of the deep learning architecture (e.g. CNN) takes input from the previous layer, processes the input, and outputs it to the next layer. The final layer is connected to the

Table 6.2: Commonly Used Problem Types in Medical Imaging with Deep Learning.

Input Image (2D or 3D or nD)	Pixel-wise prediction (pixel-classification)	**Image segmentation** **Output:** Every pixel gets one label (foreground or background)
Input Image (2D or 3D or nD)	Pixel-wise prediction (pixel-classification or regression)	**Object detection** Pixels are determined to enclose the object. This problem can be formulated as a regression problem. Unlike a classification problem where one needs to have concrete classes (e.g. cat or dog, 1 or 0, cancer vs non-cancer), in a regression problem the outcome is a continuous variable (like a coordinate system). In object detection, one may find four or more points' localization and the combination of these points will indicate where the object is located **Output:** Image with a bounding box
Input Image (2D or 3D or nD)	Image-level prediction	**Image classification** This is a standard deep learning problem, where an image is classified into a certain labelled output **Output:** Class label (cancer vs non-cancer)

n, number of input dimensions.

output (true label), differences between predicted and true labels are back-propagated, and the deep learning architecture's hyperparameters are updated accordingly until the algorithm converges.

- *Evaluation.* The first step in evaluation is to quantitatively define what success looks like. What will practitioners see if the application is successful? Which metrics are important for your problem definition? All the quantitative metrics defining the success criteria of the application should be clearly defined. For all the metrics of success, the critical and widely accepted method of an evaluation strategy starts with data splitting. In the deep learning model development stage, the dataset is often split into three parts, with separate sets used for *training*, *validation*, and *testing*. The main reason for separating the dataset is that machine learning models tend to memorize the training data instead of learning representative patterns.
- The *training dataset* is used to fit the machine learning model between input data and the desired labels (i.e. surrogate truths such as tumour malignancy status of an observed tumour on a radiology scan, or ground truths such as biopsy-proven histology). One example could be the tumour malignancy status of an observed tumour on a radiology scan, where the true information is coming from actual biopsy tissue. Another example is a radiologist-drawn organ or pathology location on a radiology scan versus a machine-predicted organ or pathology location, where the radiologist drawing is considered as the ground truth. All model parameters are updated by considering the error rate on the training set.
- The *validation set* is used for hyper-parameter selection or choosing the best-trained model. The final performance of the trained model is evaluated on the test set, which should be unseen and never used in training and validation. In addition, it is now a requirement to include a *test dataset* from a completely different source so that generalization of the algorithm can be better assessed. The generalization capacity of a deep learning model is proven by success on the test dataset, which includes unseen examples (examples that are not used in training and validation sets).

6.2 Challenges and Failures in Healthcare AI from a 'Building Blocks' Perspective

A challenge of every clinical deep learning application is that posed by non-standard and non-normalized data that may have inherent artifacts and noise. The design of most clinical AI applications starts with data acquisition. The collected data must be pre-processed by computer software. This step includes normalization of the data (image intensities), standardization, and filtering out the noisy samples.

A lack of comprehensive evaluation of medical data and resultant AI models is a significant problem. The retrospective datasets used by private corporations to develop their algorithms are rarely shared, making them inaccessible to the clinical community that intends to use the AI applications in patient care. AI model development in clinical practice often uses retrospective methodologies, and is based on datasets with small sample sizes. This can lead to selection and spectrum bias, such as models constructed to ideally fit a certain dataset (also known as *overfitting* or memorization of training data instead of learning representative patterns), but this fit is not replicated for other datasets. To adapt software to changing patient demographics, continuous reevaluation and calibration of algorithms should be the standard. There is now a growing understanding of the need to build algorithms for broader populations that account for subgroups.

Another challenge relates to algorithm trustworthiness [7]. The most popular deep learning models follow a black-box approach, where the model takes the input and makes a prediction without showing the basis for such a prediction. This can be extremely hazardous in high-risk healthcare applications. On the other hand, there are some models that allow human interaction (human in the loop) or produce interpretability maps or explainability layers to show users how the decision is made internally. This transparency is critical to the adoption of AI, especially in healthcare.

6.3 Conclusion

AI is changing the landscape of clinical medicine. The success of AI algorithms in clinical medicine is often attributed to three pillars: large-scale data for learning, the choice of an appropriate algorithm (learners), and optimization algorithms. These building blocks are the same for almost every AI application. This chapter briefly explains these blocks, and identifies the unique difficulties for the incorporation of AI into medicine in the future.

KEY INSIGHTS

- **AI is rapidly diffusing through healthcare systems to support clinical medicine and outpatient services.**
- **Machine learning and deep learning fall under the general umbrella term of AI. Deep learning architectures are complex, as they are designed to mimic human actions and solve complicated programs.**
- **The buildings blocks of deep learning algorithms – including those employed in clinical medicine – include large-scale data collection and labelling, selection of appropriate AI algorithms, and system optimization and evaluation.**
- **AI algorithms for clinical medicine must not only be evaluated for accuracy and efficiency, but also from the perspectives of generalization and trustworthiness.**

References

1. Ruffle JK, Farmer AD, Aziz Q. Artificial intelligence-assisted gastroenterology: promises and pitfalls. American Journal of Gastroenterology 2019;114(3):422–428.
2. Alom MZ, Taha TM, Yakopcic C et al. The history began from AlexNet: a comprehensive survey on deep learning approaches. CoRR. 2018;abs/1803.01164. http://arxiv.org/abs/1803.01164.
3. Krizhevsky A, Sutskever I, Hinton GE. *ImageNet Classification with Deep Convolutional Neural Networks*. Advances in Neural Information Processing Systems, vol. 25. Red Hook, NY: Curran Associates; 2012.
4. Simonyan K, Zisserman A. Very deep convolutional networks for large-scale image recognition. 3rd International Conference on Learning Representations, San Diego, CA, May 7–9, 2015. https://www.robots.ox.ac.uk/~vgg/research/very_deep.
5. Szegedy C, Liu W, Jia Y et al. Going deeper with convolutions. 2015 IEEE Conference on Computer Vision and Pattern Recognition (CVPR), 2015, pp. 1–9. https://doi.org/10.1109/CVPR.2015.7298594.
6. He K, Zhang X, Ren S, Sun J. Deep residual learning for image recognition. 2016 IEEE Conference on Computer Vision and Pattern Recognition (CVPR), 2016, pp. 770–778. https://doi.org/10.1109/CVPR.2016.90.
7. Cutillo CM, Sharma KR, Foschini L et al. Machine intelligence in healthcare—perspectives on trustworthiness, explainability, usability, and transparency. *NPJ Digital Medicine* 2020;3(1):1–5.

7

Expert Systems for Interpretable Decisions in the Clinical Domain

Syed Muhammad Anwar

University of Engineering and Technology, Taxila, Pakistan

Sheikh Zayed Institute for Pediatric Surgical Innovation, Children's National Hospital, Washington DC, USA

Learning Objectives

- Understand the basic components required to implement and apply an expert system.
- Understand the role of expert systems in various domains of clinical medicine.
- Summarize the successful application of machine learning into clinical practice.
- Identify the major challenges in the implementation of deep learning into clinical practice.
- Outline a roadmap for how expert systems can overcome these challenges.

7.1 Introduction

This chapter highlights some of the recent challenges with adopting AI systems, particularly deep learning, into clinical medicine, and provides a perspective on how rule-based expert systems are already being put into clinical practice.

7.2 Deep Learning in Clinical Medicine

In recent years there has been an upsurge in the development of machine learning–based clinical diagnostic systems. Deep learning algorithms can overcome the need for significant human resources by their ability to learn appropriate decision-level rules directly from data (see Chapter 6). For example, a recent systematic review and meta-analysis demonstrated that deep learning models are now able to perform at a level equal to human experts in most medical imaging tasks [1]. While this is a big achievement for machine learning, the clinical adoption of such advanced models has been slower than anticipated. For example, the performance of deep learning models in tumour segmentation can be very accurate and sometimes rival a human expert. However, a clinical diagnosis based on this segmentation still requires human (expert) experience and knowledge, including information about the tumour type, size, and clinical significance.

AI in Clinical Medicine: A Practical Guide for Healthcare Professionals, First Edition. Edited by Michael F. Byrne, Nasim Parsa, Alexandra T. Greenhill, Daljeet Chahal, Omer Ahmad, and Ulas Bagci.
© 2023 John Wiley & Sons Ltd. Published 2023 by John Wiley & Sons Ltd.
Companion website: www.wiley.com/go/byrne/aiinclinicalmedicine

One challenge with applying deep learning models to clinical medicine is that most of these models are used in a black-box manner. The typical workflow for a deep learning algorithm involves providing data to the model(s) to achieve a certain desired output. However, the human interacts with the model only at the input and output stages. The deep learning model identifies features and learns patterns that are present in the data. Once the model is trained to make an inference, there is no clear explanation provided (with a mathematical and statistical justification) as to why or how the model makes a certain decision. In other words, black-box design means that the decisions that are made by deep learning algorithms are not transparent or explainable at a human level. The lack of explainability in deep learning algorithms is one of the main reasons for their lack of adoption into clinical medicine.

7.3 Interpretability versus Explainability

Although the terms interpretability and explainability are often used interchangeably, it is important to clarify the difference between the two. Interpretability is about the model itself, where a human can understand the working mechanism of it. Explainability arises through a decision mechanism, where the decisions made by a model can be explained in the same manner that a domain expert (such as a clinician) explains the decision (such as a clinical diagnosis).

For high-risk applications, such as in healthcare, it is important to have more transparent AI models [2]. An interpretable model refers to a system that can describe a cause-and-effect relationship. In particular, the decision (for example, in an automated tumour diagnosis system) needs to be interpretable, rather than presented as a binary outcome. Clinical AI models should be explainable, providing a detailed description of how a particular decision is made. Explainability can be at the model level as well as posthoc, where supplementary outcomes are used to explain why the model made a certain decision. AI models that are explainable provide both transparency and accountability.

7.4 Expert Systems in the Clinical Domain

Expert systems were developed as early as 1970 [3] and represent the first successful implementation of AI in real life. In simple terms, an expert system is a computer program with the ability to help a user make a decision. These systems comprise three major components: (i) the human expert from whom the knowledge is transferred to the computer program; (ii) the resulting knowledge base; and (iii) the inference module that brings intelligence to the computer program. Traditionally, the majority of expert systems used for clinical applications were *rule based*. For example, a simple rule for a blood pressure (BP) monitoring system would be: if the systolic BP is lower than 120 mmHg, then the condition is normal; if the BP is greater than 120 mmHg, the condition is pre-hypertension; and if the BP is greater than 140 mmHg, the condition is hypertension. Expert systems share inherent similarities to human-level decision-making. In most cases, the rules governing a rule-based system are determined by a domain expert (such as a clinician). In this way, expert systems act as agents to transfer expert knowledge to a computer algorithm. Expert systems are deployed in many types of computer programs to efficiently respond to events in real time, taking some of the decision-making burden off the end-user. It must be noted that expert systems are not meant to replace humans, but are designed to assist them to improve productivity and performance.

Expert systems have a long history of success in clinical medicine applications. Some of the widely used examples include MYCIN and CADUCEUS. MYCIN is an early expert system that was designed to assist clinicians in diagnosing and selecting therapies for bacterial infections [4]. CADUCEUS, developed in the early 1980s, was an evolution of MYCIN that was used to assist in diagnosing a larger number of diseases [5]. An advantage of expert systems is that they are explainable and hence more trustworthy than the more popular deep networks. Expert systems are also inherently more suited for interpretability, and they also utilize domain expert knowledge in the form of a knowledge base.

7.4.1 The Role of Human Experts in Clinical Medicine and Expert Systems

Clinical medicine is highly dependent on medical knowledge and expertise. Every day, medical professionals make high-risk decisions that can directly or indirectly affect a human's life. Such decisions are made based on domain-specific medical knowledge, clinical expertise, and experience. From an AI perspective, decisions made by clinical experts are interpretable by stakeholders involved in the process, which could include patients as well as other clinicians. Human experts play a major role in building the knowledge base, by transferring their knowledge to the computer program. For AI to see more uptake in clinical medicine, future systems need to be intelligent, have a strong knowledge base, and be understandable or interpretable.

7.4.2 Knowledge Base

The central component of an expert system is the knowledge base. This base includes high-quality domain-specific knowledge such as factual and experiential knowledge. This knowledge is represented in the form of conditional rules, which are similar to computer algorithms that use the 'IF-THEN-ELSE' programming construct to search, select, or eliminate the conditions from the decision mechanism. IF-THEN-ELSE is a high-level program language statement that compares two or more sets of data and tests the results. *IF* the results are true, the *THEN* instructions are taken; if not, the *ELSE* instructions are taken. One of the challenges in creating a rule-based expert system is to correctly identify the *rules* for each specific domain. While a stronger knowledge base enhances the performance of the expert system, it can be difficult to build and maintain, especially considering the diverse nature of clinical conditions and challenges presented therein.

7.4.3 The Inference Engine

The rules established by the knowledge base are used by the inference engine to apply logic constructs in order to make a decision. Once identified, these rules are hardwired into the expert system, resulting in a brittle system. This type of system is not intelligent, in that it cannot mimic human decision-making. For such a system, any change would require a significant effort.

One solution is to introduce diversity into the algorithm. Use of a fuzzy-based logic model allows truth values to be represented at varying levels within the range of '0' to '1', instead of a Boolean representation (0 or 1) where truth is normally represented as '1'. This continuous representation of values allows the expert system to deal with uncertainty (for example, a true value of 0.9 is more certain than a true value of 0.8, since the former is closer to 1). These fuzzy systems need detailed investigation and verification prior to implementation.

7.5 Roadmap to Knowledge-Driven Deep Learning

Recent studies have highlighted different strategies to overcome some of the past challenges of AI in clinical medicine:

- The incorporation of domain knowledge with convolutional neural network architecture achieved a more stable performance and a faster convergence than CNNs alone – for example, in prostate cancer detection [6]. Although data-driven models have achieved significant performance in segmenting prostate cancer lesions, embedding prior domain knowledge will permit more robust performance.
- The performance of expert systems could be improved by using knowledge-driven deep learning. Although a fuzzy expert system was proposed for the detection of chronic kidney disease [7], significant effort was required to identify the key parameters and then to define the fuzzy rules.

Expert systems are inherently explainable, but constructing the rules required for a clinical situation is overwhelmingly complicated and time-consuming, and once these rules are infused into the knowledge base, changing them would require a significant effort. Meanwhile, deep learning–based systems lack the necessary explainability to be used in high-risk contexts such as medical decision-making. One solution to this is to create a learnable knowledge base [8]. While there are studies where the knowledge base is learnt from the data, this still only incorporates data-driven knowledge.

A step forward would be to fuse expert knowledge (coming from the domain expert) into the data-driven models [9]. This could in turn optimize the inference stage of the expert system, making it more explainable.

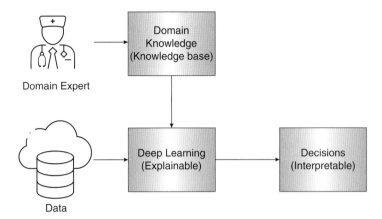

Figure 7.1: A workflow for mixed intelligence systems using a knowledge base and deep learning for interpretable decisions in the clinical domain.

Here we present the building blocks for establishing a mixed intelligence system, which consists of an expert system that includes a strong knowledge base and integrates a deep learning algorithm with the ability to learn patterns from data. We propose a three-step process for future expert systems in clinical medicine, illustrated by the generic workflow in Figure 7.1:

- **Step 1:** Drive expert knowledge from the domain expert to create knowledge graphs (which semantically define the relationship between knowledge entities) for generating the knowledge base. (A knowledge graph is a knowledge base that uses a graph-structured data model or topology to integrate data.)
- **Step 2:** Use deep learning that discovers patterns in a data-driven paradigm to learn significant features.
- **Step 3:** Fuse the knowledge base to refine features, and hence have explainable AI models for healthcare applications.

While these proposed steps need further exploration and validation, we hypothesize that such systems would allow faster clinical adoption of AI.

Establishing a comprehensive set of rules for more complex rule-based expert systems is where deep learning–based algorithms have been proven to be very useful.

Creating a hybrid of deep learning models and expert systems is one approach to overcoming some of the recent challenges of deep learning applications in healthcare. This approach includes increasing the involvement of a domain expert (in this case, a clinical specialist) who adds domain expert knowledge to create the knowledge base. The knowledge base embodies high-quality domain-specific knowledge that is interpretable and can be used to make inferences from the deep learning models. This permits deep learning models to be more explainable, overcoming one of the key challenges of deep learning in healthcare.

7.6 Potential Applications of Mixed Intelligence Systems

The following three applications illustrate where expert systems combined with knowledge-driven deep learning may prove to be beneficial to clinical medicine while overcoming some of the challenges of interpretability. These examples illustrate how domain expertise is necessary to take these algorithms to the next level.

7.6.1 Personalized Surgical Treatment Planning

Detailed pre-operative planning and risk analysis is necessary to ensure the best outcomes, especially for high-risk surgical procedures. Depending on the procedure, this can be a very time-consuming and laborious task. Automated image analysis algorithms applied to pre-operative imaging can suggest potential intra-operative surgical strategies for each given individual. However, these AI-recommended surgical approaches must be verified by the surgeon based on their knowledge and experience. The fusion of data-driven knowledge (from pre-operative X-rays) and expert knowledge (from the surgeon) could promote personalized surgical treatment planning.

7.6.2 Survival Prediction

Making an overall survival prediction for patients diagnosed with a serious medical condition is a challenging task that requires medical experience and expertise. For example, when making a survival prediction for a patient with a brain tumour, the clinician is required to integrate data from a number of sources including X-rays, lab reports, demographic information, and response to therapy. To make an accurate overall survival prediction, an expert system would require a knowledge base comprising a diverse set of entities, including tumour features, demographics, and domain expertise. Combining knowledge-driven deep learning with expert systems would permit such a system to be adapted for clinical use.

7.6.3 Radiotherapy Planning

Careful radiotherapy planning is necessary to minimize radiation exposure. While machine learning is used for automated planning in tumour treatment, the incorporation of expert systems that utilize automated inference and the knowledge base would lead to better patient outcomes.

7.7 Conclusion

To summarize, conventional expert systems require significant effort to appropriately identify features and rules. Data-driven approaches, particularly deep learning, can permit the selection of appropriate parameters from the data. However, domain knowledge is necessary to make improved decisions related to the task at hand. Fusing expert systems with deep learning approaches could be a major step towards developing successful AI algorithms for clinical medicine, and may help address some of the major barriers, including trustworthiness, interpretability, fairness, and adoption into clinics.

KEY INSIGHTS

- ■ **Recent AI developments, particularly the development of data-driven deep learning models, have opened vast avenues of research that could significantly improve the role of technology in healthcare.**
- ■ **For AI to see more uptake in clinical medicine, future systems need to be intelligent, have a strong knowledge base, and be understandable or interpretable.**
- ■ **Fusing expert systems, which incorporate expert knowledge from clinical experts, with data-driven knowledge learnt from clinical data would be a major step towards developing successful AI algorithms for clinical medicine, and may address some of the major barriers that have prevented adoption in the past.**

References

1. Liu X, Faes L, Kale AU et al. A comparison of deep learning performance against healthcare professionals in detecting diseases from medical imaging: a systematic review and meta-analysis. *Lancet Digital Health* 2019;1(6):e271–e297.
2. Anwar SM. AIM and explainable methods in medical imaging and diagnostics. In: Lidströmer N, Ashrafian H (eds), *Artificial Intelligence in Medicine*. Cham: Springer; 2021, 1–10. https://doi.org/10.1007/978-3-030-58080-3_293-1
3. Liao SH. Expert system methodologies and applications—a decade review from 1995 to 2004. *Expert Systems with Applications* 2005;28(1):93–103.
4. Van Melle W. MYCIN: a knowledge-based consultation program for infectious disease diagnosis. *International Journal of Man-Machine Studies* 1978;10(3):313–322.
5. Pople HE. CADUCEUS: an experimental expert system for medical diagnosis. In: Winston PH, Prendergast KA (eds), *The AI Business*. Cambridge, MA: MIT; 1984, 67–80.
6. Sobecki P, Jóźwiak R, Sklinda K, Przelaskowski A. Effect of domain knowledge encoding in CNN model architecture—a prostate cancer study using mpMRI images. *PeerJ* 2021;9:e11006.
7. Hamedan F, Orooji A, Sanadgol H, Sheikhtaheri A. Clinical decision support system to predict chronic kidney disease: a fuzzy expert system approach. *International Journal of Medical Informatics* 2020;138:104–134.

For additional references please see www.wiley.com/go/byrne/aiinclinicalmedicine.

8

The Role of Natural Language Processing in Intelligence-Based Medicine

Maryam Panahiazar[1], Nolan Chen[2], Ramin E. Beygui[1], and Dexter Hadley[3]

[1] *UCSF School of Medicine, University of California, San Francisco, CA, USA*

[2] *Electrical and Computer Engineering, University of California Berkeley, Berkeley, CA, USA*

[3] *Division of Artificial Intelligence, Departments of Clinical and Computer Sciences, University of Central Florida, College of Medicine, Orlando, FL, USA*

Learning Objectives

- Become familiar with a few important and common natural language processing (NLP) techniques in healthcare.
- Understand the role of AI technologies such as deep learning in intelligence-based medicine.
- Review a use case to illustrate some limitations, challenges, opportunities, and potential solutions in women's health.
- Appreciate the future of AI in healthcare.

8.1 Introduction

Natural language processing (NLP) is the branch of AI that enables computers to understand and interpret human speech and language. Several promising applications of NLP in healthcare include supporting clinical decision making, improving clinical documentation, preventing diseases, and predicting outcomes. Clinical data, including notes and reports, are increasingly generated and stored in electronic medical records (EMR). The challenges in big-scale data management, processing, and reusability highlight the urgent need to develop a novel and expandable AI infrastructure to enable healthcare providers to access knowledge for individual patients, and allow for better decision-making and outcomes.

AI in Clinical Medicine: A Practical Guide for Healthcare Professionals, First Edition. Edited by Michael F. Byrne, Nasim Parsa, Alexandra T. Greenhill, Daljeet Chahal, Omer Ahmad, and Ulas Bagci.
© 2023 John Wiley & Sons Ltd. Published 2023 by John Wiley & Sons Ltd.
Companion website: www.wiley.com/go/byrne/aiinclinicalmedicine

NLP has numerous potential applications in healthcare. Several novel NLP platforms available for public use are offered through Google, Microsoft, Facebook, and IBM. This chapter briefly discusses a few NLP techniques applicable to healthcare using these platforms. We highlight the possibilities, promises, and challenges in NLP by describing a clinical use case.

8.2 Introducing a Few Common and Important Natural Language Processing Techniques in Healthcare

NLP leverages AI to help analytical systems understand unstructured data. We will describe a few well-known NLP techniques to give the reader a foundation in NLP. *Named entity recognition* (NER) is an information-extraction technique that segments named entities as real-world objects (e.g. medication, symptom) into predefined categories (e.g. heart disease medications, cancer medications). *Classification* or *text categorization* is used to analyse text data and assign label tags to different clauses based on pre-defined categories (e.g. identifying at-risk patients based on specific test results). *Topic modelling* is used to classify a collection of documents and group them based on particular words with a specific topic (e.g. a group of documents that explain the patient's history). *Optical character recognition* (OCR) is a method that a computer can use to read a printed text and convert it to a digital format (e.g. scanning the prescription note and turning it into a text file). The *Stanford CoreNLP toolkit* is an extensible pipeline that provides core natural language analysis. It provides most of the common core NLP steps, from *tokenization* (a way of separating part of the text into smaller units called tokens) to *coreference resolution* (a technology for consolidating the textual information about an entity). For example, coreference resolution can be used to know and uncover the relationships between all medications and symptoms for a patient from the discharge summary [1,2].

8.3 Summary of State-of-the-Art Platforms for Natural Language Processing in Healthcare

Even though NLP still has many challenges to resolve, health systems and researchers are able to utilize the platforms that use NLP techniques to solve healthcare problems. Several state-of-the-art NLP platforms are available for public use through Google [3], Microsoft [4], Facebook [5], and IBM [6]. We define these platforms on three levels – those requiring no understanding, those requiring basic understanding, and those requiring more detailed understanding of computer programming. Existing platforms make the use of NLP possible at any level of computing knowledge. In the following section, we introduce several platforms.

8.3.1 Microsoft Azure Text Analytics

This platform is designed to mine unstructured text such as clinical notes and clinical reports using text analysis (`https://docs.microsoft.com/en-us/azure`) [4]. No specific AI expertise is needed to use this platform. In Azure, several services provide NLP capabilities, including Azure Databricks, Microsoft Cognitive Services, and Azure with Spark. One can choose between these services based on different parameters, such as pre-built model, low-level or high-level NLP capabilities, and data size. One can classify medical terminology using domain-specific, pre-trained models and ontology. Ontology in medicine fields can be used to explain terms and relationships between them (e.g. part of the body, medication, and subset of related medications; `https://bioportal.bioontology.org`). Using text analytics, one can find, classify, and define relationships between medical concepts such as diagnosis, symptoms, and drug dosage and frequency. Microsoft Azure is user-friendly for all levels of experience. It uses many NLP techniques, such as a tokenizer for splitting the text into words or phrases; entity extraction to identify subjects in the text; part of speech detection to place a text as a verb, noun, participle, and verb phrase; and sentence boundary detection to detect complete sentences within paragraphs of the text.

8.3.2 Google AutoML Natural Language Classifier

A natural language classifier (NLC) enables users to build and deploy custom machine learning models that analyse documents, categorize them, and identify entities within them (`https://cloud.google.com/natural-language/automl/docs/quick-start`) [3]. AutoML NLC can train custom models for distinct tasks, including single-label classification, multi-label classification, entity extraction, and sentiment analysis. The AutoML NLC training algorithm is a black box and is performed automatically. Training a model can take several hours to complete. The required training time depends on several factors, such as dataset size, the nature of the training items, and model complexity. AutoML NLC uses early stopping to ensure the best possible model without overfitting. NLP application programming interface (API) is a machine learning tool pre-trained to perform tasks such as analysing a selected text. API has several methods for analysing and annotating text. Each level of analysis provides valuable information for language understanding. A basic knowledge of programming is needed to use AutoML NLC. The methods that have been used in natural language API include sentiment analysis, inspecting the given text, and identifying the prevailing emotional opinion within the text, primarily to determine a writer's attitude as positive, negative, or neutral (e.g. a patient's description of their stress level in a questionnaire). Entity analysis inspects the given text for known entities (e.g. common nouns such as hospital, clinic, medication) and returns information about those entities. Syntactic analysis extracts linguistic information, breaking up the given text into a series of sentences and tokens (usually word boundaries), providing further analysis on those tokens. Content classification analyses text content and returns a content category for the content (e.g. category describing the diagnosis).

8.3.3 IBM Watson Natural Language Classifier

Using the IBM Watson NLC service, one can train a model to classify text according to defined classes. The Watson service in IBM Cloud uses machine learning algorithms to return the top-matching pre-defined classes for text inputs [6]. It analyses text to extract meta-data from content such as concepts, entities, emotion, relations, sentiment, and more. The NLC service learns from users' data and can return information for text on which it was not trained. Using the IBM NLC is very straightforward, and one needs little programming knowledge to set up a straightforward classifier configuration. A classifier configuration defines related information to the NLC instance on IBM Cloud. It also specifies the classifier target fields. A classifier field is a field group in API that contains the name of a classifier configuration and a classifier input field. The view suggestions button is displayed next to a classifier field. The classifier input field in API contains the text input that NLC interprets and classifies. It is typically a description field. Classifier target fields are fields in the API set where a user chooses suggestions for a classifier field. The standard user interface (UI) is very straightforward (https://www.ibm.com/docs/en/opw/8.1.0?topic=guide-getting-started-standard-ui).

8.3.4 Facebook's fastText

This is a popular library for text classification, and is an open-source project on GitHub (GitHub is a host platform for collaboration and version control). The library can be used as a command-line tool or a Python package (www.python.org) as a programming language. Therefore, basic programming knowledge is needed for straightforward commands [5]. After installing the tools, the next step is to obtain data and start the text classification following the step-by-step process, including splitting the data into training and testing sets. After the model is trained, it is ready to test and take some questions to classify different sentences with a label (e.g. How does one treat patients with high cholesterol? Possible label: cardiovascular disease). Within other platforms, fastText can train with millions of examples of text data in less than 10 minutes over a multi-core central processing unit (CPU), and can perform predictions on unseen raw text (https://fasttext.cc).

8.4 Use Case Project for Natural Language Processing – Approaches and Challenges

This section demonstrates the use of NLP platforms to empower data labeling and annotation of EMR data to facilitate deep learning on cancer images. We explain the problems and possible solutions to make it more meaningful and practical for the reader.

Breast cancer is a leading cause of cancer death among women in the United States. Screening mammography effectively reduces breast cancer mortality, but carries a significant burden of unnecessary recalls and biopsies. Deep learning using mammography images has seen enormous success in breast cancer screening for prevention and prediction. In 2015, deep learning significantly outperformed humans on image classification – finding and predicting cancer from images – with more than 95% accuracy [7,8]. AI techniques can be used to better classify, predict, and find existing cancer and thus reduce overdiagnosis (resulting in a decreased recall and biopsy rates). AI can also help to improve early detection of interval cancers. Interval cancers are primary breast cancers diagnosed in women who have had a negative screening result. In these cases, there is usually no recommendation for recall or further analysis. Nevertheless, some women do develop cancer between screening tests.

We aimed to analye pathology reports from the EMR to extract labels that contain information related to the diagnosis, as determined by examining cells and tissues. A pathology report is a document that contains the diagnosis determined under a microscope by examining cells and tissues. These labels extracted from the pathology report will be used to annotate large-scale mammography images for deep learning in our future work. A crucial factor in the success of deep learning is the availability of large-scale labeled data, which is hard to obtain. As part of our previous studies [9,10], we demonstrated the feasibility of a framework using machine learning and text-mining models to derive pathological diagnosis from free-text breast pathology reports to be used to annotate images for deep learning processing. About 7000 records of women (mean age 51.8 years)and ~10,000 (9787) reports were extracted from an in-house pathology database at the University of California, San Francisco (UCSF). The 'final diagnosis' section was considered in the analysis. All mammograms from 2000 to 2016 were selected and 3099 outcomes were manually labelled by an expert as Bilateral(-), Left(+), Right(+), and Bilateral(+). Bilateral(+) means both breasts positive for cancer [10]. Examples of pathology reports are shown in Figure 8.1.

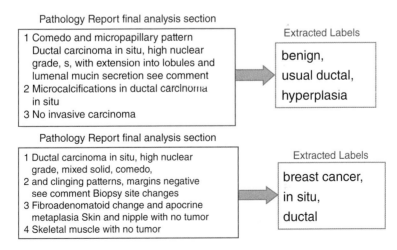

Figure 8.1: Examples of pathology reports with extracted labels. The terms like hyperplasia, in situ, andductal are breast cancer terminologies.

Source: Adapted from [7].

In this study, the Google AutoML NLC was accessed via the online Web UI for each step, from creating a database to training and testing the model. The AutoML model was used to extract labels from pathology reports with NLP techniques. AutoML NLC can train custom models for single-label classification, entity extraction, and sentiment analysis. For this study, we used single-label classification that allows a document to be assigned labels as in the following steps: (i) pre-processing; (ii) creating a dataset; (iii) training the model; (iv) testing the model; (v) using the prediction model. After our model was successfully trained, we analysed our documents in a Google Cloud Storage bucket for prediction. Training and testing datasets were uploaded to the Web UI to create a Google Cloud dataset as two CSV files. Google AutoML NLC does not accept multiple entries with identical text (as some of the pathology reports in our training set were completely identical in their wording), so we could not use our training set as is in Google AutoML. To remedy this issue, we appended a number to the end of the duplicated pathology reports (for clarity, these were separate reports from distinct biopsy specimens).

The pathology reports for this study were identically worded but amended to make them different enough so that Google AutoML would accept them while preserving a similar function in the model's training. For example, if we had three reports with the text 'benign tissue', we would leave the first occurrence of 'benign tissue' as is, and the second would be changed to 'benign tissue2' and the third to 'benign tissue3'. Google AutoML NLC will not train on a dataset if there are fewer than 10 entries in any category, so categories with very few entries were changed to a general category of 'other'. In cases where the categories with fewer than 10 entries were more general than those with more than 10 entries, the entry was replicated and assigned to each specific category. For example, for 'in situ', each report with a breast cancer label was duplicated. The reports were assigned the categories of 'breast cancer, in situ, ductal' and 'breast cancer, in situ, lobular'. These are just a few examples of problems and possible solutions. The Google AutoML NLC training algorithm is a black box and performed automatically. Training a model can take several hours. The required training time depends on several factors, such as the size of the dataset, the nature of the training items, and the complexity of the models. Google AutoML NLC uses early stopping to ensure the best possible model without overfitting. For classification models, the average training time was around 6 hours, with a maximum time of 24 hours.

While the labels we used, such as 'breast cancer, ductal, in situ' have three parts, the labels themselves are a single label, and the algorithms were trained with the three-part labels as a single-label string of text. So, in essence, the algorithms do not know that the labels have multiple parts, and the algorithm predictor only selects a single label, which happens to be a string with three parts. Another important distinction is how Google AutoML and Microsoft Azure refer to the model names. In Microsoft Azure, the Multiclass Logistic Regression refers to the idea that there are more than two possible prediction classes, making it multiclass logistic regression instead of the standard logistic regression case with only two possible prediction classes. In Google AutoML, single- versus multi-label refers to the number of labels the predictor needs to

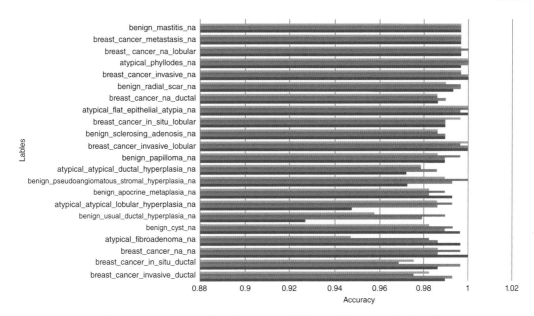

Figure 8.2: Accuracy performance for Azure and Google AutoML for all labels of pathology reports.

choose for each inputted pathology report, which is one, due to the single-string labels used for this project. Thus we used single-label prediction in Google AutoML. Google AutoML NLC also provides automatic calculation of precision and recall statistics; however, for consistency of this analysis, we did not use this calculation. Instead, we used the trained model to predict labels for our pre-made testing set that we used for testing all the other algorithmic models. Google AutoML NLC allows label prediction either manually through the Web UI or via an application programming interface (API). Due to the large volume of test cases, we used the Python API to access our trained model, and had it predict the most likely label for each member of the pre-made testing set. In the resulting trained model, classifications for the testing set are obtained by entering the pathology reports of the testing set and parsing the output (Figure 8.2).

8.5 Conclusions

This chapter provides a brief overview of a few NLP techniques applicable to health-care using current state-of-the-art platforms such as Google ML, Microsoft Azure, Facebook fastText, and IBM Watson. A clinical scenario in breast cancer was used to highlight the opportunities and challenges in using AI Platforms in medicine. It is important to highlight how NLP technologies can be deployed in clinical practice for healthcare provider to provide new public health insights using existing medical data and clinical notes. This technology assists the provider in decision-making for disease prevention, prediction, and improving clinical outcomes.

KEY INSIGHTS

- With knowledge of basic NLP techniques, such as named entity recognition (NER), text classification or text categorization, topic modelling, and optical character recognition, healthcare professionals can play a key role in advancing AI in medicine.
- Existing NLP platforms are accessible to users with different levels of experience in programming and AI knowledge. These platforms include Google ML, Microsoft Azure, Facebook fastText, and IBM Watson.
- There are already examples of clinical application of NLP to label existing data in electronic medical records using open-source platforms. While it is important to recognize and address limitations, NLP has a lot to offer for the advancement of technology in healthcare.

Conflicts of Interest

The authors declare that they have no conflict of interest. The authors acknowledge all open source platforms in this chapter.

References

1. Manning CD, Surdeanu M, Bauer J et al. The Stanford CoreNLP natural language processing toolkit. In: *Proceedings of 52nd Annual Meeting of the Association for Computational Linguistics: System Demonstrations*. Baltimore, MD: Association for Computational Linguistics; 2014, 55–60. http://www.aclweb.org/anthology/P/P14/P14-5010.
2. Houssein EH, Mohamed RE, Ali AA. Machine learning techniques for biomedical natural language processing: a comprehensive review. *IEEE Access* 2021;9:140628–140653. https://doi.org.10.1109/ACCESS.2021.3119621.
3. Google Cloud. *AutoML Natural Language Beginner's Guide*, 2020. https://cloud.google.com/natural-language/automl/docs/beginners-guide.
4. Microsoft Azure. *Natural Language Processing Technology*, 2021. https://docs.microsoft.com/en-us/azure/architecture/data-guide/technology-choices/natural-language-processing.
5. Young JC, Rusli A. Review and visualization of Facebook's fastText pretrained word vector model. 2019 International Conference on Engineering, Science, and Industrial Applications (ICESI), 2019, 1–6. https://doi.org/10.1109/ICESI.2019.8863015.
6. IBM. *IBM Watson Natural Language Classifier*, 2021. https://www.ibm.com/docs/en/opw/8.1.0?topic=ui-watson-natural-language-classifier.
7. O'Mahony N, Campbell S, Carvalho A et al. Deep learning vs. traditional computer vision. In: Arai K, Kapoor S (eds), *Advances in Computer Vision*. Advances in Intelligent Systems and Computing, vol 943. Cham: Springer, 2019, 128–144. https://doi.org/10.1007/978-3-030-17795-9_10.

For additional references please see www.wiley.com/go/byrne/aiinclinical medicine.

III

AI Applied to Clinical Medicine

Frontline Care Specialties

Medical Specialties

Surgical Specialties

Diagnostic Specialties

9

AI in Primary Care, Preventative Medicine, and Triage

Yasmin Abedin[1], Omer F. Ahmad[2],
and Junaid Bajwa[3,4]

[1] *Computer Science, University College London, London, UK*

[2] *Wellcome EPSRC Centre for Interventional and Surgical Sciences (WEISS), University College London, London, UK*

[3] *Microsoft Research (Global)*

[4] *NHS, UK*

Learning Objectives

- Understand current applications of AI in primary care, preventative medicine, and triage.
- Explore potential future applications of AI in primary care, preventative medicine, and triage.
- Evaluate the challenges faced in implementing AI in primary care.

9.1 Introduction

Healthcare provision in primary care settings has undergone many changes in recent years, all of which have been further accelerated during the COVID-19 pandemic. The adoption of platforms to digitize the patient journey, such as requesting an appointment online, accessing a doctor virtually, and mobile communications, has the potential to improve the efficiency and accessibility of primary care. Although many primary care physicians (PCPs) have begun to leverage online and mobile technologies to communicate with their patients, the use of AI technology in primary care settings is limited.

PCPs are often described as the 'gatekeepers' in healthcare systems, and are the first medical professionals to see patients with non-emergency health problems. Gatekeeping means that patients must see a PCP to access further specialist care [1]. This means that one key challenge PCPs face is in being able to triage patients effectively so that issues needing imminent treatment can be dealt with promptly, and those who have less urgent problems are managed efficiently and appropriately. PCPs also play a key role in managing patients with long-term chronic conditions, which involves both mental and physical aspects of healthcare. In addition to the

AI in Clinical Medicine: A Practical Guide for Healthcare Professionals, First Edition. Edited by Michael F. Byrne, Nasim Parsa, Alexandra T. Greenhill, Daljeet Chahal, Omer Ahmad, and Ulas Bagci.
© 2023 John Wiley & Sons Ltd. Published 2023 by John Wiley & Sons Ltd.
Companion website: www.wiley.com/go/byrne/aiinclinicalmedicine

high pressures of the clinical role, PCPs have a mounting level of bureaucratic pressure, particularly in the USA where patient encounters need clear documentation and clinical codes for legal, auditing, and billing purposes.

The UK's Academic Health Science Network (AHSN) released a 'state of the nation' report in 2018 based on a survey conducted by National Health Service (NHS) England and the Academic Health Science Network AI Initiative to provide an overview of AI healthcare activity and to investigate the potential for AI to contribute to improved care. It specifically investigated the use of remote diagnostics and monitoring capabilities across different points of care. Results showed that 67% of solutions reported are delivering services in hospitals, with only 39% of solutions being delivered in community or primary care [2]. This finding highlights a gap between hospitals and primary care in remote diagnostics and monitoring, considering that the majority of patients with chronic disease are managed in the community by PCPs. However, the move to digital-first primary care consultations poses an opportunity to further incorporate advanced technologies in primary care. From accurate triage systems to intelligent consultation transcription services leveraging natural language processing (NLP), patient consultations can be streamlined to reduce the administrative burden on doctors and enable them to focus on the patient and their care plan. Primary healthcare is at an exciting point in time where the technology infrastructure is being laid for further advancements to take place.

9.2 Primary Care

9.2.1 Current Applications

Arguably one of the biggest changes to primary care healthcare delivery has been the mass adoption of telemedicine during the global pandemic. The *Oxford Medical Dictionary* defines telemedicine as 'the use of information technology in the diagnosis and treatment of patients' [3]. Traditionally in primary care medicine, the doctor will see the patient face to face before giving a diagnosis and management plan, and potentially providing a prescription. However, COVID-19 rendered this infeasible, and healthcare providers needed to immediately implement alternatives to minimise the risk of viral transmission for both healthcare workers and patients, while still trying to ensure appropriate access.

Prior to the pandemic, several companies were already working on building platforms to improve accessibility to medical care, for example Livi (www.livi.co.uk), PushDoctor (www.pushdoctor.co.uk), and Babylon Health (www.babylonhealth.com). Babylon Health, for example (also known as 'GP at hand'), is a UK-based company founded in 2013, which has since expanded internationally across the USA, parts of Africa, East Asia, and the Middle East. Babylon Health provides healthcare services through its website or mobile applications. GP at hand was introduced in London in 2017 to provide patients with the ability to have a video consultation with an NHS PCP within two hours of booking. Many other companies have since been formed to provide remote consultation tools for doctors to incorporate into their existing practice – for example, AccurX (`www.accurx.com`) and Visionable (`https://visionable.com`). The benefits of investments in this area prior to 2020 meant that some of the technological infrastructure was in place to support the demand for telemedicine during the COVID-19 pandemic. The pandemic also encouraged additional investments to be made into these technologies (and other digital innovations) to support continuity of access.

9.2.2 Emerging Role of AI

To further improve the efficiency of telemedicine, AI is also becoming embedded into various points of the patient pathway.

9.2.2.1 The Patient

The very first step for a patient receiving medical care is to decide whether their problem requires medical input. Many people resort to online search engines to find health information and advice. However, this presents a very real risk of the patient obtaining misleading or irrelevant information. Various AI-based symptom checker tools have been developed with validated medical information and can provide patients with a suggested diagnosis and next steps. Ada (`https://ada.com`) is a company based in Germany providing an intelligent symptom checker and personalised assessment report via a mobile application across Europe, Africa, and South America. This process serves an important role in flagging to the patient when they need urgent treatment, when they would benefit from a face-to-face consultation, or when they can self-manage their symptoms at home.

9.2.2.2 The PCP

AI is also being embedded to support PCPs in making diagnoses. A key challenge in primary care medicine is being able to recognize symptoms and diagnose conditions across all domains and specialities of medicine. With the amount of medical knowledge and research ever-growing, PCPs are finding it increasingly difficult to offer expertise to patients that matches that of specialists.

Dermatology provides examples of use cases where AI can help to bridge the gap between speciality medicine and primary care. Due to limited access to dermatologists, only 28% of skin presentations are assessed by a dermatologist [4]. Therefore, PCPs must be able to confidently assess and manage skin conditions. As an exemplar, computer vision AI is providing support to PCPs to help in the diagnosis of skin diseases. A study in 2021 evaluated an AI-based tool using convolutional neural networks, which assists with interpreting clinical images of dermatological conditions and providing diagnoses through skin condition likelihood scores. It found that PCPs receiving AI assistance had 10% higher agreement with diagnoses made by a dermatologist panel compared to those who received no AI assistance [5].

9.2.2.3 Treatment

Another point of the patient pathway seeing improvements through AI innovation is the delivery of treatment – for example, therapy for mental health conditions. One example is cognitive behavioural therapy (CBT), a type of talking therapy for diagnoses such as depression and anxiety. CBT guides patients in altering their thinking patterns to improve their symptoms [6]. Access to face-to-face psychological therapies is difficult for most people due to two main reasons: a private therapist is expensive and, in the USA, almost 40% of people live in areas with a shortage of mental health professionals [7]. In recent years, a surge of chatbots has leveraged AI technology to guide patients through reframing their thought patterns. Woebot (`https://woebothealth.com`) is a popular CBT therapy application that uses AI to process user responses in order to 'learn' responses from users' free-text answers. It also allows users to track and visualize patterns in their mood, and removes the long process of waiting for a one-to-one session with a suitable therapist.

9.2.3 Future Applications

The mounting bureaucratic pressure on PCPs is another area of focus for technological overhaul. An area of exciting potential is the automation of administrative tasks such as note-taking during consultations. 'Dragon Ambient eXperience' (`https://www.nuance.com/healthcare/ambient-clinical-intelligence/see-the-dragon-ambient-experience.html`) is an intelligent patient transcription tool developed by Nuance and Microsoft using NLP [8]. It listens to doctor–patient conversations while providing workflow, knowledge, and task automation, allowing clinical documentation to write itself within the electronic health record (Figure 9.1). Automating clinical documentation closes the gap between clinical conversation and documentation, freeing up time for doctors to increase their level of patient engagement, and also removes the need to focus on the administrative tasks surrounding patient consultations. Although this software does not aim to ultimately change the care received by the patient, it has huge potential to

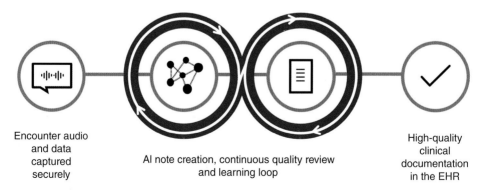

Encounter audio and data captured securely

AI note creation, continuous quality review and learning loop

High-quality clinical documentation in the EHR

Figure 9.1: Schematic demonstrating how NLP is enabling information within the clinical record to write itself. EHR, electronic health record.

Source: Dr Yasmin Abedin.

revolutionise the doctor's experience of a consultation by saving time both during and after the consultation, reduce physician burnout, and improve the patient experience. If doctors have more time to focus on their patient rather than ever-increasing administrative processes, it is beneficial for all involved.

9.3 Preventative Medicine

9.3.1 Current Applications

At the simplest level of abstraction, the traditional model of healthcare involves a patient developing a problem and the doctor or broader clinical team (including pharmacists, nurses, healthcare assistants, and other allied health professionals) providing a solution. As medical knowledge and care have advanced, doctors and clinical professionals have gained an increased understanding of the causes of many common healthcare problems. This knowledge has led to a shift in how healthcare is perceived: medicine is moving from a 'diagnose and treat' to a 'recognize and prevent' model of healthcare.

Wearable technology companies, such as Fitbit (acquired by Google in 2021) and Garmin, as well as others with wearable offerings, such as Apple and Samsung, have been at the forefront in democratizing the ability of patients to manage and track different aspects of their health. Exercise is the primary use case in the area of wearable technology, with devices allowing users to track their activity level, heart rate, and calorie expenditure. The goal of improving awareness of exercise habits is to encourage patients to make improvements to their lifestyles. The benefits of exercise are supported by overwhelming evidence, mainly in correlation with a reduced risk of developing chronic conditions such as heart disease, type 2 diabetes, stroke, and some cancers (particularly in 'activated' consumers and patients who feel confident and are willing to take a proactive role in managing their health).

Ensuring patient safety in their place of home is a critical part of preventing further complications. Approximately 35% of people above the age of 65 have one or more falls per year [9]. With many elderly people living alone, falling at home can lead to fractures, a long lie, subsequent kidney injury, and multi-organ consequences. Smartphone applications have been developed with intelligent fall detection and to provide automatic alerts to emergency services to ensure that patients who fall receive care immediately. This technology uses an accelerometer to measure acceleration forces when the fall occurs, a gyroscope to detect orientation, and an advanced machine learning algorithm trained to distinguish a fall from activities of daily life.

'Wellness medicine' is an area that has seen growth, particularly sleep science. Sleep is a critical biological process and is well known to underpin good health. A company called 'Emerald' (https://emeraldinno.com) has developed a wireless, sensory, and machine learning platform for remote monitoring of sleep, breathing, and behaviour. Developed at MIT, Emerald has applications in various disease areas, including sleep disorders, musculoskeletal disorders, pulmonary disease, and neurological disease [10]. These developments allow unobtrusive tracking of sleep at scale, which can both benefit the patient in understanding their habits and aid in the diagnosis of a sleep disorder, as well as medical research through data collection, which can facilitate studies exploring the interplay between sleep, good health, and well-being.

9.3.2 Future Applications

With the widespread adoption of digital healthcare records, the next step is to leverage this vast pool of data to enable data-driven healthcare provision for patients and improved clinical outcomes. A big opportunity in preventative medicine is the use of deep learning for the early detection and prevention of chronic diseases. Often patients display a myriad of symptoms before they are diagnosed with a specific condition. These can be subtle, such as cancers showing weight loss and fatigue, or more overt, such as cognitive decline in the progression towards Alzheimer's disease. Machine learning analysis of patient records is currently underutilized. Reasons for this include data protection concerns and the challenges associated with the integration of heterogeneous, high-dimensional data (a dataset with a high number of features). A growing number of academic research papers in this area highlights that this underutilization will soon change. A 2020 review found that the use of AI to analyse electronic health records has increased over the past years, with deep learning being the method of choice [11]. As research in this area intensifies, personalized predictions based on an individual patient's history may become an integral part of their medical care.

Other more specific areas where preventative medicine innovation has potential for impact is in remote monitoring of important metrics, such as blood pressure. Valencell, a US-based biometric technology company, announced a cuffless blood pressure device that could be worn on the finger as a ring, and on the wrist like a watch. This technology has been validated in a clinical study to demonstrate it meets the relevant standards, and is in the process of clearance by the US Food and Drug Administration (FDA) [12]. Passive blood pressure monitoring can ultimately help patients at risk of high blood pressure to reduce their risk of mortality through early detection of hypertension.

Type 1 diabetes (T1DM) is an example of a chronic health condition where AI has the scope to both improve quality of life and prevent complications, such as diabetic ketoacidosis. In standard T1DM insulin therapy, patients take insulin doses according to a specific regimen, with additional correction doses being added if their blood glucose is abnormally high. This requires patients to closely monitor their blood sugar, which can be a huge burden, particularly for younger patients. T1DM management has shown huge progress since the development of continuous glucose monitors. These monitors provide real-time blood glucose measurements and trend data to help patients keep their blood glucose within normal limits. Incorporated with insulin delivery devices, the administration of insulin can be automated using algorithms to automatically adjust the insulin dose necessary. Management of T1DM is being advanced further through the development of decision support systems (DSS). DSS are tools that can help patients and their doctors refine their treatment plan by automatically analysing the patient's data and providing personalized recommendations (Figure 9.2). With the integration of

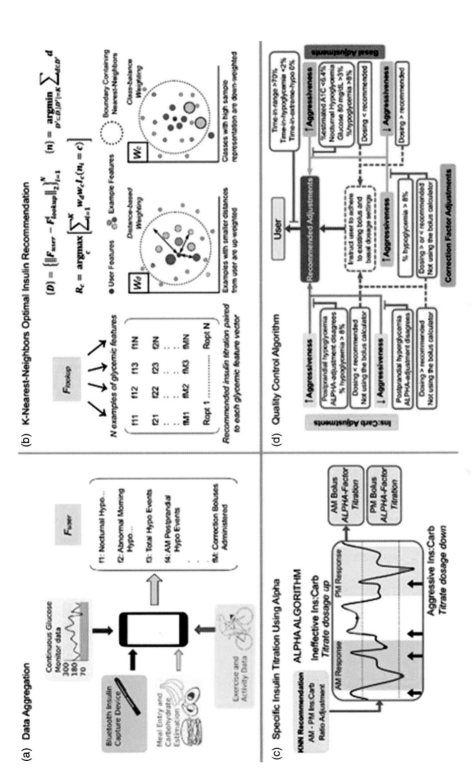

Figure 9.2: A decision support system (DSS) framework to provide patient-specific insulin doses. (a) Patient data is collated and processed to extract features (F_{user}) such as insulin, meal, and activity data needed to titrate insulin doses. (b) The patient's features (F_{user}) are matched to the closest examples in a look-up table (F_{lookup}) using the K-nearest neighbours (KNN) algorithm. The distance between user features and the examples in the look-up table, together with other measures, are used to produce an output by the KNN algorithm, which is a final insulin dosage recommendation, R_c. (c) For the recommendations produced by the KNN-DSS, the ALPHA algorithm assigns an aggressiveness factor that titrates carbohydrate ratios and correction factors to optimize time in the target blood glucose range, and reduce time in hypoglycaemia. (d) A quality control algorithm is used to ensure that KNN-DSS recommendations adhere to physician standards.

Source: Tyler NS et al., 2020 / Springer Nature.

activity monitors, a large dataset is available to train machine learning models for the development of therapy personalization and holistic T1DM management. For example, patients can be notified of their risk of exercise-induced hypoglycaemia and be advised to consume carbohydrates to prevent this [13].

9.4 Triage

9.4.1 Current Applications

The convenience and efficiency of virtual care have meant that PCPs are facing rising levels of pressure, as they are now speaking to many more patients in a single day compared to the previous model of first arranging face-to-face consultations. Furthermore, the World Health Organization has estimated a projected shortfall of 18 million healthcare workers – mostly in low- and lower-middle-income countries – by 2030 [14]. Thus, AI must support productivity and enable safer working practices, including effective triaging, without compromising the quality of the care provided.

The most commonly used online consultation platform in the UK is eConsult [15] (`https://econsult.net`), which offers digital consultations and triaging tools to PCPs to help manage ever-increasing access issues, and provides a data-driven approach to demand management. Chatbots using NLP have also been pivotal in triaging patients. Chatbots can simulate human dialogue, providing patients with an experience that feels close to speaking with healthcare workers. Babylon Health has implemented an AI-powered triage chatbot within its platform to provide patients with potential diagnoses and next steps.

Very specific medical issues can be difficult for general chatbots to triage, so other AI tools including decision trees are sometimes employed. For example, musculo-skeletal (MSK) issues are a very common complaint in primary care, with approximately 20% of the population suffering from an MSK-related condition [16]. Phio is a web application providing at-home triage for MSK pain using clinical decision trees to guide patients through an assessment. The results of this assessment can help to effectively and efficiently prioritise which patients need immediate attention from a human physician.

Microsoft has developed a chatbot (the Azure Health Bot, `https://azure.microsoft.com/en-us/services/bot-services/health-bot`) that can be licensed by organizations to deploy their own AI-powered, customized, conversational, compliant (General Data Protection Regulation [GDPR]/Health Insurance Portability and Accountability Act [HIPAA]) healthcare experience at scale. Over the last year, the Health Bot has delivered close to 1 billion messages to over 80 million people across 25 countries [17]. This allows healthcare providers to access advanced technology without the high investment costs that in-house development often requires.

The ability of a chatbot to perform tasks traditionally performed by clinical staff represents a significant improvement in operational efficiency. Furthermore, it helps patients avoid unnecessary visits, saving the time of both doctors and patients.

9.4.2 Future Applications

Chatbots are currently used to triage patients. However, chatbots may potentially feature as virtual medical assistants for PCPs as well as patient carers in some situations in the future. An AI-powered assistant would be able to understand speech and text, as well as additional inputs such as images and video. A virtual assistant in this setting could potentially serve as 24-hour carer for the patient, with the ability to actively monitor the patient and perform symptom checks. Sensely (`www.sensely.com`) is a company that is building a virtual medical assistant able to use different inputs to assess the user's symptoms. The virtual assistant can check symptoms and triage, but also can track health metrics such as weight, conduct health-risk assessments, and monitor chronic conditions.

The integration of wearables with chatbots to provide personalized, evidence-based virtual care for patients will help with preventing complications, and provide doctors with a medical history should complications occur. Patients can receive a personalized experience, and enjoy the peace of mind that they are receiving 24/7 monitoring.

9.5 Challenges

Telemedicine has the potential to improve the accessibility of healthcare for patients. However, the shift towards telephone and video consultations has raised concerns around three key areas:

- Patients have concerns about receiving suboptimal care compared to in-person consultations where a physical exam is possible. In primary care, many issues can be resolved via phone or video. However, for complex issues, virtual consultations can lengthen the waiting time for patients to receive necessary treatment by requiring further in-person visits to their doctor.
- Doctors are facing the challenge of conducting consultations that they have not been trained to do with electronic health record (EHR) software that has often not been optimized for patient care delivery. The very recent changes to primary care consultations mean that most, if not all, practising doctors did not receive training on conducting virtual consultations. Medical school teaches that what the patient says is a small part of the medical history. A large proportion of information can be gained from observing the patient in addition to the physical examination. Removing this ability but expecting doctors to provide the same standard of care is a difficult challenge, and one that must be addressed by medical bodies. EHR software has frequently been optimized for reimbursement and medical billing rather than patient care, with limited interoperability between different EHR vendors [18]. This represents a major challenge for the development of robust AI models. Moreover, physicians are often dissatisfied with EHR software, which only exacerbates the issue of poor-quality data entry.

Ethical issues surround the use of technology and AI in providing care. Healthcare access disparities may be exacerbated across vulnerable populations such as ethnic minorities, the elderly, and those with low socioeconomic backgrounds, due to a digital divide. (This is discussed in detail in Chapters 39 and 40.) A recent study from a New York City health system found that demographic factors, including race and age, were significantly predictive of telehealth use [19]. Patients over the age of 65 had the lowest odds of using telehealth, and Black and Hispanic patients had a lower odds of using telehealth than their white or Asian counterparts. This finding highlights the potential danger that certain patients will be unable to access healthcare when they need it, further widening health gaps in society. With more development and greater adoption of digital tools by healthcare staff, our society must accept the responsibility to improve technological literacy in this population group and ensure equality in access to healthcare services. The AI systems themselves must also be fair and inclusive by using representative and diverse sample data to ensure appropriate predictions for the target population.

KEY INSIGHTS

- **Primary care has faced dramatic changes accelerated by the COVID-19 pandemic with the mass adoption of telemedicine and digital-first primary care consultations.**
- **Symptom checkers and triage tools using NLP technology may provide patients with an effective and efficient way of accessing reliable clinical advice.**
- **AI has the opportunity to remove some administrative pressures on medical professionals through the automation of clinical documentation.**
- **Wearable technology supports patients in taking control of their health, with intelligent insights and analytics to support improved behavioural change. Real-time biometric tracking allows automated treatment delivery for certain conditions such as T1DM.**
- **Widespread adoption of digital healthcare records provides an opportunity for deep learning to support early detection and management of chronic diseases.**
- **Virtual medical assistants pose an opportunity for patients to receive a personalized experience and 24/7 monitoring.**
- **Key considerations include the need for appropriately heterogeneous and equitable datasets upon which any AI is trained; the change in workflow required to reliably adopt AI at scale into any clinical practice; and AI systems being secure, and respecting privacy.**

Conflicts of Interest

Dr Junaid Bajwa is an employee of Microsoft.

References

1. Blinkenberg J, Pahlavanyali S, Hetlevik Ø, Sandvik H, Hunskaar S. General practitioners' and out-of-hours doctors' role as gatekeeper in emergency admissions to somatic hospitals in Norway: registry-based observational study. *BMC Health Services Research* 2019;19(1):1–2.
2. Academic Health Science Network. Accelerating Artificial Intelligence in Health and Care: Results from a State of the Nation Survey, 2018. https://wessexahsn.org.uk/img/news/AHSN%20Network%20AI%20Report-1536078823.pdf.
3. *Oxford Concise Medical Dictionary.* Oxford: Oxford University Press; 2010. https://www.oxfordreference.com/view/10.1093/acref/9780199557141.001.0001/acref-9780199557141-e-9930.
4. Feldman SR, Fleischer AB Jr, Williford PM, White R, Byington R. Increasing utilization of dermatologists by managed care: an analysis of the national ambulatory medical care survey, 1990–1994. *Journal of the American Academy of Dermatology* 1997;37(5):784–788.
5. Jain A, Way D, Gupta V et al. Development and assessment of an artificial intelligence–based tool for skin condition diagnosis by primary care physicians and nurse practitioners in teledermatology practices. *JAMA Network Open* 2021;4(4):e217249.
6. NHS. *Overview – Cognitive Behavioural Therapy (CBT),* 2019. https://www.nhs.uk/mental-health/talking-therapies-medicine-treatments/talking-therapies-and-counselling/cognitive-behavioural-therapy-cbt/overview.
7. KFF. *Mental Health Care Health Professional Shortage Areas (HPSAs),* 2021. https://www.kff.org/other/state-indicator/mental-health-care-health-professional-shortage-areas-hpsas/?currentTimeframe=0&sortModel=%7B%22colId%22:%22Location%22,%22sort%22:%22asc%22%7D.

For additional references and Further Reading, please see www.wiley.com/go/byrne/aiinclinicalmedicine.

10

Do It Yourself: Wearable Sensors and AI for Self-Assessment of Mental Health

Harish RaviPrakash[1] and Syed Muhammad Anwar[2,3]

[1] AstraZeneca, Waltham, MA, USA

[2] University of Engineering and Technology, Taxila, Pakistan

[3] Sheikh Zayed Institute for Pediatric Surgical Innovation, Children's National Hospital, Washington, DC, USA

Learning Objectives

- Gain an understanding of the current state of the art in wearable sensors for mental well-being.
- Discuss wearable devices that are available off the shelf and could aid in mental health analysis.
- Identify the role of various physiological processes in identifying acute and perceived stress.
- Examine the application of machine learning in mental health, and the self-assessment of health using AI-based software and data from wearable sensors.

10.1 Introduction

Mental health conditions affect an individual's mood, thinking, and behaviour [1]. Mental health disorders are common, present in up to 25% of adults in the USA [2]. The most common conditions include clinical depression, anxiety, schizophrenia, and bipolar disorder, of which depression is the leading cause of disability worldwide with over 264 million affected [3]. Substance use and mental health disorders are often comorbid, with an over 45% prevalence rate of bipolar disorder with substance use, and over 40% prevalence rate for major depression with substance use [4]. Suicide is the second leading cause of death in people between the ages of 15 and 24 years in the USA, and with the onset of the COVID-19 pandemic there has been an increase in the number of people exhibiting signs of depression, suicidality, and substance use [5]. Interpreting a person's state of mind can thus be crucial in

AI in Clinical Medicine: A Practical Guide for Healthcare Professionals, First Edition. Edited by Michael F. Byrne, Nasim Parsa, Alexandra T. Greenhill, Daljeet Chahal, Omer Ahmad, and Ulas Bagci.
© 2023 John Wiley & Sons Ltd. Published 2023 by John Wiley & Sons Ltd.
Companion website: www.wiley.com/go/byrne/aiinclinicalmedicine

providing mental healthcare at an early stage, to potentially limit substance use and prevent suicidal and other similarly damaging thoughts.

Several portable devices were developed with state-of-the-art technology to monitor stress and mental health symptoms. The development process broadly includes bio-marker identification for mental health symptoms, and the development of precise and accurate diagnostic algorithms. Heart rate, respiration rate, oxygen saturation, and neural activity are among the biomarkers used to monitor health symptoms [6]. Wearable devices allow the real-time collection of data and subsequent data analysis, and then provide relevant user feedback. Wearable devices are popular for activity tracking and heart rate monitoring [7], and while the adoption of wearable devices for mental health monitoring has been slower, the availability of wearable electroen-cephalography (EEG) [8] and photoplethysmography (PPG) sensors [9] is increasing. In this chapter, we review the current technologies for monitoring mental health and their associated machine learning algorithms, and propose a roadmap for the design of an efficient wearable device for personalized mental health tracking and diagnosis.

10.2 Psychological Health Assessment Tools

Multiple methods can be used to assess mental health status, particularly mental health conditions involving acute and chronic stress. While low amounts of stress are generally beneficial, chronic stress can trigger a multitude of health conditions, including depression and cardiovascular disease. Self-reported questionnaires and psychologist interviews are the most frequently used methods for quantifying perceived stress levels. For questionnaire-based assessment, the perceived stress scale (PSS) is a self-reported questionnaire that provides a measure of global perceived stress, but is limited by the potential for user bias. Stress assessment by an expert psychologist has its own challenges, such as social stigma, cost, and availability. Significant effort has been expended to develop reliable self-assessment of stress, excluding the human bias, with performance as close as possible to an expert psychologist.

Other physical measures used for stress quantification include facial and emotional analysis. For example, facial photographs have been used for detecting human emotions, where image processing techniques are deployed to detect facial features that correspond to emotional responses [10]. However, the reliability and cost (in terms of hardware and data processing) associated with these techniques may limit large-scale adaptation. For stress assessment during daily life, a wearable solution based on physiological observations could be highly beneficial.

10.3 Modalities for Mental Health Assessment

To obtain a comprehensive understanding of a patient's mental state, primary care physicians can order standard cognitive tests – including the mini mental state exam-ination and the Montréal cognitive assessment [11] – which evaluate memory, attention span, language function, and judgement. Another method involves EEG and the analyses of its frequency bands, which are compared with appropriate age-matched normative EEG databases to identify deviations from the norm and deduce clinical correlates. Functional magnetic resonance imaging (fMRI) methodology plays a key role in modern psychiatric research, and can be used to analyse the changes in activation in brain regions that are associated with different illnesses in order to understand the neural basis of mental illness and to translate the findings to other modalities [12].

The increase in the number of wearable devices and mobile health applications allows for monitoring of physiological activity (such as the use of EEG) in daily life, in comparison to the 'snapshot' provided by an fMRI or clinical EEG, where a visit to a dedicated facility is required. For example, the emergence of wearable EEG headsets and smart watches has enabled observation and logging of various physiological signals such as heart rate variability [13] and galvanic skin response (GSR) [14] during routine, day-to-day activities. Wearable personal devices enable the collection of large-scale data. Such data can be used to train deep learning algorithms to identify and monitor stress [13–15]. An EEG signal and its frequency domain representation are shown in Figure 10.1. As demonstrated in Figure 10.1a,

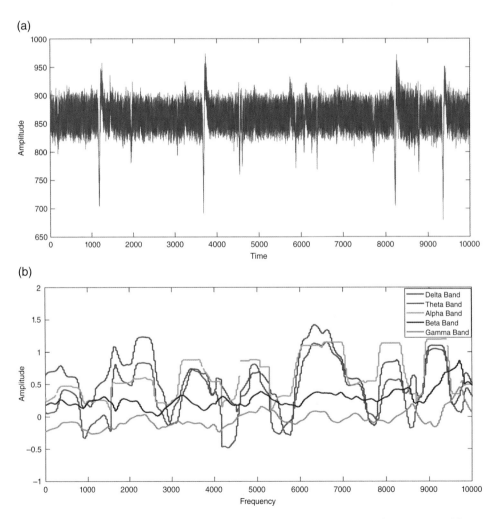

Figure 10.1: Sample electroencephalogram (EEG) signals. (a) Raw EEG data acquired from electrode placed on the scalp. (b) Frequency domain representation including alpha, beta, gamma, theta, and delta bands.

the raw EEG signal has a noise-like representation, and appropriate features – such as frequency bands – need to be extracted in order for this information to be useful. Similarly, other physiological signals including those acquired from heat, GSR, and PPG need to be broken down and extracted.

10.4 Machine Learning for Mental Health Diagnosis – Wearable Sensors and AI

Accurate, reliable, and fast algorithms are necessary for the real-time diagnosis of mental health disorders. Several machine learning algorithms, and more recently deep learning–based algorithms, were developed to diagnose mental health illness accurately and rapidly. These algorithms can be trained using the combined multi-modal data generated from different wearable devices (such as EEG) and smart watch sensors (such as heart rate, accelerometer, respiratory rate etc.).

A brief summary of recent studies using machine learning for mental health assessment is presented in Table 10.1.

Table 10.1: Recent work in mental health diagnosis using machine learning approaches with different modalities of data. CNN, convolutional neural networks; EEG, electroencephalography; HER, electronic health records; fMRI, functional magnetic resonance imaging; NN, neural networks; RNN, recurrent neural networks; SVM, support vector machine.

Study	Modality	Illness	Type of algorithm	Results
Sharma et al. [19]	Self-reports	Depression	XGBoost	Identified blood and urine biomarkers such as triglycerides, neutrophil granulo-cytes, and others as indicative of depression
Yan et al. [20]	fMRI	Depression	SVM	Identified connections in the frontoparietal, default mode, and visual networks indica-tive of depression
Poletti et al. [21]	Lab reports	Depression	Elastic net	Identified immune inflammatory signa-tures as indicative of bipolar and unipolar depression
Nemesure et al. [22]	EHR	Anxiety	XGBoost	Identified vaccination status as most predic-tive of anxiety
Jacobson et al. [23]	Actigraph	Anxiety	Auto-Encoder	Identified individuals at risk of deterioration based on wearable movement data

Table 10.1: (Continued)

Study	Modality	Illness	Type of algorithm	Results
Zheng et al. [24]	EHR	Suicide risk	Deep NN	Stratified patients into different risk groups
Kim et al. [25]	Social media	Mental illness	CNN	Proof of concept of using social media content for early detection of mental illness
Penchina et al. [17]	EEG	Anxiety	RNN	Helped identify anxiousness states in EEG
Coutts et al. [18]	Smart watch	Mental illness	RNN	Utilized heart rate variability to effectively predict mental health
Saeed et al. [26]	EEG	Stress	SVM	Identified temporal alpha symmetry as a potential biomarker for stress classification

Some AI algorithms described in this table use extreme gradient bosting (XGBoost), decision tree–based models designed for speed and performance. Other algorithms that highlight the relative importance of certain features (lab tests, time-series data, etc.) are then used for further training. This helps to improve the interpretability and adoption of algorithms. Machine learning algorithms have also been developed into mental health screening tools in primary care [16]. The recurrent neural network is a type of algorithm that works best for data and time-based signals such as EEG [17] or smart watch–based approaches [18].

10.4.1 Smart Watches for Mental Health Assessment

Different researchers have used smart watches to assess sleep quality, aversive emotions, depression, and stress:

- Research has suggested that sleep quality is correlated with psychological well-being [26]. Smart watches and actigraphs can record sleep information, so the identification of sleep stages from wearable devices has been an important topic [27,28]. Herlan et al. used electrodermal activity (EDA) features for sleep detection, and ultimately observed differences in sleep stages between healthy subjects and subjects with sleep disorders [29].
- Engelniederhammer et al. explored the relationship between personal space infringement and emotions using a smart band that captured EDA and skin temperature, and observed that aversive emotions were experienced by people when their personal space was crossed [15].

Zanella-Calzada et al. used motor activity signal data such as activity counts from a smart watch to detect episodes of depression [30]. Narziev et al. extended this premise further and combined the activity information along with mood and sleep information to classify depression category [31]. Silva et al. explored stress in a slightly different setting, using a smart band to monitor skin conductance, body temperature, HRV, and other measurements, and used this to detect stress in Portuguese medical students [32]. In a larger study, Pakhomov et al. used the heart rate from the PPG sensor of a smart watch to help identify periods of stress encountered by the wearer [33]. The authors found that the heart rate recorded by the smart watch was elevated during periods of stressful events, suggesting that smart watches could be used in the natural environment to identify psychosocial stressors.

Off-the-shelf devices that currently monitor physiological signals that can aid in monitoring mental health include the Fitbit® Sense (which captures EDA as well as heart rate; Google, Mountain View, CA, USA) and the Apple® (Cupertino, CA, USA) and Samsung® Galaxy (Suwon, South Korea) watches (with stress monitor apps to record heart rate data, for example), and can be used with a number of mental health apps on smart phones, such as Calm [34].

10.4.2 Electroencephalography for Mental Health Assessment

Researchers have also developed novel wearable EEG devices to track real-time mental states. Unlike smart watches, which are sleek and compact, EEGs are bulkier devices. Therefore, for them to be widely adopted as wearables, a well-designed headband or headset design is necessary. Headset-type EEG devices can measure EEG signals not only from the prefrontal cortex but also from the parietal, temporal, and occipital cortices, enabling more comprehensive estimation of one's mental health status [35]. Off-the-shelf devices of the headset variety include the NeuroSky® MindWave (San Jose, CA, USA) and Emotiv® Insight (San Francisco, CA, USA).

Wearable EEGs in the form of a headband are available from multiple vendors, and come with proprietary machine learning algorithms that track cognitive states and changes by analysing the raw data in real time. These include the Emotiv EPOC^X and InteraXon Muse™ (Toronto, Canada). To better understand the applicability of wearable EEGs, Richer et al. identified generalized entropy-based measures to differentiate mental states (neutral, focused, and relaxed) using the commercially available Muse Headband [36]. Entropy-based methods utilize uncertainty associated with random variables to quantify information content within the data.

Time domain analysis of a signal analyses changes that occur over a period of time, while *frequency domain analysis* is concerned with changes in a signal in various frequency bands and is used to analyse the repetitions of a signal.

Researchers have also developed novel wearable EEG devices to work around proprietary software bottlenecks, such as cost and the difficulty in adapting a software to meet varying application requirements. Arpaia et al. proposed a two-electrode device, and trained an SVM on differences in signals to classify stress conditions with over 90% accuracy [37]. Ahn et al. developed a novel three-electrode device to record both EEG and electrocardiogram (ECG) signals in real time, and *frequency domain* features were used with an SVM model to detect stressor situations with over 87% accuracy [8]. Frequency domain is an analysis of signals or mathematical functions, in reference to frequency, instead of time. The authors identified that the computed alpha band power symmetry is significantly different between stress and stress-free conditions, as was the ratio of low- to high-frequency power from HRV measurements. Arsalan et al. identified stressors in public speaking scenarios using a multimodal approach [38]. The authors combined wearable EEG (Muse headband)–based frequency domain features with GSR and PPG–based *time domain features* to train an SVM classifier, and achieved an accuracy of over 96%. The performance improvement observed in effectively utilizing multiple modalities and multi-domain features suggests the need to explore multimodal approaches to monitor mental health in real time. The availability of wearable EEG devices and the ability to extract and model the captured features using machine learning approaches opens the door for real-time monitoring of mental health.

10.5 Discussion and Future Roadmap

While there have been several approaches to using wearable devices for the detection and monitoring of mental health in real time, only a select few are clinically applicable. We propose the roadmap in Figure 10.2 to create an efficient AI-driven system that can be used clinically in mental health assessment.

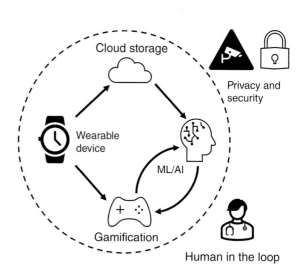

Figure 10.2: Roadmap for an efficient AI-driven real-time mental health self-assessment system.

10.5.1 Data from Wearable Devices and Smart Phones

Wearable devices, such as smart watches, are convenient accessories in our daily life and they provide an opportunity to acquire and use physiological data to appropriately assess aspects of health, including stress.

We propose two methods for efficient data collection:

- Record activity patterns and physiological data using smart watches and smart phones. More detailed data can be collected using wearable EEG headbands to record brain activity.
- Develop games or other incentives to elicit the measurement and recording of a baseline stress response as well as responses to other physiological stimuli. This would enable machine learning models to be trained to delineate between stress and normal conditions. This type of initiative will need collaboration between game design engineers, psychologists, and psychiatrists.

10.5.2 Machine Learning for Data Analysis

The collected data can be processed using advanced machine learning algorithms, including deep learning, and then utilized to predict stressful conditions. Existing studies can be employed to identify the key features to be included from EEG electrodes and frequency bands. The machine learning algorithms more suited for this challenging task should be able to use multimodal data and decision-level fusion techniques, which work to combine the decisions taken by multiple classifiers to reach a common final decision.

10.5.3 Human–Computer Interaction for Stress Management

For addressing day-to-day stress, an AI-driven stress management system can be designed that not only predicts stress level, but also facilitates stress management. To achieve these objectives, we propose using gamification with a human–computer interaction-based design. Gamification is a method where designers incorporate game dynamics in a non-gaming setting, for example game mechanics such as a reward-based system to help manage stress conditions. This could include challenges with different levels, wherein the score and/or time provides an indication of the stress level. The predictions from the machine learning framework can guide the gamification process to generate scenarios that can aid in mitigating human stress. For such a design, a collaborative approach between computer scientists and psychologists will be required.

10.5.4 Privacy Challenges and Solutions

Privacy is one of the major challenges with accessing personal data. The recent success of edge computing involving cloud-based products has the potential to address this challenge. For example, the AI-driven stress assessment and management solution could be hosted on a cloud platform. The computing capability of smart phones and cloud computing can be combined to run sophisticated AI algorithms. Physiological and activity data can be transmitted through a secure cloud that only the user would have access to. Recent advances in cloud-based security can ensure that such a product is safe and protected from a breach of personal privacy.

10.5.5 Human in the Loop

While a properly trained AI-based algorithm may predict an individual's stress level, it is pivotal that these processes have safeguards in place. This is especially important in cases of diagnosis of severe health conditions, as there are psychological, emotional, monetary, and social consequences. The mental health status of users must be interpreted with great accuracy and responsibility. As such, it is still important to ensure that experts are appropriately consulted or kept in the loop. Expert knowledge should be acquired at all stages of the design and implementation of projects, and any system should be programmed to inform or consult a healthcare provider when required. For example, while a chatbot designed to evaluate stress-related responses can identify that a person has a certain level of stress, this must be verified by a psychologist who has interacted with the individual. In our proposed roadmap, we suggest including experts at all stages of the design.

KEY INSIGHTS

- **As an alternative to self-reported mechanisms, stress assessment can be accurately achieved through the interpretation of physiological signals obtained from fixed devices or wearable sensors.**
- **Machine learning can be used to make reliable stress-level predictions.**
- **The availability of wearable EEG devices and the ability to extract and model the captured features using machine learning approaches opens the door for real-time monitoring of mental health.**
- **Privacy is an important consideration in stress assessment applications that rely on the use of shared data.**
- **For automated stress assessment applications to be successful, they must include feedback to the user to help them mitigate stress.**

References

1. Mayo Clinic. *Mental Illness – Symptoms and Causes*, 2019. https://www.mayoclinic.org/diseases-conditions/mental-illness/symptoms-causes/syc-20374968.
2. Johns Hopkins Medicine. *Mental Health Disorder Statistics*, 2021. https://www.hopkinsmedicine.org/health/wellness-and-prevention/mental-health-disorder-statistics.
3. World Health Organization. *Depression*, 2021. https://www.who.int/news-room/fact-sheets/detail/depression.

4. Pettinati HM, O CP, Dundon WD. Reviews and overviews mechanisms of psychiatric illness current status of co-occurring mood and substance use disorders: a new therapeutic target. *American Journal of Psychiatry* 2013;170:23–30.
5. American Association of Suicidology. *Facts and Statistics*, 2021. https://suicidology.org/facts-and-statistics.
6. Rosman L, Gehi A, Lampert R. When smartwatches contribute to health anxiety in patients with atrial fibrillation. *Cardiovascular Digital Health Journal* 2020;1(1):9–10. https://doi.org/10.1016/j.cvdhj.2020.06.004.
7. Isakadze N, Martin SS. How useful is the smartwatch ECG? *Trends in Cardiovascular Medicine* 2020;30(7):442–448.

For additional references and Further Reading please see www.wiley.com/go/byrne/aiinclinicalmedicine.

11

AI in Dentistry

Lyudmila Tuzova[1,2], Dmitry Tuzoff[1,3],
and L. Eric Pulver[1,4]

[1] Denti.AI Technology Inc., Toronto, ON, Canada

[2] Georgia Institute of Technology, Atlanta, GA, USA

[3] Steklov Institute of Mathematics, St Petersburg, Russia

[4] Adjunct Instructor Indiana University Dental School IN, USA,
Oral & Maxillofacial Surgeon Private Practice. Indiana University
Dental School, Indianapolis, IN, USA

Learning Objectives

- Understand current trends for AI in dentistry: what is the focus of research?
- Review several use cases and application opportunities.
- Gain a basic understanding of AI regulations in the USA that may influence how dentistry adopts this technology.
- Discuss some of the key challenges for AI in dentistry.
- Present a roadmap for the future of AI in dentistry.

11.1 Introduction

Dentistry is an attractive area for the application of AI. Recently, there has been a significant rise in interest in dental AI applications in both academia and industry. The powerful algorithms behind AI can significantly impact all aspects of the clinical workflow. Potential applications include computer-aided detection and diagnosis, patient management, auto-population of electronic medical records, detection and measurement of anatomical structures, and computer-aided design and manufacturing. AI applications can assist dental professionals in decision-making, risk assessment, treatment planning, and continuous monitoring. The opportunities for AI in dentistry look very promising. However, AI in dentistry is still far from being widely adopted.

The questions this chapter considers are: What opportunities are there for AI in dentistry? What challenges are there for AI in dentistry?

11.2 Current Trends: What Is the Focus of Research?

The adoption of AI technologies has been slower in dentistry than in other medical fields, despite an increase in awareness within the dental industry. The difficulty in accessing dental data can partly explain this dynamic.

AI in Clinical Medicine: A Practical Guide for Healthcare Professionals, First Edition. Edited by Michael F. Byrne,
Nasim Parsa, Alexandra T. Greenhill, Daljeet Chahal, Omer Ahmad, and Ulas Bagci.
© 2023 John Wiley & Sons Ltd. Published 2023 by John Wiley & Sons Ltd.
Companion website: www.wiley.com/go/byrne/aiinclinicalmedicine

Developing a high-quality AI product requires a lot of representative samples obtained from multiple sources – but dental images and patient data are not easily accessible for research and product development purposes.

Actively explored areas of AI research vary widely within dentistry [1–3]. The dental topics that are most frequently addressed in academic research, as determined by the total number of citations [4], include teeth detection and numbering, detection of most prevalent pathological findings (such as caries lesions and apical periodontitis), orthodontics assessment, and assessing periodontal diseases. Other applications include using AI for dental materials design and manufacturing, detecting cysts and tumours, detecting root fractures, robotics, and virtual reality (VR) [5,6].

Most recent studies (~75%) are focused on applying AI for image interpretation tasks. For imaging-based studies, dental radiographs prevail. Cone-beam computed tomography (CBCT) and panoramic radiographic modalities generate almost the same amount of interest, followed by intraoral radiographs. Despite the increasing popularity of CBCT, panoramic radiographs remain very popular and are widely used by dentists in many countries [1,3].

TOP 15 RECENT DENTAL AI APPLICATIONS PAPERS RANKED BY THE NUMBER OF CITATIONS

Information about cited papers was retrieved using Dimensions.AI [4] to get insight into the most frequently researched topics in dentistry. The following search criteria and keywords were used:

- *Titles or abstracts contain the following keywords*: ("artificial intelligence" OR "neural network" OR "neural networks" OR "machine learning" OR "deep learning" OR "AI" OR "CNN" OR "Convolutional") AND ("dentistry" OR "dental" OR "teeth" OR "CBCT" OR "panoramic" OR "periapical" OR "bitewing" OR "intraoral" OR "extraoral")
- *Years of publication*: 2010–2021.

The papers were then ranked by the number of citations, and the top 100 relevant publications were included in the analysis. Although not a perfect predictor of research quality, citations reflect the general interest in the area:

- Lee J-H, Kim D-H, Jeong S-N, Choi S-H. Detection and diagnosis of dental caries using a deep learning-based convolutional neural network algorithm. *Journal of Dentistry* 2018;77:106–111.
- Miki Y, Muramatsu C, Hayashi T et al. Classification of teeth in cone-beam CT using deep convolutional neural network. *Computers in Biology and Medicine* 2017;80:24–29.
- Lee J-H, Kim D-H, Jeong S-N, Choi S-H. Diagnosis and prediction of periodontally compromised teeth using a deep learning-based convolutional neural network algorithm. *Journal of Periodontal & Implant Science* 2018;48(2):114.

- Krois J, Ekert T, Meinhold L et al. Deep learning for the radiographic detection of periodontal bone loss. *Scientific Reports* 2019;9(1):8495.
- Ekert T, Krois J, Meinhold L et al. Deep learning for the radiographic detection of apical lesions. *Journal of Endodontics* 2019;45(7):917–922.e5.
- Tuzoff DV, Tuzova LN, Bornstein MM et al. Tooth detection and numbering in panoramic radiographs using convolutional neural networks. *Dentomaxillofacial Radiology* 2019;48(4):20180051.
- Chen H, Zhang K, Lyu P et al. A deep learning approach to automatic teeth detection and numbering based on object detection in dental periapical films. *Scientific Reports* 2019;9(1):3840.
- Murata M, Ariji Y, Ohashi Y et al. Deep-learning classification using convolutional neural network for evaluation of maxillary sinusitis on panoramic radiography. *Oral Radiology* 2019;35(3):301–307.
- Tuan TM, Ngan TT, Son LH. A novel semi-supervised fuzzy clustering method based on interactive fuzzy satisficing for dental x-ray image segmentation. *Applied Intelligence* 2016;45(2):402–428.
- Hiraiwa T, Ariji Y, Fukuda M et al. A deep-learning artificial intelligence system for assessment of root morphology of the mandibular first molar on panoramic radiography. *Dentomaxillofacial Radiology* 2019;48(3):20180218.
- Jung S-K, Kim T-W. New approach for the diagnosis of extractions with neural network machine learning. *American Journal of Orthodontics and Dentofacial Orthopedics* 2016;149(1):127–133.
- Xu X, Liu C, Zheng Y. 3D tooth segmentation and labeling using deep Convolutional Neural Networks. IEEE Transactions on Visualization and Computer Graphics 2019;25(7):2336–2348.
- Ariji Y, Yanashita Y, Kutsuna S et al. Automatic detection and classification of radiolucent lesions in the mandible on panoramic radiographs using a deep learning object detection technique. Oral Surgery, Oral Medicine, Oral Pathology and Oral Radiology 2019;128(4):424–430.
- Poedjiastoeti W, Suebnukarn S. Application of convolutional neural network in the diagnosis of jaw tumors. *Healthcare Informatics Research* 2018;24(3):236–241.
- Prajapati SA, Nagaraj R, Mitra S. Classification of dental diseases using CNN and transfer learning. In: *2017 5th International Symposium on Computational and Business Intelligence (ISCBI)*. New York: IEEE; 2017, 70–74.

11.3 Use Cases and Application Opportunities

Examining active areas of dentistry AI research, it appears that there are already promising technologies incorporating AI in real-world dental settings, either in clinical studies or commercial opportunities. Examples of automated functions include:

- *Identifying and marking potential pathological findings.* AI can assist dental professionals in detecting various types of pathological conditions, such as

(a)   (b)

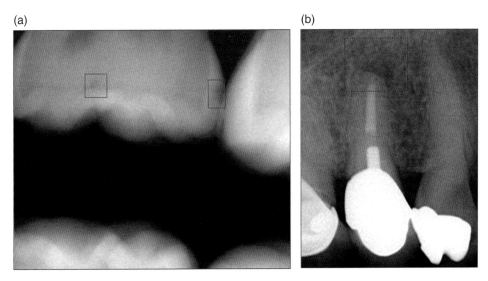

Figure 11.1: (a) Examples of caries decay detected on various tooth surfaces. (b) Examples of apical lesions detected.

Source: Denti.AI.

caries, apical lesions, cysts, and tumours (Figure 11.1). Dental images contain a lot of information that must be rapidly assessed at the time of the patient visit. Highlighting suspicious regions decreases the chance of missing important pathology.

- *Detecting dental structures, past treatments, and assessing periodontal status.* AI can automatically identify dental structures and landmarks, such as teeth, bone levels, and cementoenamel junction (CEJ) points. AI can also identify and mark various pre-existing conditions and results of previous treatment such as crowns, fillings, implants, and endodontic treatment, as well as missing teeth. Results of automated interpretation can be used as an initial step in the patient examination and, once confirmed, for automated dental charting. Figure 11.2 shows an example of such automation.
- *Orthodontics.* AI can he applied to various orthodontics tasks. It is already used in the industry for aligner design and treatment monitoring (Figure 11.3). Trained on real-life cases, AI software helps to create aligners that produce more predictable and effective treatment results while decreasing orthodontists' chair time.
- *Automated dental charting.* Filling dental charts is a time-consuming and tedious procedure that is often done incompletely. However, this task is very important for the long-term success of the practice and for ensuring strong patient outcomes. Inaccurate or incomplete charting also has implications for quality assurance and potential medico-legal ramifications. By helping dental professionals with more efficient and accurate processes, AI will allow them to focus more on treatment planning, procedures, and interactions with their patients. In addition, automated charting will produce more complete charts to help monitor patients' conditions in a more consistent and

(a)   (b)

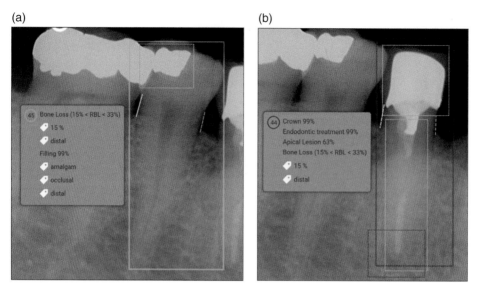

Figure 11.2: (a) An example of automatically detected tooth, filling, and bone level marks, showing a potential bone loss on a distal surface according to American Academy of Periodontology (AAP) staging. (b) An example of automatically detected tooth, treated canal, crown, and bone level marks, showing signs of an apical lesion and bone loss on a distal surface. The AI's findings are accompanied by percentages of the degree of confidence.

Source: Denti.AI.

(a)   (b)

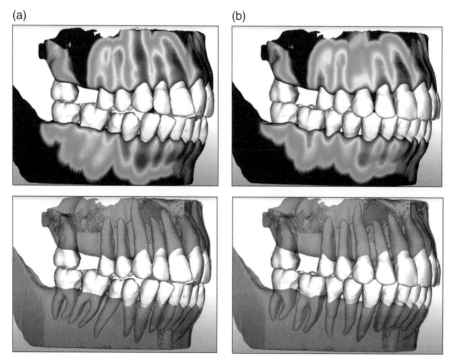

Figure 11.3: (a) A patient's conditions before treatment as automatically segmented by AI using a cone-beam computed tomography (CBCT) image. Top: a colour map created by AI shows the distance between roots and the bone surface; bottom: each individual root's angulation and length are visualized. (b) The same patient's conditions after treatment.

Source: Courtesy of Marina Domracheva, 3D Predict.

standardized way and perform timely recalls. Figure 11.4 shows an example of a clinical workflow that can be achieved with the help of AI.

- *Voice-activated periodontal charting.* AI applications can also be applied to natural language processing tasks. One example of commercially available applications is voice-automated periodontal charting. This software frees hygienists' hands while doing periodontal measurements. The chart is filled automatically by processing various voice commands, an example of which is demonstrated in Figure 11.5.

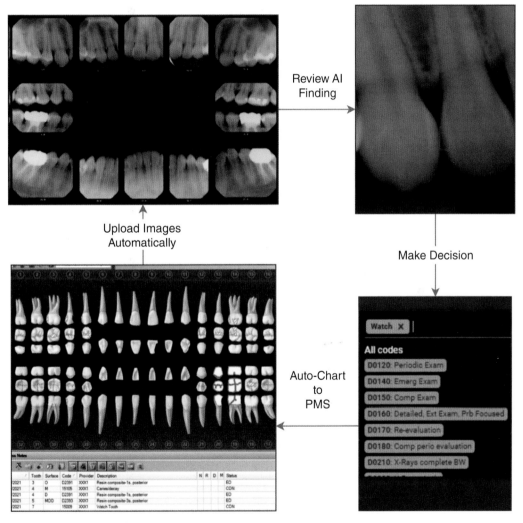

Figure 11.4: An example of dental charting workflow automation: patients' images are uploaded automatically from a practice management system (PMS) to the AI software; a dental professional reviews images with AI predictions shown as an aid, makes adjustments if necessary, and chooses treatment plan options. The conditions, diagnoses, and treatment codes are automatically exported to the PMS.

Source: Denti.AI.

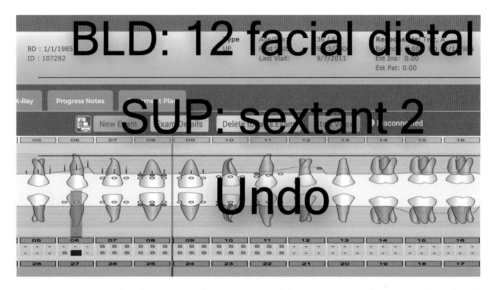

Figure 11.5: An example of automated processing of the sequence of commands: 'Bleeding on twelve distal facial', 'Suppuration on sextant two', 'Undo'.

Source: Denti.AI.

▪ *Computer-aided design and manufacturing.* Although there is a great interest in developing products to assist dental professionals in a clinical environment, AI technologies are not limited to this area. For example, generative adversarial networks or GANs are being used to design dental crowns. Figure 11.6 shows an AI-generated crown. The AI algorithm helps create unique restorations that accurately reflect the anatomy of the patient and are natural looking. Automation in this area solves tasks that are otherwise time-consuming and labour intensive.

▪ *CBCT analysis.* With the growing number of CBCT images, computer-assisted CBCT visualization is becoming increasingly important. CBCT analysis is difficult and time-consuming. Modern AI and computer vision algorithms can automatically segment various dental structures and provide highly detailed

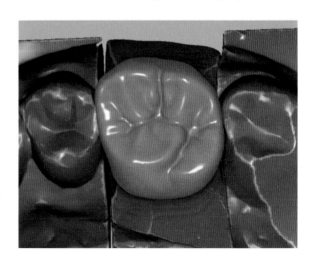

Figure 11.6: Crown automatically generated using generative adversarial networks (GANs).

Source: Courtesy of Sergei Azernikov, Glidewell Dental.

(a)

(b)

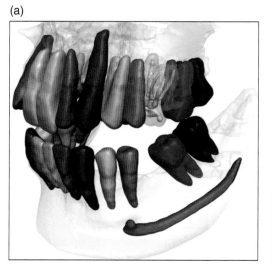 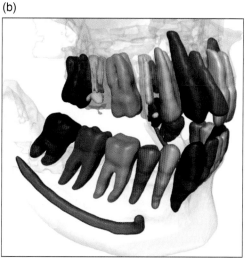

Figure 11.7: An example of automatically segmented dental structures for cone-beam computed tomography (CBCT) images and visualization of the results in 3D. Colours match identified tooth numbers. (a) A challenging case of multiple root canals and an example of a correctly detected missing tooth. (b) An additional viewing perspective.

Source: Denti.AI.

3D visualizations for assessment and treatment planning. Dental professionals can review 3D images from different viewpoints with the important anatomical structures automatically segmented. Figure 11.7 shows an example of a visualization generated automatically from a CBCT image. AI can also help identify abnormalities, including cases not presented on two-dimensional X-rays. Automatic detection of abnormalities on CBCT can increase the chance that patients are referred earlier to specialists for efficient treatment.

- *Patient education.* By allowing dentists to share the dental findings in a visual manner, AI helps engage patients in the decision-making process and increase overall trust. AI may help shift the focus of dental care to a more proactive approach. Identifying problems earlier and being able to show the issue to the patient will enable the dental professional to recommend preventative procedures, and will help with patient acceptance when treatment is necessary.
- *Outside of the dental chair.* The computer-assisted analysis is not limited to the dental chair. The results of the computer-aided analysis can be used for:
    - *Quality control and statistics*: more consistent and standardized charting information enables retrospective analysis, statistics, and quality monitoring.
    - *Insurance claim reviews*: the results of the automated analysis can be used to assist clinics and insurance companies in preparing and validating insurance claims.
    - *Teledentistry*: AI-based solutions open more opportunities for remote treatment monitoring, triage, and patient education.

11.4 AI and Dentistry Regulations in the USA

The real-world application of AI in dentistry is still in its early stages, and regulatory requirements might explain why, or at least part of the reason why. Muehlematter et al. reviewed the current dynamics in approvals of AI-based medical devices in different medical fields [7]. According to their report, the number of AI and machine learning–based medical devices approved in the USA by the Food and Drug Administration (FDA) increased from 9 in 2015 to 77 in 2019. Similarly, the number of *Conformité Européenne*–marked devices in Europe increased from 13 in 2015 to 100 in 2019. Approval does not necessarily mean that all these products enter the market, but reflects the level of activity in the industry and the readiness of regulatory bodies to accept an emerging technology.

Although the overall number of approved and cleared devices in the medical field is growing quickly, the regulatory approval progress in dentistry has been slower. The regulatory requirements for using AI-based dental products vary greatly depending on the intended use; on whether the AI software is a part of hardware medical device or is a standalone application performing medical functions without being a part of a hardware medical device (Software as a Medical Device, or SaMD) [8]; and whether it is being marketed to dental providers or insurers. Some products may not require approval, some require limited performance testing, and some must pass rigorous clinical testing procedures before entering the market.

The use of SaMD products is growing fast. Considering the unique characteristics of this type of medical device entity, much effort is concentrated on developing regulatory frameworks for SaMD classification, evaluation, and quality control [8].

A number of exciting start-ups in dentistry have been working hard on developing and obtaining clearances for their AI SaMD products and showed significant progress in 2021–2022. Examples of the dental SaMD products that have already been cleared or approved by the FDA include automated dental charting (Denti. AI), computer-aided detection of caries (Carestream Dental, Overjet, Pearl, Videa), cephalometric landmark detection for orthodontal assessment (Dentsply Sirona, Ewoosoft), and periodontal bone level assessment (Overjet). More products and features are appearing on the market every few months.

11.5 Challenges

Despite having huge support, interest, and effort from academic research, industry, and providers, AI within oral healthcare has not become mainstream. Reasons already discussed include limited data accessibility and rigorous regulatory procedures. In addition, other factors also play a role, including the following:

- *Annotating data is a long and expensive process.* For machine learning–based applications relying on dental images, the number of annotated images plays a crucial role as machine learning algorithms require a lot of data to learn patterns. Annotating radiographs by hand is a tedious and time-consuming task and requires individuals with a high level of qualification and experience.

- *Inadequate record-keeping.* The current low quality of record-keeping, including the lack of data [9], can be challenging for AI applications requiring dental records. For example, patient diagnoses are almost never recorded in the dental charts. Instead, dental records are almost only filled with treatment codes, and only about 50% of past treatment records are complete.
- *Disagreement between experts.* To evaluate AI-based imaging software, a reference standard (or ground truth) needs to be established. Dental images are naturally hard to interpret, and disagreement between experts is widespread: dental images show a great amount of information, may vary in quality, and contain numerous edge-case scenarios. Sometimes the disagreements between experts may be attributed to differences in experience and training, at other times they may be explained by the limitations of the imaging technologies, inconsistencies in standards and interpretation, or differences in clinical contexts and applications. Figure 11.8 shows one example of such disagreement in the definition of bone level and CEJ point locations.
- *Dentists require more context.* When interpreting dental images, clinicians use non-obvious information, such as the correlation between different pathologies, jaw symmetry, and adjacent teeth conditions. They also often compare multiple X-ray images during a patient's evaluation. Although AI can utilize this information, accounting for these factors makes the task harder for software developers.

11.6 Roadmap to the Future

Implementing AI in the dental industry is challenging for all parties involved: regulatory bodies, dental providers/clinics, and AI product developers. The regulations and standards are constantly changing, and AI developers must explore new technologies, all the while having a deep understanding of the oral healthcare field.

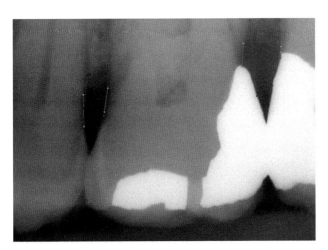

Figure 11.8: An example of systematic disagreement in establishing the reference standard. The differences in locating the bone level and cemento-enamel junction points on restored surfaces by two dentists (green and red lines).

Source: Denti.AI.

At the same time, dental clinics need to adjust their workflows and provide feedback to AI developers, while acting as ambassadors for the new technology. All stakeholders must be open to being active participants within the product life cycle.

AI in the oral healthcare field is still a 'work in progress'. The following topics are actively discussed in the community:

- *Continuous software improvement* [8]. Machine learning algorithms are designed to continuously learn from new data. However, current regulatory procedures require 'locking' the software for the product to be marketed, limiting the AI's ability to continually learn and improve performance from new observations. Ongoing discussions within the industry are taking place on how new approval procedures can be implemented to speed up the delivery of the updated software.
- *More clinical studies*. Many research studies now focus on assessing how AI software performs alone or how the software compares to dental professionals. Being an important step of software assessment, so-called standalone studies are limited in their ability to predict how AI products will impact dental professionals' performance while using AI.
- *Real-world software testing* [9]. Clinical studies that have been performed are mostly done retrospectively in 'laboratory' conditions. However, many factors may influence the performance of the software in real-world applications. Instead, feasibility clinical studies may help assess the technology in a real-world application, and get early feedback from practitioners on how the technology provides value and ways it can be improved.
- *Continuous evaluation* [8,9]. Currently, most performance evaluation steps are done before an AI product moves to the market. However, AI-based software may perform differently depending on the changing environment. Continuous real-life monitoring will likely be an essential part of the AI-based product life cycle.
- *Reliability of performance assessment* [2,9–11]. Presently, the evaluation of AI-based software is not well defined or transparent. Creating independent data sources will help standardize software and make the performance evaluation results more reliable.

From a technological and application point of view, there are numerous directions of development, including:

- *Training machine learning algorithms using multi-source input* [9]. Many products utilize limited sources of information (e.g. a single image of a patient) as an input for machine learning–based software. More advanced technologies that consider different input sources and modalities may advance the quality of the products.
- *Unsupervised and semi-supervised learning* [9]. Many products rely on the 'supervised learning' paradigm, when machine learning learns from well-defined x–y pairs, where x is input data and y is a 'true' label. However, setting

the reference standard for imaging-based applications is expensive and not without its problems. Using unsupervised or semi-supervised techniques can help improve software performance without annotating all the data, and can also uncover important insights along the way.

- *Other applications and AI technologies* [5.6]. AI capabilities go far beyond the discussed applications. Robotics, VR, and teledentistry are additional areas where technology and medicine can focus attention.

Despite the challenges, AI in dentistry may eventually bridge the gaps between academia, industry, dental providers, and policymakers. These interdisciplinary dynamics should benefit the patient. Introducing AI can help all parties set common ground for patient care standards. It will likely lead to a standardized and high-quality product development life cycle, more reliable performance assessment, and better-defined standards of care and diagnosis. More accurate medical records will improve quality control, monitor patients' conditions, and open more research opportunities. Finally, tailored visualizations will allow patients to become an active part of the decision-making process and help to increase their overall level of trust in their oral healthcare provider.

KEY INSIGHTS

- **Although at a slower rate compared to other medical fields, AI in dentistry has seen a rapid growth in interest in recent years. The diversity of publications reflects the numerous potential opportunities of AI technology in dentistry. The application of AI for computer-aided radiograph interpretation in the fields of general dentistry, orthodontics, and periodontics is among the most popular topics of research.**
- **AI can be applied or is currently being used in a wide range of tasks executed within and beyond the dental chair. The main benefits that AI provides in this area include an increase in transparency and trust by engaging patients in decision-making, an increase in interaction and communication with patients during the visit, help in visualization and analysis of complex structures, digitalization of patients' data and record-keeping, a decrease in the chance of missed pathology, and better patient outcomes.**
- **The overall number of approved or cleared medical devices is growing fast, which shows that the industry is gaining more confidence and trust in the technology. At the same time, dentistry is slower than many other medical fields in reaching the market. Only a few AI-based dentistry devices have been approved or cleared in the USA by the FDA at this time. Examples, as detailed in the text, include computer-aided detection of caries, cephalometric landmark detection for orthodontal assessment, and periodontal bone level assessment.**

■ Although it demonstrates promising results, applying AI in dentistry is not without challenges. Some of the challenges include the long and expensive process of annotating data, inadequate record-keeping, strict regulatory requirements, inconsistency, and a high level of disagreement between experts.

■ An interdisciplinary approach and a joint effort from academia, industry, and regulatory bodies are required to reach a transparent, reliable, and trustworthy way of applying AI to dentistry. Some of the main directions for discussion and improvement include the development of a regulatory framework for delivering AI that is continuously learning and improving, a focus on real-world and continuous technology assessment, and an increase in transparency and the robustness of technology development and validation. From a technological point of view, research and development areas are far from being exhausted, both in existing applications and in new areas, such as robotics and virtual reality.

Conflicts of Interest

Dmitry Tuzoff, Lyudmila Tuzova, and Eric Pulver have a commercial interest in a product or service mentioned in this chapter.

References

1. Schwendicke F, Golla T, Dreher M, Krois J. Convolutional neural networks for dental image diagnostics: a scoping review. *Journal of Dentistry* 2019;91:103226.
2. Hwang J-J, Jung Y-H, Cho B-H, Heo M-S. An overview of deep learning in the field of dentistry. *Imaging Science in Dentistry* 2019;49(1):1–7.
3. Hung K, Montalvao C, Tanaka R, Kawai T, Bornstein MM. The use and performance of artificial intelligence applications in dental and maxillofacial radiology: a systematic review. *Dentomaxillofacial Radiology* 2020;49(1):20190107.
4. Digital Science. *Dimensions* (software), 2018–. Available from `https://app.dimensions.ai`, accessed under licence agreement.
5. Joda T, Bornstein MM, Jung RE, Ferrari M, Waltimo T, Zitzmann NU. Recent trends and future direction of dental research in the digital era. *International Journal of Environmental Research and Public Health* 2020;17(6):1987. `https://doi.org/10.3390/ijerph17061987`.
6. Grischke J, Johannsmeier L, Eich L, Griga L, Haddadin S. Dentronics: towards robotics and artificial intelligence in dentistry. *Dental Materials* 2020;36:765–778. `https://doi.org/10.1016/j.dental.2020.03.021`.
7. Muehlematter UJ, Daniore P, Vokinger KN. Approval of artificial intelligence and machine learning-based medical devices in the USA and Europe (2015–20): a comparative analysis. *Lancet Digital Health* 2021;3(3):e195–e203.

For additional references please see `www.wiley.com/go/byrne/aiinclinical medicine`.

12

AI in Emergency Medicine

Jonathon Stewart[1,2,3], Adrian Goudie[1], Juan Lu[2,3], and Girish Dwivedi[2,3,4]

[1] *Emergency Department, Fiona Stanley Hospital, Murdoch, WA, Australia*

[2] *Harry Perkins Institute of Medical Research, Murdoch, WA, Australia*

[3] *Medical School, University of Western Australia, Crawley, WA, Australia*

[4] *Department of Cardiology, Fiona Stanley Hospital, Murdoch, WA, Australia*

Learning Objectives

- Gain an appreciation of the scope of current research concerning AI in emergency medicine.
- Develop an understanding of the challenges of using AI in emergency medicine.
- Develop an awareness of how AI may impact emergency medicine in the future.

12.1 Introduction

This chapter aims to give a broad overview of the current state of AI use in emergency medicine and its future possibilities. It highlights recent relevant advances and achievements in multiple fields that show the possibilities, promises, and challenges of using AI in emergency medicine. The breadth of emergency medicine and the growing popularity of AI across multiple fields and industries mean that giving a complete overview of all possible implications of AI in emergency medicine is not feasible. We encourage interested readers to review the extensive online reference list for further details of the research that supports the statements made in this chapter.

12.2 Prehospital

The influence of AI in emergency medicine may begin even before patients arrive at the emergency department (ED). Emergency medical services (EMS) personnel must use the limited information available 'in the field' to accurately risk-stratify patients, begin initial treatment, and ensure transport to an appropriate centre. AI has already been applied in the prehospital setting to routinely collect information and vital signs [1–4]. Nederpelt et al. developed a deep neural network–based field AI triage model to predict outcomes in gunshot victims [4]. Trained on a retrospective database of 29,816 patients, the model required only basic information that is readily available in the field. A simplified version of their model (using only gunshot wound anatomical location, vital signs, and age as inputs) was able to predict shock (area under the receiver operating characteristic curve [AUROC] 0.88), early massive transfusion (AUROC 0.85), and the need for major surgery (AUROC 0.79). This proof-of-concept model supports the idea that AI could assist with in-field triage and ensure the transfer of gunshot victims to an appropriate trauma centre.

AI used in the pre-hospital setting may allow for more accurate pre-hospital risk stratification in general. AI models can use pre-hospital information to predict the need for hospital admission or critical care admission with greater accuracy than conventional triage and early warning scores [5,6]. Kang et al. developed and validated a deep learning algorithm to predict the need for critical care using only information available to EMS personnel such as patient demographics, initial vital signs, chief complaint, and symptom onset [5]. They used a retrospective dataset of almost nine million patients to train their model. The predictive performance of their deep learning model (AUROC 0.867) outperformed the performance of conventional triage tools, including the National Early Warning Score (AUROC 0.741) and the Modified Early Warning Score (MEWS; AUROC 0.696). Future AI-based models may be used to create a generalizable pre-hospital triage tool that can accurately predict the severity of a patient's condition and their clinical course.

12.3 Cardiac Arrest

Early recognition of cardiac arrest and activation of emergency medical services are the first steps in the chain of survival [7]. Blomberg et al. developed and evaluated an AI-based speech recognition model to identify calls for out-of-hospital cardiac arrest (OHCA) [8]. Their model more accurately and rapidly identified calls for OHCA than did humans; however, when tested in a randomized control trial, the use of this system did not improve dispatcher recognition of OHCA [8]. Outcomes from cardiac arrest remain poor, and prognostication is challenging. The application of AI-based techniques to routinely collect data may allow for a more accurate prediction of patient-orientated outcomes including neurologically intact survival, and enable earlier prognostication than current practice [9–11]. AI may be used to better identify those most likely to benefit from intensive therapeutic intervention and those in which further intervention is futile [12].

Opportunities to apply AI in novel ways include the analysis of ventricular fibrillation waveforms to predict survival with good neurological outcomes and using electroencephalogram data to predict carotid blood flow during cardiopulmonary resuscitation (CPR) [13–14]. Identifying a return to spontaneous circulation (ROSC) can be challenging, as pulses may be weak and difficult to palpate. AI algorithms that incorporate end-tidal carbon dioxide can help improve the performance of pulse detection and more accurately identify ROSC [15]. AI has also been used to accurately classify rhythms from defibrillators used in OHCA into pulseless electrical activity or pulse-generating rhythm [16].

12.4 Triage

Triage presents a unique opportunity to deploy AI-based tools to improve ED efficiency and effectiveness. Currently, a trained triage nurse triages patients in the ED, but patients may have to wait hours before an emergency doctor makes a disposition decision. Unwell patients, such as those with sepsis, must be accurately identified at ED triage. Early identification and treatment improve sepsis outcomes. Kim et al. developed a machine learning model for the prediction of septic shock within 24 hours of ED arrival for adults with suspected infection [17]. Baseline machine learning models that used only age and vital signs outperformed existing risk scores, including the quick sepsis-related organ failure assessment (qSOFA) (AUROC 0.813) and MEWS (AUROC 0.790). Ensemble classifiers achieved the best performance (AUROC 0.902). Neural networks with only one or two layers outperformed deeper models. Including chief complaint and laboratory findings in the machine learning models improved the AUROC to 0.924. Adding more advanced natural language processing of free-text triage data improves predictive performance [18,19].

Incorporating novel parameters may also improve model performance. Chiew et al. found that a machine learning model that included heart rate variability as an input outperformed conventional risk-stratification tools in the prediction of 30-day in-hospital mortality among suspected sepsis patients in the ED [20]. Using AI-based models in ED triage may provide clinical decision support and assist with the early identification of important clinical conditions. AI-based models could give a useful initial prediction at triage, then improve this prediction as more data become available. Such models are likely to be implemented into clinical practice in the near future.

Acute stroke is another significant cause of health burden that benefits from early recognition and treatment. Sung et al. developed a machine learning–based stroke-alert trigger that used clinical features, medical history, vital signs, and risk factors to identify patients with suspected stroke at ED triage [21]. The best-performing machine learning model (AUROC 0.898) outperformed commonly used rule-based algorithms such as the Face Arm Speech Test (FAST; AUROC 0.770) and Balance, Eyes, FAST (BE-FAST; AUROC 0.753).

The integration of AI into triage may help in multiple other ways. Early identification of patients requiring investigations or admission would assist with patient flow and demand management. Applied to structured clinical data acquired at the time of triage, AI has accurately predicted adult and paediatric patients' disposition, length of stay, need for intensive care, clinical outcomes, and mortality [22–30]. These AI-based predictions have outperformed clinicians' predictions and conventional scoring tools [23,26,28,30–32]. Natural language processing has advanced significantly over recent years. When applied to free-text notes, AI can predict disposition [33]. Combined with structured clinical data, these subjective free-text notes can improve model performance [19,34]. AI can also predict patient wait times [35–37]. In a simulated setting, an AI model was able to auto-transcribe a conversation at triage and give the appropriate triage score [38].

12.5 Monitoring

AI may be applied to patient vital sign monitors in the ED to allow for earlier identification of patients in septic shock while reducing false alarms [39,40]. Advances in computer vision and signal processing may significantly change how patients are monitored, in particular through non-invasive monitoring [41–44]. The compensatory reserve measure (CRM) is a promising example of a novel monitoring technique based on machine learning [45]. Haemorrhage in trauma is often amenable to life-saving intervention; however, it may not be clinically evident or well reflected in traditional vital signs until later in a patient's clinical course when sudden decompensation occurs [46]. CRM is a continuous monitoring technology that combines feature extraction and machine learning analysis of arterial pulse waveforms generated from standard pulse oximetry to predict a patient's physiological reserve and identify which patients are at risk of developing decompensated shock [45]. In a prospective observational study of 89 trauma patients, the CRM achieved a significantly higher sensitivity than systolic blood pressure (83% vs 26%) in predicting the need for post-traumatic haemorrhage intervention [46]. Convertino et al. validated a colour-coded visual analogue dashboard for a CRM monitor [47]. The device displayed the patient's CRM as red (less than 30%), yellow (30–59%), or green (60% or greater), with the odds of haemorrhage increased 12-fold for those patients with a CRM in the red zone.

AI may also improve the consistency and convenience of non-invasive monitoring. Computer vision algorithms have been combined with thermal imaging cameras and have been used to accurately determine respiratory rate [48]. Cuff-less blood pressure (BP) monitoring has been achieved through applying AI to electrocardiogram (ECG) and finger photo-plethysmograph data [41–44]. It is also now possible to extract pulse waves from facial videos and use these pulse waves to estimate the presence of atrial fibrillation, heart rate variability, and other physiological indices [49].

12.6 Electrocardiogram

The ECG is an inexpensive, common, and non-invasive investigation. Large, labelled datasets have facilitated extensive AI research in this area [50]. ECG machines often already incorporate non-AI algorithms for ECG analysis; however, AI-based algorithms appear to be more accurate in identifying abnormal ECGs [51]. Smith et al. compared an algorithm using a deep neural network (DNN) to a currently used algorithm for 12-lead ECG analysis [51]. The DNN was trained on approximately 130,000 ECGs that had been annotated by expert interpreters. The DNN contained over 20 million parameters and 1.6 million neurons. The accuracy of the DNN for finding a major abnormality on the ECG was 92.2%, and the accuracy of the currently used algorithm was 87.2% with comparable sensitivity and improved specificity. The DNN also had a significantly higher rate of accurate ECG interpretation (72.0% vs 59.8%) [51].

AI has been applied to ECG analysis to identify lead misplacements and identify a range of pathologies, including left ventricular hypertrophy and hypertrophic cardiomyopathy [52–54]. AI algorithms have demonstrated the ability to successfully detect myocardial ischaemia, localize the culprit lesion, and predict which patients require urgent revascularization [55–58]. In addition, AI algorithms have identified novel ECG features that improve detection of non-ST-elevation myocardial infarction (NSTEMI) [56].

AI algorithms have at times outperformed clinicians in recognizing pathology and can also identify features that are usually considered difficult or impossible to identify on ECG, such as age and sex, mitral regurgitation, aortic stenosis, left ventricular mass, pulmonary hypertension, or left ventricular dysfunction [59–65]. AI has been applied to the ECG to predict cardiac arrest and unexpected intensive care unit (ICU) admission [66]. AI models can accurately estimate serum electrolytes and identify disturbances of potassium, sodium, and calcium based on ECG [67–69]. Increasingly, AI-based ECG algorithms can explain their decisions, or at least highlight sections of the ECG that are most influencing their conclusions [70,71].

12.7 Imaging

12.7.1 X-Ray

Medical imaging interpretation has become a significant focus of AI research, given the success of computer vision algorithms and the abundance of labelled imaging data. Integrating AI into radiology workflows could allow radiologists to supply earlier reports of critical images to emergency physicians or augment the emergency physicians' own interpretation of images [72–74].

AI can now accurately detect important abnormalities on chest X-rays such as pneumothorax, pleural effusion, consolidation, and pneumoperitoneum [72]. Kao et al. developed and deployed an AI-based automated radiology alert system for the detection of pneumothorax on chest X-rays [75]. The AI-based system was run in parallel with their manual (radiological technologists–led) alert system to assess diagnostic accuracy. The AI-based system reduced the mean emergency physician alert time from 8.45 minutes to 0.69 minutes [75]. The AI system had a higher sensitivity (0.837 vs 0.256) but a worse positive predictive value (0.686 vs 1.000) than the manual system [75]. AI may also be applied in novel ways, such as classifying cardioembolic stroke and non-cardioembolic stroke based on chest X-rays [76].

Fractures are occasionally missed by emergency physicians, presenting an opportunity for AI. AI-based systems can accurately detect and highlight fractures on a variety of X-rays with an accuracy comparable to radiologists or orthopaedic specialists [73, 77–80]. The addition of AI to detect fractures can improve emergency physician diagnostic accuracy without decreasing reading speed [80,81].

12.7.2 Computed Tomography

AI can accurately identify pathology on computed tomography (CT) of the head, including intracranial haemorrhage [82]. Arbabshirani et al. used AI to analyse CTs of the head and then reprioritize 'routine' head CT studies as 'stat' on real-time radiology worklists if the AI algorithm detected intracranial haemorrhage. This was prospectively implemented for three months. During this implementation, the median time to diagnosis was significantly reduced from 512 minutes to 19 minutes, and 94 of the 347 'routine' studies were reprioritized to 'stat', with 60 of these 94 having intracranial haemorrhage identified by the radiologist [82].

AI-based algorithms are also able to identify pulmonary embolism (PE) on a CT pulmonary angiogram (CTPA) [83]. Schmuelling et al. implemented an AI-based PE detection algorithm [84]. They found that while the AI algorithm performed well, it did not result in an improvement in clinical performance measures such as reduced time to anticoagulation and patient turnaround times in the ED [84]. Deep learning–based reconstruction of CTPA images achieved greater image quality with thinner slices and lower radiation dosing when compared to alternative reconstruction techniques [85].

12.7.3 Ultrasound

Point-of-care ultrasound is increasingly used by emergency physicians to answer clinically relevant questions. AI-based techniques are helping to overcome hardware limitations and enhance the image quality obtained by less expensive handheld probes. Focused cardiac ultrasound is becoming a standard of care and may be enhanced through applications of AI [86]. Asch et al. used over 50,000 echocardiographic studies to train a machine learning algorithm to automatically estimate left ventricular ejection fraction (LVEF) [87]. Their algorithm did not require image segmentation and instead 'mimics a human expert's eye'. Though only tested on 99 patients, they showed that automated estimation of LVEF was feasible and accurate, achieving a sensitivity of 0.90 and specificity of 0.92 for a detection of ejection fraction of less than 35%. AI-enabled ultrasound devices are also able to guide cardiac image acquisition and identify common user errors such as foreshortening [86–89]. AI algorithms have shown good agreement with experts in visually estimating inferior vena cava collapsibility [90]. Additionally, AI can accurately identify vessels, bones, tendons, and nerves on upper-limb ultrasound and label them with bounding boxes [91]. AI algorithms can also enhance the needle tip and predict the needle path to assist with ultrasound-guided intravenous access [92].

12.8 Patient Assessment and Outcome Prediction

12.8.1 Sepsis

Making predictions based on limited and imperfect information is a core part of both emergency medicine and AI. The majority of AI research in emergency medicine focuses on prediction [93]. Outcomes in sepsis are improved by early detection and treatment. However, the onset can be insidious, making detection challenging.

AI models have been able to use clinical and laboratory data to predict sepsis onset ahead of time, or identify sepsis, and have outperformed both clinicians and currently used risk stratification scores in predicting sepsis-related morbidity and mortality in adults and children [17,20,28,94–106]. Recently, sepsis-detection AI models have become more interpretable. Zhang et al. have developed an ED sepsis prediction algorithm that can show the contribution of individual medical events to the final prediction [107].

AI-based sepsis alerts have been implemented in hospital wards and ICUs, with mixed results. AI-based alerts may not change management decisions and often occur after clinical interventions (such as starting antibiotics) have already been initiated [108–110]. Despite this, others have reported improved patient-orientated outcomes, including mortality and length of stay, following the implementation of AI-based sepsis alerts [106–111].

Chen et al. developed and implemented a real-time interactive AI-based model to predict sepsis and other adverse outcomes in adult ED patients with pneumonia [94]. The AI based model outperformed current risk-stratification tools, with a lower risk of sepsis in the group who used the AI-based prediction model than those who did not [94]. However, only 12.3% of the clinicians used the AI-based prediction when available [94].

12.8.2 Chest Pain

Chest pain is a common ED presentation, and clinicians and researchers have been interested in applying AI to chest pain since the early 1990s [112]. Distinguishing potentially life-threatening causes of chest pain from the benign can be challenging, so risk stratification is important. AI-based techniques that are integrated into health information systems have demonstrated that they can outperform conventional scoring tools at risk-stratifying patients into high-risk and low-risk chest pain, diagnosing acute coronary syndrome, predicting major adverse cardiovascular events, and predicting mortality [113–116]. However, Hollander et al. remind us that AI-based techniques may be rejected by emergency physicians if the results are not timely and do not change patient management [117]. Despite implementing an AI model that had previously achieved high accuracy in the diagnosis of acute myocardial infarction into practice, this was shown to change the emergency physician disposition decision in less than 1% of cases during the real-time use of the model in the implementation period [117]. Despite 70% of emergency physicians believing the model to be accurate in a follow-up survey, less than 10% of physicians stated that they used the model in their decision-making, as the AI-generated data were presented too late, or the results 'confirmed clinical suspicion but did not alter it' [117].

12.9 Departmental Management

AI may assist the emergency physician in dealing with the complex and competing demands of managing a busy ED. AI based models have been used to forecast future ED demand [118]. Such models can integrate multiple data sources for example, weather data and calendar data, to improve the accuracy of their performance [119].

By predicting the likelihood of ED re-presentation or hospital readmission, AI models may identify patients who are at a high risk of repeat presentation following discharge from the ED or hospital [120–123]. Accurate early identification of these patients would allow for interventions that may avoid readmission and also reduce demand on EDs.

Emergency medicine physicians experience a high rate of burnout [124]. Preliminary work has suggested that on-shift physiological monitoring of emergency physicians through wearable sensors may be able to detect stress, potentially allowing earlier intervention [125].

AI-based techniques have also demonstrated an ability to automatically determine patients' eligibility for clinical trial enrolment, and in doing so reduce screening time [126].

12.10 Public Health: Opioid Overdose and Disease Outbreaks

As an important interface between the health system and the public, the ED is where important public health data are collected. AI-based systems that use ED data to monitor Australian state-wide self-harm presentations and assist with suicide-prevention efforts are currently being planned [127]. By combining data from the ED with multiple other sources, AI may also be able to automatically identify high-level emerging patterns in illicit drug use [128]. AI models have also been used to predict risk of opioid overdose and the identification of low-risk subgroups that have minimal risk of overdose [129].

Novel applications of AI to social media data have been used to forecast disease outbreaks. AI algorithms were used to analyse Twitter discussions of COVID-19 among emergency physicians and found that these discussions correlated with, and may even precede increases in COVID-19-related hospital bed utilization [130].

12.11 Success in Implementing AI in the Emergency Department

Despite a large number of studies assessing AI in healthcare, only a small number of AI implementation studies have been conducted to date, and relatively few examples describing the successful implementation of AI in the ED exist [93,95,131].

General principles of successful AI implementation were reported by Liu et al., who described Chi Mei Hospital's (Taiwan) experience of developing and implementing fifteen AI systems into clinical practice [132]. They advise that AI projects should be implemented gradually and seamlessly, without increasing complexity in the care process or increasing staff workload. AI models should not be compulsory, and healthcare workers should be able to choose whether they use the AI's suggestions. Projects must deliver obvious and concrete benefits, and departmental consensus must be obtained about which projects are pursued. Finally, executive support, appropriate funding, staff training, and dedicated AI analysts were also identified as key elements to successful AI implementation [132].

Petitgand et al. examined the implementation of an AI-based decision support system in a Canadian ED, focusing specifically on the question of physician and nurse adoption [133]. They highlight the importance of considering the interconnectedness between technical, human, and organizational factors when implementing AI systems and the importance of addressing the end-users' specific assumptions and expectations about AI.

More research on AI implementation in the ED is needed, as research based on patients who are admitted to the hospital may not translate well to patients in the ED.

12.12 Challenges

Numerous technological, clinical, human, economic, legal, and ethical challenges must be overcome if AI is to be successfully integrated into patient care, but a full discussion of these is beyond the scope of this chapter [131,134–138].

12.12.1 Evidence is Still Lacking

Strong evidence demonstrating that AI improves patient care is still lacking [24,131,139]. Relatively few high-quality randomized control trials have been conducted to assess if AI implementation leads to improvements in patient-orientated outcomes [95,131,139]. Many AI studies still lack a validation phase, and there is some concern that AI research is suffering from a reproducibility crisis [24,140].

12.12.2 Potential Bias and Discrimination

A strength of AI is its ability to detect patterns that humans cannot; however, this may lead to AI discriminating against patients in unpredictable ways. For example, AI can accurately identify a patient's race from chest X-rays or ECG [141,142].

12.12.3 AI Fragility

AI may be more fragile than some people imagine; for example, changing just a single pixel in an image can lead to misclassification [143]. The performance of an AI algorithm for detecting inferior vena cava collapsibility on ultrasound deteriorated when faced with studies from novel ultrasound machines of both higher and lower image quality than the training machine [144]. Modern algorithms may not always yield better results, and AI may not outperform conventional risk-stratification techniques [145,146].

12.12.4 Physician Deskilling

Increased reliance on automated interpretations may lead to deskilling. Although Chi Mei Hospital has introduced AI medical image interpretation, it has discouraged (and even prohibited) medical interns or and resident physicians from using it for this reason [132].

12.12.5 Human Challenges

The implementation of AI algorithms into practice is influenced by complex human factors. The real-world performance of AI may not match the results reported in retrospective research papers, and there is the risk of AI-based systems being used before they are appropriately validated. AI-based tools may not change patient management, may increase staff workload, and may generate clinically meaningless alerts. This could lead to emergency physician and staff disillusionment with AI-based technology and rejection of these systems.

12.13 Future Possibilities

Grant et al. described AI in emergency medicine as having surmountable barriers and revolutionary potential [147]. Gutenstein suggested that if designed carefully, AI will allow the emergency physician to avoid the limiting factor of their own cognition and better match their performance to their intentions [148].

A likely use for AI in the near future is the enhancement of existing risk-stratification scores. For example, the qSOFA score uses a patient's mental status, respiratory rate, and blood pressure to predict mortality. Kwon et al. demonstrated that despite both using the same variables as inputs, a machine learning–based qSOFA score was superior to the conventional qSOFA score in predicting three-day mortality [97]. A more precise quantification of a patient's risk could allow for more personalized care. Hybrid risk stratification models that capture and integrate the physician's assessment with AI may become more common and lead to increased performance over either one alone [23,149]. AI algorithms are likely more able to accurately model the complex relationship between a patient's physiological, clinical, and laboratory data and use this to better predict outcomes and direct management [150].

Some examples are:

- AI models may accurately identify patients at triage who are likely to require admission or critical care.
- When integrated with existing clinical processes, AI may relieve the burden on emergency physicians through earlier and automated mobilization of appropriate resources.
- AI-based models offer to augment the capabilities of the emergency physician, such as through enhancing their radiological skills.
- Advanced monitoring that can predict deterioration ahead of time may ensure that at-risk patients are admitted faster to the ICU or to medical wards.
- Wearable monitoring devices may create a safety net for patients who are waiting to be seen or who are discharged home.

For these advantages to be realized, health systems must develop robust, repeatable, and clinically acceptable frameworks for AI implementation and monitoring. Larger and more complex AI models that can be trained and validated on patient data from different hospitals without compromising patient privacy are emerging [151]. Model explainability will likely be highlighted as an ongoing need; however, this may be reduced over time, with some research already showing that physicians are willing to trust a well-performing model even in the absence of explainability [152].

Over the coming years, there will likely be a greater emphasis on teaching AI-related skills in medical schools and emergency medicine specialist training, allowing future physicians to better understand AI technologies and their implementation [147]. There will also likely be more emphasis on the implementation of research and randomized control trials to attempt to demonstrate the benefit of AI to patients.

Emergency medicine is at times chaotic, and emergency physicians often deal with patients who are afraid and vulnerable. AI will not replace the necessary and empathetic human connection between the emergency physician and the patient. At its best, AI may permit cognitive offloading, enhance risk stratification, and improve departmental efficiency, which will allow emergency physicians more time to care for and communicate with their patients.

12.14 Chapter Limitations

The research that informed this chapter has limitations that have not been explicitly discussed. Though prospective and implementation research is slowly emerging, most studies described in this chapter are retrospective. AI research has been ongoing for decades; this chapter focuses on recent research and does not provide historical context.

KEY INSIGHTS

- **Making predictions based on limited and imperfect information is a core part of both emergency medicine and AI.**
- **Robust evidence of AI implemented into clinical practice improving patient-orientated outcomes is lacking.**
- **More research on AI implementation in the ED is needed, as research based on patients who are admitted to the hospital may not translate well to patients in the ED.**
- **In the short term, AI applications may focus on improving risk-stratification tools, improving workflows, and allowing earlier identification of unwell patients.**
- **AI is a tool, not a replacement for physicians, and at the end of the day the physician still must make the final decision.**

References

1. Chen L, Reisner AT, McKenna TM, Gribok A, Reifman J. Diagnosis of hemorrhage in a prehospital trauma population using linear and nonlinear multiparameter analysis of vital signs. *2007 29th Annual International Conference of the IEEE Engineering in Medicine and Biology Society*. Lyon: IEEE; 2007, 3748–3751. http://ieeexplore.ieee.org/document/4353147.

2. Chen L, McKenna TM, Reisner AT, Gribok A, Reifman J. Decision tool for the early diagnosis of trauma patient hypovolemia. *Journal of Biomedical Informatics* 2008;41(3):469–478.

3. Liu NT, Holcomb JB, Wade CE et al. Development and validation of a machine learning algorithm and hybrid system to predict the need for life-saving interventions in trauma patients. *Medical & Biological Engineering & Computing* 2014;52(2):193–203.

4. Nederpelt CJ, Mokhtari AK, Alser O et al. Development of a field artificial intelligence triage tool: confidence in the prediction of shock, transfusion, and definitive surgical therapy in patients with truncal gunshot wounds. *Journal of Trauma and Acute Care Surgery* 2021;90(6):1054–1060.

5. Kang D-Y, Cho K-J, Kwon O et al. Artificial intelligence algorithm to predict the need for critical care in prehospital emergency medical services. *Scandinavian Journal of Trauma, Resuscitation and Emergency Medicine* 2020;28(1):17.

6. Shirakawa T, Sonoo T, Ogura K et al. Institution-specific machine learning models for prehospital assessment to predict hospital admission: prediction model development study. *JMIR Medical Informatics* 2020;8(10):e20324.

7. Cummins RO, Ornato JP, Thies WH, Pepe PE. Improving survival from sudden cardiac arrest: the 'chain of survival' concept. A statement for health professionals from the Advanced Cardiac Life Support Subcommittee and the Emergency Cardiac Care Committee, American Heart Association. *Circulation* 1991;83(5):1832–1847.

For additional references and Further Reading please see www.wiley.com/go/byrne/aiinclinicalmedicine.

AI in Respirology and Bronchoscopy

Kevin Deasy[1], Henri Colt[2], and Marcus Kennedy[1]

[1] *Cork University Hospital, Cork, Ireland*
[2] *University of California, Irvine, CA, USA*

13

Learning Objectives

By exploring the following topics, our goal in this chapter is to provide readers with a better understanding of research and clinical applications of AI in bronchoscopy:

- Innovative research using AI in bronchoscopy:
  - Computer-aided diagnostics in white light and autofluorescence bronchoscopy.
  - Computer-aided diagnostics in endobronchial ultrasound.
  - Machine learning in pathology.
- Current clinical applications of AI in bronchoscopy:
  - Lung nodules and bronchoscopy gene classification – AEGIS and Precepta®.
  - Automated airway segmentation.
  - Navigation bronchoscopy.
  - Robotics and augmented reality.

13.1 Introduction

Bronchoscopy entails a visual exploration of the tracheobronchial tree in order to inspect and obtain specimens from the airways, lungs, and mediastinum. The first bronchoscopes used more than 100 years ago were rigid tubes through which an optical lens rigid telescope could be passed. Such rigid bronchoscopy is still used today. Technological advances in fibreoptics, distal video chip technology, hybrid visualization processes, digitalization, and now AI have revolutionized the field, allowing physicians better access with greater accuracy and in a more minimally invasive fashion to even the most peripheral bronchial and pulmonary regions.

Because bronchoscopy operates at an interface between multiple investigative modalities, each of its facets (exploratory, diagnostic, and therapeutic) is subject to the favourable advances of new technologies. Integrated hybrid imaging, for example, is a recent breakthrough that allows proceduralists to use an array of imaging modalities that have progressed from simple fluoroscopy to endobronchial

AI in Clinical Medicine: A Practical Guide for Healthcare Professionals, First Edition. Edited by Michael F. Byrne, Nasim Parsa, Alexandra T. Greenhill, Daljeet Chahal, Omer Ahmad, and Ulas Bagci.
© 2023 John Wiley & Sons Ltd. Published 2023 by John Wiley & Sons Ltd.
Companion website: www.wiley.com/go/byrne/aiinclinicalmedicine

ultrasound and hybrid imaging with electromagnetic navigation that uses pre-procedural computed tomography (CT) scans to create a three-dimensional (3D) virtual airway map to guide inspection and catheter/probe access to peripheral lung tissues. Coupled with advances in histo-cytological diagnostics, genetics, and molecular medicine, as well as new tissue ablative technologies, the field is undergoing an exciting evolutionary flux, made even more exciting by the recent incorporation of machine learning and AI.

In this chapter, our discussion will focus on two areas: (i) current innovative AI research within bronchoscopy; and (ii) current clinical applications where AI is used to enhance accurate diagnosis and to access airway lesions and lung nodules in the peripheral lung parenchyma.

13.2 Brief Overview of AI and Machine Learning

AI, including machine learning, relies on neural networks to interpret and process defined inputs. A neural network is a combined system of hardware and software based on the operation of the human neural system. In bronchoscopic applications, a specific type of neural network called a convoluted neural network (CNN) is used for image recognition and processing of per pixel data. Powerful image processing and AI use deep learning to perform generative and descriptive tasks capable of processing images and video. In computer vision, for example, deep CNNs have become a technique of choice [1]. A particular contributor to deep learning research is the widespread development and availability of complex graphics processing units (GPUs) and GPU-computing libraries such as Cuda and OpenCL. GPUs are extremely useful at processing tasks in parallel, in part because they have a significant order of magnitude greater thread-execution capability compared to central processing units (CPUs). (GPUs have more cores – hundreds – with higher throughput and are good for processing multiple parallel tasks, able to perform thousands of operations at once. CPUs have much fewer cores – typically less than eight – and perform best in serial processing of low-latency tasks, but processing only a handful of operations at once.) GPUs have sparked a worldwide AI boom. Using currently available hardware, deep learning on GPUs is typically 10–30 times faster than on CPUs. They are a key part of modern supercomputing and are woven into the essential fabric of new hyperscale data centres. They have become essential accelerators of tasks from encryption to networking to AI.

Today's consumers experience the power of machine learning every day. They use increasingly powerful applications on smart phones, for example, to photograph objects in the real world, such as plants and insects, then use deep learning algorithms to quickly identify and classify them as if by magic. Many applications not possible only years ago now leverage AI and advanced camera technology to perform complex real-time analysis and object recognition. Augmented reality software incorporates machine learning, using the camera to overlay and interpret planes in the environment in real time and as part of simple measurement tools. In bronchoscopy, using similar technologies, software can combine this with real-time 3D overlays of anatomical structures automatically interpreted by software that is pre-trained by machine learning. Continued training allows these tools to further process depth perception and build dynamic overlays of geometry in order to interpret airway findings, such as anatomy and airway lesions, without the need for pre-procedural imaging.

13.3 Innovative Research Using AI in Bronchoscopy

13.3.1 Computer-Aided Diagnostics in White Light and Autofluorescence Bronchoscopy

Medical imaging research has exploded exponentially in the last seven years [1]. Prior to 2014, we found fewer than a dozen publications in the field. In 2020, the number of articles for that year alone rose to 2495, and by November 2021 we identified a further 2315 using a PubMed search using the terms 'medical imaging', 'deep learning' and 'neural networks', 1999–2021. Most articles pertain to radiological imaging and segmentation, but there are substantial developments in object detection classification.

One area of focus is the development of augmented imaging with real-time projection of highlighted anatomy or abnormal lesions. Matava et al. developed and evaluated a CNN (Figure 13.1) capable of identifying and classifying airway anatomy in real time [2]. They use a clinical dataset of 775 laryngoscopy and bronchoscopy videos to train and test three CNNs to identify vocal cords and tracheal rings. Their best results used the ResNet and Inception CNNs; after transfer learning, they achieved a specificity of 98.5% and 97%, with sensitivities of 86.5% and 89.2%, respectively. They were able to process live video feeds at 5 frames per second (fps) with

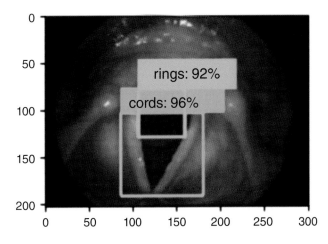

Figure 13.1: Vocal cords (green bounding box) and tracheal rings (blue bounding box) and their respective confidence levels.

Source: Matava et al. (2020) Springer Nature.

ResNet and 10 fps with Inception. The practical usability of these techniques could extend to real-time airway inspections with overlaid anatomy labelled for the bronchoscopist. It might also be able to automatically highlight and suggest abnormalities based on real-time image interpretation of abnormal airway lesions.

Other research is addressing disease processes. For instance, lung cancer begins when abnormal lesions develop in healthy bronchial epithelium. These abnormal lesions have dysplastic potential to evolve into carcinomas or can presuppose the presence of more distal tumours. Investigations that can detect early bronchial lesions may be helpful for screening patients, particularly when coupled with the search for biomarkers signalling lung cancer risk (see the discussion of AEGIS and Precepta later in the chapter). Using autofluorescence bronchoscopy (AFB) in conjunction with conventional white light bronchoscopy (WLB), investigators were able to double the detection rate of dysplasia and carcinoma-in-situ [3]. AFB highlights differences between normal bronchial mucosa and that of developing lesions. Some studies show that AFB has higher sensitivity than WLB for suspicious lesions [4]. However, the rate of false positives is high, often due to unintended contact between the bronchoscope and the airway during coughing (for this reason, many suggest performing procedures under general anaesthesia). Coupled with the requirement to scan and interpret images from the entire airway, this procedure is now used regularly in only a few centres [5]. Patient selection is a confounding factor, and it is noteworthy that, to date, no bronchoscopic modality has demonstrated added benefit to conventional lung cancer screening programs.

Experts agree that the identification and interpretation of endobronchial lesions discovered during bronchoscopy are operator dependent and tied to experience and knowledge, both of which have significant inter-operator variability. CNNs were proposed to enhance computer-aided diagnosis (CADx) using both white light and autofluorescence bronchoscopy. Feng et al. described the use of machine learning to aid in CADx of WLB images for lung cancer [6]. The hypothesis was that CADx might provide adequate accuracy through quantitative textural analysis of bronchoscopic imaging before a pathological diagnosis. This would help physicians make treatment decisions in severely symptomatic patients. The researchers used image composition transformation from the RGB (red, green, blue) colour space to the HSV (hue, saturation, value) colour space. They examined images from 34 patients with WLB images of confirmed tumours, and derived 13 grey-level co-occurrence matrix textural features from each of the three individual channels, allowing 42 textural features of the white light image to be evaluated. They tested whether this could distinguish malignant types. Their CADx system achieved an accuracy of 86% for differentiating tumours. Previous research was comparable in the RGB colour space, and achieved an accuracy of 80% for differentiating normal bronchial mucosa from bronchitis or airway tumours [7]. These results suggest that CADx can help differentiate lung cancer subtypes using bronchoscopic images and rapidly provide precise information for clinicians before final pathological results become available. Whether these technological advances will improve bronchoscopic detection of cancer and ultimately patient outcomes requires investigation.

There has also been research to harness machine learning for AFB. Chang et al. proposed an automatic AFB analysis approach to analyse an entire video stream of data [8]. The authors used computer-based image analysis, machine learning, and deep learning to detect informative AFB video frames in a video stream in three stages: video processing, frame classification, and lesion analysis. A combination of trained support vector machines (SVMs) and CNNs was used to interpret datasets and analyse informative frames. Using pre-trained algorithms, investigators successfully identified 99.5% of the informative data in the video, with more than 97% of lesion frames correctly identified. The combined false-positive/false-negative rate was less than 3%. These results demonstrate that deep learning can complement AFB to improve diagnostic capacity.

13.3.2 Computed-Aided Diagnostics in Endobronchial Ultrasound

Endobronchial ultrasound (EBUS), including radial and linear ultrasound, is an effective and efficient, minimally invasive procedure used to diagnose lung cancer, infections, and other diseases causing enlarged lymph nodes in the chest. Despite initial resistance from both medical and surgical specialties, and a reluctance by many hospital administrators to invest in EBUS systems, its current acceptance and widespread applicability make EBUS a paradigm for successfully introducing innovative technologies in chest medicine [9].

Initially, EBUS involved the interpretation of images from an ultrasound probe passed through the working channel of a bronchoscope. Around 2007, the first linear array convex probe scopes (CP-EBUS) were developed. CP-EBUS provides a view that is parallel to the shaft of the bronchoscope; the angle of view is 90° and the direction of view is 35° forward oblique. Radial probe EBUS (RP-EBUS) provides high-definition, 360° images of the airway wall and surrounding structures. The major advantage of CP-EBUS over RP-EBUS is the ability to guide real-time sampling using needle aspiration. By incorporating the ultrasound probe at the tip of the bronchoscope, real-time imaging became possible for guiding biopsy of mediastinal nodes and peri-bronchial masses. Numerous meta-analyses confirmed that EBUS-guided transbronchial needle aspiration (EBUS-TBNA) has high sensitivity and specificity for lung cancer [10–12], and EBUS-TBNA has become standard of care, even if not always standard of practice, as part of lung cancer staging and diagnosis. CP-EBUS is perhaps the most important advancement in bronchoscopy in the last 15 years.

EBUS has the potential for further development by leveraging machine learning to interpret findings. Starting with RP-EBUS for the interpretation of peripheral lung masses, Chen et al. described the use of a hybrid neural network combining CNN and SVM [13]. They used data augmentation to expand the size of training data, then utilized the CNN CaffeNet for feature extraction, before employing an SVM classifier to distinguish benign from malignant lesions. Transfer learning was applied to fine-tune CaffeNet (Figure 13.2), which allowed their CNN to become

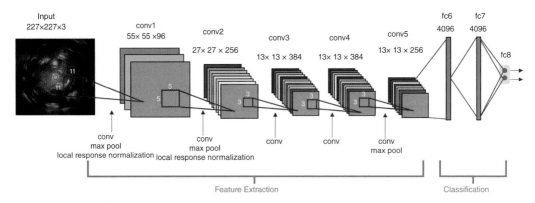

Figure 13.2: Structure of CaffeNet showing radial probe endobronchial ultrasound (RP-EBUS) input.

Source: Chen, Chia-Hung et al. (2019) / with permission of Elsevier.

more data specific, thus achieving reasonable accuracy with their system: differentiating 164 cases (56 benign and 108 malignant lesions) with 85.4% accuracy. This deep learning algorithm outperformed conventional texture-based methods.

Research using CP-EBUS showed that strain elastography, a recently available technique used for tissue characterization, can help differentiate and diagnose intrathoracic benign and malignant lymph nodes (LNs) by reflecting the relative stiffness of tissues [14]. Elastography allows the interpretation of ultrasound to assess the relative stiffness of tissues. Imaging is non-invasive and can be viewed as a colour map, or measured as a shear wave velocity. The operator exerts repeated, slight pressure on the probe while examining the lesions. Elastography can then quantify the elasticity of the tissues by measuring their deformation, and present it in various forms of colour. Evidence demonstrates the value of strain elastography in differentiating benign from malignant LNs. The endoscopist can select and target LNs and possible metastatic sites within the LN for biopsy according to strain elastography during EBUS-TBNA. In one study, Zhi et al. used machine learning to accurately select images from a video stream of EBUS strain elastography [15]. Their algorithm for automatic image selection (Figure 13.3) shows the capability of machine learning to help select stable and high-quality representative images from EBUS strain elastography videos. Accuracy of this machine learning algorithm was 78.02–83.52%, compared with 80.22–82.42% for an expert group. While there is the potential to diagnose intrathoracic lymphadenopathy, more work is needed, including how to use deep learning to process and categorize LNs based on their strain morphology.

13.3.3 Machine Learning in Pathology

Airway samples, including cytological aspirates from EBUS-TBNA, must be assessed by trained cytologists to confirm specimen adequacy and content. Results typically take days to process and report. Rapid onsite evaluation (ROSE) is performed in some institutions, allowing for real-time cytological assessment. However, this

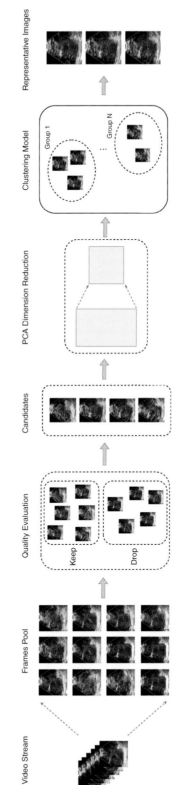

Figure 13.3: Automatic representative images selection model for strain elastography videos.

Source: Zhi, Xinxin et al. 2021 / Frontiers Media SA / CC BY-4.0.

requires some technical coordination onsite, which is not feasible in many institutions. The development of machine learning techniques is ongoing to automatically assess cytology samples in real time. AI has, of course, been used for the microscopic examination of histo-cytopathology images, with PAPNET for cervical cancer being the most well-known screening application. A solution for real-time interpretation of cytology would help EBUS-TBNA operators optimize sampling to increase the diagnostic yield of the initial EBUS procedure, help avoid repetitive invasive procedures, and reduce time to diagnosis and staging of lung cancer.

AI has had remarkable success in medical image analysis owing to the rapid progress of deep learning algorithms. Multiple researchers have promising results using AI to analyse lung cancer cytology [16–18]. Teramoto et al. developed a deep convolutional neural network (DCNN) to examine cytology of lung cancer and to differentiate cytology (Figure 13.4) into adenocarcinoma, squamous cell carcinoma, or small cell carcinoma [16]. Using their pre-trained DCNN, 70% of lung cancer cells were classified correctly and had 85.6% accuracy when differentiating small cell from non-small cell lung cancer. Further work by Teramoto et al. showed that they could use AI to distinguish between malignant and benign cytology with an

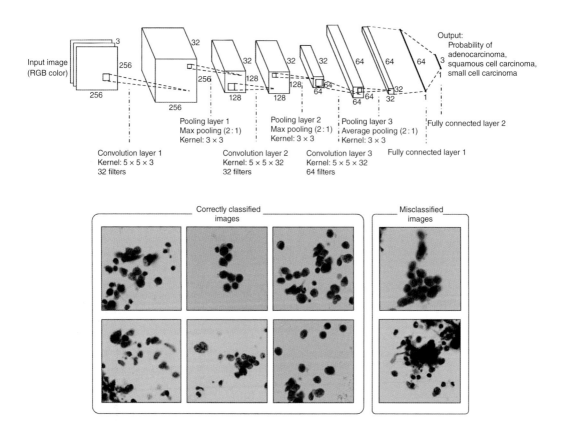

Figure 13.4: Automated classification of lung cancer types from cytological images using deep convolutional neural networks.

Source: Teramoto et al. 2017 / Hindawi / CC BY-4.0.

accuracy of 85.3% by combining DCNN with a progressive generative adversarial network [17]. Asfahan et al. specifically developed a proof-of-concept study to show the application of AI in the bronchoscopy suite for EBUS-TBNA. They used a CNN to classify images of EBUS-TBNA smears in the bronchoscopy suite and looked at 441 cytology images. Their goal was to classify any cytology images showing either adequate lymphocytes (>40 per high-powered field), granuloma, or malignant cytology. The overall accuracy of their model was 92.4%. More importantly, their model had a sensitivity of 96.1% and a specificity of 93.3% in differentiating adequate from inadequate smears. Results from these studies highlight how CNNs can be used for cytodiagnosis, and demonstrate their potential to serve as adjuncts for procedures such as EBUS-TBNA when ROSE is not available.

13.4 Current Clinical Applications of AI in Bronchoscopy

13.4.1 Lung Nodules and Bronchoscopy Gene Classification – AEGIS and Precepta

Bronchoscopy for lung nodules, although safe, is hampered by a sensitivity that significantly varies depending on the location and size of the lesion of concern. Patients with non-diagnostic bronchoscopy present a challenge for clinicians because decisions must be made regarding management and referrals for additional invasive procedures. One goal of lung nodule management, therefore, is to make an early accurate diagnosis of malignant nodules while decreasing the need for invasive procedures to diagnose benign nodules. Overall, however, the diagnostic yield of bronchoscopy ranges from 5% to 76% (median 31%), depending on the location and size of the lesion [19]. Findings from the Airway Epithelial Gene Expression in the Diagnosis of Lung Cancer AEGIS-1 and AEGIS-2, two multicentre prospective sub-studies enrolling current or former smokers undergoing bronchoscopy for suspected lung cancer, showed that a negative classifier score in patients with an intermediate (10–60%) pre-test probability of lung cancer and a non-diagnostic bronchoscopy result decreased the post-test probability of lung cancer to less than 9%, supporting a more conservative diagnostic approach [20].

Machine learning enabled the AEGIS trials to develop and validate the Percepta® Genomic Sequencing Classifier (GSC; Veracyte, San Francisco, CA, USA). The classifier leveraged a 'field of injury' concept to identify genomic changes associated with lung cancer in either current or former smokers. The supposition is that patients in this cohort with lung cancer have changes in gene expression throughout their airways. These changes occur as a result of direct endobronchial and genetic damage due to smoke exposure, raising the risk of lung cancer. Percepta GSC is an ensemble of machine learning models (Figure 13.5; elastic net logistic regression, support vector machine, and hierarchical logistic regression), which combine genomic and clinical features, as well as their interactions, to achieve high negative and positive

(a)   (b)

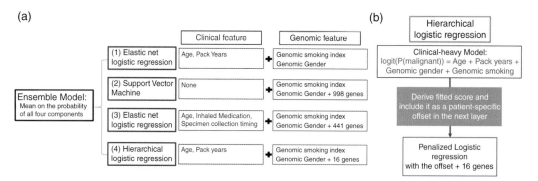

Figure 13.5: Genomic sequencing classifier structure showing (a) overall structure of the Ensemble model and (b) detailed structure of the hierarchical logistic regression component. *Source:* Choi Y et al. 2020 / Springer Nature / CC BY-4.0.

predictive values for risk classification of indeterminate lung nodules. The system was trained on more than 1600 samples from four different independent cohorts. It utilizes whole-transcriptome mRNA sequencing of transcripts from 1232 genes from bronchial brushings to reclassify the pre-test risk of malignancy to either a higher- or lower-risk profile in lung nodules of current or former smokers. The GSC works to inform decision-making in patients, particularly those with intermediate pre-test probability of lung cancer. In this cohort, it down-classified the risk of primary lung cancer to low with a 91% negative predictive value (NPV) to help avoid additional invasive procedures, or alternatively up-classified the risk to high with a 65% positive predictive value (PPV) to inform the next intervention steps [21]. Furthermore, the system can classify low to very low risk with an NPV of greater than 99% and high to very high risk with a 91% PPV. The clinical management decisions using GSC were evaluated, showing that down-classification of nodule malignancy risk with the GSC decreased additional invasive procedures without delaying time to diagnosis in those with lung cancer [22].

13.4.2 Navigation Bronchoscopy

In many institutions today, a patient's journey into the bronchoscopy suite begins with the physician's review of the results of pre-procedural imaging. There has been rapid progress in the world of thoracic imaging when it comes to machine learning and interpretation of diagnostic classification imaging sequences. This is particularly useful for lung nodule analysis and characterization of radiological diagnoses such as in interstitial lung diseases. While these topics are outside the remit of this chapter, a comment about the processing of thoracic cross-sectional imaging is warranted because of increased use of what has become known as 'navigation bronchoscopy', the use of technology to help the bronchoscopist accurately navigate the complex branching structure of the lower airways. This technology lends itself well to deep machine learning.

13.4.3 Automated Airway Segmentation

Airway segmentation is the generation of a 3D airway model representing the airways of a lung from CT imaging. Traditional airway-segmentation techniques use threshold intensities to identify and map the lumen of an airway based on its typical appearance on a CT. This relies on the different attenuation of an airway from the bronchial wall and lung parenchyma. However, as the distal airways propagate a combination of the resolution of CT imaging, volume effects and movement artifacts affect airway segmentation. This results in 'leaks', which consequently lead to missed small airways or distorted architectural results on the 3D model. Anyone with interests in airway segmentation can begin with free open-source software such as CustusX [23] or 3DSlicer [24] with their airway-segmenting application programming interface (API).

Creating a gold standard airway-segmentation system using proprietary software with algorithms incorporating tubular structure detection still requires expert manual augmentation of the semi-automatic output. This usually requires 1–2 hours per segmentation [25]. AI can be used to enhance the accurate detection of patient anatomy, and the implementation of deep machine learning through CNNs is the current basis for identifying small airways in the peripheral lung and surrounding anatomy. This has allowed the progressive development and training of CNNs to establish more accurate segmentation techniques (Figure 13.6), with remarkable progress in the precision and accuracy of airway segmentation and navigational bronchoscopy. However, a major limitation common to all guided virtual bronchoscopy is the inherent use of cross-sectional CT imaging performed sometimes weeks to months in advance of the procedure. (Virtual bronchoscopy is a computer-generated 3D rendering using CT imaging to produce an interactive viewport of the tracheobronchial tree and endobronchial views that simulate the findings at conventional bronchoscopy.) Additionally, CT images performed during the planning phase for virtual navigation bronchoscopy are acquired in a fully awake patient at maximal inspiration. Changes in anatomy are therefore inevitable in the bronchoscopy suite when the patient is either sedated or ventilated. This is called CT-to-body divergence and is critical to understanding that virtual targets may not be in the same location as real lesions.

(a)   (b)   (c)   (d)

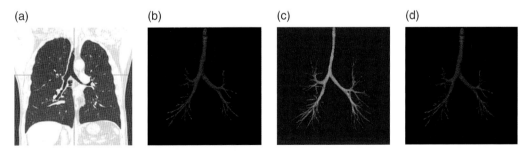

Figure 13.6: Optimized deep-airway segmentation. (a) A thoracic computed tomography scan. (b) Initial airway. (c) Result of 2.5D convoluted neural network. (d) Result of manual segmentation.

Source: Yun et al. 2019 / ELSEVIER.

13.4.4 Robotics and Augmented Reality

Some proprietary software overcomes this divergence. Machine learning helps to further fuse navigation modalities and allows continuous tracking of the broncho-scope in positions relative to actual anatomy. This is especially true with robotic bronchoscopy. Examples of robotic systems with advanced capabilities include the MONARCH® Platform from Auris Health (Redwood City, CA, USA; Figure 13.7) and Ion™ from Intuitive (Sunnyvale, CA, USA; Figure 13.8). The MONARCH Platform combines three distinct navigation modalities (electromagnetics, optical pattern recognition, and robotic kinetic data) that enable it to localize the broncho-scope during the procedure and provide the bronchoscopist with accurate positional feedback. Intuitive (best known for da Vinci™) has developed Ion, a robotic-assisted bronchoscopy system. Its PlanPoint™ software incorporates machine learning tech-nology to optimize the segmentation of complex airway anatomy, followed by precise planning of the endoscopic procedure using proprietary robotic bronchoscopy tech-nology. The display console is designed to allow views of multiple modalities including RP-EBUS, fluoroscopy, and live endoscopy on a single display.

LungVision™ from Body Vision Medical (Campbell, CA, USA; Figure 13.9) is a standalone platform built using AI-driven tomography to deliver augmented fluo-roscopy. This system incorporates next-generation augmented reality made possible by deep learning. It is Food and Drug Administration (FDA) approved for use in the USA and applies machine learning to allow real-time visualization of targeted nodules or soft tissue lesions using a standard C-arm during bronchoscopy.

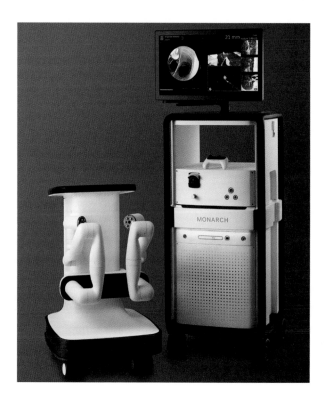

Figure 13.7: MONARCH® Platform. ©2021 Auris Health.

Source: http://www.aurishealth.com/monarch-platform.

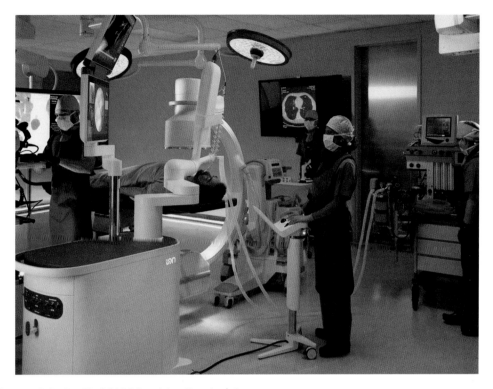

Figure 13.8: Ion™. ©2021 Intuitive Surgical, Inc.

Source: http://www.intuitive.com/en-us/products-and-services/ion.

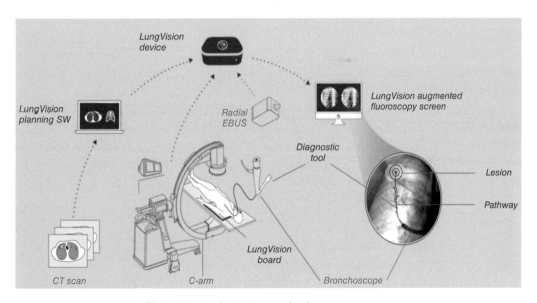

Figure 13.9: LungVision™. ©2021 Body Vision Medical.

Source: Hogarth D. Kyle 2018 / Future Medicine Ltd.

Dynamic registration overcomes CT-to-body divergence and accurately identifies a lesion's location by fusing intraprocedural fluoroscopy with a real-time tomographic reconstruction from standard fluoroscopy. This is termed C-arm–based tomography (CABT). CABT compensates for respiratory motion and airway distortion caused by accessory biopsy instruments. In a 200-patient prospective multicentre study of the LungVision augmented fluoroscopy system, the diagnostic yield was 78% [26]. Yields range from 75% to 87.4% in other, smaller studies [27–29]. The benefit of LungVision is its ability to use basic fluoroscopy imaging augmented by machine learning not only to visualize nodules, which are augmented and highlighted, but also to visualize the bronchoscope and biopsy tools navigating to the nodule location. The goal is to facilitate greater confidence and accurate tissue sampling at a lower cost than electromagnetic navigation bronchoscopy (ENB) or robotic bronchoscopy platforms.

13.5　Final Word

The goal of some forward-thinking bronchoscopists is to fuse augmented reality with traditional bronchoscopy or robotic-assisted procedures using AI to provide dynamic intraprocedural recognition of airways and target lesions. In our opinion, an ideal product would include an integrated approach to robotic bronchoscopy and augmented hybrid imaging modalities. While we do not favour or endorse any particular technology, we believe that one step in this direction is provided by Body Vision.

Applications and future innovation will inevitably include endobronchial optical imaging detection and tracking, allowing anatomy and airway abnormalities to be highlighted and categorised dynamically in real time. Clearly, promising work is already taking place for several applications, and the next piece of the puzzle lies in the area of diagnostics that incorporate automatic interpretation of cytology or pathology specimens in real time. Genomic diagnostics, such as Percepta, already help stratify risks in patient cohorts. We can only hope that, with more knowledge and the implementation of results from gene research, these diagnostic tools will become increasingly accurate as larger datasets for training future deep learning. The paradigmatic shift to incorporate technologies that use AI and deep learning modalities into daily practice is sure to occur as more practitioners gain access to more powerful processors that drive more complex calculations and use new advances in affordable computational power. Exciting times are ahead.

KEY INSIGHTS

■ **AI research innovations such as CADx to differentiate lung cancer subtypes and the use of deep learning to complement autofluorescence bronchoscopy are promising, but require further investigation as to whether they will improve bronchoscopic detection of cancer and ultimately patient outcomes.**

- **Research is underway to enhance EBUS with machine learning, deep learning, and CNNs to allow faster and more accurate diagnosis.**
- **Machine learning has enabled a GSC to inform decision-making in patients at risk for lung cancer by decreasing additional invasive procedures without delaying time to diagnosis in those with lung cancer.**
- **Other areas of innovation in bronchoscopy include automated airway segmentation, navigation bronchoscopy, robotics, and augmented reality.**

References

1. Litjens G, Kooi T, Bejnordi BE et al. A survey on deep learning in medical image analysis. *Medical Image Analysis* 2017;42:60–88.
2. Matava C, Pankiv E, Raisbeck S, Caldeira M, Alam F. A convolutional neural network for real time classification, identification, and labelling of vocal cord and tracheal using laryngoscopy and bronchoscopy video. *Journal of Medical Systems* 2020;44(2):44.
3. Lam S, MacAulay C, Hung J et al. Detection of dysplasia and carcinoma in situ with a lung imaging fluorescence endoscope device. *Journal of Thoracic and Cardiovascular Surgery* 1993;105(6):1035–1040.
4. Chhajed PN, Shibuya K, Hoshino H et al. A comparison of video and autofluorescence bronchoscopy in patients at high risk of lung cancer. *European Respiratory Journal* 2005;25(6):951–955.
5. Liu Z, Zhang Y, Li YP et al. Clinical relevance of using autofluorescence bronchoscopy and white light bronchoscopy in different types of airway lesions. *Journal of Cancer Research and Therapeutics* 2016;12(1):69–72.
6. Feng PH, Lin YT, Lo CM. A machine learning texture model for classifying lung cancer subtypes using preliminary bronchoscopic findings. *Medical Physics* 2018;45(12):5509–5514.
7. Benz M, Rojas-Solano JR, Kage A et al. Computer-assisted diagnosis for white light bronchoscopy: first results. *Chest* 2010;138(4):433A.

For additional references and Further Reading, please see www.wiley.com/go/byrne/aiinclinicalmedicine.

14

AI in Cardiology and Cardiac Surgery

Lin Gu

RIKEN AIP, Tokyo, Japan

The University of Tokyo, Tokyo, Japan

Learning Objectives

- Understand how AI is most likely to advance the field of cardiology and cardiac surgery.
- Be familiar with the current progress of cardiac AI and how it might change this clinical area.
- Be aware of the potential risks and limitations of implementing cardiac AI into clinical medicine.
- Prepare to embrace AI-enabled tools to expand clinical abilities and deliver accurate and prompt diagnosis.

14.1 Introduction

Let us imagine the following scenario. A 40-year-old man wakes up from sleep due to a momentary episode of chest pain. After noticing the flashing heart rate variability warning on his smart watch, he takes an electrocardiogram (ECG) by placing his finger on the watch. After 30 seconds, a US Food and Drug Administration (FDA)–approved health management app detects atrial fibrillation and recommends that he see his physician. In the online appointment arranged by his smart phone, his physician, who has received the ECG and past medical history, sends him to undergo additional tests to assess his cardiac health. During the magnetic resonance imaging (MRI) exam, the voice of the system instructs him to adjust his position to ensure that his ascending aorta is in the optimal location for imaging. With multiple modality data in hand, the physician confirms AI's prediction that intervention would benefit the patient's medical outcome and prescribes a treatment that was specifically recommended for the patient by AI. After the patient watches the surgical team using augmented reality (AR) to plan and practise the procedure on the virtual heart model automatically

AI in Clinical Medicine: A Practical Guide for Healthcare Professionals, First Edition. Edited by Michael F. Byrne, Nasim Parsa, Alexandra T. Greenhill, Daljeet Chahal, Omer Ahmad, and Ulas Bagci.
© 2023 John Wiley & Sons Ltd. Published 2023 by John Wiley & Sons Ltd.
Companion website: www.wiley.com/go/byrne/aiinclinicalmedicine

reconstructed from his computed tomography (CT) scan, he experiences a reduction in his anxiety and stress. During the operation, the surgeon manipulates the AI-equipped robot to perform minimally invasive cardiac procedures. Meanwhile, the operating room AI collects all of the data to recommend the postoperative support necessary to reduce the patient's hospital readmission risk.

Half of this science fiction scenario is real, while the other half will very likely come true.

Cardiovascular disease represents the leading cause of morbidity and mortality in the world. Given the pervasive success of AI in the field of medicine, AI represents a unique opportunity to revolutionize the field of cardiology and cardiac surgery. In this chapter, we review the emerging role of AI in the fields of cardiology and cardiac surgery, and discuss the potential risks and limitations of AI in this space. It is only with a deep understanding of both advantages and risks that clinicians can confidently apply AI for the benefit of their cardiac patients.

14.2 Cardiology Imaging and Electrophysiology

14.2.1 Acquisition and Reconstruction

AI has the potential to enable automatic scanning while providing high-resolution data to allow the physician to assess both the anatomical and physiological condition of the coronary arteries. In nuclear cardiology, AI algorithms have been used to perform automatic motion correction, image reconstruction, tomographic oblique reorientation, and resultant clinical decision support. For example, Siemen's AIDAN system uses ALPHA technology and algorithms to mitigate patients' respiratory motion during positron emission tomography (PET) acquisition. Both MRI and CT include AI algorithms to attenuate motion artifacts due to cardiac and respiratory motion. The FDA has already approved several products that improve CT acquisition using deep learning models, and these will likely be the common devices in every hospital.

14.2.2 Quality Control

Automated quality control aims to standardize imaging acquisition by checking whether the acquired images meet a defined imaging standard. The measurement quality of MRI, CT, and ultrasound procedures can be variable due to differences in both acquisition devices and operating procedures. By automatically evaluating the acquired image, AI could provide the operating physician with instructions about the proper operating procedure and also feedback on imaging quality, so that the operator can decide if the acquired images meet the standard for diagnosis. Just like the example of the individual with chest pain at the beginning of this chapter, an AI quality control module could prevent the operator from missing basal and apical slices during MRI procedures. AI quality control could also assist the operator by confirming the location of the ascending or descending aorta. For ultrasound procedures, an AI-based quality control function could ensure that image quality criteria are achieved on zoom, gain, and organ coverage. In addition, it could reduce the contact between the operators and cardiac patients, thus limiting the risk of disease transmission during COVID-19 or other pandemics.

14.2.3　Cardiac Image Segmentation

Cardiac image segmentation (partitioning of the image into regions such as the left ventricle, right ventricle, and coronary arteries) provides quantitative measures like myocardial mass and wall thickness. AI will save cardiologists from the tedious manual work of delineating specific anatomical or pathological structures on CT and MRI images. AI has already achieved improvements in the MRI segmentation of the myocardium. However, the accurate segmentation of the thin walls of the right ventricle and extreme basal and apical slices is still challenging. Detailed information about the geometry and shape of these structures should be incorporated into algorithms to increase the ability to delineate more robustly these weak visible boundaries from an MRI. An alternative solution is to directly estimate the segmentation from under-sampled k-space data in an end-to-end way. This is still an open question that needs further research.

14.2.4　Cardiac Imaging and ECG Biomarkers

AI has been used to estimate anatomical and functional biomarkers from cardio-vascular imaging and ECGs, such as quantitative analysis for coronary artery diseases (CAD) and atherosclerosis. HeartFlow has received the first FDA clearance to estimate fractional flow reserve (FFR) from coronary computed tomography angiography (CCTA) in a non-invasive manner. This is a major improvement over the invasive FFR that requires a coronary catheterization. Several class II and III medical devices have also received FDA or National Medical Products Administration (NMPA, China) approval to extract FFR estimation, wall shear stress (WSS), and coronary artery scoring data from CCTA. RuiXin FFR, a NMPA class III software system, can estimate the key haemodynamic biomarkers from a CCTA non-invasively. This is an important tool for physicians to decide whether a patient needs intervention. The FAME study (Fractional Flow Reserve vs Angiography for Multivessel Evaluation) showed that FFR information eliminates a third of the lesions that might have been stented if physicians use the angiography alone, and results in better outcomes [1]. The estimated CT-FFR, WSS, and axial plaque stress (APS) measurements are shown in Figure 14.1. A multicentre prospective study demonstrated that the sensitivity, specificity, and accuracy of FFR calculated by this system are equivalent to the standard invasive wire-based FFR [2].

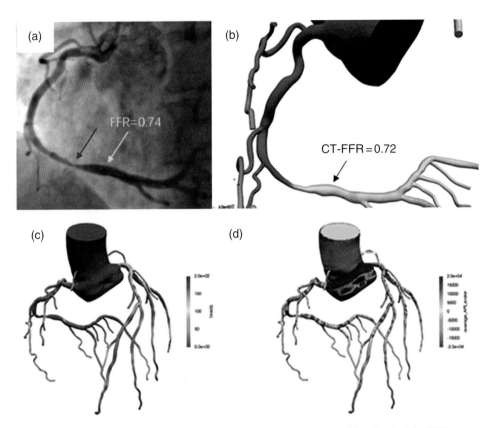

Figure 14.1: Haemodynamic biomarkers automatically estimated by the RuiXin-FFR system from coronary computed tomography angiography (CCTA). The images show a patient who suffers from coronary stenosis. (a) Coronary angiography and the measured fractional flow reserve (FFR; shown by the yellow arrow and the number 0.74) from the invasive pressure wire. The red arrow points to the stenosis (80%). (b) Non-invasive CT-FFR estimation 0.72, indicating a myocardial ischaemia. (c) Wall shear stress (WSS) estimation. High WSS shows a higher risk of plaque rupture, whereas low WSS is associated with the formation of plaques. The bar shows WSS from 0 to 50. (d) APS simulates haemodynamic stress acting on stenotic lesions. The bar ranges from 20,000 to –20,000. Image provided courtesy of RuiXin.

There are several other potential AI applications with respect to cardiac biomarker measurements:

- Currently, coronary plaques can be directly characterized using coronary artery calcium scores. AI systems could be used to calculate this score from the CCTA, which may reduce both false-positive results and inter-observer variability. Convolutional neural network (CNN) algorithms will likely directly quantify coronary artery classification and Agatston scores from CT scans.
- Additional AI biomarker applications include obtaining highly standardized quantitative parameters such as perfusion deficits, ischaemic changes, and ejection fraction changes between stress and rest conditions. For example, an FDA-approved commercial AI software, Cedars-Sinai quantitative perfusion

SPECT (QPS), could be used to obtain this information from single proton emission computed tomography (SPECT) data.

- A unique advantage of AI is its ability to extract subtle characteristics that can easily be overlooked by human eyes. AI could assist physicians, especially junior faculty, when diagnosing complex or subtle conditions that require a high level of knowledge or up-to-date expertise. For example, the QT/QTc interval must be carefully monitored to avoid the risk of pro-arrhythmia caused by dofetilide, an effective antiarrhythmic medicine. A proof-of-concept study has shown that deep learning could make a superior prediction of plasma dofetilide concentrations by assessing morphological changes on the surface ECG (beyond the QT interval), compared to the analysis of the QT interval alone.
- AI could be used with commercially available SPECT and PET image viewing software to assist physicians in identifying hypo-perfused myocardial tissue by automatically comparing images with a normal myocardial perfusion distribution.
- AI could also identify subtler spatial-temporal abnormalities in cardiac motion by tracking the time series of cardiac MRI, CT, or ultrasonography. Motion features could be estimated to predict survival and other diseases such as myocardial infarction and heart failure (HF) with preserved ejection fraction and ventricular dyssynchrony.

14.2.5 Large-Scale Population Screening

AI techniques enable the screening of ambulatory data to improve population health. Thanks to the prevalence of affordable individual devices, cost-effective population screening is now a reality. The challenge in reviewing this population-scale data lies in the level of expertise required as well as the sheer volume of data. Now with AI technologies, these data could be automatically reviewed and interpreted with reasonable accuracy and speed. The first success of this type of approach was demonstrated in a study that used an AI network to classify skin cancer [3]. This was achieved with a level of competence comparable to board-certified dermatologists. The study demonstrated that a dermatology assist app can identify skin conditions from a photo taken with a phone.

In the cardiology field, Apple collaborated with Stanford Medicine to evaluate whether its AI algorithm could detect potential arrhythmias from heart rate measurements collected by the Apple Watch. The study demonstrated that the AI-detected atrial fibrillation coincides with an ECG-confirmed one; the classification of atrial fibrillation via the watch reached a 99.3% specificity rate and 96.9% sensitivity [4]. These outcomes could result in an individual being triaged to see a cardiologist or an electrophysiologist. As a result, Apple has obtained FDA clearance for the ECG feature of its watch. Integrating ambulatory-obtained ECGs directly into the clinic, like the independent warning in the initial case scenario, is not yet possible, since there is still the risk of false-positive results. However, these techniques are rapidly evolving and show strong potential to improve population health by screening underdiagnosed conditions and stratifying the risks using these low-cost wearable devices.

14.3 Solutions for Specific Tasks

14.3.1 Cardiac Diagnostics

AI offers considerable promise in integrating large volumes of data, including multiple complementary data across modalities, to quickly provide definitive and essential diagnostic information. These diagnostic tools could effectively assist medical experts in interpreting results to a standardized high level of performance, while minimizing subjectivity as well as intra- and inter-user variation. One study involving 1501 patients reported that the XGBoost AI algorithm could deliver an overall diagnostic accuracy of 85% when classifying intermediate coronary artery lesions having an FFR of ≤0.80 [5]. Specifically, this angiography-based algorithm uses 28 features including 24 computed angiographic features extracted from angiographic lumen diameter measurements along the centreline, and four clinical features (age, sex, body surface area, and involved segment). The diagnostic performance for identifying lesions indicates the potential to reduce the need for pressure wires and the risk of procedural complications in the future.

Another study extracted three types of quantitative imaging parameters – perfusion deficits, ischemic changes, and ejection fraction changes – from stress SPECT MPI data [6]. A support vector machine (SVM) algorithm combined these three parameters and reported a more accurate diagnosis compared to using each parameter individually. When incorporating both clinical variant and total perfusion deficit (TPD) data, the SVM algorithm performance was shown to be more accurate, compared with one of two expert readers. In a multicentre (nine sites) study including 1638 patients without known CAD, AI demonstrated an advantage in automatically interpreting SPECT MPI data compared with TPD data [7]. Using raw and quantitative polar maps of MPI data, deep CNNs have shown a higher area under the curve (AUC) in predicting obstructive disease compared with TPD (per patient: 0.80 vs 0.78; per vessel: 0.76 vs 0.73: $p < 0.01$). Another study including 44,959 patients evaluated the ability of AI to identify asymptomatic left ventricular dysfunction [8]. Trained on ECG data alone, the CNN was able to recognize ventricular dysfunction for AUC, sensitivity, specificity, and accuracy of 0.93, 86.3%, 85.7%, and 85.7%, respectively.

AI allows the integration of multiple complementary data across modalities for a proper diagnosis in real time. Acute coronary syndrome is typically identified by a biomarker, ST segment, from ECGs. A timely evaluation of ECGs is critical to initiate reperfusion therapy, especially for patients suffering from an ST-elevation myocardial infarction (STEMI). However, rapid diagnosis of these patients is limited by the availability and performance of a 12-lead ECG. With an FDA-approved attachment like Kardia Mobile (AliveCor®, Mountain View, CA, USA) or ECG Check

(Cardiac Designs®, Round Rock, TX, USA), a smartphone app can reliably obtain an ECG reading and accurately predict STEMI. The accuracy of this innovation compares favourably with the gold standard 12-lead ECG [9]. Standard speakers and smart phones can help save a patient from cardiac arrest. Trained on real-world labelled 911 audio recordings of cardiac arrests, the SVM could identify agonal breathing, a typical sign of cardiac arrest, in real time. This proof-of-concept contactless system demonstrates the potential of community devices such as Amazon Echo in identifying an unwitnessed cardiac arrest for the initiation of cardiopulmonary resuscitation (CPR).

14.3.2 Risk Scoring and Prevention

Preventative intervention can dramatically minimize the risk of HF or hospitalization. Before performing an actual intervention, it is necessary to identify the risk factors and their non-linear association with the CAD risk to determine the proper intensity and cost of intervention. However, current risk scoring systems are often too cumbersome for efficient bedside use at point-of-care situations. Instead, an AI risk calculator could serve an important role by recommending less drug therapy and reducing the number of missed cases among low-risk individuals.

The American College of Cardiology/American Heart Association (ACC/AHA) pooled cohort equations risk calculator is the most common tool used to conduct cardiac risk stratification based on nine risk factors [10]. Using these same data, one SVM trained on the data from 6459 participants collected in a 13-year study outperformed the ACC/AHA risk calculator [11]. This was due, in part, to SVM's ability to utilize non-linear relations. A random forest-based machine learning algorithm was developed in one study involving 6814 participants [12]. This made use of 735 variables from multiple risk factors, including the non-traditional ones such as imaging, ECG, and serum biomarkers. This model also improved upon the established risk scores by decreasing the Brier score by 10–25%.

Using electronic health record (EHR) data, the L1-regularized logistic regression and random forest models are found to be able to accurately predict incident HF, especially imminent (<6 months) HF. AI could also prevent hospital readmissions of HF patients. Reducing readmission is associated with decreased short- and long-term mortality in certain situations. Deep learning algorithms have been reported to predict which patients will require readmission with AUCs from 0.63 to 0.71. Remote monitoring that measures pulmonary artery pressure to reduce HF hospitalization has already been evaluated [13]. Although this work is promising, a more careful study of AI-enabled hospitalization prediction and prevention methods is needed for efficacy and safety.

14.3.3 Prototypes and Precision Medicine

AI enables physicians to go beyond guideline-directed medical therapy to prescribe optimal treatments according to each patient's condition. Unsupervised clustering analysis has successfully classified chronic HF patients into several novel pheno-types that show different prognoses and responses to therapies, based on their HF preserved ejection fraction. AI can use novel and even non-traditional data such as genomic and circulating proteomic signatures as well as quantitative features from images or ECG data to help identify unique patient phenotypes, novel therapeutic targets, or predictive and prognostic biomarkers. Some potential applications include the use of a retinal fundus image to predict HF risk, even in the absence of other clinical information, or an AI-based voice analysis on a smart phone to indepen-dently characterize CAD risk factors. AI has the potential to break some accepted paradigms and open the door for several new digital biomarkers.

14.3.4 Unstructured Electronic Health Record Understanding and Generation

Existing clinical decision support (CDS) systems are constrained by the limited access to structured data within the EHR. Natural language processing (NLP) tools allow automated inputs to CDS systems, by extracting the information from unstruc-tured clinical narratives in EHRs. For example, MedTagger software (Open Health Natural Language Processing Consortium), an NLP infrastructure, has been imple-mented in the Mayo Clinic to tackle large volumes of high-complexity data. The feasibility of this system was validated on patients with peripheral artery disease (PAD). The NLP system processed the clinical narrative notes retrieved from the EHR system for automatic ascertainment of PAD. This has greater accuracy than billing code algorithms, demonstrating the potential of NLP for efficient assessment of PAD as well as improved care by CDS [14].

After a patient examination, an AI-driven system such as Syntermed Emory Toolbox could automatically generate the patient report. Already approved by the FDA, it provides natural language interpretation using over 230 rules. A study involving 1000 CAD or ischaemia patients found that there are no significant dif-ferences between the Syntermed-generated reports and the reports from nine cardiac specialists [15].

14.4 Cardiac Surgery

14.4.1 Augmented Reality and Virtual Reality

Combining virtual reality (VR) and augmented reality (AR) with AI has demon-strated value in cardiac surgery. VR/AR could assist surgeons in planning a heart intervention in a structurally immersive and intuitive environment, which would give the surgeons confidence and their patients reassurance. The EchoPixel True 3D system has received FDA approval to render individual patient anatomy into a VR format. This system can display the existing DICOM data in a life-sized VR object. SentiAR has developed an AR procedural guidance system that allows sur-geons to view, measure, and manipulate a patient's anatomy in a holographic display.

14.4.2 Robotic Surgical Systems

For targeted coronary revascularization, an AI-based system allows the intervention team to remotely monitor and control the equipment. Advantages of this approach include the reduction of ionizing radiation exposure to the cardiologist when performing an intraoperative angiography. For example, Corindus, a Siemens Healthineers company, received FDA clearance to develop its CorPath GRX platform for robotic-assisted coronary interventions. The robotic system allows the operator to navigate complex anatomies consistently and predictably with automated procedural movements. Verb Surgical integrates AI into its surgical robots to notify interventional cardiologists of potential issues during a procedure, driving more successful surgical outcomes.

14.5 Remaining Challenges

The gap between the large number of cardiac tools that are currently being developed in academic research and the relatively small number of practical AI clinical solutions is partially due to some of the stringent regulations from regulatory authorities. The lag between development and implementation is also due to data bias, training data availability, and transparency, constraints that need to be overcome. Data bias has been repeatedly reported in other fields and is described in Chapters 39 and 40. The black-box nature of deep learning further accentuates the consequences. For example, if a particular subgroup of people is less likely to be given a heart transplant for any reason, the subsequent AI analyses may incorrectly predict that this subgroup is less likely to benefit from transplant treatment, and so AI may be unlikely to recommend this lifesaving intervention in this patient population. Fortunately, cardiac disease is a field that is traditionally rich in data compared to other fields. However, until the availability of large and detailed training data, many tasks such as segmentation, which require precise annotation on the anatomical structure or pathologies, are conducted by medical experts, which is both time-consuming and expensive.

14.6 Conclusion

The innovations discussed in this chapter are just a small sample of potentials for the application of AI in cardiology and cardiac surgery. Although cardiac AI has been approved and implemented to read CCTA imaging, it is still far away from science-fiction scenarios where cardiovascular physicians, surgeons, or interventionalists would be replaced by machine learning algorithms. Instead, AI will merely assist physicians by complementing and reinforcing human intellect, experience, and activity. For example, AI may allow physicians to achieve better patient outcomes with less effort while helping them to maintain high levels of up-to-date expertise.

AI could collaborate with medical experts to expand their skills and improve the quality of care. Compared to a fully automated diagnosis tool, keeping the doctor in the loop would eventually lead to faster and more accurate patient treatments. Cardiologists and cardiac surgeons who are familiar with AI need to help drive innovation rather than passively waiting for AI-based cardiothoracic technologies to become available.

KEY INSIGHTS

- **While AI research in cardiology is progressing at a fast pace, its translation into actual clinical practice is relatively limited.**
- **AI is already changing cardiology in the areas of cardiovascular imaging and ECG.**
- **AI will take centre stage in improving population cardiac health by triaging underdiagnosed people to see their physician.**
- **The future of AI-enabled robotic surgical systems in cardiac disease is exciting.**
- **AI has the potential to open the door for new cardiac digital biomarkers.**
- **Limitations include data bias, limited training data, and lack of transparency.**

References

1. Tonino PA, De Bruyne B, Pijls NH et al. Fractional flow reserve versus angiography for guiding percutaneous coronary intervention. *New England Journal of Medicine* 2009;360(3):213–224.
2. Tang CX, Wang YN, Zhou F et al. Diagnostic performance of fractional flow reserve derived from coronary CT angiography for detection of lesion-specific ischemia: a multicenter study and meta-analysis. *European Journal of Radiology* 2019;116:90–97.
3. Esteva A, Kuprel B, Novoa RA et al. Dermatologist-level classification of skin cancer with deep neural networks. *Nature* 2017;542(7639):115–118.
4. Avram R, Ramsis M, Cristal AD et al. Validation of an algorithm for continuous monitoring of atrial fibrillation using a consumer smartwatch. *Heart Rhythm* 2021;18(9):1482–1490.
5. Cho H, Lee JG, Kang SJ et al. Angiography-based machine learning for predicting fractional flow reserve in intermediate coronary artery lesions. *Journal of the American Heart Association* 2019;8(4):e011685.
6. Arsanjani R, Xu Y, Dey D et al. Improved accuracy of myocardial perfusion SPECT for the detection of coronary artery disease using a support vector machine algorithm. *Journal of Nuclear Medicine* 2013;54(4):549–555.
7. Betancur J, Commandeur F, Motlagh M et al. Deep learning for prediction of obstructive disease from fast myocardial perfusion SPECT: a multicenter study. *JACC Cardiovascular Imaging* 2018;11(11):1654–1663.

For additional references and Further Reading, please see www.wiley.com/go/byrne/aiinclinicalmedicine.

15

AI in the Intensive Care Unit

Dipayan Chaudhuri[1,2] and Sandeep S. Kohli[3,4]

[1] *Division of Critical Care, Department of Medicine, McMaster University, Hamilton, ON, Canada*

[2] *Department of Health Research Methods, Evidence and Impact, McMaster University, Hamilton, ON, Canada*

[3] *Division of Critical Care, Department of Medicine, Oakville Trafalgar Memorial Hospital, Oakville, ON, Canada*

[4] *Department of Medicine, McMaster University, Hamilton, ON, Canada*

Learning Objectives

- Understand the AI methodology that is being used to address problems in the intensive care unit (ICU).
- Understand how clinical scoring systems could be improved using AI.
- Recognize how AI could be used to improve the management of sepsis.
- Understand how reinforcement learning could automate ICU decision-making.
- Understand how deep learning could optimize ICU resource management.
- Identify the limitations for the use of AI in the care of a critically ill patient.

15.1 Introduction

The intensive care unit (ICU) is a highly monitored and therefore data-rich environment. Intensivists, or physicians who specialize in the care of critically ill patients, face the daily challenge of making decisions based on the interpretation of constantly changing streams of data from both structured and unstructured sources. Structured data sources in the ICU include a patient's list of medical conditions, medications, serial vital sign metrics, laboratory data, fluid input/output measurements, mechanical ventilator parameters, life-support system requirements, therapeutic interventions, electrocardiography (ECG), and blood gas variables. Unstructured data include radiology reports, subjective bedside observations of clinical status, verbal conversations with family and allied caregivers, nursing notes, and a sub-specialist's notes in the medical record.

Managing this complexity of data in the ICU is not a new problem, so it is of no surprise that integrated computer systems to monitor critically ill patients were first developed in the 1970s [1]. Since then, computer programs of increasing sophistication have been deployed to assist with specific tasks in the ICU, including blood gas interpretation [2], cardiac rhythm interpretation [3], and mechanical ventilator management [4]. Despite these advances, the ICU can still be described as a 'data rich,

AI in Clinical Medicine: A Practical Guide for Healthcare Professionals, First Edition. Edited by Michael F. Byrne, Nasim Parsa, Alexandra T. Greenhill, Daljeet Chahal, Omer Ahmad, and Ulas Bagci.
© 2023 John Wiley & Sons Ltd. Published 2023 by John Wiley & Sons Ltd.
Companion website: www.wiley.com/go/byrne/aiinclinicalmedicine

information poor' (DRIP) environment, a term first used in 1982 to define organizations that did not effectively utilize the data they collect to achieve their intended outcomes [5]. Applying AI to analyse the vast amounts of data stored in an ICU's electronic medical record (EMR) could address this problem by revealing insights that improve patient outcomes and ICU resource management. This chapter will introduce our current understanding of AI in the ICU setting, including a summary of which AI methods are being used to address the most common clinical problems, and a broad overview of AI's impact on sepsis. The current limitations and future opportunities for the use of AI in the ICU will also be discussed.

15.2 AI Methodology in the ICU

Although often used interchangeably in the critical care medicine literature, the terms AI and machine learning are not the same. AI has traditionally been used to describe a technology that mimics the intelligence of a sentient being, whereas machine learning is a subtype of AI that uses computer algorithms to analyse a dataset for patterns and relationships (creating a 'model') without using conventional programming logic. The latter approach has been historically used in most ICUs to perform simple tasks, from binary logic being used to trigger alarms for heart rates that are too fast or slow, to the identification of abnormal blood gas measurements.

Machine learning can further be broken down into several subtypes. In supervised machine learning, labelled data points (composed of inputs or 'features', and related outputs or 'labels') are provided to a computer, and a model is created to identify correct and incorrect outputs using algorithms that improve their performance with increasing amounts of data; that is, they 'learn'. An example would be the use of a set of patients' symptoms, vital signs, and corresponding lab values (i.e. features) to create a model that correctly identifies a patient with sepsis (i.e. the label). Once the model can predict who has sepsis to an accepted level of performance, it would be considered 'trained'. It is then tested on previously unseen datasets to verify its ability to identify patients with sepsis.

If a model is created with unlabelled data – namely, when it is unknown whether the patient has sepsis, yet the model is still able to correctly cluster patients with sepsis from those without the condition through previously unknown relationships in the data – it is called 'unsupervised' machine learning. This is often achieved by a series of artificial neurons called a neural network, which analyse complex datasets for hidden or previously unknown relationships through processes that mimic the function of a human brain [6]. When neural networks are composed of three or more layers, they can be used to support deep learning. Deep learning will be reviewed in a later section of this chapter.

A less common subtype of AI worthy of mention because of its emerging use in ICU research is reinforcement learning. In reinforcement learning, the computer acts as an 'agent', making decisions within a defined 'state', or environment of changing variables, to optimize reward. Such a model is said to be learning, because it evaluates the performance of each step it takes by determining the impact on the overall state, allowing itself to improve via trial and error. Once a solution is defined for a given state and action, it is referred to as a policy [7]. Outside of the ICU, reinforcement learning was proven to mimic sentient-like capacity for making complex decisions in a now well-known set of experiments where a trained agent was used to play a strategy board game called Go, beating a professional human player for the first time in history [8]. 'Alpha Go' would examine the position of stones on the board at any given time and, using its learnt policy, would decide where to place the next stone to maximize its chance of winning [8]. Because an ICU patient is in a constantly changing state, and almost every action has some demonstrable impact on measurable patient outcomes (neutral, good, or bad) that can be used to further train a reinforcement learning model, this type of AI could be a powerful method for clinical decision support in the ICU of the future.

15.3 Clinical Scoring Systems

The tasks of estimating disease severity and predicting outcomes are important for benchmarking ICU quality, gauging efficacy of treatments, and stratifying an individual patient's risk to determine optimal resource allocation. Many clinical scoring systems have been developed over the years to perform these functions, and most use data collected from the first day, or few days, of ICU admission to determine severity and predict length of stay or death. However, most intensivists do not use scoring systems outside of clinical trials, as they are often too complicated to use in practice. They also tend to be derived from data of specific populations, limiting their generalizability or applicability for dissimilar cohorts of patients [9]. Lastly, they are plagued by performance inaccuracy, as every intensivist can share an anecdote of a patient fully recovering despite their clinical score predicting a 100% chance of death during their ICU stay, and vice versa.

A commonly used and well-validated tool that is mired by these limitations is the APACHE (Acute Physiology and Chronic Health Evaluation) scoring system. First described in 1981 [10], it was devised using data from American hospitals and is therefore of unproven accuracy in other patient populations. Moreover, while its latest iteration (APACHE IV) has improved performance, it relies on the measurement and input of 129 different variables [11], making it a highly complex and cumbersome score to use.

To overcome these challenges, researchers have turned to AI. Because of increasingly powerful and available processing power, and emerging access to large, curated datasets such as the open-source MIMIC (Medical Information Mart for Intensive Care) database [12], researchers now have an easier job of creating and testing models that may improve upon currently validated scoring systems. In a recently published systematic review, Syed et al. identified more than 60 publications that have used MIMIC data to derive an AI-based model, albeit most were narrow in focus as they looked solely at the prediction of sepsis, septic shock, and death [13]. Their review also revealed that the most common algorithms used to create models from this ICU database were support vector machines (SVM), random forest (RF), and a deep learning algorithm called long short-term memory (LSTM).

Interestingly, only a few authors chose to use unstructured data (nursing notes, etc.) as an input in their model [13]. This observation may highlight one of the limitations to the use of AI in the ICU setting, as many of the data relied upon on a day-to-day basis to support clinical decisions are unstructured, and building models that omit these data may limit their utility. Until methods are devised to efficiently capture and structure these data, AI-based scoring systems may prove to be no more accurate than their more traditional counterparts. As Mamdani and Slutsky point out, the solution to this problem may be to accept ICU data in their real-world, imperfect state, rather than spending significant resources to ensure they are in a more ideal state before they are used in a machine learning model [14].

Shillan et al. took a broader view in their systematic review, uncovering more than 250 papers that have used machine learning to analyse routinely collected ICU data, nearly half being published since 2015 [15]. Again, they found that SVM and RF were the most common algorithms, although neural networks (24.8%) and classification/decision trees (21.6%) were also frequently used [15]. Like Syed et al., they identified the accurate prediction of complications as the most commonly addressed use case. However, they also uncovered a significant sample size problem, as only 2% of the studies used data on more than 100,000 patients [15].

It is known that 'overfitting' tends to occur when machine learning models are built on small sample sizes, as the AI learns the training data so well that it does not perform nearly as well when applied to unseen data. The sample size issue poses yet another limitation to the application of AI in ICU, as an individual ICU will not create enough data to build a valid model, so digital infrastructure is needed to build large databases that collate data from multiple hospital ICUs. Unfortunately, this has proven to be easier said than done because of data privacy and security issues [15]. The scarcity of large ICU datasets has created another problem, as algorithms must be validated using independent data to gain acceptance by the clinical community, and only a small number of studies have done this to date [15].

If healthcare institutions do find ways to overcome the sample size issue, by sharing data for instance, the potential of AI to improve upon existing clinical scoring systems has been clearly demonstrated. In a recent study, the ICU records of more than 400 hospitals and 200,000 patients across the USA were compiled to create a collaborative research database that was used to evaluate new models for predicting length of stay and mortality [16]. Three RF models were devised, two regressors for predicting length of stay and mortality, and one classifier for predicting a binary outcome of survival or death. The outputs of these models were then compared to APACHE IV/IVa-derived predictions using the same database. The most striking finding was the very high accuracy observed for the binary classification task, which was 96% for in-hospital mortality and 99% for ICU mortality.

Although this model will need subsequent validation using an independent dataset, the ethical implications of a binary mortality classifier with extremely high fidelity are worth considering. Would an intensivist rely on this AI-based prediction to justify withholding of life-support interventions in the name of futility? What effects would this information have on patients and their family members, if offered well in advance of their predicted deterioration? Such issues need to be worked out before AI-based clinical scoring systems with extremely high accuracy are validated and deployed in real-world settings.

15.4 Improving Sepsis Recognition with AI

ICUs are high-mortality settings, and an important driver of this burden is sepsis. Prior to the COVID-19 pandemic, sepsis impacted more than 1.7 million people in the USA and was the major cause of death in US hospitals, accounting for 270,000 deaths per year. It was also the leading cause of 30-day hospital readmissions, costing more than $2 billion per year [17]. Unfortunately, sepsis can be an elusive diagnosis, as the common signs and symptoms of sepsis are often absent or overlap with other conditions. For instance, not all patients with sepsis present with a fever, and serum leucocytosis – which is often used to infer the presence of sepsis – can also be caused by non-infectious conditions. Accurate and early identification of sepsis has therefore been a focus of researchers, as goal-directed resuscitation and antibiotics have been proven to reduce mortality [18]. Several early warning systems (EWS) have been validated and deployed en masse over the last few years to perform this function using EMR data.

Yet, despite their increasing ubiquity, EWS tend to rely on clinical and laboratory parameters that develop later in the evolution of the sepsis syndrome; that is, when the initiation of treatments may no longer improve patient outcome. Several investigators have tried to address this problem using AI. By leveraging the trove of data available in a hospital's EMR, AI algorithms are being developed that are searching for hidden patterns of clinical parameters that may help identify sepsis before its clinical recognition. Interestingly, much of this work has been done outside the ICU in the emergency room (ER), where patients may first present with community-acquired infections that can evolve into sepsis.

To this end, researchers in the UK have developed a machine learning model based on logistic regression to predict the risk of sepsis using an adult patient's first set of recorded vital signs and laboratory values in the ER. Their algorithm was validated against external data from another hospital's ER, performing at a reasonable level given the reported C-statistic for severe sepsis of 0.81 [19]. Note that a C-statistic equal to 1.0 indicates that the model is perfect at classifying outcomes, whereas a value of 0.5 essentially makes the prediction equal to a coin flip. In contrast, continuous vital sign measurements in a paediatric ICU were used to devise an algorithm that could identify severe sepsis up to eight hours before the clinically deployed EMR-based EWS [20]. Also using continuous ICU data, but relying instead on the hidden information contained within the waveforms of blood pressure and ECG tracings, Mollura et al. built a model consisting of multiple decision trees (i.e. a bagged tree classifier) to identify sepsis within the first hour of ICU stay [21]. Although this model was built on MIMIC data, and requires independent and prospective validation, it is fascinating to note that laboratory parameters were not used. In an era of constrained resources, where access to laboratory data is often delayed, AI models

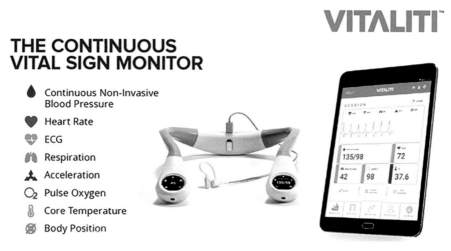

Figure 15.1: The Vitaliti™ continuous vital sign monitor and user interface. Image included with the permission of Cloud Dx Inc.

such as this one hold significant promise. With the emergence of advanced wearable technologies that can measure multiple continuous waveforms with the accuracy of bedside monitors [22], AI algorithms utilizing raw waveforms could help usher in a new era of ICU-level monitoring in almost any setting, including a patient's home (see Figure 15.1).

One limitation of the Mollura et al. study is that the analysis of physiological waveforms still represents a fundamental reliance on structured data. As Horng et al. point out, perhaps the insights held within unstructured data sources are the key to unlocking the true potential of AI [23]. To demonstrate this possibility, they sought to determine if the addition of assessments entered by clinicians as free text into the EMR could help automate the identification of infections in the ER. This investigation utilized data from more than 230,000 patients to build an SVM model that was based upon structured data for identifying infections [23]. They found that augmenting this algorithm with a bag-of-words model to classify free text significantly improved its performance, a finding that was consistent across their training, validation, and test datasets (area under the curve [AUC] of 0.86). While this work was retrospective, the potential for natural language processing (NLP) to facilitate the use of unstructured data by AI is worthy of note.

15.5 Reinforcement Learning in ICU

Emerging evidence suggests that beyond early sepsis recognition to facilitate more rapid initiation of therapy, the ongoing management of sepsis can also be improved through AI. In a fascinating experiment conducted by Komorowski et al. and reported in *Nature Medicine*, an AI agent (named the 'AI Clinician') was built using a reinforcement learning model to automate the fluid and vasopressor management of patients with sepsis [24]. To create the model, a training dataset was derived from the MIMIC-III database using patient time-series data, treatment doses, and patient outcomes. Treatment decisions were separately analysed and classified into discrete actions, and the reward of each option was quantified. The model then identified the treatments that optimized reward, or patient survival, to create the policy that would be followed by the AI.

To evaluate the performance of the AI Clinician, its policy was pitted against the performance of actual treatment decisions (i.e. the clinician's policy) using a validation dataset, again derived from the MIMIC-III database. This approach is termed 'off-policy' evaluation and is an important step to determine the safety of a reinforcement learning model before real-world deployment. Ultimately, after further evaluation against an independent dataset comprising more than 79,000 unique ICU admissions, the investigators found that their AI Clinician performed very well. What particularly stood out was that mortality was lowest when the clinician's actual treatments matched those chosen by the AI [24]. This is certainly a breakthrough finding. Not only did they demonstrate the potential for AI to automate the management of a complex medical problem like sepsis, their model also shed light on where real-world clinicians go wrong in their treatment of sepsis. That said, for the medical community to embrace an AI directing treatment, prospective evaluation in a randomized trial against usual care will be vital to give it credibility in a real-world setting.

If AI clinicians developed by reinforcement learning do eventually gain credibility through randomized control trials, it is conceivable that they could one day replace intensivists at the bedside. Before arriving at this conclusion, it is important to consider the viewpoint of Garnacho-Montero and Martin-Loeches, who recently opined that an AI will not replace physicians in the management of sepsis because septic patients are heterogeneous, and to treat them with expertise requires the formulation of an overarching clinical impression that includes a deeper knowledge of the patient's personal attributes, including their physical exam findings and medical history [25]. Although there is arguably a path where these facets of clinical evaluation will one day be digitized as data that could be used to inform an AI, that path is arduous. A more realistic view of AI's role in the future of critical care was recently articulated by Komorowski, who is in fact one of the principal investigators of the aforementioned AI Clinician experiment: 'I would argue that concerns around AI taking over the jobs of physicians can be dispelled. Awareness, multi-tasking, flexibility, and communication skills are human capabilities that no AI has achieved or seem likely to achieve anytime soon. Instead, I foresee that AI will remain in the co-pilot seat, improving our workflow and instilling more rationality into our practice' [26].

15.6 Deep Learning in ICU

Although deep learning is becoming the standard of care for improving the accuracy and efficiency of imaging tasks in radiology, its application in the specialty of critical care is still in its infancy. However, deep learning has the potential to address complex problems in the ICU that may not be solvable by conventional machine learning. Delirium is a good example. Patients who become delirious in ICU are known to have worse outcomes. Moreover, it is a poorly understood disorder that is notoriously difficult to treat [27]. Davoudi et al. hypothesized that a deep learning model, powered by a novel, low-cost monitoring platform that collected previously unattainable data on a patient's affect and emotional state, could be used to identify the environmental factors that impact delirium [28]. Their platform comprised a camera and technologies that collectively captured information on patient motion, facial expressions, ambient light, and sound levels. Figure 15.2a depicts their sensor set-up in situ, and the corresponding data collected are in Figure 15.2b.

With this novel sensor platform, the investigators conducted a small, prospective pilot study in patients with and without delirium to determine if they could detect

(a)

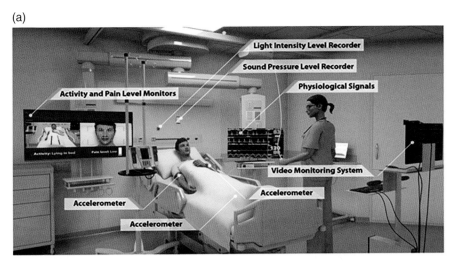

(b)

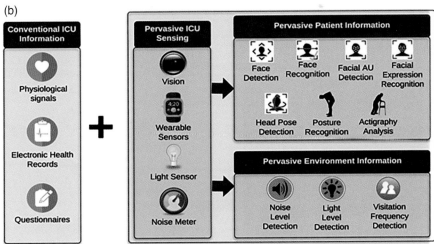

Figure 15.2: (a) The Intelligent ICU system includes wearable accelerometer sensors, video monitoring system, light sensor, and sound sensor. (b) The Intelligent ICU pervasive information is provided by performing face detection, face recognition, facial action unit detection, head pose detection, facial expression recognition, posture recognition, extremity movement analysis, sound pressure level detection, light level detection, and visitation frequency detection. Face Detection Icon, Face Recognition Icon, Facial AU Detection Icon, Facial Expression Recognition Icon, and Head Pose Detection Icon. © iStock.com/bitontawan [28].

differences in their pain, functional status, and environmental exposure. For all recruited patients, traditional clinical data were collected from the EMR. The monitoring system then collected data continuously for one week, amassing more than 50 million video frames, a portion of which were annotated with ground truth labels for patient face and posture to train the deep learning models.

Previously validated computer vision and deep learning techniques were then used for face recognition, facial expression analysis, head pose detection, and for quantifying the number of visitors in the room at any one time. The researchers also uniquely leveraged facial recognition data to localize anatomical joint and limb positions and used these estimates to develop their own convolutional neural network for detecting patient posture. Interestingly, they discovered that delirious patients were sensitive to light but not to noise. This finding certainly has implications for the management of patients with delirium in ICU, and more work is needed to understand this observation. More importantly, Davoudi et al. demonstrated that autonomous monitoring of patient behaviour and environment can be achieved using deep learning models and a simple set of low-cost sensors [28]. Although one could argue that additional sensors would offer little value to an ICU clinician, given the added data burden they represent, AI could make them very useful in the ICU of the future by automatically distilling the data into clinically impactful information.

Another enticing use case for deep learning in critical care medicine is in ICU resource management. COVID-19 placed unprecedented strain on ICUs across the world, as many exceeded their bed capacity during the pandemic. Motivated to address this problem, Chung et al. [29] developed a neural network that predicted which patients with COVID-19 would require ICU admission with a reported accuracy of 96.9%. Their work was also insightful, as they reported metrics to quantify the trustworthiness of their model, postulating that transparency would facilitate its broader adoption by the clinical community. Figure 15.3 depicts their novel approach to model design.

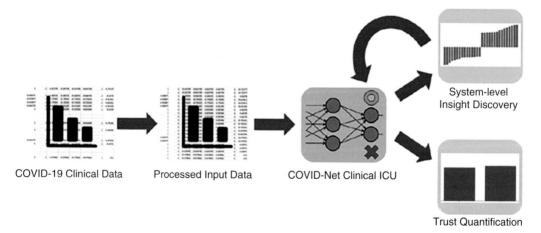

Figure 15.3: Overview of transparent, trust-centric design methodology for COVID-Net Clinical ICU [29]. Used with the permission of Dr Alexander Wong.

15.7 Limitations and Future Directions

Prior to the COVID-19 pandemic, it was estimated that more than five million patients were admitted to ICUs across the USA every year, at an annual cost of more than $100 billion [17]. Clearly, opportunities exist for AI to reduce this burden. However, among the list of Food and Drug Administration (FDA)-approved AI-enabled medical devices, most are approved solely for use in radiology [30]. Not a single technology is classified under the specialty of ICU.

There are several reasons for this. As previously touched on, there is a lack of large and complete ICU datasets to both train and independently validate new models. Where models have successfully gone through this process, the evaluation is invariably retrospective. Prospective studies are needed in real-world settings to both ensure their safety and confirm their equivalency and/or superiority against the standard of care. Moreover, machine learning models using reference populations are prone to bias if certain groups are under-represented, and to a lack of generalizability if applied to other populations. The black-box problem has also surfaced as an obstacle in critical care medicine. As pointed out in *Lancet Respiratory Medicine*, machine learning and neural networks have been described as a black box, where data goes in and predictions or decisions come out, with little understanding as to how they were made [31]. The UK National Health Service has been a leader in recognizing the need to solve this problem, publishing a code of conduct for the use of data-driven technologies in healthcare that emphasized the need for transparent machine learning models [32]. Ultimately, AI must be 'explainable' for it to be successfully deployed and scaled in the ICU, as it must be trusted by all stakeholders in the healthcare ecosystem, from regulators, payers, privacy commissions, and clinicians, to patients and their families.

KEY INSIGHTS

- **Supervised, unsupervised, deep, and reinforcement learning are all methods of machine learning being used by researchers to solve problems and perform tasks in the ICU. But as of the time of writing, no algorithms have been approved by the FDA for use in the ICU.**
- **Machine learning can improve the accuracy of clinical scoring systems used in the ICU to predict patient outcomes.**
- **Machine learning models for the early recognition of sepsis are improved when free-text data within the EMR are digitized using NLP and included in the model. Unstructured data sources may be the missing ingredient for AI models to truly reach their predictive potential in the ICU.**
- **Reinforcement learning agents could be trained to reduce treatment errors and automate clinical decision-making in the ICU.**

- Deep learning models could unlock the information collected from cameras and novel sensing devices in the ICU, and these data may then be used to solve complex problems like delirium.
- Access to large datasets is needed to develop AI models in the ICU. Furthermore, prospective trials – which test AI models against standards of care – and trustworthy/explainable algorithms are needed for AI to find its place as a useful tool in the ICU.

Conflicts of Interest

Dipayan Chaudhari has no conflicts of interest to disclose. Sonny Kohli is the co-founder and chief medical officer of Cloud DX, a publicly traded company that has created an advanced continuous vital sign monitoring wearable.

References

1. Gardner RM, Scoville OP, West BJ et al. Integrated computer systems for monitoring of the critically ill. *Proceedings of the Annual Symposium on Computer Applications in Medical Care* 1977;1:301–307.
2. Gardner RM, Cannon GH, Morris AH, Olsen KR, Price WG. Computerized blood gas interpretation and reporting system. *IEEE Computer* 1975;8:19–25.
3. Frost DA, Yanowitz FG, Pryor IA. Evaluation of a computerized arrhythmia alarm system. *American Journal of Cardiology* 1977;39:583–587.
4. Gutierrez G. Artificial intelligence in the intensive care unit. *Critical Care* 2020:24(1):101.
5. Peters TJ, Waterman RH. *In Search of Excellence: Lessons from America's Best-Run Companies.* New York: Harper & Row; 1982.
6. Holmgren G, Andersson P, Jakobsson A et al. Artificial neural networks improve and simplify intensive care mortality prognostication: a national cohort study of 217,289 first-time intensive care unit admissions. *Journal of Intensive Care* 2019;7:44.
7. Liu S, See KC, Ngiam KY et al. reinforcement learning for clinical decision support in critical care: comprehensive review. *Journal of Medical Internet Research* 2020;22(7):e1847.

For additional references please see www.wiley.com/go/byrne/aiinclinical medicine.

16

AI in Dermatology

Albert T. Young[1], Jennifer Y. Chen[2,3], Abhishek Bhattarcharya[4], and Maria L. Wei[2,3]

[1] Department of Dermatology, Henry Ford Health, Detroit, MI, USA

[2] Department of Dermatology, University of California, San Francisco, CA, USA

[3] Dermatology Service, San Francisco VA Health Care System, San Francisco, CA, USA

[4] School of Medicine, University of Michigan, MI, USA

Learning Objectives

- Review current and upcoming clinical applications of AI in dermatology.
- Recognize potential sources of bias when evaluating dermatology AI models.
- Understand barriers and the path to clinical implementation.

16.1 Introduction

Dermatology is well suited for clinical applications of AI because it is a visually based specialty. If implemented effectively, AI may expand both the access to and the quality of dermatological care, but potential risks exist. Here, we describe the history of AI in dermatology, current and upcoming clinical applications, and important considerations for clinical implementation.

16.2 History of AI in Dermatology

Much of AI in dermatology involves the automated diagnosis of skin lesions from images, with efforts dating back to 1987 [1]. Subsequent models performed similarly to dermoscopy (i.e. use of a handheld magnifier) for the diagnosis of melanoma in experimental settings, but had uncertain external validity [2]. AI technology prior to the advent of deep learning in 2012 was limited by relatively small datasets and the need for labour-intensive feature engineering – that is, manually distilling images into colour, texture, and shape features for classification – in order to create each new model.

The modern deep learning era of AI in dermatology was launched with the use of deep convolutional neural networks (CNNs) to classify skin cancer, with a performance similar to that of 21 board-certified dermatologists [3]. In comparison with previous feature engineering approaches, deep learning allowed models to 'learn' the most relevant features for a prediction task without specific human

AI in Clinical Medicine: A Practical Guide for Healthcare Professionals, First Edition. Edited by Michael F. Byrne, Nasim Parsa, Alexandra T. Greenhill, Daljeet Chahal, Omer Ahmad, and Ulas Bagci.
Companion website: www.wiley.com/go/byrne/aiinclinicalmedicine

guidance. A major achievement was the compilation of a dataset of 129,450 images – two orders of magnitude larger than previous datasets – to train the CNN [3]. Since then, human-level performance has been convincingly demonstrated in experimental settings [4,5]. However, AI has generally fallen short of dermatologist performance in real-world practice [6–8], and has also been shown to be inferior to collective decision-making by a group of dermatologists in terms of diagnostic accuracy [9].

Recent AI technology advances include the ability of models to analyse clinical data such as demographic information and medical history, in addition to image data [10–12]; to identify and evaluate multiple lesions at once from wide-field images [13,14]; and to learn from whole slide images without the need for expensive pixel-wise manual annotations [15]. Studies to assess the robustness of models and barriers to their clinical use are now in progress [4,16,17].

Currently, there are no US Food and Drug Administration (FDA)-approved AI-based medical devices or algorithms in dermatology [18,19]. One AI system (FotoFinder® Moleanalyzer Pro, FotoFinder Systems, Inc., Columbia, MD, USA) for dermoscopic diagnosis has been market approved in Europe and performed comparably to dermatologists in a setting simulating store-and-forward teledermatology (i.e. asynchronous, as opposed to real-time teledermatology) [20] and in a prospective clinic setting [21].

16.3 Potential Clinical Applications

AI has been applied to the diagnosis of many skin disorders, including melanoma [3,20,22], non-melanoma skin cancer [3,13], onychomycosis [23], rosacea [24], erythema migrans [25,26], herpes zoster [27], cutaneous lupus [28], alopecia areata [29], psoriasis and eczema/atopic dermatitis [24,30], and pressure ulcers [31]. While early models focused on skin cancer, several AI models are now able to classify up to 174 disease classes [6,7,10,32,33]. Here, we discuss clinical applications that may soon become available, organized by the setting in which they will be primarily used (Figure 16.1).

16.3.1 Patient-Directed Screening and Monitoring

The widespread use of smart phones facilitates the direct use of AI applications by patients for screening or monitoring. AI models can run on smart phones, preserving privacy by keeping health information from leaving one's personal device [34]. Proof of concept for automated smart phone risk assessment has been established: an AI model trained on patient smart phone–generated images performed comparably to general practitioners for classifying whether pigmented lesions are at lower versus higher risk [35]. Another model has increased the sensitivity of malignancy diagnosis by 23 non-medical professionals from 47.6% to 87.5% without a loss in specificity [6].

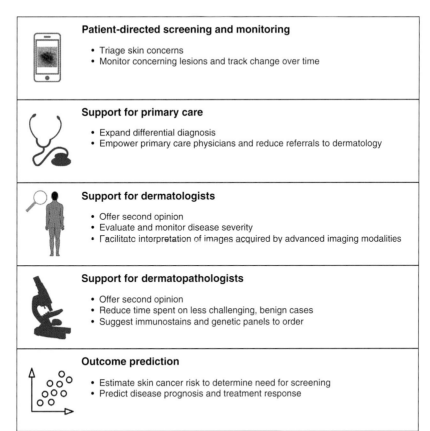

Figure 16.1: Potential clinical deployments of AI in dermatology.

Sources: Jmarchn / Wikimedia / CC BY-SA 3.0 (man from behind); Danil Polshin / Wikimedia / CC BY-SA 3.0 (scatter graph).

Apart from screening, AI may also facilitate the monitoring of lesion change over time [36]. AI may work synergistically with applications designed for self-examination and documentation of moles [37,38]. AI may also aid in the cosmetic evaluation of user-taken selfies for commercial purposes [39].

16.3.2 Supporting Skin Exams in a Primary Care Setting

AI will be able to help primary care practitioners better diagnose skin disease, triage referral to dermatology, and initiate therapy. Clinical decision support tools may be embedded in the electronic health record (EHR) and may reduce referrals to dermatology and support treatment initiation for inflammatory disorders by the referring clinician [40].

An AI model, developed using cases referred by primary care for teledermatology consultation, achieved a top 3 accuracy of 93% and top 3 sensitivity of 83% across 26 skin conditions representing 80% of cases seen in primary care [10], which was non-inferior to dermatologists and superior to primary care physicians (PCPs) and nurse practitioners. If deployed in a primary care setting, such a model can help PCPs arrive at a more accurate primary diagnosis, as well as prompt consideration of other diagnoses.

VisualDx, a currently available mobile app, allows healthcare providers to search an image library of skin conditions by inputting clinical features or by taking a photo of the skin lesion or rash (available with the DermExpert add-on) [41]. However, no data have been published assessing its use.

16.3.3 Support for Dermatologists

AI can also provide second opinions to dermatologists to enhance their diagnostic and treatment capabilities. AI may help dermatologists better triage teledermatology referrals [10] and improve performance during face-to-face visits [42]. Even when AI performance falls short of dermatologists' performance, dermatologists can still benefit from the applications because AI and humans make different patterns of errors; for example, AI is better at evaluating certain ambiguous images, while humans are less likely to be misled by suboptimal image quality such as blurriness or shadows, though this has not yet been systematically studied (Figure 16.2) [6].

Not only can AI assist dermatologists with diagnosis, it can also make basic clinical management recommendations based on images, for example in predicting whether a lesion should be excised [43] or whether the patient should be treated with a steroid, antibiotic, antiviral, or antifungal [6]. Such models are not yet able to replicate the dermatologists' expertise in selecting treatments that are optimized for each patient's unique preferences and circumstances, but this remains an intriguing future application.

AI may also one day be used by dermatologists to evaluate and monitor disease severity, for example by automating the assessment of alopecia [29], eczema [44], nevi [45], and psoriasis [46,47]. While still in their infancy, these tools promise more objective measurement of disease compared to clinical assessment tools that have imperfect inter- and intra-rater reliability, such as the Psoriasis Area and Severity Index (PASI) [46]. This capability would be useful to assess treatment response and disease progression. Currently, none of the reported AI models can reliably predict the probability that a benign lesion will evolve into a malignancy; the development of such a model requires prospectively collected datasets to allow longitudinal assessment of lesion evolution [48].

Aside from helping analyze conventional clinical images, AI may facilitate the use of advanced imaging modalities by decreasing the need for extensive training and experience [49]. For example, AI can automatically detect the dermal-epidermal junction, a critical step in acquiring images with reflectance confocal microscopy (RCM), a non-invasive imaging technique for skin cancer diagnosis requiring additional specialized training for image assessment that is not currently widely available [50]. AI models that analyse RCM images are also under development [51].

Dermatologists incorrect

Dermatologists correct

AI incorrect

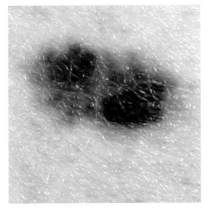

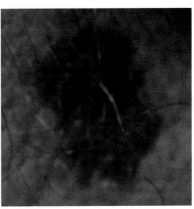

- Pathologic diagnosis: **nevus**
- Dermatologists: 93% recommend biopsy
- AI: 17% probability of malignancy, recommend biopsy

- Pathologic diagnosis: **melanoma**
- Dermatologists: 100% recommend biopsy
- AI: 6% probability of malignancy, recommend observation

AI correct

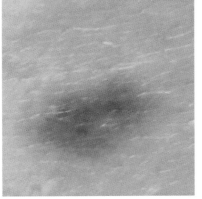

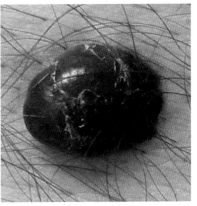

- Pathologic diagnosis: **nevus**
- Dermatologists: 64% recommend biopsy
- AI: 6% probability of malignancy, recommend observation

- Pathologic diagnosis: **melanoma**
- Dermatologists: 100% recommend biopsy
- AI: 82% probability of malignancy, recommend biopsy

Figure 16.2: Examples of images in which an AI model agrees or disagrees with dermatologists.

16.3.4 Support for Dermatopathologists

AI has the potential to support dermatopathologists, particularly in recognizing skin cancers that can be difficult to diagnose, such as early melanomas, by supporting the growing use of digital whole slide imaging [52]. Several AI models have been developed for the automated diagnosis of melanoma [11,53–57]. Two have performed comparably to pathologists in experimental settings [53,56], though these comparisons are limited by the evaluation of only a partial [53] or single [56] haematoxylin and eosin (H&E)–stained slide, whereas in clinical practice pathologists may request additional immunohistochemistry staining or clinical information. Performance did not improve when CNNs combined the acquired images with basic patient data (age, sex, anatomical site of the lesion) [11].

AI has also been studied for the diagnosis of basal cell carcinoma (BCC) from whole slide images [15,58,59]. Campanella et al. demonstrated that by ranking slides according to the probability of malignancy, a CNN could allow pathologists to exclude roughly 68% of slides while maintaining 100% sensitivity for BCC [15]. Notably, this study also pioneered weakly supervised multiple instance learning approaches that had two advantages over conventional fully supervised learning: (i) no need for labour-intensive pixel-level annotation of slides into diseased versus non-diseased regions; and (ii) better generalizability [15]. Kimeswenger et al. subsequently incorporated 'attention' (a technique that mimics cognitive attention) to automatically detect regions of a histological image most relevant for BCC diagnosis, and found that the CNNs and pathologists recognize BCCs based on different histological patterns [58]. Another potential application for this AI methodology is screening out negative slides in Mohs micrographic surgery [59].

Apart from suggesting diagnoses, AI has had some success in predicting sentinel lymph node status [60] and visceral recurrence and death [61] based on routine histology of primary melanoma tumors. Theoretical applications of AI include the automated detection of mitoses, the suggestion of tumour margins, the evaluation of immunostaining results, the suggestion of which immunostaining panels to order, and the suggestion of gene panels to order [62]. AI has successfully predicted specific mutations based on H&E-stained slides in lung adenocarcinoma [63], but so far has had limited success in predicting mutations in melanoma [64].

16.3.5 Outcome Predictions

Apart from its many image-based applications, AI may be used to predict various dermatological outcomes [65]. While the US Preventive Services Task Force (USPSTF) has concluded that evidence is insufficient to assess the balance of risks versus benefits of skin cancer screening in the general population by clinician visual examination [66], an Australian guideline [67] has recommended screening those at highest risk with sequential digital dermoscopy. AI support of image analysis might increase the benefit of skin cancer analysis in patients stratified by risk of skin cancer.

AI models have been developed to predict an individual's risk of developing melanoma [68–71] or non-melanoma skin cancer [71–75] based on EHR data and/or genetics. One study developed disease risk scores using 103,008 '23andMe' customers for which those in the highest percentile of risk had a 5.2, 8.1, and 12.9 times risk increase relative to the middle percentile for developing BCC, squamous cell carcinoma (SCC), and melanoma, respectively [71]. The disease risk score comprised 32 risk factors (selected after testing hundreds of candidate predictors), including age, sex, a polygenic risk score, family history, susceptibility (e.g. degree of skin pigmentation), personal history of skin lesions, exposures (e.g. sun exposure), and miscellaneous variables (e.g. body mass index) [71]. Overall, the models explained

21.6%, 20.0%, and 19.8% of the phenotypic variance of BCC, SCC, and melanoma, respectively [71]. Interestingly, the polygenic risk score explained only 1.5–3% of the variance in skin cancer risk [71]. Such models have the potential to identify high-risk patients who should undergo skin cancer screenings, but their predictive value is limited by inherent randomness in cancer development, and their clinical utility has yet to be demonstrated.

For inflammatory skin disorders, studies have used AI to predict response to biological therapy in psoriasis [76] and future severity of atopic dermatitis in children [77]; limitations include small sample size and subjectivity of measurements. Additionally, AI has been used to predict the risk of developing psoriatic arthritis in psoriasis patients using 200 genetic markers, achieving over 90% precision among the top 5% of patients predicted to develop psoriatic arthritis.

16.4 The Path to Clinical Implementation

AI will have a major impact on dermatology in the coming years and must be implemented with rigorous quality checks to reduce the risk of harm. The American Academy of Dermatology (AAD) has released a position statement on what is termed 'augmented intelligence' or AuI to guide clinical implementation [78]. In this statement, the AAD emphasized the need to have high-quality and minimally biased training sets, early engagement and collaboration of stakeholders, and maximal transparency regarding AuI models' decision-making and data.

16.4.1 Necessary Elements for Dermatology AI Model Validation

Careful validation of AI models is essential prior to their clinical use. Existing models should be vetted using computational 'stress tests' to ensure adequate performance in real-world settings where there may unfavourable conditions [4]. First, models should be validated on large external datasets, since studies report that relying only on internal validation results tends to overestimate performance [4,32]. The reasons for lower performance on external validation include non-representative training sets and data leakage between training and test sets during model development [32]. Few studies detail the performance of AI models on external validation, because such models are not made public; Han et al. have set an outstanding example by allowing submission of external images to their models at https://modelderm.com, to receive diagnostic predictions [6,13,79]. In addition, there is a need for public benchmark datasets such as the melanoma classification benchmark [80] and accessible databases such as DataDerm, the clinical data registry of the AAD [81].

Furthermore, models should be tested for their robustness to differences in image quality and transformations such as image rotation, brightness and contrast manipulation, adversarial noise, and artifacts such as ink markings and rulers [4,16,82–85].

An advantage of CNNs is their ability to automatically determine the most relevant features of an image for classification. However, a disadvantage is that the CNN training can introduce unexpected biases. For example, CNNs may inadvertently learn an association between melanoma and surgical skin markings [84] or scale bars [85], increasing the false-positive rate of benign nevi by approximately 40%; how these associations are learnt is unknown, but may be due to imbalances in the distribution of the artifact in melanoma versus nevus training images. Modelling uncertainties may help users assess when models are more likely to be wrong [86], and more interpretable CNNs may help users pinpoint what information the CNNs rely on to make decisions [58].

None of the currently available smart phone apps intended for use by laypersons to assess skin lesions has demonstrated sufficient performance or generalizability to recommend its use [87]. Some of the challenges include a selection bias introduced by the limited choice of lesion types as well as high-quality curated images and inadequate follow-up to identify false-negative results [88]. Of note is that the CE (Conformité Européenne) certification, given to two flawed apps (SkinVision and TeleSkin's skinScan app), may be inadequate to protect users from the risks of using smart phone diagnostic apps; in contrast, the FDA has a stricter assessment process [88].

Ultimately, AI must measurably improve health outcomes to gain widespread acceptance. To our knowledge, no published randomized control trials (RCTs) of AI applications in dermatology exist. When examining the few RCTs of AI models that exist, there are significant concerns regarding overestimation of the benefit of AI in the clinical setting due to the retrospective in silico nature of most studies, small clinician samples for comparison, poor reporting, and high risk of bias [89,90]. Future RCTs of AI in dermatology should refer to the SPIRIT-AI (Standard Protocol Items: Recommendations for Interventional Trials-Artificial Intelligence) [91] and CONSORT-AI (Consolidated Standards of Reporting Trials-Artificial Intelligence) [92] guidelines, which set out minimum requirements for reporting trial protocols and results (as described in Chapter 42).

16.4.2 Algorithmic Bias and Health Equity

AI has the potential to worsen health inequities if not implemented correctly through the introduction of pre-existing and emergent biases (as described in Chapters 39 and 40). For instance, one of the largest and most used open-source databases for pigmented skin lesions, the International Skin Imaging Collaboration (ISIC) archive, contains data from lighter-pigmented individuals in the USA, Europe, and Australia [93]. A prospective diagnostic accuracy study that compared an AI model against other non-invasive imaging techniques excluded people with darker-pigmented skin (Fitzpatrick phototype III or higher), limiting its generalizability [21]. Although melanoma is more common in lighter-pigmented individuals, patients with darker pigmentation often present with more advanced disease and have lower survival outcomes compared to their lighter-pigmented counterparts [94]. The predictive capability of machine learning models, especially for image-based classifications, is often dictated by the quality of the content of the dataset on which they are trained. If the data are skewed, the outcomes from the model will propagate the bias, for instance in the case of unbalanced representation of skin pigmentation in datasets used for melanoma prediction.

16.4.3 Patient and Clinician Attitudes towards AI in Dermatology

AI tools must gain the support of patients and clinicians to be useful. In surveys of patients in dermatology, most patients support the use of AI as a clinical decision-support tool for clinicians or as a direct-to-patient tool (e.g. a smart phone app), but few support its use as a standalone system [95,96]. This preference, to keep humans in the loop, reflects patient attitudes towards clinical AI and AuI more broadly [78,97]. Perceived benefits of AI include more accurate diagnosis, increased diagnostic speed, and increased healthcare access; concerns include increased anxiety, loss of human interaction, and less accurate diagnosis (e.g. resulting from low-quality photos taken in variable light) [96]. Clinicians are also generally receptive to AI tools, as long as they are used to assist, but not replace, their practice. In a survey answered by 121 dermatology fellows, 64% believed AuI would positively influence their practice; however, the response rate of 3.9% limits the interpretability of these results. Survey respondents reported that they would be much more likely to biopsy a lesion not clinically concerning for cancer if an AI tool indicated a malignant diagnosis, rather than forgo a biopsy of a concerning lesion if the AI indicated a benign diagnosis [98]. Physician concerns included disruptions to the patient–physician relationship, lack of patient follow-up owing to using AI without clinician support, clinician loss of control of AI, human deskilling, and worsening of healthcare disparities [98]. These findings corroborate a survey of Chinese dermatologists, which showed that 95.4% supported AuI while only 3.4% thought AI would replace the work of dermatologists [99]. A survey of dermatopathologists showed that 72.3% believed that AI will improve dermatopathology, although their support for AI varied by the specific application [62].

16.4.4 Human–Computer Collaboration

Even in the age of rapid AI development, a clinician's ability to contextualize information for patients, offer counselling relevant to a particular case, and provide follow-up care is invaluable. Applications of AI in dermatology likely will involve human–computer collaboration, human and machine in 'perfect harmony'. One study sought to understand how clinicians with varying levels of expertise would interact with image-based AI support across different clinical workflows, for example AI as telemedicine triage versus AI as a second opinion [100]. Decision support with AI-based multiclass probabilities improved clinician accuracy from 63.6% to 77.0%, but this gain was not seen with less granular or less explicit types of decision support; that is, AI-based probability of malignancy alone or AI-based content-based image retrieval, which searches databases to retrieve similar images with known diagnoses [100]. The least experienced clinicians benefited most from high-quality AI support, but clinicians of all experience levels saw a decrease in accuracy when supported by intentionally faulty AI [100]. Explainable AI-guided teaching was also shown to be valuable, for example in guiding medical students to pay more attention to chronic sun damage in the background resulting in more accurate diagnosis of pigmented actinic keratosis [100].

KEY INSIGHTS

- AI will have a major impact on dermatology in the coming years, especially because of recent advances in deep learning for computer vision.
- This chapter provides many exciting examples of where AI is being applied to dermatology; however, the US FDA has not yet approved any AI-based medical devices or algorithms in dermatology.
- There are many challenges in validating AI models, and ultimately AI must measurably improve health outcomes to gain widespread acceptance.
- In surveys of patients in dermatology, most support the use of AI as a clinical decision-support tool for clinicians or as a direct-to-patient tool (e.g. a smart phone app), but few support its use as a standalone system.
- Future applications of AI in dermatology likely will involve human–computer collaboration.

References

1. Cascinelli N, Ferrario M, Tonelli T, Leo E. A possible new tool for clinical diagnosis of melanoma: the computer. *Journal of the American Academy of Dermatology* 1987;16(2):361–367.
2. Rajpara SM, Botello AP, Townend J, Ormerod AD. Systematic review of dermoscopy and digital dermoscopy/artificial intelligence for the diagnosis of melanoma. *British Journal of Dermatology* 2009;161(3):591–604.
3. Esteva A, Kuprel B, Novoa RA et al. Dermatologist-level classification of skin cancer with deep neural networks. *Nature* 2017;542(7639):115–118. https://doi.org/10.1038/nature21056.
4. Young AT, Fernandez K, Pfau J et al. Stress testing reveals gaps in clinic readiness of image-based diagnostic artificial intelligence models. *npj Digital Medicine* 2021;4(1):10. https://doi.org/10.1038/s41746-020-00380-6.

5. Young AT, Xiong M, Pfau J, Keiser MJ, Wei ML. Artificial intelligence in dermatology: a primer. *Journal of Investigative Dermatology* 2020;140(8):1504–1512. https://doi.org/10.1016/j.jid.2020.02.026.

6. Han SS, Park I, Eun Chang S et al. Augmented intelligence dermatology: deep neural networks empower medical professionals in diagnosing skin cancer and predicting treatment options for 134 skin disorders. *Journal of Investigative Dermatology* 2020;140(9):1753–1761. https://doi.org/10.1016/j.jid.2020.01.019.

7. Muñoz-López C, Ramírez-Cornejo C, Marchetti MA et al. Performance of a deep neural network in teledermatology: a single-centre prospective diagnostic study. *Journal of the European Academy of Dermatology and Venereology* 2021;35(2):546–553. https://doi.org/10.1111/jdv.16979.

For additional references and Further Reading please see www.wiley.com/go/byrne/aiinclinicalmedicine.

17
Artificial Intelligence in Gastroenterology

Trent Walradt[1] and Tyler M. Berzin[2]

[1] Department of Internal Medicine, Beth Israel Deaconess Medical Center, Harvard Medical School, Boston, MA, USA

[2] Center for Advanced Endoscopy, Division of Gastroenterology, Beth Israel Deaconess Medical Center and Harvard Medical School, Boston, MA, USA

Learning Objectives

- Understand the evidence supporting the use of computer-aided detection (CADe) and computer-aided diagnosis (CADx) applied to colon polyps.
- Describe the spectrum of applications of AI in gastrointestinal endoscopy.
- Understand the expected evolution of regulatory pathways for AI tools in gastroenterology.
- Identify future applications of AI in gastroenterology.

17.1 Introduction

Gastroenterologists are required to interpret a vast amount of visual data during endoscopy. Moreover, they must make clinical decisions based on these data in real time. Even among experts, there is great deal of inter-provider variability in the interpretation of these images, leading to clinical variability in recognizing and diagnosing lesions accurately during gastrointestinal (GI) endoscopy.

Computer vision, a field of AI that pertains to algorithms that 'see and interpret' visual data, represents an ideal solution to some of the challenges inherent in GI endoscopy. Numerous computer vision algorithms have been developed for computer-aided detection (CADe) and computer-aided diagnosis (CADx) of GI lesions over the past decade. Some of the first prospective randomized trials utilizing AI in medicine have been in CADe for polyp detection during colonoscopy [1]. A broad array of applications of AI in gastroenterology are being developed to augment physician performance and productivity inside and outside of the endoscopy suite. As more products become commercially available, it is important for physicians to familiarize themselves with these technologies and the evidence.

In this chapter, we will review the current applications and expected evolution of AI in the field of gastroenterology.

AI in Clinical Medicine: A Practical Guide for Healthcare Professionals, First Edition. Edited by Michael F. Byrne, Nasim Parsa, Alexandra T. Greenhill, Daljeet Chahal, Omer Ahmad, and Ulas Bagci.
© 2023 John Wiley & Sons Ltd. Published 2023 by John Wiley & Sons Ltd.
Companion website: www.wiley.com/go/byrne/aiinclinicalmedicine

17.2 Colonoscopy

17.2.1 Computer-Aided Detection

Colorectal cancer (CRC) is the third most commonly diagnosed cancer and the fourth leading cause of death worldwide [2]. Screening colonoscopy reduces deaths due to CRC through the identification and removal of pre-cancerous polyps [3]. The adenoma detection rate (ADR), the proportion of screened subjects in whom at least one adenomatous lesion is identified, is a key quality metric. Patients who undergo colonoscopy by gastroenterologists with higher ADRs generally have a lower risk of interval colon cancer (cancer diagnosed before the next surveillance examination is due) than patients who undergo colonoscopy by gastroenterologists with lower ADRs. Consequently, significant effort has been focused on applying AI and computer vision to augment physician ADR during screening colonoscopy.

The use of CADe during colonoscopy is the most mature application of AI in gastroenterology. Early efforts were designed to recognize polyps in still images based on explicitly defined features such as colour, shape, and texture [4]. Modern technologies now employ deep learning algorithms capable of analysing video to detect polyps in real time [5]. Current CADe systems signal the presence of a polyp with an alarm on the endoscopy screen (usually a hollow box), with or without an accompanying audio alarm (Figure 17.1) [5].

Seven randomized control trials (RCTs) assessing the efficacy of CADe systems on polyp detection during colonoscopy have been performed [1,6–11]. Mohan et al. published a meta-analysis evaluating the cumulative impact of six of these trials [12]. They found that using CADe during colonoscopy resulted in a significant increase in ADR (relative risk = 1.5, 95% confidence interval [CI] 1.3–1.72; p < 0.0001) when compared with standard colonoscopy. It is important to note that the increase in

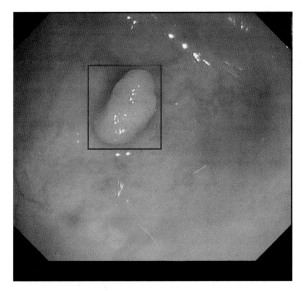

Figure 17.1: Example output from a computer-aided detection system using white light endoscopy. The visual alarm is represented by a bounded box.

Source: Tyler Berzin.

ADR seen with CADe in these studies was driven in large part by the detection of diminutive (≤5 mm) polyps. The clinical benefit of removing these polyps is an area of active debate [13]. In addition, the majority of these trials were singled-blinded, single-centre studies, which may limit the external validity of these results. Based on the published data showing increased adenoma detection, CADe technology for colon polyp detection is now commercially available in Europe, Japan, and the USA. Ongoing research will be required to evaluate both the clinical efficacy and added costs of implementing CADe for screening and surveillance colonoscopy in routine clinical practice.

17.2.2 Computer-Aided Diagnosis

A second major area of research in gastroenterology is the use of CADx to predict lesion histology during endoscopic procedures. During colonoscopy, definitively identifying hyperplastic polyps by CADx would help gastroenterologists avoid unnecessary polypectomies and could potentially reduce costs associated with pathological assessment. The American Society of Gastrointestinal Endoscopy Preservation and Incorporation of Valuable Endoscopic Innovations (PIVI) initiative proposed that a technology can be used to make the decision to leave a diminutive polyp in place if the technology can provide a ≥90% negative predictive value (NPV) for adenomatous histology ('diagnose and leave') [14]. The PIVI also posits that a technology can be used to resect and discard diminutive polyps without pathological assessment if the technology provides ≥90% agreement with histopathology for post-polypectomy surveillance intervals ('resect and discard'). Many technologies have been developed with the goal of surpassing these thresholds.

CADx systems for polyp diagnosis have been developed utilizing various endoscopic imaging approaches, ranging from routine high-definition white light endoscopy (WLE) to narrow-band imaging and magnification endoscopy (Figure 17.2).

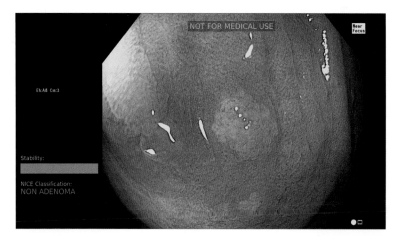

Figure 17.2: Example output from a computer-aided diagnosis system. The system predicts whether or not the lesion of interest is neoplastic. Used with the permission of ai4gi.

Thus far, six prospective, non-randomized trials have been performed to evaluate CADx for polyp diagnosis [15–20]. In 2019, Mori et al. published the largest of these trials evaluating the performance of a CADx algorithm that analysed images obtained using endocytoscopes (colonoscopes capable of 520× magnification) after application of narrow-band imaging and methylene blue staining (two advanced imaging modalities that enhance mucosal and vascular patterns) [19]. The primary outcome was whether CADx with methylene blue produced an NPV ≥90% for identifying diminutive rectosigmoid adenomas using the pathological diagnosis of resected specimens as the gold standard. The authors found that for the 250 rectosigmoid polyps in their study, using the most conservative estimate, the NPV was 93.7% (95% CI 88.3–97.1%). Thus, the point estimate of the NPV met the PIVI-2 threshold to support a diagnose-and-leave strategy. CADx has not achieved regulatory approval in most countries, but as the technology develops it is poised to play a significant role in screening and surveillance colonoscopy. This will likely manifest as hybrid CADe/CADx computer vision algorithms that will simultaneously localize polyps and provide a prediction of histology.

17.3 Esophagogastroduodenoscopy

When identified early, upper GI malignancies can often be cured via endoscopic resection or ablation. Unfortunately, pre-malignant lesions are frequently difficult to identify. For instance, up to 25% of early gastric cancer may be missed when utilizing high-definition WLE [21]. The first prospective trials applying AI to the detection of upper GI malignancies have recently been published (Figure 17.3). In 2020, DeGroof et al. developed a CADe system to detect high-grade dysplasia and early cancer in patients with Barrett's oesophagus using WLE [22]. The system achieved 89% accuracy, 90% sensitivity, and 88% specificity, outperforming 53 non-expert

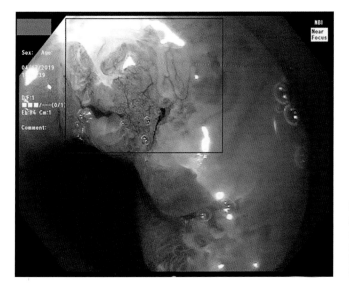

Figure 17.3: Real-time continuous AI algorithm detection of Barrett's dysplasia in a patient with short-segment Barrett's oesophagus. Used with the permission of Jason B. Samarasena.

endoscopists. In a subsequent prospective pilot study, the CADe system was used during live endoscopic procedures and correctly detected neoplasia in 9/10 patients, while producing a false positive in only 1/10 patients with non-dysplastic Barrett's oesophagus [23]. More recently, Wu et al. published a multicentre RCT evaluating the use of a convolutional neural network–based algorithm to monitor blind spots (gastric areas unobserved during esophagogastroduodenoscopy) and detect early gastric cancer [24]. In this study, 1050 patients from five hospitals were randomized to receive AI-assisted endoscopy or standard-of-care endoscopy. The AI-assisted group had significantly fewer blind spots than the standard-of-care group (mean 5.38 [standard deviation (SD) 4.32] versus 9.82 [SD 4.98]; $p < 0.001$). The accuracy, sensitivity, and specificity of the system were 84.69%, 100%, and 84.29%, respectively for detecting gastric cancer.

17.4 Video Capsule Endoscopy

Video capsule endoscopy (VCE) is an imaging modality that uses a pill-sized video camera that is swallowed and allows for the wireless transmission of video from the entire GI tract. VCE is primarily used for evaluation of the deep small bowel. Interpreting VCE, however, is a difficult and time-consuming task that requires physicians to review 40,000–60,000 frames per study. Lesion detection rates as low as 26–47% have been reported [25]. Recently, AI algorithms have been developed to aid in the interpretation of the massive amount of data generated by VCE reports. AI has been used for the detection of blood, angioectasias, ulcers, protruding lesions in the small bowel, coeliac disease, and parasites [25–29]. These efforts have the potential to dramatically decrease the workload on physicians and improve diagnostic efficiency.

17.5 Endoscopic Ultrasound

Endoscopic ultrasound (EUS) is an imaging modality in which endoscopically directed ultrasound is used to visualize the walls of the digestive tract and adjacent structures. The application of AI to EUS is still in its infancy, and current studies are based on training and testing using still images. Most AI applications for EUS have focused on pancreatic pathology. AI algorithms have been used to predict malignancy in intraductal papillary mucinous neoplasms and differentiate autoimmune pancreatitis from pancreatic ductal adenocarcinoma [30,31]. Outside of the pancreas, AI has also been applied with EUS to differentiate GI stromal tumors from benign subepithelial lesions, as well as to classify focal liver lesions as malignant or benign [32,33].

17.6 Clinical Prediction Models

Although the majority of recent AI gastroenterology research has focused on computer vision applied to endoscopic applications, other types of AI algorithms have also been used to develop a variety of clinical prediction models for gastroenterology.

For instance, Shung et al. developed a machine learning model to determine risk in patients with upper gastrointestinal bleeding (UGIB) [34]. The model was developed and internally validated using a cohort of 1958 patients who presented with UGIB to medical centres in the USA, Scotland, England, and Denmark. The model was then shown to outperform existing scoring systems when externally validated in 399 patients from Singapore and New Zealand. Ovanovic et al. recruited 291 consecutive patients from a single centre who presented with suspected choledocholithiasis and underwent endoscopic retrograde cholangiopancreatography (ERCP) [35]. They developed an artificial neural network and a multivariate logistic regression model and compared each model's ability to predict the presence of common bile duct stones on ERCP. They found the area under the receiver-operating characteristic curve was 0.884 for the artificial neural network and 0.787 for the multivariate logistic regression model. Investigators have also used AI to produce models to predict corticosteroid use and hospitalization in patients with inflammatory bowel disease, and predict the presence of lymph node metastasis in patients with T1 colorectal cancer [36–37].

17.7 Regulation

As AI technologies continue to mature, regulatory pathways must also evolve to evaluate and approve these tools. In the USA, the Food and Drug Administration (FDA) has proposed two axes for the assessment of AI-based software [38]. The first axis, risk, is based on a framework established by the International Medical Device Regulators Forum. Risk is defined by the seriousness of the disease to which a technology is applied, and the significance of the information provided by that technology. The second axis is adaptability and relates to the spectrum between 'locked' algorithms, which have fixed performance characteristics, and those designed to learn and evolve autonomously. One CADe system, GI-Genius (Medtronic, Minneapolis, MN, USA), has received regulatory approval in the USA [39]. Under the current FDA framework, any significant modification to the CADe system will require an additional approval process. Although this framework is practical for locked algorithms, it may slow the progress of AI algorithms that are rapidly iterative, or those that incorporate continuous learning. Consequently, the FDA has proposed a new system of regulation for AI technologies known as the software pre-certification program. This program aims to evaluate software developers rather than the just the software itself. Modifications to software from pre-certified developers will then be able to proceed through a streamlined review. Finally, the pre-certification program also requires that companies collect real-world data so that the FDA can monitor safety and perform streamlined reviews of modifications.

17.8 Future Directions

The field of gastroenterology has been a trailblazer in the development and prospective clinical study of AI technologies in clinical medicine. Many of the first RCTs evaluating AI technologies in all of clinical medicine are in the field of GI endoscopy

[1,6–11]. In order to promote the quality of clinical investigation in this area, Vinsard et al. proposed a set of principles for the development and testing of CADe and CADx colonoscopy studies [40]. More recently, the SPIRIT and CONSORT groups have developed reporting guidelines for clinical trials using AI interventions that are relevant to all fields of medicine (see Chapter 42) [41,42].

A key requirement for AI algorithm development for GI endoscopy is publicly available, labelled image libraries [43]. Such resources would facilitate regulatory approval of new algorithms, and comparative testing between existing systems. Although candidate libraries have been created, there will be an ongoing need for expanding the number, variety, and usability of high-quality GI endoscopy image sets [44,45]. Professional societies will likely lead the way in developing standards for labelling, sharing, and storing endoscopic images and videos to create large, multi-institutional datasets. Of note is that all AI applications, not just image-based ones, rely heavily on the availability of large, high-quality datasets. Thus, collecting clinical data in addition to images is crucial for the advancement of AI applications in GI.

Finally, it must be emphasized that AI has the capacity to meaningfully streamline clinical workflow in gastroenterology practice. For instance, several early efforts have the potential to automate the production of endoscopy reports by automatically measuring withdrawal time, recording bowel preparation quality, recognize and label anatomical landmarks, and identify endoscopic tools and interventions [46–48]. AI technologies will also play a role in other aspects of electronic health record data entry, data abstraction, and quality reporting. For example, while ADR is a core quality measure in gastroenterology practice, it requires abstracting data points from two locations, the colonoscopy report and pathology results, which may be stored and formatted differently. As a practical matter, this data is often collected and calculated by hand, if at all. Natural language processing applications of AI will play a role in streamlining this type of quality reporting [49]. AI technologies like these that simplify or replace repetitive, burdensome tasks are sorely needed in gastroenterology practice, and in clinical medicine in general.

KEY INSIGHTS

- AI is being employed in multiple areas of gastroenterology. The most significant progress has been seen in CADe and CADx of colorectal polyps.
- Some of the first prospective, randomized trials utilizing AI in medicine have been in CADe for polyp detection during colonoscopy. These trials have shown a significant increase in adenoma detection rate when using CADe during colonoscopy when compared with standard colonoscopy. Consequently, the first generation of CADe systems is beginning to achieve regulatory approval for use in clinical practice.
- Evidence is accruing for CADx to predict polyp histology during endoscopic procedures. Definitively identifying hyperplastic polyps

by CADx would help gastroenterologists avoid unnecessary polyp-ectomies or could potentially support a 'resect-and-discard' strategy for small polyps.

■ As AI technologies continue to mature, regulatory pathways must also evolve to evaluate and approve these tools. The FDA has proposed a new system of regulation for AI technologies, known as the software pre-certification program, that aims to evaluate software developers rather than just the software itself.

■ AI has the capacity to meaningfully streamline clinical workflow in gastroenterology practice. Applications include automating the production of endoscopy reports and using natural language processing to streamline data collection.

Conflicts of Interest

Tyler Berzin has served as a consultant for Wision AI, Fujifilm, and Medtronic. Trent Walradt has no conflicts of interest to disclose.

References

1. Wang P, Berzin TM, Glissen Brown JR et al. Real-time automatic detection system increases colonoscopic polyp and adenoma detection rates: a prospective randomised controlled study. *Gut* 2019;68(10):1813–1819.
2. Bray F, Ferlay J, Soerjomataram I et al. Global cancer statistics 2018: GLOBOCAN estimates of incidence and mortality worldwide for 36 cancers in 185 countries. *CA: A Cancer Journal for Clinicians* 2018;68(6):394–424.
3. Nishihara R, Wu K, Lochhead P et al. Long-term colorectal-cancer incidence and mortality after lower endoscopy. *New England Journal of Medicine* 2013;369(12):1095–1105.
4. Maroulis DE, Iakovidis DK, Karkanis SA, Karras DA. CoLD: a versatile detection system for colorectal lesions in endoscopy video-frames. *Computer Methods and Programs in Biomedicine* 2003;70(2):151–166.
5. Bilal M, Glissen Brown JR, Berzin TM. Using computer-aided polyp detection during colonoscopy. *American Journal of Gastroenterology* 2020;115(7):963–966.
6. Gong D, Wu L, Zhang J et al. Detection of colorectal adenomas with a real-time computer-aided system (ENDOANGEL): a randomised controlled study. *Lancet Gastroenterology and Hepatology* 2020;5(4):352–361.
7. Liu P, Wang P, Glissen Brown JR et al. The single-monitor trial: an embedded CADe system increased adenoma detection during colonoscopy: a prospective randomized study. *Therapeutic Advances in Gastroenterology* 2020;13:1756284820979165.

For additional references and Further Reading please see www.wiley.com/go/byrne/aiinclinicalmedicine.

18

AI in Haematology

Paulina B. Szklanna[1,2,3], Luisa Weiss[1,3], Brian Mac Namee[4], Rehman Faryal[5], Barry Kevane[1,5,6], Fionnuala Ní Áinle[1,5,6], and Patricia B. Maguire[1,2,3,7]

[1] ConwaySPHERE, Conway Institute, University College Dublin, Dublin, Ireland

[2] AI Healthcare Hub, Institute for Discovery, University College Dublin, Dublin, Ireland

[3] School of Biomolecular & Biomedical Science, University College Dublin, Dublin, Ireland

[4] School of Computer Science, University College Dublin, Dublin, Ireland

[5] Department of Haematology, Mater Misericordiae University Hospital, Dublin, Ireland

[6] School of Medicine, University College Dublin, Dublin, Ireland

[7] UCD Institute for Discovery, University College Dublin, Dublin, Ireland

Learning Objectives

- Recapitulate the basic knowledge of haematology and haematological diseases.
- Understand the current thinking, testing, and best practice in the field of haematology.
- Comprehend the history and current novel applications of AI in haematology.
- Identify and address the challenges associated with the implementation of AI-driven solutions into haematology.

18.1 Introduction

Haematology is a diverse field of medicine encompassing both the clinical and laboratory aspects of blood disorders. Dominated by the examination of the morphology of blood cells in the mid-twentieth century, haematology has recently expanded its horizons into more specialized subdivisions, including general haematology, haemato-oncology, thrombosis and haemostasis, and transfusion medicine. Modern haematology is now strongly integrated across current medical practice, forming deep inter-disciplinary links with many other specialties.

At the core of a normal human adult blood system lies a hierarchical organization of blood cells, with its upper echelons occupied by haematopoietic stem cells with their perpetual self-renewal and differentiation abilities, and its base comprising terminally differentiated and functional blood cells (Figure 18.1). This hierarchical framework provides a differentiation roadmap of haematopoiesis in a stepwise

AI in Clinical Medicine: A Practical Guide for Healthcare Professionals, First Edition. Edited by Michael F. Byrne, Nasim Parsa, Alexandra T. Greenhill, Daljeet Chahal, Omer Ahmad, and Ulas Bagci.
© 2023 John Wiley & Sons Ltd. Published 2023 by John Wiley & Sons Ltd.
Companion website: www.wiley.com/go/byrne/aiinclinicalmedicine

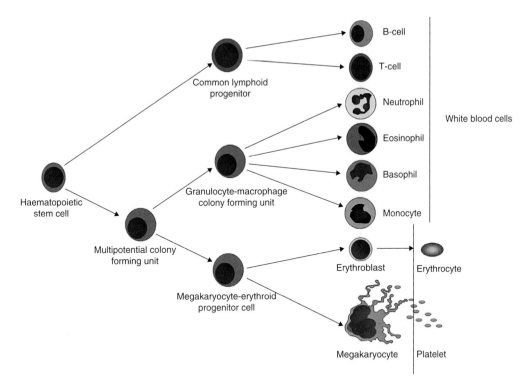

Figure 18.1: Hierarchical blood cell organization. At the core of a normal human adult blood system lies a hierarchical organization of blood cells produced during haematopoiesis in the bone marrow. All types of blood cells originate from haematopoietic stem cells that sequentially differentiate into erythrocytes, platelets, and white blood cells (WBCs). Platelets, best known for their role in haemostasis, also play a key role in immune regulation, wound healing, and thromboinflammation. WBCs encapsulate a variety of different cell types, which together are the cornerstone of the immune system. The main function of erythrocytes is oxygen transport.

process from progenitors (haematopoietic stem cells) to mature blood cells such as erythrocytes and B cells. Disruption of the normal blood system at any level of the hierarchy may result in malignant processes, anaemia, and bleeding disorders.

Unlike other organ systems in the human body, the haematological organ system is well connected and intercalated with other body systems, due to its fluidity through an established network of vessels, and provides a medium for its cellular components to act and respond to pathological insults. Apart from cellular components of its system such as red blood cells (RBCs), white blood cells, and platelets, its fluid-phase components include coagulation factors, natural anticoagulants, and proteins of the fibrinolytic system, which play a significant role in coordinating and executing varied responses in events of pathological insult.

Haematological responses are a common manifestation of many haematological (sepsis, disseminated intravascular coagulopathy [DIC], leukaemia) and non-haematological diseases. Early detection of abnormal haematological parameters provides an important insight into these various clinical circumstances. A better understanding of haematology has also helped shape, for example, some of the current practices in other medical fields, including obstetric medicine. Normal pregnancy is associated with changes to the haematological system, favouring a more procoagulant phenotype during pregnancy; and women with acquired bleeding disorders, such as von Willebrand factor or coagulation factors deficiency, face an increased risk of post-partum haemorrhage [1]. These haematological changes, alongside dysregulation of angiogenic and inflammatory mediators (including placental growth factor and various interleukins), are enhanced in pregnancy disorders such as pre-eclampsia [2]. Quantification of such blood-based biomarkers in these clinical settings has helped to improve both foetal and maternal outcomes [3].

18.2 Current Thinking, Testing, and Best Practice in Haematology

Within the last decade there has been a significant shift in the management of blood disorders, based on a better understanding of underlying pathophysiological processes and improved diagnostics, leading to more personalized treatment strategies and overall better patient outcomes. Perhaps the greatest advancements have been made in the setting of haematological neoplasms, where therapies can be broadly categorized into targeted treatments encompassing immunotherapies with monoclonal antibodies (such as rituximab) or specific protein inhibition, for example tyrosine kinase inhibitors and cytotoxic chemotherapies. While these have all been extensively studied and are widely approved in the clinic, several pre-clinical studies and clinical trials are currently underway assessing the use of chimeric antigen receptor (CAR) T cell [4] or CAR–natural killer cell therapies, currently approved for treatment of acute lymphoblastic leukaemia, for example [5,6].

Besides haemato-oncological malignancies, one of the very resource-intensive domains under haematology is the management of aberrant clotting or thrombosis. Cardiovascular diseases, including myocardial infarction, stroke, and venous thromboembolism, currently account for one in three deaths worldwide [7]. Connected by a common underlying denominator, thrombosis, the treatment of acute and the secondary prevention of recurrent events frequently entail anticoagulation. Over the last decade, the approval of direct oral anticoagulants (DOACs) conferred a paradigm shift in the treatment of thrombosis. Besides presenting similar if not superior efficacy compared with warfarin, DOACs also indicate more favourable bleeding profiles [8], resulting in DOACs currently now being prescribed for anticoagulation in preference to warfarin, unless contraindicated.

Management of bleeding disorders such as haemophilia has also been revolutionized with the introduction of long-acting recombinant clotting factors and antibody-based non-substitutional therapies such as emicizumab. In addition, recent advancements in gene therapies indicate promising results in the treatment of haemophilias, but also sickle cell disease and thalassaemias, dramatically increasing quality of life for these patients [9].

18.3 The Implementation of AI in Haematology

The first application of AI to haematological laboratory diagnostics was described over 25 years ago, when peripheral blood interpretation, immunophenotyping, and bone marrow reporting were combined to classify and diagnose haematological malignancies, achieving accuracy (correct classification of 94/100 cases) similar to a physician's interpretation (correct classification on 99/100 cases) [10]. Later, Golub et al. [11] applied AI to RNA microarray data from known leukaemia cases, with signal-to-noise ratio ranking, neighbourhood-based methods, and self-organizing maps enabling successful distinction of acute myeloid and acute lymphoblastic leukaemia. This was the first study to classify such leukaemia subtypes based on a combination of microarray data, bioinformatics, and AI, revolutionizing leukaemia diagnosis, and paving the way towards molecular-based diagnostic systems. Nowadays, such gene expression datasets are commonly used in both supervised (class prediction) and unsupervised (class discovery) learning approaches, allowing for a genome-wide approach and an efficient diagnostic and prognostic platform for blood-based cancers such as leukaemia [12,13].

Improvements in computer vision and image analysis have also been extensively applied to haematopathology for identification and segmentation of cells alongside feature extraction and classification. A specific type of artificial neural network that takes advantage of the spatial arrangement of data, called a convolutional neural network (CNN), has proved to be highly accurate in classification of differentiation and recognition of blood cells [14,15]. CNN models have also been used in radiology to distinguish between normal bone and lytic lesions on computed tomography (CT), or to detect bone marrow involvement in acute myeloid leukaemia [16,17].

18.4 Current Applications of AI in Haematology

The recent advances in the field of AI have inspired its use in more widespread areas of medicine and haematology, with the successful application of simple and complex models in microfluidics, blood cell classification, diagnosis, and haematological malignancies. Simple models like decision trees, random forests, or supported vector machines have all now been elegantly applied. These models usually rely on numerical data, for instance full blood count (FBC) data, which are easily obtained and hold a myriad of vital health information. One recent example is the use of recursive partitioning as well as classification and regression trees to assess FBC data to demonstrate consideration of the neutrophil to lymphocyte ratio (NLR) as well as the white cell count for the detection of suspected bacteraemia during pregnancy and the post-partum period [18].

Intriguingly, a recent study evaluated routinely tested blood parameters for their utility to differentiate among 43 haematological diseases (including, among others, several forms of anaemia, leukaemia, and haemorrhagic conditions). Utilizing the 61 most frequently tested blood parameters, a random forest model outperformed a support vector machine model and could predict an individual patient's top five most probable diseases with 86% accuracy, highlighting the usefulness of routine laboratory parameters as potential pathological 'fingerprints' [19]. This study highlights the importance of machine learning models in identifying FBC patterns to provide higher diagnostic accuracy compared with interpretation based on reference ranges. Furthermore, FBCs and other haematological parameters have been used in diagnosis and risk stratification of several other disorders, such as enabling prediction of disease severity [20,21] and mortality [22] in hospitalized COVID-19 patients, with area under the receiver operating characteristic (AUROC) ranging from 0.92 to 0.99 using a variety of models including decision tree, gradient boosting, and extreme gradient boosting (XGBoost) models. An XGBoost model based on blood test results from 15,176 neurological patients was also utilised for the diagnosis of brain tumour, achieving a sensitivity of 96% and specificity of 74% upon validation with 283 patients [23]. Further incorporation and validation of AI approaches will lead to a fundamental disruption of differential disease diagnosis.

The high rates of occurrence of heterogeneous data in haematology have also motivated the usage of more complex machine learning models. In the case of low-grade Hodgkin's lymphoma, the five most predictive radiomic features extracted from positron emission tomography (PET) scans were used in a support vector machine–based classifier. This approach revealed higher predictive accuracy (AUC = 95.2%) for refractory disease than the current gold standard diagnosis of metabolic tumour volume or total lesion glycolysis (AUC = 78%) [24]. Similarly, the intricate problem of prediction of infection in patients newly diagnosed with chronic lymphocytic leukaemia (CCL) was addressed by an ensemble algorithm composed of 28 machine learning algorithms with a combined positive predictive value of 72% [25]. Infections in patients with CCL are a major cause of morbidity and mortality, and the ability to identify patients at risk will have a positive impact on their treatment outcome.

Aside from that, novel developments of computer vision, powered by deep learning, have also been applied in haematology with high rates of success. Achi et al. [26] used histology images to train a CNN network for the automated detection of lymphoma. Following training and validation on 2320 images, their CNN model was tested on 240 images where, for each test set of 5 images, the predicted diagnosis was combined from the prediction of 5 images. This model achieved a diagnostic accuracy of 95% for image-by-image prediction and 100% for set-by-set prediction [26]. This study, although preliminary, highlights the advantage of incorporation of automated diagnostic screening into the pathological workflow to augment efficiency. Similarly, image-based CNN models have been used to classify diverse shapes of RBCs in an automated manner in sickle cell anaemia with high accuracy [15], and an objective image analysis-based scoring algorithm has been also used to successfully differentiate diffuse B-cell lymphoma subtypes [27]. Clinically useful, automated AI-based solutions for cell classification have been of major interest in the field, and the application of a novel AI-based digital imaging system for cell recognition and classification in peripheral blood smear analysis was recently granted Food and Drug Administration (FDA) approval [28].

18.5 Considerations and Challenges for AI in Haematology

The considerations and challenges facing AI in haematology are akin to those associated with AI generally in medicine, mainly that very few models translate into the clinical setting and have been used to make genuine decisions about patient care. This discrepancy between the development of a scientifically sound algorithm and the usage of a created model to offer real value to the patient is defined as the AI chasm. Therefore, many important challenges and questions, including crossing this chasm and the interpretability of the final model, need to be considered prior to its utilization in healthcare. Careful consideration of these challenges will help to create a list of necessary and desirable components of the final solution that will be a guidepost throughout the process [29].

In haematology, a large volume of heterogeneous patient data is routinely generated, leading to a 'data rich, information poor' dilemma, where the volume and complexity of the data exceed our ability to extract meaningful knowledge. This heterogeneity affects the informativeness of each data point, and therefore feature selection is often employed in machine learning in haematology. Features of importance can be selected deliberately in a manual feature selection based on domain knowledge, or algorithmically using principal component analysis or correlation-based filtering [30]. Aside from simplifying the model, feature selection also helps to avoid overfitting and reduces training time.

Another important challenge is the lack of big datasets, especially with the rarity of some haematological diseases and the difficulty and/or expense of developing large databases [30]. To counteract small sample sizes, data augmentation (altering of training data to increase variability) or regularization (application of a penalty to the model as it increases in complexity) can be applied. The challenge of big datasets in haematology can also be addressed by utilizing domain expertise in the modelling process. This might be achieved using active learning [31], weak supervision [32], and semi-supervised learning [33], as well as explainable machine learning approaches that allow a model to be tuned based on input from domain experts [34]. Small sample sizes may also affect model validation, and a k-fold cross-validation resampling procedure can be applied where the available dataset size is insufficient for splitting in order to evaluate the model.

An additional challenge for the integration of AI in haematology (and healthcare research overall) is that of missing data resulting from irregular data collection, no patient follow-up, and lack of standardization in protocols or equipment used [30]. Sometimes these missing data can be statistically interpolated or imputed with a constant value. Missing data can often be informative, and this informative 'missingness' can be incorporated into a prediction model [30,35]. Therefore, careful thought and consideration need to be given to missing data and the potential effect on the model.

Considering the previously mentioned heterogeneity of data, the selection of an appropriate model is crucial. In haematology, supervised models, where the label is assigned and predictions are compared to the outcomes, are most often used. These models range from a simple logistic regression or decision tree, through more complex models such as support vector machine, gradient boosting, or random forest, to advanced, deep learning models such as convolutional neural networks, recurrent neural networks, or deep Boltzmann machine [29]. Unsupervised models, where labels are not assigned and the model itself identifies similarities and patterns, are less frequently used in haematology.

Yet the ultimate challenge will be to cross the AI chasm and create real-world applications of AI in haematology in order to improve patient care. To achieve this, the final model should easily integrate into the clinical workflow and achieve clinical trust by predicting clinically meaningful outcomes with appropriate, patient-orientated endpoints. The ability to understand how individual variables contribute to the predicted outcome and inclusion of appropriate metrics (such as positive predictive value, negative predictive value, and AUROC) will all be important in the clinical scenario [30,36]. Extensive testing of models on several internal and external cohorts of patients will bolster clinical trust, making it more likely for AI to be integrated as part of standardized patient care.

18.6 The Future of AI in Haematology

The incredible rate at which data are generated in the field of haematology encourages the use of novel AI-based solutions as clinically useful tools to facilitate minimally invasive and quick disease diagnosis, as well as to drive personalized treatment strategies. The creation of such solutions to answer important clinical questions and ultimately improve patient outcomes requires large centralized databases. These are merged with state-of-the-art analytical services that will capture, integrate, and analyse anonymous data from thousands of patients from high-quality multidisciplinary sources, such as those recently achieved in patients with haematological malignancies [37].

The opportunities for AI in haematology extend beyond the creation of comprehensive, large-scale datasets. Applications to date of AI in haematology highlight the possibilities associated with the future integration of AI-powered algorithms into haematology guidelines worldwide. With the introduction of high-throughput methodologies and an exponential increase of available information, the field is primed to integrate novel applications of AI with the aim to promote personalized interventions and enhance treatment. New applications, capable of assimilation of the patient's data, have the potential to support patients in self-management of their health, ultimately allowing for more meaningful doctor–patient interactions [38]. In fact, the potential of AI-based applications in haematology is virtually endless and the only remaining question is: how far can we go?

KEY INSIGHTS

■ **Over the last decade, multiple advances in the field of haematology have led to more personalized treatment strategies and overall better patient outcomes.**

■ **Simple and complex AI methodologies, especially computer vision, are being applied to many facets of haematology, including microfluidics, blood cell classification, diagnosis, and haematological malignancies.**

■ **Despite the exponential increase in the number of AI models in haematology-focused research, very few models have crossed the divide between development and implementation into clinical practice.**

■ **The field is primed to integrate novel applications of AI with the aim to drive personalized interventions and enhance treatment.**

References

1. Patel P, Balanchivadze N. Hematologic findings in pregnancy: a guide for the internist. *Cureus* 2021;13(5):e15149.
2. Kelliher S, Maguire PB, Szklanna PB et al. Pathophysiology of the venous thromboembolism risk in preeclampsia. *Hamostaseologie* 2020;40(5):594–604.
3. Duhig KE, Myers J, Seed PT et al. Placental growth factor testing to assess women with suspected pre-eclampsia: a multicentre, pragmatic, stepped-wedge cluster-randomised controlled trial. *Lancet* 2019;393(10183):1807–1818.
4. Wang M, Munoz J, Goy A et al. KTE-X19 CAR T-cell therapy in relapsed or refractory mantle-cell lymphoma. *New England Journal of Medicine* 2020;382(14):1331–1342.
5. Liu E, Marin D, Banerjee P et al. Use of CAR-transduced natural killer cells in CD19-positive lymphoid tumors. *New England Journal of Medicine* 2020;382(6):545–553.
6. Yu S, Li A, Liu Q et al. Chimeric antigen receptor T cells: a novel therapy for solid tumors. *Journal of Hematology & Oncology* 2017;10(1):1–13.
7. World Health Organization. *Cardiovascular diseases (CVDs)*, 2021. https://www.who.int/en/news-room/fact-sheets/detail/cardiovascular-diseases-(cvds).

For additional references and Further Reading please see www.wiley.com/go/byrne/aiinclinicalmedicine.

19

AI and Infectious Diseases

Alanna Ebigbo and Helmut Messmann

Internal Medicine III, Department of Gastroenterology and Infectious Diseases, University Hospital Augsburg, Augsburg, Germany

Learning Objectives

- Understand the global threat posed by infectious diseases.
- Understand the significance of antimicrobial resistance.
- State the major infectious diseases involved in regional or global outbreaks.
- Discuss the possible applications of AI in the diagnosis and treatment of infectious diseases.
- Understand the utility of AI for the pre-emptive and early recognition of regional or global disease outbreaks.
- Understand the possible application of AI in the management of antimicrobial resistance.

19.1 Introduction

Infectious diseases (IDs), such as tuberculosis, HIV, and malaria, continue to pose a significant health challenge for affected world regions. Decades of research have not been able to sufficiently control these global health issues. Antimicrobial drug resistance, pathogen mutation, vaccine escape mutations, and ineffective drugs have made it challenging to control morbidity and mortality. Numerous epidemics and pandemics, including the Ebola virus disease epidemic of 2012 and the COVID-19 pandemic, highlight the devastating impact IDs have had on healthcare systems and national economies.

AI systems can harness and process large amounts of data to combat ID on various levels. In this chapter, we will highlight the following applications of AI in ID:

- Disease outbreaks and surveillance.
- Disease diagnosis.
- Prediction and control of antimicrobial resistance.
- Disease treatment.

AI in Clinical Medicine: A Practical Guide for Healthcare Professionals, First Edition. Edited by Michael F. Byrne,
Nasim Parsa, Alexandra T. Greenhill, Daljeet Chahal, Omer Ahmad, and Ulas Bagci.
© 2023 John Wiley & Sons Ltd. Published 2023 by John Wiley & Sons Ltd.
Companion website: www.wiley.com/go/byrne/aiinclinicalmedicine

In addition, we will use practical examples in HIV, malaria, tuberculosis, Zika, and COVID-19 to demonstrate how AI can be used in the setting of ID prevention and control.

19.2 Disease Outbreaks and Surveillance

Disease outbreaks, such as the Zika virus outbreak in southern America, usually have a high morbidity and mortality rate within a short period. When a disease outbreak is limited to a region or country, it is termed epidemic, and the spread of a disease across geographical boundaries is a pandemic. Every disease outbreak usually has an epicentre from which the disease pathogen spreads to other areas. The COVID-19 pandemic probably had its epicentre in Wuhan, China, in December 2019. The coronavirus, SARS-CoV-2, then spread to the rest of the world within a few weeks, leading up to the World Health Organization's (WHO) proclamation of a pandemic in February 2020. The origin of the disease pathogen and the mechanism of its spread are important elements in the fight against an epidemic or pandemic. However, the factors influencing its spread may be difficult to comprehend.

Surveillance systems at national and international levels produce vast amounts of data, for example on the initial appearance of disease symptoms, incidence rates across regions, reproductive number, and spread pattern. Many factors, including geographical effects, demographics, population densities, and travel behaviour, will directly or indirectly affect the development and spread of an outbreak. The challenge is to predict and identify an outbreak swiftly to curb the further spread of disease. In the past, disease outbreaks were often ongoing for weeks or even months before health authorities officially recognized the situation. Even though the data that would enable pre-emptive identification and comprehension of an epidemic or a pandemic are available on various databases, the challenge is to harness and understand the enormous amounts of data being generated. Here, AI comes into play and can be used to better understand the mechanisms regarding the onset and spread of an epidemic or pandemic. With AI, disease tracking platforms can predict when and where the next disease outbreak is expected to happen. AI can also use data from social media platforms and internet searches to identify a pandemic development or disease spread at an early stage. This approach has been used to prospectively predict dengue outbreaks, and to track and predict influenza outbreaks with high accuracy compared with observed data. Also, prediction models using AI algorithms and other data collected by satellite sensors and data measured onsite, such as rainfall, have been used to estimate dengue virus outbreaks, and to predict malaria and Zika virus outbreaks with high accuracy.

For contact tracing and identification of strategies to block the further transmission of disease, complex data can be processed by AI algorithms to assist in the containment of a disease outbreak.

19.3 Disease Diagnosis

Many AI systems have been applied in the image and pattern recognition domains. Deep learning has been applied to the assessment of chest X-ray and computed tomography (CT) images in the diagnosis of pneumonia, tuberculosis, or pulmonary nodules. In addition, AI algorithms can optimize the workflow by filtering pathological from non-pathological images, thereby prioritizing image analysis.

Community- and hospital-acquired pneumonia poses a significant challenge for physicians and radiologists. Chest X-rays are the standard tools for diagnosing pneumonia; however, considering the vast numbers of X-rays being performed, additional tools to aid clinicians and radiologists will benefit patients and healthcare providers. Also, radiological signs of pneumonia are not always obvious and can be missed or misinterpreted during the assessment of images. Finally, expert radiologists may not be readily available for image evaluation, especially in low-resource settings. AI systems using convolutional neural networks (CNNs) have been shown to successfully diagnose pneumonia on chest X-ray images at a level exceeding that of practising radiologists. Various studies have shown that deep learning algorithms with CNNs can efficiently detect COVID-19 in chest X-ray images.

Figure 19.1 shows the model development workflow of an AI-based detection system for rapid COVID-19 pneumonia screening based on chest X-ray images [1]. After retrospective collection of relevant chest X-ray images, the data were split into two development strategies: an 80% : 20% training and validation strategy, and a 70% : 20% : 10% training, validation, and testing strategy. These two strategies demonstrate the efforts required when trying to extract the maximum benefit from a limited dataset. The second strategy, as opposed to the first, includes 10% 'unseen' data; that is, data that were not used for training, thereby mimicking the clinical deployment scenario. The model development workflow involves the introduction of different clinical detection scenarios, including two-, three-, and four-class detection scenarios. Finally, model training and optimization drive the process of transfer learning as well as hyperparameter tuning. Transfer learning makes use of pretrained base AI architectures, which are necessary when data availability is limited. In hyperparameter tuning, the optimal values, which will result in maximal performance of the model, are determined.

Figure 19.2 shows the visualization of the model prediction of COVID-19 pneumonia on chest X-ray images using overlaid heat or activation maps. Features detected on input images by the model are highlighted using gradient-based visualization (Grad-CAM). Grad-CAM visualizations improve the readability of the output provided by the model, and are important for the explainability of the results.

For pulmonary tuberculosis (PTB), some studies have investigated the application of artificial neural networks (ANNs) for the prediction of infection as well as the differentiation between PTB and non-tuberculous mycobacterial disease (NTMD) in chest X-ray and CT images. PTB and NTMD can have similar manifestations in radiological imaging. The early diagnosis of PTB or NTMD can prevent potentially unnecessary treatments with the risk of adverse reactions and unnecessary

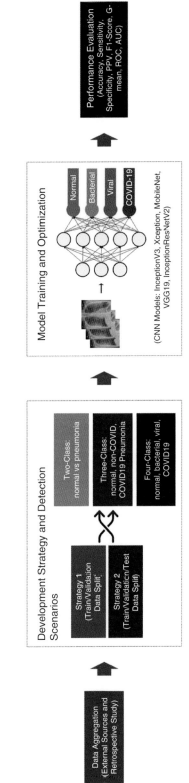

Figure 19.1: Model development workflow. This AI-based detection system permits rapid COVID-19 pneumonia screening based on chest X-ray images using a strategy to maximize the limited data available.

Source: [1] / PLOS / CC BY-4.0.

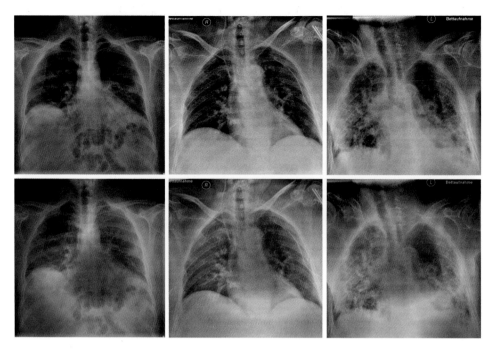

Figure 19.2: Grad-CAM for three chest X-ray images of patients with the diagnosis of COVID-19 pneumonia. The first row shows the original chest X-ray; the second row shows the overlaid activation map on the original image.

Source: [1] Baltazar et al. (2021), PLOS ONE.

healthcare costs. Also, AI has been used to predict mycobacterial resistance against the standard drugs rifampicin, pyrazinamide, isoniazid, and fluoroquinolones.

Malaria remains a global threat and mainly affects poorer countries with high child mortality rates. The diagnosis of malaria requires time, expertise, and resources. AI algorithms have been developed and shown to successfully detect red blood cells with malaria parasites using data from holographic microscopy.

Other applications for AI in diagnosing IDs include diagnosing surgical site infection, the rapid diagnosis of infection in the emergency unit, and the distinction between bacterial and viral infections [2–4].

19.4 Prediction and Control of Antimicrobial Resistance

Antimicrobial resistance (AMR) in parasites, viruses, and bacteria is rising and poses a global health challenge. The WHO has listed specific threats, most notably including the following pathogens:

- *Escherichia coli* and *Klebsiella pneumoniae* resistant to third-generation cephalosporins and carbapenems.

- Multiresistant *Staphylococcus aureus.*
- *Neisseria gonorrhoeae* with increased resistance to third-generation cephalosporins.
- Multi/extended-resistant tuberculosis.
- Malaria with resistance to artemisinin or artemisinin combination treatments.
- Drug-resistant HIV.

AI has been investigated in various ways to tackle the problem of AMR. New amino acid compounds, so-called peptides, have been recognized as potential antibiotics in situations where standard therapies have failed. AI can be used to predict the degree of antimicrobial activity of a peptide in a particular situation or setting. AI simulations and forecasts have shown excellent accuracy in differentiating between peptides with and without sufficient antimicrobial activity. In addition to evaluating known peptides for antimicrobial activity, ANNs can also assist in developing new peptides or combinations of peptides and run in silico tests or forecasts of antimicrobial activity.

Large-scale data from antimicrobial resistance surveillance systems can be preprocessed with the aid of so-called dashboards. These are data collection systems with the capacity to integrate and process large amounts of heterogeneous data, and finally produce information that can be used to make predictions, analyse trends, and guide policymaking. For example, data from surveillance systems of antimicrobial resistance within a geographical region can be collected and aggregated within a dashboard. Finally, the output can be implemented at various levels of healthcare, from the primary healthcare providers to the governmental bodies and policymakers.

AI systems can be applied to antibiotic stewardship programmes to aid clinicians in the more correct, personalized, and tailored prescription of antimicrobial treatment, while considering clinical and microbiological data. Decision-support systems can propose an antibiotic regimen based on the body temperature, infection sites, symptoms/signs, and possible antibacterial spectrum. Shen et al. constructed a model that has the ability to propose treatment based on patient symptoms, history, antibacterial spectrum, and drug–drug interactions [5]. The model was evaluated using receiver operating characteristic (ROC) analysis on randomly selected real medical records. The area under the ROC (AUROC) curve was 0.8991, demonstrating the potential that such systems may have.

AI models can reduce the utilization of antibiotics by distinguishing between symptoms caused by pathogens from non-infectious causes and systemic inflammatory response syndrome. With a random forest approach, clinical predictors can be identified, which can result in a more rapid diagnosis than standard laboratory variables.

Finally, AI algorithms can predict the development of AMR in the individual patient based on medical history, patient characteristics, and electronic health record data.

19.5 Disease Treatment

The effectiveness of any antimicrobial or antiviral treatment depends mainly on adherence to treatment, as frequent omission of treatment doses, such as in anti-retroviral therapy (ART) for HIV infection, can lead to viral resistance. Treatment of HIV is a long-term process and involves regular measurements of viral load. It is crucial to ensure that ART is taken correctly, and that adherence to treatment remains high. AI can assist physicians and patients by keeping track of adherence to ART and by motivating patients. This can be achieved by analysing refill data from pharmacies or implementing a monitoring device attached to standard medical bottles that records the time and date when the bottle is opened. Data analysis using AI can correctly predict the risk of virological failure and reduce the necessity of frequent viral load counts, thereby saving time and resources.

Sepsis is a possible complication of bacterial infection with a high mortality rate. Identifying patients at risk of development of sepsis may be difficult; however, it could have a significant impact on the mortality rate and also on the overall cost of treatment. Timely and appropriate antimicrobial treatment of sepsis is a strong predictor of survival. AI models have been developed and validated to accurately predict the onset of sepsis up to 12 hours before clinical prediction, which in turn can positively affect the onset of antibiotic treatment in this patient group. Based on a total of 65 clinical, patient history and laboratory parameters, Nemati et al. retrospectively developed the Artificial Intelligence Sepsis Expert (AISE) algorithm for early prediction of sepsis [6]. For prediction of sepsis 4–12 hours before onset, AISE achieved AUROC in the range of 0.83–0.85. Such systems could improve the mortality and overall survival rate of sepsis.

AI algorithms have been evaluated as decision-support systems to determine the optimal choice of an antibiotic or antiviral treatment regimen while considering factors such as microbial resistance, patient characteristics, demographic data, and medical history. Such clinical decision-support systems will have the ability to reduce the probability of or prevent the development of antimicrobial resistance, adverse effects, and treatment failure [1,7,8].

19.6 Conclusion

This chapter has demonstrated the potential of AI applications in the diagnosis and treatment of IDs. On a global scale, AI systems may open up new and innovative possibilities for healthcare systems to recognize ID outbreaks early, and enable more effective preventative or containment measures. However, there remain significant limitations to the real-life applications of most AI systems. Roberts et al. performed a systematic review of articles that describe new machine learning models for the diagnosis or prognosis of COVID-19 from chest X-ray or CT images [7]. In this review of more than 2000 studies, only 62 studies were included in the final analysis. None of these studies was identified by the authors as potentially useful in clinical prac-tice, due to methodological flaws or underlying bias. However, if harnessed correctly, the immense computing abilities of AI systems will have the potential to assist healthcare providers and health organizations in improving disease prognosis and outcome.

KEY INSIGHTS

- Infectious diseases continue to pose a significant threat to global health.
- AI can predict impending disease outbreaks by utilizing Big Data provided from national or international surveillance systems or even social media platforms.
- Antimicrobial resistance can have a negative impact on the prognosis of IDs.
- AI can assist in managing antimicrobial resistance by supporting clinical decisions and antibiotic stewardship programmes.

References

1. Baltazar LR, Manzanillo MG, Gaudillo J et al. Artificial intelligence on COVID-19 pneumonia detection using chest xray images. *PLOS ONE* 2021;16(10):e0257884.
2. Samareh A, Chang X, Lober WB et al. Artificial intelligence methods for surgical site infection: impacts on detection, monitoring, and decision making. *Surgical Infections* 2019;20(7):546–554. http://doi.org/10.1089/sur.2019.150.
3. Kirubarajan A, Taher A, Khan S, Masood S. Artificial intelligence in emergency medicine: a scoping review. *Journal of the American College of Emergency Physicians Open* 2020;1(6):1691–1702. https://doi.org/10.1002/emp2.12277.
4. Agrebi S, Larbi A. Use of artificial intelligence in infectious diseases. *Artificial Intelligence in Precision Health* 2020;415–438. https://doi.org/10.1016/B978-0-12-817133-2.00018-5.
5. Shen Y, Yuan K, Chen D et al. An ontology-driven clinical decision support system (IDDAP) for infectious disease diagnosis and antibiotic prescription. Artificial Intelligence in Medicine 2018;86:20–32. https://doi.org/10.1016/j.artmed.2018.01.003.
6. Nemati S, Holder A, Razmi F et al. An interpretable machine learning model for accurate prediction of sepsis in the ICU. Critical Care Medicine 2018;46(4):547–553. https://doi.org/10.1097/CCM.0000000000002936.
7. Roberts M, Driggs D, Thorpe M et al. Common pitfalls and recommendations for using machine learning to detect and prognosticate for COVID-19 using chest radiographs and CT scans. *Nature Machine Intelligence* 2021;3:199–217. https://doi.org/10.1038/s42256-021-00307-0.

For additional references and Further Reading please see www.wiley.com/go/byrne/aiinclinicalmedicine.

20

AI in Precision Medicine: The Way Forward

Prasun J. Mishra

American Association for Precision Medicine (AAPM), Belmont, CA, USA

Agility Pharmaceuticals and Precision BioPharma Inc., Belmont, CA, USA

Learning Objectives

- Understand the concept of precision medicine and AI-related applications.
- Review barriers to, and examples of, precision medicine.
- Understand the role of molecular biology (omics) in stratifying populations within precision medicine.
- Appreciate the barriers and siloes in the quest to implement precision medicine.
- See the path forward for proper implementation of precision medicine.

> *And that's why we are here today because something called precision medicine gives us one of the greatest opportunities to offer new medical breakthroughs that we have ever seen. (President Barak Obama, 2015,* `https://obamawhitehouse.archives.gov/precision-medicine`*)*

20.1 Precision Medicine: The Future of Healthcare

President Obama's words from the inauguration of the Precision Medicine Initiative (PMI) represent a defining moment in the history of medicine, as they highlighted one of the significant advances in healthcare to date: precision medicine. Precision medicine is 'an emerging approach for disease treatment and prevention that takes into account individual variability in genes, environment, and lifestyle for each person' (Precision Medicine Initiative, `https://medlineplus.gov/genetics/understanding/precisionmedicine/initiative`). Unlike the traditional one-size-fits-all approach, the precision medicine approach allows more accurate classification of patients into various subgroups based on their genetic make-up to stratify responders, non-responders, and toxic responders. The field advocates the delivery of the right drug to the right patient in the right dose by the right mechanism at the right time.

AI in Clinical Medicine: A Practical Guide for Healthcare Professionals, First Edition. Edited by Michael F. Byrne, Nasim Parsa, Alexandra T. Greenhill, Daljeet Chahal, Omer Ahmad, and Ulas Bagci.
© 2023 John Wiley & Sons Ltd. Published 2023 by John Wiley & Sons Ltd.
Companion website: www.wiley.com/go/byrne/aiinclinicalmedicine

20.1.1 Why Precision Medicine?

Today, most medical care is based on the expected response in an average patient, but we know that there is no such thing as an average patient. It is important that we move away from the one-size-fits-all paradigm towards developing more precise methods to prevent and treat diseases. Through a better understanding of the patient population, preventative and therapeutic interventions can be focused on those who will benefit, sparing the side effects for those who will not.

20.1.2 A Historical Perspective

Historically, the evolution of precision medicine began with the advent of the pharmacogenetics field, where we all studied the inherited differences in drug metabolic responses. With the rise of omics, pharmacogenetics evolved into pharmacogenomics. We studied all the many different genes and gene signatures to determine drug behaviour and to improve the efficacy of a drug. Later, the clinical application of pharmacogenomics and pharmacogenetics was referred to as tailored medicine, individualized medicine, and personalized medicine [1,2]. The term 'personalized medicine' stirred some concerns about where we would find the resources to develop customized medicines for each patient. Although it was called personalized medicine, the intention was never to create drugs or medical devices for each patient. Instead, it allowed individuals to be classified into sub-populations based on their sensibility to a specific treatment. The field eventually evolved to encompass several other factors, and hence the broader and now well-accepted moniker 'precision medicine' was coined to describe the field accurately. Today, precision medicine considers an individual's family history, medical genetics, lifestyle, and environmental factors to deliver personalized care.

20.1.3 Examples of Precision Medicine

There are many classic examples of precision medicine, as the concept is not entirely new, from testing *Braf V600* mutations before treating melanoma patients with vemurafenib to screening for *BCR-ABL* gene rearrangements before treating with imatinib (Gleevec). More recently, we are delivering T cell-specific chimeric antigen receptor T cell therapy (CAR-T) to patients. These are just a few examples of the success of precision medicine in clinical practice.

Historically, the National Research Council for National Academies was given the task of examining the field of precision medicine and providing recommendations as to where the field should be heading. In 2011, the committee recommended building a knowledge network, where data from basic molecular sciences, population sciences, and clinical discovery will be fed into information columns to create a taxonomic classification [3]. Today, several hospitals have built this integrated engine where data from computational health, digital health, ethics and engagement, omics, and imaging are being fed into a knowledge network. In this knowledge network,

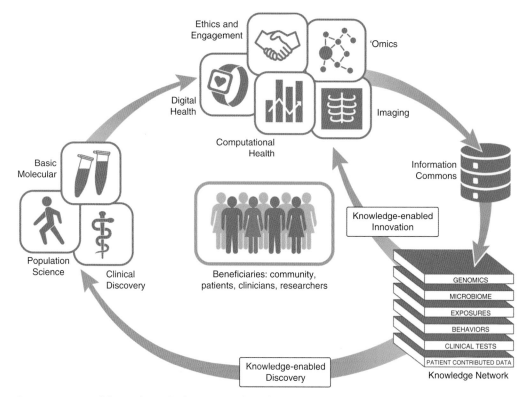

Figure 20.1: Building a knowledge network and taxonomical classifier to predict the individualized treatment options accurately.

Source: The Regents of the University of California.

various datasets such as omics, exposures, microbiome, behaviours, clinical tests, and patient-contributed data are layered. Integrated analysis is done to gain insights into integrated biology to allow for knowledge-enabled innovation. This knowledge network, in turn, also provides data for knowledge-enabled discovery, and is then utilized for basic molecular, population science, and clinical discovery to further perfect the system (see Figure 20.1).

20.1.4 Barriers and Scientific Challenges

Several barriers need to be overcome to fulfil the promise of precision medicine. A survey by PwC in 2017 identified that the top three barriers were unstable or non-secure legal and regulatory frameworks (92%), lack of access to relevant data (58%), and limited ability to integrate data sources (31%) [4].

Furthermore, there are various scientific challenges. Taking a few examples from the cancer field that has led the precision medicine revolution, the first problem is tumour heterogeneity. A patient may have many different lesions in the body, each arising from different clonal cells constituting a tumour. Also, the tumour itself is heterogeneous and is made of different clones, and other sections have a very different genomic profile [5]. The second problem is tumour evolution. Tumours in the early stages have different sets of genetic drivers. If the tumour relapses after treatment, an entirely different set of gene mutations will drive tumour growth; however, these relapse-causing mutations are present in low frequency in primary tumours [6]. This leads to anticipation-based chemotherapy in patients. The third challenge is that cancer mutations are very high in number, and mutation rates across cancers are not uniform [7].

As we learn more, our view of cancer is constantly changing. Using the example of lung cancer, we traditionally classified three kinds of lung cancer: squamous, large cell, and adenocarcinoma. Then in 1987 we learnt the role of *KRAS,* and in 2004 the role of *EGFR* gene mutations in driving lung cancer. To date, several other genes identified have included *EML4-ALK, HER2, BRAF, MET, AKT1, MAP2k1,* and *PI3KCA*. Despite this growing knowledge, much more needs to be learnt, and there are many other unknown genes yet to be discovered that drive lung cancer progression. The more we learn, the more we realize that cancers are more complex than we initially thought [8].

Another black box is the potential of the non-coding region or so-called junk DNA. It is well known that genetic variations in the non-coding region of a gene can result in over- or under-representation of the target gene, and confer drug sensitivity or resistance gain or loss of a gene function [1,2]. The majority of sequencing tests tend to ignore the non-coding regions. Another challenge is oncogene bypass [11], activating another gene when inhibiting a particular pathway. Finally, a further challenges we are facing is the accuracy and reproducibility of lab-developed tests. The Food and Drug Administration (FDA) has intervened in this, and precisionFDA focuses on developing precise drug diagnostic combinations (`https://precision.fda.gov`).

20.2 The Way Forward

With new advances and sequencing technologies, the cost and time to sequence a human genome have been dramatically reduced, and have even defied Moore's Law. We now have excellent reference genomes to align a newly sequenced genome, distinguishing signal from noise. Today, when patients are presented in the clinic, their molecular profiling includes sequencing, multi-omics, and imaging. Patients are then stratified into different groups based on their data, and assigned to personalized treatment regimens.

20.2.1 Gene Variant Analysis in the Context of Each Patient's Disease

A clinical example of patient-specific analysis to find the most appropriate therapeutic option is presented in Figure 20.2. Three patients presented themselves in the clinic; all three have mutations in a single gene, *BRAF*. The first patient is a melanoma patient with a *BRAF V600* mutation. The second and third patients are colorectal cancer patients, one with a *BRAF V600* mutation and the other with a *BRAF D594G*

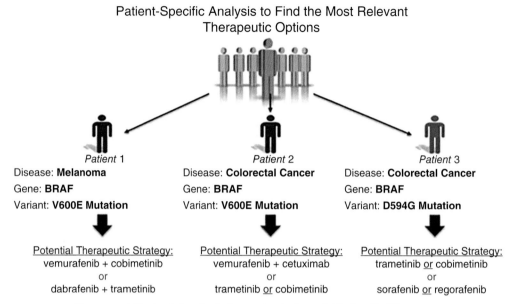

Figure 20.2: Gene variant analysis in the context of each patient's disease to suggest personalized treatment.

Source: [12]: Courtesy of Dr. Pravin Mishra.

mutation. Based on their genome profile, cancer type, and type of mutations, we can now prescribe different medications to them. For melanoma patients, treatment would be vemurafenib and cobimetinib, or dabrafenib and trametinib. For colorectal cancer patients with a *BRAF V600E* mutation, we would use vemurafenib plus cetuximab, trametinib, or cobimetinib. The colorectal cancer patient with *BRAF D914G* mutations could be treated with trametinib, cobimetinib, sorafenib, or regorafenib. This is an example of gene variant analysis in the context of each patient's disease.

20.2.2 Integrating Datasets

As per the recommendations of the National Research Council of the National Academies, we are getting better at integrating various layers of datasets, similar to Google Maps. As in Google Maps, different geographic information system (GIS) layers are now organized by geographical positioning, and similar things can be done for the omics datasets. We can integrate several layers such as exposomes, genome, epigenome, microbiome, microRNA data, imaging, and other types of patient data. Different layers can be put together to generate a better picture of the patient's disease. This has been a focus of the author's research, where we have integrated multi-omics, clinical, and real-world data together. We can create an information standard and a knowledge network to understand individual patient data better. Physicians can prescribe meaningful drugs or drug combinations to a patient so that the right medications can be prescribed to the right patients at the right time.

20.2.3 Addressing the Challenge of Data Siloes

Through the PwC survey we know that the availability of data and data integration are major barriers that we have to overcome [4]. Typically, patient data remain siloed behind different institutional firewalls. Some of this is due to safety, some to Health Insurance Portability and Accountability Act (HIPAA) compliance, and other firewalls are due to institutional policies. We have to find a way to incentivize institutions to share data in a HIPAA-compliant way, and create integrated shared datasets to further the vision of precision health. We have to encourage a consortium model of data sharing and research. One example is GA4GH, the Global Alliance for Genomics and Health, which allows data sharing and enables more collaborative research between academia, biotech pharma, and pharma companies. The consortium also governs the shared intellectual property (IP). Another example is the American Association for Precision Medicine (AAPM), which has also formed consortiums and has provided IP governance to the community to share the data and co-innovate collectively.

20.2.4 Cost and Affordability

Moving forward, the affordability and cost of precision medicine will also drive individual decisions. In order to address this we have to tap into economies of scale to bring down the prices associated with precision medicine. As a community, we have to reduce the cost associated with multi-omics. Moreover, we have to work with payers to make these tests covered/reimbursable by insurance companies so that patients can avail themselves of the benefits of precision medicine without worrying about the costs.

20.3 Benefits of Precision Medicine in the Clinical Care Pathway

Precision medicine provides multifaceted benefits at all stages of the clinical care pathway. In early clinical development, precision medicine can help identify patients who respond most appropriately to a particular therapeutic. These results can help stratify populations in later-phase trials. A precision medicine approach can enrich study populations using predictive biomarkers during patient recruitment and enrolment, which may improve efficacy signals while reducing drug development costs and timelines. Even post-approval, precision medicine insights can be used to optimize treatment decisions, and ensure that the right drug is used to treat the right patient at the right time. In this way, we can impact all three stages of the clinical care pathway – that is, prevention, diagnostics, and treatment – to deliver improved health-related outcomes and better patient health [13].

20.4 Investing in Precision Medicine–Based Drugs Is the Future of Drug Development

The pharmaceutical industry has realized that investing in precision medicine–based drugs is the future of drug development. It helps stratify a specific patient population that responds to a particular medicine. Evidence to date suggests that precision medicine–based drugs are highly likely to get approved by the FDA. Precision medicine imparts the ability to distinguish responders from non-responders or toxic responders, thereby enhancing the likelihood of success of a specific clinical trial.

Moreover, several studies have now demonstrated that precision medicine has faster approvals based on fewer and smaller trials. For example, in 2017 about 30% of new drugs or new drug approvals were precision medicine based and had some biomarker components associated with them. Furthermore, approximately 48% of the precision medicines in our study qualified for the FDA's breakthrough therapy designation [14].

Additionally, FDA approval of companion diagnostic (CDx) assays has gone up every year in the past decade [15]. The total number of approvals by the end of 2020 was 44. A complete list of over 485 unique drugs is available with pharmacogenetics in labels on the FDA website (`https://www.fda.gov/drugs/science-and-research-drugs/table-pharmacogenomic-biomarkers-drug-labeling`).

20.5 Healthcare Stakeholders and Their Role in the Success of Precision Medicine

Healthcare stakeholders have an important role to play in the success of precision medicine. Governments, policymakers, research institutions, the biomedical science community, patient advocacy groups, and regulatory bodies all have to work together to deliver the promise of precision medicine. The AAPM has, for example, taken a stand to facilitate dialogue around the four Ps of precision medicine: Predictive, Preventative, Personalized, and Participative. The patients' providers and public health planners (government and payers) must all work together to deliver improved outcomes and reduce costs.

20.6 AI, Big Data, Wearables, and Real-World Data

Advancements in data analytics, artificial intelligence, machine learning, and deep learning have recently presented a new opportunity to take precision medicine to the next level. Deep learning algorithms can now diagnose diabetic retinopathy [16] and skin cancer lesions [17] at physician-level performance. Through natural language processing, AI also integrates radiology reports with 91% accuracy [18].

Wearable devices tracking our vital health signs provide a great source of real-world data (RWD) and real-world evidence (RWE). Computers, mobile devices, wearables, and other biosensors currently gather significant amounts of health-related data. RWD holds enormous potential to diagnose and treat patients better, and also to design and conduct clinical trials and studies in the healthcare setting to answer questions previously thought infeasible. In addition, with the development of new sophisticated, AI-driven analytical capabilities, we can better analyse these complex datasets and apply the results of our analyses to medical product development and approval [19]. These technological advances are pushing the field at a rapid pace by helping with some of the data analytics challenges that we are facing in precision medicine.

The US government's *All of Us* initiative creates a research cohort of approximately one million American volunteers sharing their genetic data, biological samples, and lifestyle information, all linked to their electronic health record system (EHR). *All of Us* is pioneering a new science model that emphasizes engaged participants, responsible data sharing, and privacy protection (`https://allofus.nih.gov`). This can be a goldmine for people interested in solving the problem of what makes individuals sick in the first place.

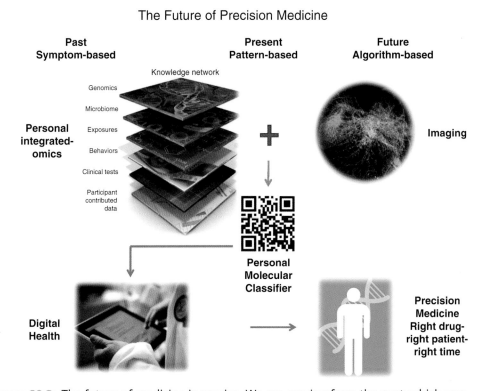

Figure 20.3: The future of medicine is precise. We are moving from the past, which was symptom-based medicine, to the present, pattern-based treatment, and towards the future, algorithm-based medicine. Courtesy of Prasun Mishra.

20.7 Future Perspective

Precision medicine's future looks bright as medicine will be specific, and inexact medicine will make its way out of routine clinical practice. We are moving from the past with symptom-based medicine, to the present with pattern-based treatment, and towards the future with algorithm-based medicine (see Figure 20.3). Soon the time will come when drugs and algorithms will be launched together. Ideally, when a patient presents in the clinic, personalized, integrated omics will be performed along with imaging. These integrated datasets can be analysed using AI tools to build a personalized molecular classifier. The classifier can be compared with existing reference datasets to create a unique treatment profile for the physician who, via digital health, can deliver the promise of precision medicine to the patient – namely, *the right drug to the right patient at the right time.*

It is important to note that safety and digital privacy need to be of the highest priority. The US Genetic Information Nondiscrimination Act (GINA) provides robust protection to Americans against discrimination based on their genetic information regarding health insurance and the environment. A law like GINA should be considered by other countries moving towards scaling up precision medicine.

KEY INSIGHTS

- ■ **The road to precision medicine has not been smooth; however, AI supports the current and future implementation of precision medicine.**
- ■ **Precision medicine has notable examples of success in oncology applications.**
- ■ **Stakeholders from across the board (patients, healthcare providers, payers, and governments) must come together to make precision medicine a reality in routine clinical practice.**
- ■ **Ethical considerations must remain one of our top priorities when working with patient data.**

References

1. Mishra PJ, Bertino JR. MicroRNA polymorphisms: the future of pharmacogenomics, molecular epidemiology and individualized medicine. *Pharmacogenomics* 2009;10(3):399–416.
2. Bertino JR, Banerjee D, Mishra PJ. Pharmacogenomics of microRNA: a miRSNP towards individualized therapy. *Pharmacogenomics* 2007;8(12):1625–1627.
3. National Research Council. *Toward Precision Medicine: Building a Knowledge Network for Biomedical Research and a New Taxonomy of Disease.* Washington, DC: National Academies Press; 2011. https://doi.org/10.17226/13284.

4. PwC. *Capitalizing on Precision Medicine*, 2017. `https://www.strategyand.pwc.com/de/en/industries/health/capitalizing-precision-medicine.html`.
5. Gerlinger M, Rowan AJ, Horswell S et al. Intratumor heterogeneity and branched evolution revealed by multiregion sequencing. New England Journal of Medicine 2012;366(10):883–892.
6. Alexandrov LB, Nik-Zainal S, Wedge DC et al. Signatures of mutational processes in human cancer. *Nature* 2013;500(7463):415–421.
7. Vogelstein B, Papadopoulos N, Velculescu VE et al. Cancer genome landscapes. *Science* 2013;339(6127):1546–1558.

For additional references and Further Reading, please see `www.wiley.com/go/byrne/aiinclinicalmedicine`.

21
AI in Paediatrics

Darren Gates and Iain Hennessey
Alder Hey Children's Hospital, Liverpool, UK

Learning Objectives

- Describe how AI can help address the shortcomings of current evidence-based practice in paediatric medicine.
- Give examples of successful AI deployments and outcomes.
- Understand some of the unique challenges for AI adoption in this field.
- Outline potential future AI applications unique to paediatrics.

21.1 Introduction

Paediatrics is one of the most difficult fields in healthcare for applying AI, due to the wide size range, unique physiology, psychology, and intellectual function of children. A prematurely born neonate weighing less than a can of soda presents a vastly different scenario to an adolescent! In addition, the relatively small dataset to train AI models, the propensity to rare diseases, increased aversion to risk when dealing with children, and reduced commercial return from paediatric applications are all factors that compound the difficulty in creating viable AI clinical tools in paediatrics. Nevertheless, in many ways paediatrics has been at the forefront of exploring the potential for AI in healthcare, driven by the inherent need to innovate in the care of such a wide spectrum of patients and diseases. The ability to make even small changes in the health and wellness of a child will have an enormous impact on the health of our future populations and must be realized.

21.2 The Use of AI in Paediatrics

A growing number of publications have described AI applications in paediatrics, particularly in the last five years (Figure 21.1).

In 2017, Kokol et al. published a bibliometric approach, tracking key themes across the last two decades [1]. Early rule-based systems were used for survival

AI in Clinical Medicine: A Practical Guide for Healthcare Professionals, First Edition. Edited by Michael F. Byrne, Nasim Parsa, Alexandra T. Greenhill, Daljeet Chahal, Omer Ahmad, and Ulas Bagci.
© 2023 John Wiley & Sons Ltd. Published 2023 by John Wiley & Sons Ltd.
Companion website: www.wiley.com/go/byrne/aiinclinicalmedicine

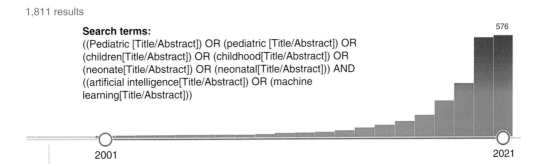

1,811 results

Search terms:
((Pediatric [Title/Abstract]) OR (pediatric [Title/Abstract]) OR
(children[Title/Abstract]) OR (childhood[Title/Abstract]) OR
(neonate[Title/Abstract]) OR (neonatal[Title/Abstract])) AND
((artificial intelligence[Title/Abstract]) OR (machine
learning[Title/Abstract]))

576

2001   2021

Figure 21.1: Results of a PubMed search, September 2021.

prediction in pre-term birth and cancer, followed by more sophisticated logistic regression models widening the focus to paediatric infection, seizures, and genetics. After 2013, machine learning techniques emerged with applications in mental health, respiratory illnesses, and epilepsy. They highlighted that the initial focus on classification has more recently shifted to predictive models. Using thematic analysis, six themes were identified, ranging from the use of AI in brain mapping to pattern recognition, developmental disorders, emergency care, and oncology gene profiling. Current work appears to focus on risk stratification and early diagnosis. As with the rest of the AI space, the biggest hurdle is still successful deployment in a clinical setting. Several paediatric institutions are, however, driving the early adoption of AI tools with direct organizational and clinical utility.

Hospital optimization projects have been shown to be low risk and easier to implement. Ehwerhemuepha et al. at the Children's Hospital of Orange County (CHOC) published their statistical learning model for unplanned seven-day readmissions at their institution [2]. They utilized features such as demographics, medications, previous history of healthcare use, severity of illness and acuity, and certain psychosocial factors to predict the risk of readmission. Their model achieved an area under the curve (AUC) of 0.778 (95% confidence interval 0.763–0.793). While most of the factors were deemed to be unmodifiable directly, the prediction is being used to facilitate discussions with parents about how readmission might be avoided and/or facilitating ongoing care for the child at home, improving their overall healthcare experience. Previous work by the same authors, to reduce 30-day readmission risk, is similar to other published works in adults that offer early return on investment by reducing any associated financial penalties.

Similar optimization tasks have been used for predicting emergency department activity and 'Was Not Brought' (used instead of 'Did Not Attend' for paediatric groups) episodes in the UK's NHS, and this is helping to address problems associated with access to healthcare. This is a unique consideration in paediatrics, as whether a patient attends an appointment is not primarily controlled by the child but by the responsible parent/guardian and may have important safeguarding implications. Tackling underlying social deprivation, with access to transport or consideration of time away from work, may also need addressing to truly improve health outcomes.

Indeed, markers of healthcare inequalities, including different types of deprivation, have frequently been the most useful features in these machine learning models. Identifying and anticipating these problems not only improves hospital efficiency, but allows caregivers to provide holistic care to the family prior to a clinical consultation.

CLINICAL VIGNETTE

Consider the challenge of monitoring a 600 g premature infant post laparotomy for necrotizing enterocolitis in the bedspace next to a 60 kg teenager following blunt abdominal trauma from a road traffic accident (Figure 21.2).

Clearly, in this paediatric intensive care unit (ICU) example, the difference in normal heart rate (ranging from 60 to 160+ bpm), blood pressure (ranging from a mean of 35 to 65 mmHg), and response to intervention will vary widely. AI algorithms aimed at spotting early deterioration will need to accommodate such heterogeneity. This is likely to require clustering of similar patients across collaborative datasets, increased fidelity of data capture, and federated learning techniques.

Progress has been made in developing data-driven alarm limits to reduce fatigue for staff in this setting, although these have yet to gain clinical acceptance and widespread adoption.

(a)   (b)

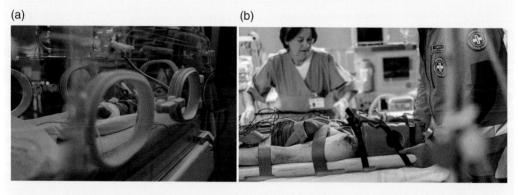

Figure 21.2: The range of patients in the paediatric intensive care unit (a) Jana Richter / Getty Images (b) Jana Richter / Getty Images.

Another route to early AI adoption is the use of digital agents to improve patient experience. The task of relieving fear and anxiety is a central tenet of paediatric practice by explaining in terms understandable to the child and family what will happen, and how we are trying to make things better. In the UK, a health and care thinktank known as The King's Fund has emphasized the essential role that improving patient experience plays in overall quality of care.

Based on this, Alder Hey Children's Hospital in Liverpool, UK, entered a research and development collaboration with the Science and Technology Foundation Council's high-precision computing facility, known as the Hartree

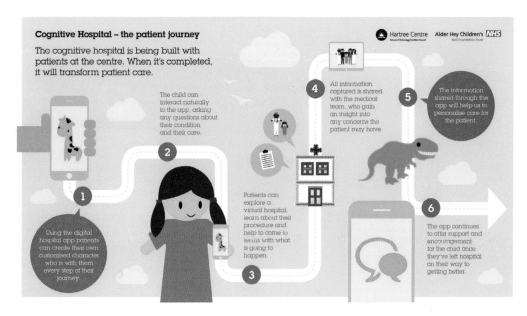

Figure 21.3: Alder Hey Innovation – cognitive hospital concept.

Centre, to develop a vision around the future 'cognitive hospital' (Figure 21.3). This imagined the potential for a hospital to 'sense' and 'feel' what was happening within it, with the ability to 'think' and 'respond' 24 hours a day, 7 days a week. The first step in this journey was to utilize the IBM Watson platform to develop an engaging chatbot known as Oli (Figure 21.4) to guide patients and families through their hospital journey. In addition to gathering the types of questions that matter most to patients, sentiment analysis can give an indication of how they are feeling, something that has been used to improve clinical pathways and patient resources.

CLINICAL VIGNETTE

When engaging with an AI agent, a child may disclose too much information or expect a response that (currently) only a human can provide. Without appropriate context, they may accept inadequate advice or fail to escalate their concerns. To build confidence in such systems, designers need to consider to which group of patients their tools are targeted, the process of onboarding and consent, the range of developmental capabilities catered for, and appropriate ways of handing over to human agents when necessary.

Early warning scores have been used in many hospitals to identify deterioration, and also to support decision-making in escalating levels of care. However, since they are currently based on population rather than patient-specific data, they are

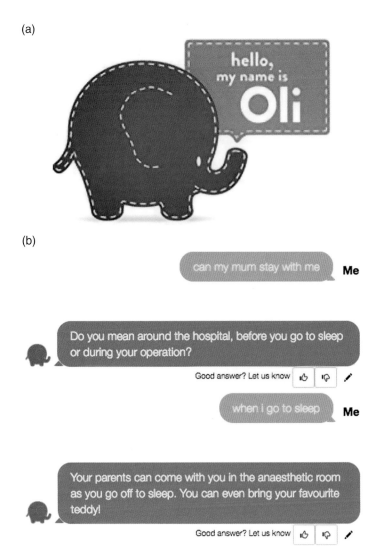

Figure 21.4: (a, b) Alder Hey Innovation – AI digital assistant.

Source: Alder Hey Children's NHS Foundation Trust.

more suited for risk adjustment to compare clinical outcomes rather than predictions for individual patients [3]. Seminal work in neonatal heart rate variability showed the potential to predict the early onset of sepsis on a patient-specific basis, with a reduction in pre-term infant mortality. The impact of increased investigations and interventions on the overall delivery of care has been evaluated in subsequent work.

In the paediatric critical care setting, other real-time predictive modelling tools have now been developed to stratify the risk of significant clinical events, such as cardiopulmonary arrest. For example, the IDO2 index, developed by Etiometry, uses a combination of known physiological mechanics and statistical models to provide a continuous risk estimation of inadequate oxygen delivery – a fundamental principle in critical care. It received US Food and Drug Administration (FDA) clearance for medical use in 2016, and it has now expanded to both neonatal and adult ICU settings. More recently, Etiometry has released a similar tool to determine the likelihood that the patient is experiencing inadequate ventilation of carbon dioxide (IVCO2 index). While early external validation showed that the tool did not perform better than an older modified Low Cardiac Output Syndrome Score, there are nonetheless several perceived benefits such as continuous availability of the prediction, baseline adjustments targeted to individual patients (selectable risk index thresholds), and explainability of the score (measurement contributions), all of which offer advantages to clinical workflow. Further validation is required to confirm clinical impact.

At the time of writing, while more than 40 AI applications are CE (Conformité Européenne) marked for thoracic radiology, none has been specifically developed for the paediatric population [4]. Transfer learning will be valuable to adapt algorithms for common tasks such as detecting pneumothorax or line positions, but the spectrum of pathology in paediatrics is different and will require specific training data for more advanced problems. Efforts to utilize AI to reduce the risk of radiation exposure have shown promising results, and are among many reasons why further focused work in this vulnerable group is required. Children are not 'mini adults', and have both a different disease spectrum and a different set of vulnerabilities in the radiological setting. Davendraligam et al. have written a comprehensive review of current and possible use cases, demonstrating how an enhanced paediatric radiology service could operate in the future [5].

While cohorts for training data are usually relatively small in paediatrics, in a paper published in *Nature Medicine*, Liang et al. demonstrated a proof-of-concept AI-based system trained on 1.4 million paediatric patient visits to diagnose common paediatric diseases [6]. Using natural language processing techniques, they built a disease classifier to predict a clinical diagnosis for each encounter by analysing the presenting complaint, history of illness, clinical examination, laboratory testing, and PACS (picture archiving and communication systems) reports, and by mimicking the hypothetical-deductive reasoning used by physicians. The F1 scores were very close to or exceeded 90%. While there is potential bias from commonly encountered conditions in the training data, this is not dissimilar to an individual physician's own bias based on personal experience, and may help to broaden their consideration of differential diagnosis given the larger dataset. Such a tool may be utilized in triage or decision support, particularly in places where access to healthcare providers is limited. However, this would need further validation about the impact on workflow and transferability to different clinical settings.

21.3 Challenges for AI in Paediatric Healthcare

There are several unique challenges for AI in paediatric healthcare. Datasets are generally smaller and more dispersed, providing consent is more complicated, and ethical considerations more nuanced. Innovation in paediatric healthcare is also relatively under-resourced, requiring advocates to drive engagement and commercial investment.

In analysing 20 national AI strategies, UNICEF found that most only make a cursory mention of children and their specific needs. While its review is larger than just healthcare, there is a clear need to promote AI that can contribute to better health outcomes without compromising children's rights. UNICEF promotes three foundations for child-centred AI that resonate well with the ambition in healthcare: (i) protection – do no harm; (ii) provision – do good; and (iii) participation – include all children. As important as the need to protect children's healthcare data from abuse is the need to share such data to benefit everyone, and to include children and young people in this shared goal.

Initiatives such as the PICU Data Collaborative at the Children's Hospital of Los Angeles (CHLA) have started to build aggregated datasets from multiple institutions to help achieve the Big Data needed to train more robust and transferable models. Similar efforts are being realized in Trusted Research Environments in Europe such as the paediatric datasets now available through the Health Data Research UK's Innovation Gateway. In recent years, PhysioNet has added new paediatric physiological signal datasets to its researcher-accessible platform. The principles of safe people, safe projects, safe setting, safe data, safe outputs, and safe return will all be crucial to maintain public confidence as paediatric AI applications diversify.

Paediatricians are very used to the concept of the 'art of medicine', applying the often sparsely available evidence to individual patients. Frequently, this involves drawing on the knowledge of experienced physicians who have seen similar scenarios before. AI offers the ability to encapsulate such knowledge from large datasets and make it accessible to a wider group of colleagues, but, for it to be acceptable to many paediatricians, it will need to clearly demonstrate how it facilitates this valued process. Similarly, the wider sociotechnical aspects of deployment are particularly important in paediatric healthcare. Clinical interactions and workflow are often more complex, involving multidisciplinary teams, parents/guardians, and children in various parts of decision-making. To support wider adoption, those developing AI tools need to consider how to make them explainable to each member of this diverse group.

It is perhaps surprising to learn that 'rare diseases' disproportionately affect children, with approximately 80% having an underlying genetic or genomic cause. The World Economic Forum has estimated that one in three paediatric hospital beds is occupied by children with a rare disease. However, the genotypes and phenotypes are diverse, with cases distributed across the globe. This exemplifies the problem of relying on local experience or evidence-based medicine drawn from small cohorts of patients to guide care. Integrated data sources and federated learning systems have been proposed to overcome the geographical barriers in these cases, and to reap the diagnostic, clinical, and personal benefits of advancing AI techniques in orphan diseases. The burgeoning potential of AI applications in the field of genomics will arguably have its greatest impact within neonatal and paediatric care.

The turning point came when he was diagnosed with an ultra-rare genetic variant, thanks to the 100,000 Genomes Project in England. There is no recognized treatment [yet], but suddenly we have a means of finding other families like ours. Most of them live thousands of miles away, but at least we are now able to find out more about what may lie ahead. (Parent of a son with a rare disease, quoted in World Economic Forum White Paper 'Solving Rare Disease Report 2020', www.weforum.org)

21.4 Future Directions

It is anticipated that AI in paediatrics will continue to impact healthcare delivery and patient experience ahead of the gradual development of more clinical bedside tools. New insights into determinants of health, subtypes of chronic conditions such as asthma, diabetes, or obesity, and methods to engage and empower young people in their care are expected in the short to medium term. Unique problems in paediatrics such as safeguarding and violence against children are particularly valuable areas for future work.

With only an estimated 500 children's hospitals internationally, resolving data sharing and processing is critical to empowering AI development at scale in paediatrics. Edge computing, federated learning, and swarm learning techniques will enable the level of data privacy and security required for organizations to collaborate, including across sociopolitical boundaries. New architectures to capture and store information, such as the patient digital twin (a virtual representation of a physical object or system such as a patient), will be a further leap forward to facilitate wider research and innovation.

KEY INSIGHTS

- **The spectrum of disease affecting children and young people is different to that of adults, demanding focused AI development to harness its potential.**
- **The heterogeneity of data and relatively small cohorts for training are key challenges to overcome.**
- **Rare diseases disproportionately affect children, and AI techniques and genomics are finally helping to address this issue.**
- **Future impact is expected from edge computing, federated learning, and digital twin technologies.**

References

1. Kokol P, Završnik J, Blažun Vošner H. Artificial intelligence and pediatrics: a synthetic mini review. *Pediatric Dimensions* 2017;2(4). https://doi.org/10.15761/PD.1000155.
2. Ehwerhemuepha L, Pugh K, Grant A et al. A statistical-learning model for unplanned 7-day readmission in pediatrics. *Hospital Pediatrics* 2020;10(1):43–51.

3. Olive MK, Owens GE. Current monitoring and innovative predictive modeling to improve care in the pediatric cardiac intensive care unit. *Translational Pediatrics* 2018;7(2):120–128.

4. Schalekamp S, Klein WM, van Leeuwen KG. Current and emerging artificial intelligence applications in chest imaging: a pediatric perspective. *Pediatric Radiology* 2021. https:// doi.org/10.1007/s00247-021-05146-0.

5. Davendralingam N, Sebire NJ, Arthurs OJ, Shelmerdine SC. Artificial intelligence in pae-diatric radiology: future opportunities. *British Journal of Radiology* 2021;94(1117):20200975.

6. Liang H, Tsui BY, Ni H et al. Evaluation and accurate diagnoses of pediatric diseases using artificial intelligence. *Nature Medicine* 2019;25(3):433–438.

For Further Reading please see www.wiley.com/go/byrne/aiinclinicalmedicine.

22

AI Applications in Rheumatology

Sarah Quidwai[1], Colm Kirby[1], and Grainne Murphy[2]

[1] *Department of Rheumatology, Tallaght University Hospital, Dublin, Ireland*

[2] *Department of Rheumatology, Cork University Hospital, Cork, Ireland*

Learning Objectives

- Appreciate the growing scope for use of machine learning in rheumatological diseases.
- Understand the limitations of clinical examination and the role of imaging and radiology in diagnosing and monitoring rheumatic musculoskeletal disease.
- Know the limitations of novel machine learning techniques and their applications to clinical medicine.
- Appreciate the promising use of AI in future practice as seen in the current literature.

22.1 Introduction

Rheumatology is undoubtedly one of the most rapidly evolving specialties within medicine. Recent advances in diagnostic imaging modalities and treatment paradigms have transformed a number of rheumatological diagnoses from what were once rapidly debilitating diseases into more benign entities. Novel imaging techniques have aided in the rapid diagnosis of inflammatory arthritis, while a variety of biological therapies have revolutionised patient outcomes. However, there remains a huge unmet need in terms of diagnostics and disease monitoring for a large cohort of rheumatology patients.

Determining disease activity has profound implications when deciding on the choice of treatment for individual patients, while identification of tissue damage has huge prognostic value. The presence of synovitis and tenosynovitis is hugely significant in patients with rheumatoid arthritis (RA), but clinical examination can lack sensitivity in this regard. Likewise, the presence of skin lesions in systemic sclerosis (SSc) identifies not only those who have active disease, but also those who will likely progress to end-organ damage. Here again, however, clinical examination lacks sensitivity.

Progress has been made in these areas in recent years. For example, in the ideal 'Treat-to-Target' (T2T) clinic model, where treatment is escalated until a certain

AI in Clinical Medicine: A Practical Guide for Healthcare Professionals, First Edition. Edited by Michael F. Byrne, Nasim Parsa, Alexandra T. Greenhill, Daljeet Chahal, Omer Ahmad, and Ulas Bagci.
© 2023 John Wiley & Sons Ltd. Published 2023 by John Wiley & Sons Ltd.
Companion website: www.wiley.com/go/byrne/aiinclinicalmedicine

disease activity threshold is met, bedside musculoskeletal ultrasound is used. This imaging tool will identify subclinical synovitis and tenosynovitis (Figure 22.1) and is cheap, readily available, and well tolerated. Tissue damage in the form of bone erosions can also be easily seen and signifies a patient who has had untreated, active disease. Additionally, ultrasound now supersedes temporal artery biopsy as the most sensitive tool for diagnosing giant cell arteritis (Figure 22.2). However, ultrasound is user dependent and highly variable between practitioners based on training, experience, and the quality of the ultrasound device being used. This all serves to create inconsistencies with image interpretation. These inconsistencies do not relate to ultrasound alone and can be observed in the interpretation of magnetic resonance images (MRI) and computed tomography (CT) images too. While most MRI and CT scans are reported by a general radiologist, multidisciplinary meetings involving specialist musculoskeletal radiologists will often provide a new interpretation of these same images. Finally, acquiring the requisite skill set to reliably interpret ultrasound, MRI, and CT requires significant investment of both time and money.

With this in mind, there is clearly potential for expanding the role of technology in rheumatology – in particular, the incorporation of AI into routine daily practice. Advances in graphic processors, digitalization of large sets of data, artificial neural networks, and machine learning are creating an environment of digitalized care that can overcome two substantial barriers to effective healthcare: namely, time and distance [1]. Machine learning is one of the most exciting areas in AI whereby

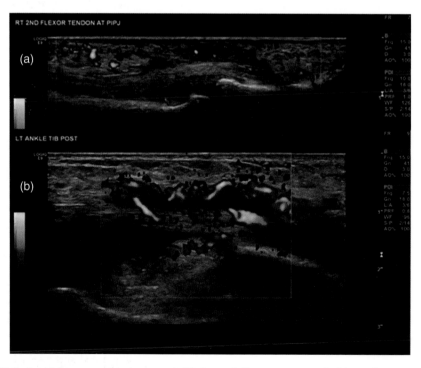

Figure 22.1: (a, b) Sonographic tenosynovitis in an inflammatory arthritis patient. Courtesy of Kirby.

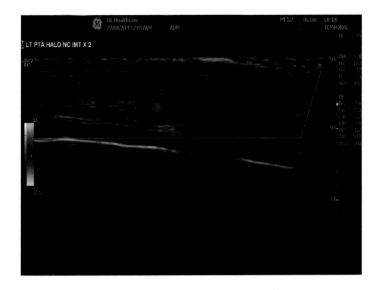

Figure 22.2: Superficial temporal artery ultrasound scan with a positive 'halo' sign, suggestive of vasculitis. Courtesy of Kirby.

machines not only undergo formal reasoning, but also improve and get 'smarter' over time. Machine learning aims to create predictive algorithmic models from data that unmask latent associations, however complex.

Rheumatology comprises a group of heterogenous multisystem disorders in which complex interactions between multiple environmental and genetic factors affect disease development and progression [2]. Applications for machine learning in rheumatology are many and are providing greater scope for precision medicine to be practised. Currently in the literature we see its use in predicting disease activity in RA patients, diagnosing synovitis and tenosynovitis on MRI, diagnosing hyaline cartilage damage on ultrasound, and potential future applications in other diseases such as SSc. In this chapter we explore machine learning and its applications in rheumatology.

22.2 Inflammation

In daily clinical practice, image interpretation is mostly performed by the physician. This is a time-consuming process that is often slowed down by physician experience and technical difficulties, so there is huge potential for incorporating AI methods. Although semi-automatic applications assist in diagnosis, machine learning allows all diagnostic steps in radiology to occur together, leading to greater consistency, while also saving time and eliminating user bias [3]. Convolutional neural networks (CNNs) are types of machine learning that contain layers of interpretation of the variables within an image (Figure 22.3).

In RA, these methods can be applied to detect disease activity in the form of synovitis and bone marrow oedema. This was first attempted using contrast-enhanced MRI to diagnose synovitis and tenosynovitis, whereby the presence and intensity of inflammatory lesion signalling can be used to automatically generate a perfusion map that both diagnoses the presence of, and quantifies the extent of, inflammation [3].

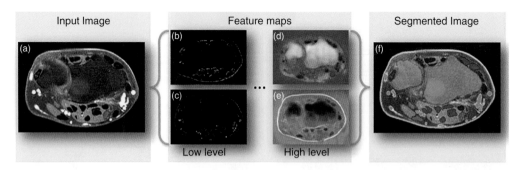

Figure 22.3: Axial magnetic resonance imaging of wrist (a) processed by a convolutional neural network (CNN), which creates 'feature maps'. It enhances transitions from dark to bright (b) or bright to dark (c) and identifies higher-level structures such as bone (d) and skin (e). Finally, the CNN combines all information into a single labelled output image (f). Courtesy of Aizenberg [5].

Tripoliti et al. showed a sensitivity of 97% in correctly diagnosing the presence of inflammation in the hand using T1-weighted MRI images, concluding that image intensity registration, mapped with time sequence, can detect synovitis and its severity with a high degree of accuracy [4]. In detecting tenosynovitis of the wrist using MRI, Aizenberg et al. concluded in their 500-patient cohort that quantitative automatic measurement using machine learning is largely consistent with visual scores, with Pearson correlation (r) of 0.90 (p < 0.0001) [5]. Another study explored the use of AI in diagnosing inflammatory tissue in the hands of patients with RA. Using contrast-enhanced T1-weighted MRI, a positive predictive ratio (PPR) of 97.71% was reported, suggesting that this automated method performs well and has high detection accuracy [4]. Limitations of these studies included the occurrence of false positives, attributed to the presence of blood vessels, and the identification of old inflammation [3]. Moving forward, it is hoped that machine learning can be applied in the realm of monitoring disease progression and damage accrual by mapping changes in synovitis and erosions over time [3].

22.3 Damage

AI is also useful for detecting damage in the form of erosions and cartilage loss. In detecting bony erosions in patients with RA, algorithms characterize the outlines of trabecular bones, comparing their shape to healthy bones. Deep learning can be applied here to determine deviations on X-rays and CT from normal parameters. CNNs can also be applied to quantify cartilage loss in RA patients using X-rays, CT, and ultrasound [3].

Recently, in diagnosing joint damage, the use of ultrasound has been shown to be more sensitive than conventional radiology. X-ray imaging assesses narrowing of the joint space, but it cannot directly visualize the hyaline cartilage. Although this is the most widely used form of imaging, for this reason its accuracy in non-weight-bearing joints such as hands and wrists has been challenged [6]. Ultrasound

(a)   (b)

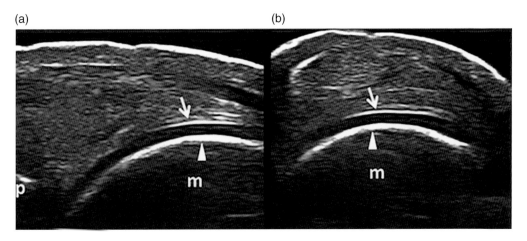

Figure 22.4: Dorsal longitudinal (a) and transverse (b) scans of the hyaline cartilage of the second metacarpal head in a healthy subject. Courtesy of Cippolletta [6].

is an excellent tool in clinical decision-making as real-time images can be obtained, identifying musculoskeletal abnormalities.

However, even with ultrasound, there are many limitations to be considered, as inter-observer bias and operator-dependent technique can decrease accuracy. AI can mitigate the potential for this by standardizing image acquisition and increasing reliability [6]. Interestingly, Cippolletta et al. developed a CNN using European League Against Rheumatism (EULAR) standardized ultrasound scans of the hyaline cartilage on metacarpal heads (Figure 22.4). The algorithm model was produced to analyse videos, not images, to reflect real-time ultrasound, and there was almost perfect replication of results between the AI algorithm and an expert sonographer's diagnosis. While not yet feasible in clinical practice, it is envisaged that incorporation of algorithms into ultrasound systems will lead to faster and more accurate diagnosis of musculoskeletal disease [6].

22.4 Disease Activity

Another useful application of AI has been in predicting disease activity in patients with RA. While certain parameters such as antibody positivity and baseline radiographic damage can help predict which patients are likelier to have a more aggressive disease course, disease activity is measured periodically at outpatient visits and only then are treatment strategies tailored accordingly. Norgeot et al. applied deep learning AI methods to predict disease activity in RA using data from the American College of Rheumatology's Rheumatology Informatics System for Effectiveness registry [7]. These data reported that 42% of patients nationally had moderate or high disease activity at their most recent visit, as measured using the Clinical Disease Activity Index [7]. Firstly, the algorithm was designed to predict a patient's most recent disease activity using demographics, inflammatory markers, and clinical features. Next, the algorithm predicted the likelihood of switching activity categories by analysing previous patterns, and within the training data this was 25%. Importantly, the model was incorrect for only 2 of the 117 patients in this study, suggesting that AI could be reliably used as a tool to make decisions regarding treatment augmentation at an earlier time point. Similarly, another algorithm using machine learning was developed to predict remission at one year in 1,204 RA patients treated with biological therapy, and accuracy ranged from 52.8% to 72.9% [8]. Together, these results suggest that deep learning models can be successfully trained to accurately predict outcomes in RA. Were these results to be reproduced in further studies, the impact could potentially be ground-breaking in the realm of personalized and individualized care, and it is likely that patient outcomes in terms of disease activity and damage accrual would substantially improve.

AI can help to create a more accurate diagnosis when multiple variables need to be considered. Variables such as symptoms, examination findings, inflammatory markers, antibody status, and radiographic findings can differ significantly between individuals with the same underlying diagnosis. A common example would be a middle-aged female who presents with psoriasis, nail pitting, and florid dactylitis in the setting of mildly raised inflammatory markers. In such a case, a diagnosis of seronegative spondyloarthropathy is reasonably straightforward, but let us compare it to another common presentation of the same disease whereby a middle-aged female presents with a seronegative polyarthralgia, unremarkable physical examination, and normal inflammatory markers. This second patient can often be initially diagnosed as having fibromyalgia, whereas in fact the underlying diagnosis is again a seronegative spondyloarthropathy, but this time presenting with predominant enthesitis.

Reed et al. developed a screening tool based on AI methods analysing a photographic image of a patient's hands, using a nine-part clinical history questionnaire and a single examination to determine the diagnosis. In this study, the algorithm was developed from 1,000 previous X-ray images of hands, and machine learning was applied to the questionnaire results. Several models were 'trained' against a rheumatologist's diagnosis, and the results were ultimately compared to a rheumatologist's diagnosis following a 45-minute consultation. The combined algorithm was able to predict inflammatory arthritis with accuracy, precision, recall, and specificity of 96.8%, 97.2%, 98.6%, and 90.5%, respectively [9].

22.5 Systemic Sclerosis

In systemic sclerosis, we are seeing a wider application of AI in recent years. Skin thickness in systemic sclerosis is considered a surrogate for disease activity, and worsening thickness generally correlates with progressing disease and multi-organ involvement. In theory, different modalities such as ultrasound, CT, and MRI (Figure 22.5) can automatically detect skin thickness directly from imaging, in stark contrast to the traditional gold standard of clinical examination, which can lack sensitivity and varies considerably between physicians. While datasets for skin fibrosis

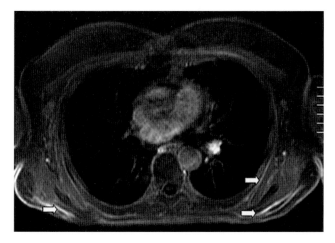

Figure 22.5: Axial post-gadolinium fat-saturated T1-weighted magnetic resonance image showing marked generalized fascial thickening (arrows) and marked gadolinium enhancement in torso due to inflammation and collagen deposition. Courtesy of Schanz [10].

(a)   (b)   (c)

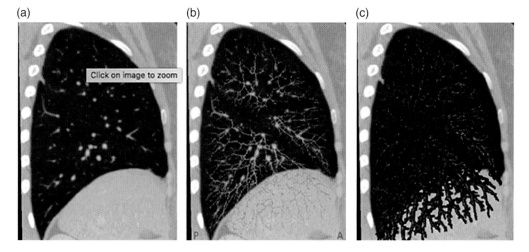

Figure 22.6: (a–c) Classification into arteries and veins using deep learning. Courtesy of Stoel [3].

require further standardization, they are likely to supersede the Modified Rodnan Skin Score, which has numerous caveats including user variability and inaccuracies due to oedema and ethnic differences [3].

New proposed areas of interest are automatic detection of vasculopathy and fibrosis, the pathological hallmarks of this multisystem disease [3]. Nailfold capillaroscopy is used to identify abnormalities in the microvasculature, and while loop width and capillary density are quantifiable by human observers, tortuosity and texture are less so. CT can identify vasculopathy by detecting abnormalities in the pulmonary vessels through quantification of the number of small and large vessels (Figure 22.6), which seems to correlate with functional impairment. Both of these imaging modalities appear to provide significant scope for implementing AI methods, as is the case with interstitial lung disease (ILD). In ILD, machine learning can be applied to automatically detect fibrosis using lung densitometry, a parameter that correlates with declining lung function [3].

Pulmonary arterial hypertension (PAH) secondary to systemic sclerosis has been shown to have a one-year mortality of up to 30%, and median survival of two to three years, if left untreated. Time from symptom onset to diagnosis is a median of two years. Introduction of a predictive algorithm using echocardiogram, pulmonary function tests, and biomarkers such as urate and NT-proBNP (N-terminal pro b-type natriuretic peptide) eliminated this diagnostic delay in the Sheffield Pulmonary Hypertension Index Project and significantly improved patient outcomes [11]. In this study, 589 of 127,815 patients were identified as having probable PAH. Of patients in the early detection cohort, 100% were alive at one year compared with 75% who were diagnosed using routine clinical practice. Survival rates at three, five, and eight years of 81%, 73%, and 64%, respectively, were seen in the screening cohort compared with 31%, 25%, and 17%, respectively, in the unscreened cohort [11].

22.6 Limitations and Future Perspectives

As a new and evolving concept, there are many limitations with the use of AI. Creating an artificial neural network is a tedious and time-consuming process. Different variables and input data need to be carefully and manually labelled with specialist input for accurate and reliable algorithmic models, and these systems too often need testing and cross-validation. The shortcomings in AI have been most starkly highlighted with IBM's 'Watson for Oncology', which had 18–98% variability in recommending treatment plans when compared to a board of oncologists. This can lead to potentially unsafe and ineffective treatment plans, and this further highlights the importance of appropriate standardization checks.

In an increasingly digitalized world, datasets are growing rapidly and AI offers a solution to analysing multidimensional data including patient histories, laboratory results, treatment, and outcomes. In an article exploring Big Data analysis techniques in rheumatic and muscular diseases (RMDs), AI methods were used in 18% of RMDs, with machine learning accounting for 97% of these AI methods [12]. Big data remain controversial, however, often conflicting with ethical principles of privacy and confidentiality.

A new era of predictive analytics and precision medicine is paving the way to the future of healthcare, helping clinicians, healthcare systems, and policymakers [2]. Further research exploring the strengths and weaknesses of AI and its role in longitudinal patient care is awaited. There will undoubtedly be a paradigm shift in how we will practise; rheumatology with machine learning will likely hasten the introduction of personalized medicine. Identification of disease activity and damage, and predictive therapeutic decisions based on forecasted disease activity scores, are likely just the beginning. Algorithmic models that will identify appropriate biological therapies for individual patients would revolutionize our approach to daily practice, result in substantial cost savings, and almost certainly improve patient outcomes.

KEY INSIGHTS

- ▪ **AI has many current applications in rheumatology.**
- ▪ **In RA, machine learning can diagnose inflammation and damage with a high degree of accuracy.**
- ▪ **In SSc, AI can quantify and monitor skin fibrosis, vasculopathy, and PAH.**
- ▪ **AI processes can save time and money and improve patient outcomes and experience.**
- ▪ **Future applications of machine learning in rheumatology potentially include real-time ultrasound interpretation and early detection of PAH in systemic sclerosis.**

References

1. Kataria S, Ravindran V. Digital health: a new dimension in rheumatology patient care. *Rheumatology International* 2018;38(11):1949–1957.
2. Kim KJ, Tagkopoulos I. Application of machine learning in rheumatic disease research. *Korean Journal of Internal Medicine* 2019;34(4):708–722.
3. Stoel B. Use of artificial intelligence in imaging in rheumatology – current status and future perspectives. *RMD Open* 2020;6(1):e001063.
4. Cipolletta E, Fiorentino MC, Moccia S et al. Artificial intelligence for ultrasound informative image selection of metacarpal head cartilage. A pilot study. *Frontiers in Medicine* 2021;8:589197.
5. Reed M, Le Souëf T, Rampono E. A pilot study of a machine-learning tool to assist in the diagnosis of hand arthritis. *Internal Medicine Journal* 2020;52(6):959–967.
6. Norgeot B, Glicksberg BS, Trupin L et al. Assessment of a deep learning model based on electronic health record data to forecast clinical outcomes in patients with rheumatoid arthritis. *JAMA Network Open* 2019;2(3):e190606.
7. Kedra J, Radstake T, Pandit A et al. Current status of use of big data and artificial intelligence in RMDs: a systematic literature review informing EULAR recommendations. *RMD Open* 2019;5(2):e001004.

For additional references please see www.wiley.com/go/byrne/aiinclinical medicine.

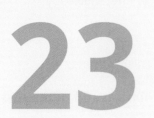

23

Perspectives on AI in Anaesthesiology

Vesela Kovacheva

Division of Obstetric Anesthesia, Department of Anesthesiology, Perioperative and Pain Medicine, Brigham and Women's Hospital, Boston, MA, USA

Harvard Medical School, Boston, MA, USA

Learning Objectives

- ▦ Describe opportunities to introduce AI technologies in anaesthesiology.
- ▦ Select the features of an AI model that are relevant for the anaesthesiologist.
- ▦ Provide examples of existing models used in peri-operative care.
- ▦ Outline the directions of future research and innovation in AI technologies for anaesthesiology.

23.1 Introduction

Anaesthesiology is a medical specialty that focuses on peri-operative patient care before, during, and after surgery. Anaesthesiologists are often involved in high-stakes medical decision-making in acute care settings. This requires a knowledge base of intensive care medicine, anaesthesiology, and pain medicine, and also the ability to analyse information from multiple patient monitoring sources. Implementing AI models can facilitate an anaesthesiologist's performance in several aspects such as pre-operative risk stratification, intra-operative maintenance of anaesthesia, and prevention of post-operative complications (Figure 23.1). Recently, several companies and institutions have worked to harness the power of AI technologies in the field of anaesthesiology and, as a result, the adoption of AI in this field is anticipated to rapidly expand in the near future.

23.2 AI in Peri-operative Patient Risk Stratification

Pre-operative planning includes the process of evaluation and optimization of patients for surgical procedures. Accurate prediction of surgical risks is needed to plan pre-operative optimization, surgical approach, and the anticipated recovery time. The American Society of Anesthesiologists' (ASA) physical status score was originally developed for statistical purposes, but is commonly used pre-operatively, and is predictive of population-based mortality. Although this score has been

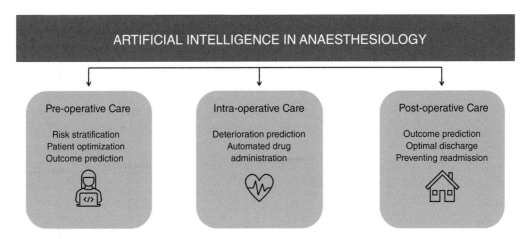

Figure 23.1: Opportunities for integration of AI technologies in anaesthesiology. These include pre-operative, intra-operative, and post-operative care.

Source: Vesela Kovacheva.

demonstrated to correlate relatively well with surgical outcomes, it does not consider several important patient-related parameters such as age, sex, and conditions such as pregnancy [1]. In addition, it does not consider the surgery type and approach. AI models have the potential to facilitate this process by incorporating the relevant patient factors and integrating information from electronic health records (EHRs). Using the EHRs of 53,000 patients, a highly precise machine learning model was able to predict the post-operative mortality with an area under the curve (AUC) of 0.93 that outperformed the ASA (AUC 0.74) and the Charlson Comorbidity Scores (AUC 0.86) [2]. A major advantage of models such as this is the immediate incorporation of predictive patient variables directly from the patient's medical record. The longitudinal integration with EHRs during the hospital admission would permit the addition of intra-operative data such as blood transfusions and hypotension episodes that can be immediately utilized to increase prediction accuracy. The ability to continuously receive real-time data would permit the model to update surgical risk predictions while in clinical use. ASA guidelines for pre-operative testing and treatment can also be incorporated into these models, optimizing evidence-based decision support by recommending the most relevant tests or strategies for patient care. This concurrent reporting may potentially save costs by avoiding unnecessary testing as well.

Future efforts need to focus on developing evidence-based decision-support systems on the best approaches for pre-operative patient optimization in order to improve surgical outcomes.

23.3 AI in intra-operative Management

During this time, the anaesthesiologist's attention is focused on maintaining an optimal level of sedation while monitoring several parameters such as blood pressure, heart rate, and fluid status. At this stage, AI tools can help by identifying deviations of these parameters from the target, and suggesting optimal interventions.

Avoiding intra-operative hypotension is critical, as even a short period of hypotension can be associated with a substantial risk of adverse events such as acute kidney injury and myocardial infarction, resulting in poor surgical outcomes and even mortality. Several machine learning models have been developed to predict intra-operative hypotension. Hatib et al. developed an algorithm that predicted the patient's risk of developing hypotension (defined as mean arterial pressure less than 65 mmHg) within the next 15 minutes [3]. The model was developed by using the data from 1334 high-fidelity arterial line waveform forms, including the subtle changes in variability, complexity, and physiological associations in the arterial pressure waveform that are undetectable to the human eye. When the model was tested on an independent group of 350 patients, it was able to predict an upcoming hypotensive event with an AUC of 0.95. This AI model is a part of a commercially available device, which is US Food and Drug Administration (FDA) approved and used in clinical practice. A randomized control trial was done on this AI algorithm that included 31 patients who had this AI model as a part of their intra-operative management and 29 control patients. The first group experienced a significantly shorter hypotension period (median 8 vs 33 minutes, $p < 0.001$) and fewer severe hypotensive events (0 vs 2) [4]. One disadvantage of using the arterial waveform is that it cannot be utilized in patients with waveform variances, including those who are breathing spontaneously or who are experiencing cardiac arrythmias. For widespread acceptance, the AI models must be compatible with the multitude of anaesthesia monitoring devices currently in use. A potential future direction will be the development of similar algorithms using routine or non-invasive devices, and coupling those with decision-support systems.

23.4 AI in Post-operative Management and Discharge Planning

In this stage, AI technologies can help by predicting post-operative complications such as pneumonia, deep venous thromboembolism, and wound infections, and facilitate discharge by predicting the discharge barriers.

In a recent study, an AI model was developed to predict the need for post-operative opioid prescription by integrating the pre- and intra-operative data from 5503 patients who underwent total hip arthroplasty [5]. The factors utilized for the prediction of prolonged post-operative opioid use were age, duration of opioid exposure, pre-operative haemoglobin, and pre-operative medications such as antidepressants, benzodiazepines, non-steroidal anti-inflammatory drugs, and beta-2 agonists. The elastic-net penalized logistic regression model achieved the best performance across discrimination (C-statistic = 0.77), calibration, and decision curve analysis. AI models such as this can be integrated into EHRs and identify patients who have high-risk patterns for opioid misuse. This may allow the anaesthesiologist to select non-opioid modes for anaesthesia and prompt the physician to include the patient in a post-operative opioid surveillance programme.

AI models can also facilitate the discharge process by early identification of patients who are ready to be discharged, and also by identifying discharge barriers. In a recent study, a machine learning model was developed to identify patients who would be ready for discharge within 24 hours and their discharge barriers [6]. This model was trained on a dataset of 15,201 patients and was compared with a baseline model using historical median length of stay to predict discharges. The model's estimated out-of-sample AUC was 0.84, and it had a higher sensitivity (52.5% vs 56.6%) and specificity (51.7% vs 82.6%) compared to the baseline model. Moreover, this model identified 65 barriers to discharge. From the group of patients who were not discharged owing to variation in clinical practice and non-clinical reasons, 128 bed-days, or 1.2 beds per day, were classified as avoidable.

23.5 Imaging and Technical Skills Aid

AI models can be utilized to augment and supplement expertise in areas of limited resources. Tools, such as an AI-enabled ultrasound [7] can help novice anaesthesiologists to perform fast and accurate intra-operative echocardiograms To develop this device, convolutional neural network models were trained and evaluated for multiple tasks using 14,035 echocardiograms obtained over a 10-year period. The model was able to compute automated ejection fraction and longitudinal strain measurements that were comparable or even superior to the manual measurements across 11 internal consistency metrics such as left atrial and ventricular volumes. AI models such as this can enable the delivery of high-quality care in regions where a specialty-trained anaesthesiologist is not available. Similar AI-enabled imaging models can be developed to identify landmarks for regional anaesthesia, and to aid in vascular access, significantly augmenting the skills of the anaesthesiologist.

23.6 Conclusion

AI is an emerging technology with great potential to augment the skills of anaesthesiologists in pre-, intra-, and post-operative settings. To be widely adopted into clinical practice, AI models need to be highly efficient, relevant, and fully integrated into the physician workflow. In such a way, the anaesthesiologist's expertise can be greatly augmented to enhance patient safety, prevent complications, and improve patient health outcomes.

KEY INSIGHTS

- **AI technologies in anaesthesiology hold tremendous potential and can integrate into all stages of peri-operative care.**
- **Pre-operatively, AI tools can accurately predict the patient's risk of complications.**

- Intra-operative decision-support AI tools can aid in personalized drug administration.
- Post-operatively, AI technologies can aid in discharge planning and optimal recovery.
- Future integration of AI models into clinical practice would enhance patient safety and improve health outcomes.

Conflicts of Interest

Vesela Kovacheva reports grants from the Foundation for Anesthesia Education and Research (FAER), Partners Innovation, Brigham Research Institute, and Connors Center First.in.Women Precision Medicine Platform, as well as consulting fees from Avania CRO.

References

1. Horvath B, Kloesel B, Todd MM, Cole DJ, Prielipp RC. The evolution, current value, and future of the American Society of Anesthesiologists Physical Status classification system. *Anesthesiology* 2021;135(5):904–919.
2. Hill BL, Brown R, Gabel E et al. An automated machine learning-based model predicts postoperative mortality using readily-extractable preoperative electronic health record data. *British Journal of Anaesthesia* 2019;123(6):877–886.
3. Hatib F, Jian Z, Buddi S et al. Machine-learning algorithm to predict hypotension based on high-fidelity arterial pressure waveform analysis. *Anesthesiology* 2018; 129(4):663–674.
4. Wijnberge M, Geerts BF, Hol L et al. Effect of a machine learning-derived early warning system for intraoperative hypotension vs standard care on depth and duration of intra-operative hypotension during elective noncardiac surgery: the HYPE randomized clinical trial. *JAMA* 2020;323(11):1052–1060.
5. Karhade AV, Schwab JH, Bedair HS. Development of machine learning algorithms for prediction of sustained postoperative opioid prescriptions after total hip arthroplasty. *Journal of Arthroplasty* 2019;34(10):2272–2277.e1.
6. Safavi KC, Khaniyev T, Copenhaver M et al. Development and validation of a machine learning model to aid discharge processes for inpatient surgical care. *JAMA Network Open* 2019;2(12):e1917221.
7. Zhang J, Gajjala S, Agrawal P et al. Fully automated echocardiogram interpretation in clinical practice. *Circulation* 2018;138(16):1623–1635.

For Further Reading please see www.wiley.com/go/byrne/aiinclinicalmedicine.

24

AI in Ear, Nose, and Throat

Jesús Rogel-Salazar[1,2,3] and Krishan Ramdoo[1,4,5]

[1] Tympa Health Technologies Ltd, London, UK

[2] Blackett Laboratory, Department of Physics, Imperial College London, London, UK

[3] Department of Physics, Astronomy and Mathematics, School of Physics, Engineering and Computer Science, University of Hertfordshire, Hatfield, UK

[4] Division of Surgery and Interventional Sciences, University College London, London, UK

[5] Royal Free Hospital, London, UK

Learning Objectives

- Gain a perspective of the state of the art in AI for ear, nose, and throat (ENT) practitioners.
- Understand current applications and the future impact of AI in ENT.
- Understand the capabilities and limitations of AI in ENT.

24.1 Introduction

Machine learning is a subset of AI focused on building applications that learn from data and improve their accuracy over time without being programmed to do so [1]. In general, the majority of the applications for ENT to which we will refer in this chapter are firmly on the machine learning side, and hence we will use the term machine learning in this chapter and AI only when it is most appropriate.

24.2 Ear, Nose, and Throat

The ability to collect data from various sources is crucial for the development of high-performance AI technologies in ENT. In the past 30 years, AI has been applied to the analysis of radiological images, audiometric data, and even the performance of cochlear implants. A review of some of these advances is presented by Crowson et al. [2], specifically for head and neck surgery. In their review, they comment on the dramatic increases in novel applications of machine learning to the ENT field in the last five years, on the promise of such applications, and also on the challenges with the implementation of machine learning tools.

AI in Clinical Medicine: A Practical Guide for Healthcare Professionals, First Edition. Edited by Michael F. Byrne, Nasim Parsa, Alexandra T. Greenhill, Daljeet Chahal, Omer Ahmad, and Ulas Bagci.
© 2023 John Wiley & Sons Ltd. Published 2023 by John Wiley & Sons Ltd.
Companion website: www.wiley.com/go/byrne/aiinclinicalmedicine

24.3 Ear

Data collection is an important step in building an AI model. In a recent study, the use of smart phone otoscopes was evaluated for the improvement of the medical learning environment, not only for training purposes but also to modernize image capture [3].

AI can also help physicians recognize conditions of the ear, and streamline referrals to specialists. By applying convolutional neural network architectures [4] with transfer learning techniques, the authors of this chapter are in the process of creating an AI model for detection of the tympanic membrane (TM) and the middle ear (Figure 24.1). The initial model provides a view of what the model considers to be (a) normal or (b) abnormal. It is then up to an ENT specialist to utilize this information in order to make the diagnosis. This work opens up the possibility of creating models that range from classification of normal versus abnormal images to the detection of more specific ailments [5–7].

In the post-operative setting, machine learning models can be used to identify factors that can influence the performance of cochlear implants [8]. Other areas include the optimization of hearing aids [9], diagnosis of vestibular disorders [10], and speech enhancement and intelligibility [11].

Another use of machine learning in ENT is for the capture of information for patient records during an examination. For example, the authors have developed standard questionnaires to capture otological patient histories. The use of natural language processing [4] can help analyse these data, and thus provide structured

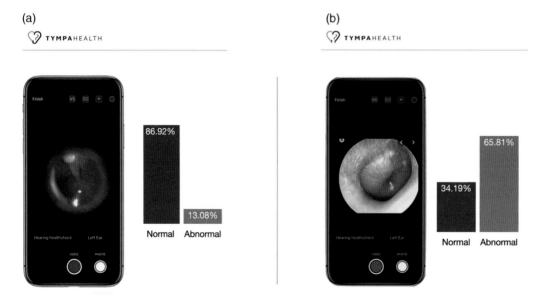

Figure 24.1: Assistive diagnostics performed by AI models created by TympaHealth to support the detection of normal and abnormal tympanic membrane and ear canal images. (a) The outcome for a typical normal image. (b) The outcome for a potential abnormality.

information to generate clinical decisions that can guide ENT specialists as well as other healthcare practitioners.

Building on studies like the ones mentioned, machine learning technology is effectively embedded into processes and platforms for the ear, improving diagnostic capabilities and ultimately hopefully improving patient outcomes. In the future, we may be able to potentially identify ear conditions by examining blood vessels on the tympanic membrane, in a similar way to how ophthalmologists can detect diabetic and hypertensive eye disease from the architecture of the blood vessels in the retina. This approach holds great promise, but whether it can be done is yet to be determined.

24.4 Nose

The application of AI in rhinology imaging techniques can be used to profile the anatomy of a given patient and to support pre-operative planning. Computer tomography (CT) is prone to errors [12], and this is an area where AI can be of support. Machine vision techniques have been successfully applied to the automatic classification of paranasal sinus anatomy, and have been shown to improve its interpretation. For example, the use of transfer learning has enabled the creation of a model to classify osteomeatal complex inflammation with an accuracy of 85% [13]. In another study, a deep learning system was used to analyse the maxillary sinus for the detection of maxillary sinusitis. The accuracy of the model was reported to be 87.5%, and the results were similar to the analyses by radiologists [14].

Another application of AI is to create a greater understanding of human olfaction and sensitivity to certain drugs. Areas of study include the physiology of pattern-based odour detection and recognition processes [15], the development of complex disease biomarkers including olfactory features [16], and odour prediction from physico-chemical properties of volatile molecules [17]. A recent study employed the use of unsupervised machine learning analysis to examine the use of aspirin for sinusitis [18]. In this case, clustering analysis divided patients into five groups based on their symptoms, and the symptoms were also compared before and after endoscopic sinus surgery for chronic rhinosinusitis. The group with the highest symptom score exhibited faster symptom improvement after surgery. Moderate non-sinonasal and mild sinonasal clusters were also reported to be associated with a lack of aspirin-sensitive history.

Healthcare trends show a move to community healthcare delivery, with specialist support provided only when needed. Conditions such as allergic rhinitis, which affects 26% of the UK adult population [19], impose a large burden on multiple secondary care rhinology clinics. A study being conducted at University College London is examining whether a rhinology history, image of the nasal mucosa, and an allergy test performed in the community would allow a patient to be treated remotely without the need to attend an initial secondary care appointment. *The role of machine learning here would be to link this information together to provide assistive diagnosis and to eventually identify specific conditions in the nose, such as rhinitis, rhinosinusitis, and polyps.* This would help with service efficiency, as the first-line treatment for patients is very simple, namely the use of nasal sprays or drops.

Since Reichert performed the first endonasal sinus surgery with a 7 mm endoscope in 1901 [20], there have been many advances in rhinology. The use of AI is expanding the capability to reach a safer and more accurate diagnosis, and better surgery outcomes, as well as a better understanding of human olfaction.

24.5 Throat

In the case of laryngology, an expert system was recently developed to assist in the diagnosis of common problems such as scratchy, burning, raw, dry, tender, or irritated throat [21]. This enables laryngologists to differentiate common throat diseases, ranging from those that are easy to recover from to others that could potentially be very harmful, such as cancers. Although a rule-based methodology may not be as advanced as supervised machine learning models, it is an excellent way to start capturing relevant information that can be used upstream in data labelling and even in testing other methods.

With recent advances in radiographical and histopathological images used in the diagnosis of cancer tissue, it has been a natural progression to use techniques such as deep learning for the assessment of breast [22] or lung tissue [23], among others. AI is now being used to classify head and neck cancers. Not surprisingly, AI is being applied to the detection of thyroid follicular lesions using supervised learning [24]. Hyperspectral imaging (HSI) is being used to train a neural network model for the detection of normal and malignant tissue areas [25]. This is a spectroscopy-based imaging modality that relies on the collection of various images at different wavelengths for the same spatial field. HSI is non-invasive and has been used in the diagnosis of diseases such as diabetic retinopathy [26]. The neural network model used for head and neck cancer achieved 96% accuracy. Although high accuracies are not the only important factor in the deployment of an AI model, the authors mention that their proposed method shows encouraging results in artifact detection and quality assessment.

AI advances have also improved vocalization analysis and viewing the vocal folds through flexible nasendoscopy and stroboscopy. As an example, vocal cord waveform disruption can be used to predict glottic malignancies [27]. In this case, a neural network model was trained to distinguish between normal and T1a glottic carcinoma vocal cord wave morphologies based on video stroboscopic images. The neural network was able to discern vibratory measures from video samples that deserved further investigation, and correctly identified malignant vocal cord pathology with 100% sensitivity and 100% specificity. If flexible naso-endoscopy could be taught to non-specialists, this would significantly reduce the cancer diagnostic waiting times.

24.6 The Future of AI in ENT

Despite significant challenges in the adoption of AI and machine learning systems, these technologies have substantial potential for transforming the field of ENT. The application of AI in clinical settings, including ENT, requires partnership between clinicians and technologists. To continue this journey into the future, it is important to consider the education and training of healthcare workforces for a digital future [28]. Another area that requires further consideration is maintaining the privacy of patient health information, balanced with machine learning and the need for large amounts of data. Finally, it is important to tackle the perception that algorithms will replace medical and clinical staff. *We firmly believe that AI advances in ENT will assist and enable healthcare professionals in continuing doing what they do best: namely, caring for patients with a human touch.*

KEY INSIGHTS

- **The application of AI in clinical settings, including ENT, requires clinicians to partner with technologists. ENT specialists should consider the opportunities to collaborate with data scientists to tackle the most relevant clinical questions.**
- **AI and machine learning support a trend to community healthcare delivery in ENT, with specialist support provided only when needed. For example, the development of models may support the early diagnosis and treatment of many common ear problems in the community, and permit accurate patient triaging for more complex issues.**
- **AI can enable the amalgamation of larger heterogeneous datasets available in ENT together with clinical expertise to improve diagnostic, treatment, and research outcomes.**
- **AI is expanding the capability to reach a safer and more accurate diagnosis, and to obtain better surgical outcomes in ENT.**

References

1. Rogel-Salazar J. *Data Science and Analytics with Python*. London: CRC Press; 2017.
2. Crowson MG, Ranisau J, Eskander A et al. A contemporary review of machine learning in otolaryngology—head and neck surgery. *Laryngoscope* 2020;130(1):45–51.
3. Schuster-Bruce JR, Ali A, Van M et al. A randomised trial to assess the educational benefit of a smartphone otoscope in undergraduate medical training. *European Archives of Oto-Rhino-Laryngology* 2020;278:1799–1804. https://doi.org/10.1007/s00405-020-06373-1.

4. Rogel-Salazar J. *Advanced Data Science and Analytics with Python.* London: CRC Press; 2020.
5. Khan M, Kwon S, Choo J et al. Automatic detection of tympanic membrane and middle ear infection from oto-endoscopic images via convolutional neural networks. *Neural Networks* 2020;126:384–394.
6. Lee J, Choi S, Chung J. Automated classification of the tympanic membrane using a convolutional neural network. *Applied Sciences* 2019;9(9):1827.
7. Tran T, Fang T, Pham V et al. Development of an automatic diagnostic algorithm for pediatric otitis media. *Otology & Neurotology* 2018;39(8):1060–1065.

For additional references and Further Reading please see www.wiley.com/go/byrne/aiinclinicalmedicine

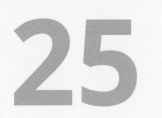

25

AI in Obstetrics and Gynaecology

Sam Mathewlynn[1,2] and Lucy Mackillop[1,2,3]

[1] Oxford University Hospitals NHS Foundation Trust, Oxford, UK

[2] Nuffield Department of Women's and Reproductive Health, University of Oxford, Oxford, UK

[3] EMIS Group plc, Leeds, UK

Learning Objectives

- Describe the status of AI development within obstetrics and gynaecology.
- Appreciate the breadth of applications of AI within obstetrics and gynaecology.
- Discuss the impact, or potential future impact, of AI on clinical care delivery within obstetrics and gynaecology.

25.1 Introduction

Both obstetrics and gynaecology are broad fields in themselves, each encompassing several sub-specialties, with numerous niches in which AI can contribute, and already has contributed, towards a changing model of care. The volume and pace of work are such that each of these areas could, in most cases, easily fill its own chapter. Consequently, the examples presented here provide an overview of AI within women's health, but do not constitute an exhaustive or detailed review.

25.2 Reproductive Medicine

The use of assisted reproduction techniques (ART) such as in vitro fertilization (IVF) or intracytoplasmic semen injection (ICSI) are increasingly common, not only to overcome subfertility, but also to address social factors, such as supporting fertility for same-sex couples. In any case, the creation and selection of a high-quality embryo are paramount to a successful procedure. There are several stages at which AI may be able to optimize the process.

25.2.1 Oocyte Selection

The selection of viable or 'competent' oocytes is key to the success of ART. In a murine model, Cavalera et al. have used a feed-forward artificial neural network (ANN) to identify competent oocytes from cytoplasmic movement analysis with an accuracy of 91%, with the potential for translation to human medicine [1].

AI in Clinical Medicine: A Practical Guide for Healthcare Professionals, First Edition. Edited by Michael F. Byrne, Nasim Parsa, Alexandra T. Greenhill, Daljeet Chahal, Omer Ahmad, and Ulas Bagci.
© 2023 John Wiley & Sons Ltd. Published 2023 by John Wiley & Sons Ltd.
Companion website: www.wiley.com/go/byrne/aiinclinicalmedicine

25.2.2 Semen Analysis

Semen analysis includes assessment of the number, motility, and morphology of sperm, usually by a highly skilled operator, but computer-aided semen analysis (CASA) is likely an area where AI will increasingly be employed. For example, Goodson et al. have shown that support vector machines (SVMs) can be used to classify human sperm into one of five motility classes based on their kinetic parameters with an overall accuracy of 89.9%, which may facilitate high-throughput analysis [2].

25.2.3 Viable Embryo Selection

Fundamental to the success of ART is the selection of a viable embryo for implantation, usually by visual inspection at the blastocyst stage. Carrasco et al. analysed 800 human embryos with known implantation data cultured in an incubator with a time-lapse system. Using a decision tree based on a recursive algorithm, they were able to select the embryos with the highest implantation potential based on morphokinetic parameters [3].

25.2.4 Assisted Reproduction Technique Outcome Prediction

ART can be an emotionally fraught process with significant health and financial implications. Provision of accurate statistics regarding the likelihood of success would help service users to make more informed decisions and would help clinicians tailor treatment to give the best chances of success. To this end, attempts have been made to predict ART outcomes using AI. Arguably the most successful strategy is presented by Güvenir et al., who achieved predictive accuracy of 84.4% using the RIMARC (ranking instances by maximizing the area under the receiver operating characteristic [ROC] curve) machine learning algorithm [4].

25.2.5 Apps for Menstrual Tracking and Ovulation Prediction

There are several consumer smart phone apps that employ AI methods to assist with menstrual tracking and prediction of ovulation, potentially providing more personalized guidance than traditional calendar-based methods. The Flo app, for example, predicts ovulation from self-entered menstrual and symptom data, and the company's website reports that this method may be up to 54.2% more accurate than conventional methods [5]. Similarly Mira, a system combining a smart phone app with an at-home hormone profile analyser, is reported by the company to be able to accurately detect a fertile window up to five days prior to ovulation [6]. Both of these examples utilize proprietary machine learning algorithms, but the specific techniques and algorithms used do not appear to be in the public domain at the time of writing. This illustrates a potential pitfall in AI advancement: progress in this field may be driven by industry, and yet may circumvent the conventional path of publication and peer review, arguably an important safety check in medical progress.

The variety and number of products available mean that it is difficult to generalize about user experience or reception among clinicians. However, an in-depth review of 85 eligible apps along with 138 publications has highlighted potential concerns around data privacy and methodological transparency, as well as problematic and potentially exclusionary assumptions about the identity and sexuality of users reflected in the design and marketing of menstrual tracking and fertility apps [7].

25.3 Early Pregnancy

An estimated 15–20% of clinically evident pregnancies end in miscarriage, and ectopic pregnancy remains an important cause of morbidity and mortality worldwide. As such, the field of early pregnancy is an important target for improvement through AI methodologies.

25.3.1 Ectopic Pregnancy

Surgical, medical, or even expectant management of ectopic pregnancy may be appropriate depending on the circumstances. De Ramon Fernandez et al. developed several decision-support models using AI methodologies to assist clinicians with the choice of initial treatment, based on prediction of which treatment would ultimately be required. The greatest accuracy, sensitivity, and specificity were achieved with a three-stage classifier SVM, yielding 96.1%, 96%, and 98%, respectively. This has the potential to reduce unsuccessful attempts at medical or expectant management [8].

25.3.2 Recurrent Miscarriage

Recurrent miscarriage, conventionally defined as three consecutive miscarriages, is often deeply traumatic for women and their families, as well as representing a diagnostic challenge since it can have several aetiologies. AI techniques have been applied to this problem by Bruno et al., who aimed to stratify patients into risk classes using an SVM machine learning algorithm, in order then to direct them towards the correct therapeutic approach. They were able to achieve accuracy of 81.9% using inputs of 43 different features, thus demonstrating a proof of concept for the future use of AI in the investigation and management of recurrent miscarriage [9].

25.4 Antenatal Care

The delivery of appropriate care during pregnancy is an important determinant of maternal and perinatal outcomes. This includes a range of approaches, including screening for pregnancy complications, attempts to predict adverse events, and the management of pre-existing or evolving conditions (such as diabetes mellitus or hypertensive disorders of pregnancy). Antenatal care therefore affords many opportunities for AI to play a role.

25.4.1　Screening for Chromosomal Abnormalities

Screening for chromosomal and genetic abnormalities in early pregnancy allows the selection of patients for invasive testing (amniocentesis or chorionic villus sampling), proactive management of the identified condition, as well as affording women the choice about whether to continue or terminate the pregnancy.

Neocleous et al. demonstrated that AI could offer an alternative method of predicting trisomy 21 and other aneuploidies. Using a multilayer feed-forward ANN with an input of ultrasound and biochemical markers at 11–13 weeks' gestation, they were able to achieve sensitivity and specificity for trisomy 21 of 97.1% and 99.5%, respectively. This represents an improvement compared with more traditional statistical methods such as the 'combined test', which can detect about 90% of cases with a false-positive rate of approximately 5%. Therefore, AI has the potential to reduce the need for invasive testing, which inherently carries some degree of risk for the mother and baby [10].

Non-invasive prenatal diagnosis (NIPD), based on the detection of cell-free foetal DNA (cffDNA) in maternal blood, is a relatively new technique that represents a low-risk alternative to invasive testing in some circumstances. Uses of NIPD include the detection of trisomy, foetal sex determination, and rhesus D genotyping. The ability to use NIPD for the detection of single-gene disorders would enhance its utility and further reduce the need for invasive tests. Rabinowitz et al. applied a Bayesian machine learning approach and were able to achieve NIPD of monogenic diseases. They were able to further improve on accuracy by accounting for differences in the length distribution of cffDNA fragments and were the first to predict insertion–deletions. This work represents the basis for the development of comprehensive NIPD for a wide range of monogenic diseases [11].

25.4.2　Prediction of Pre-eclampsia

Pre-eclampsia remains a major cause of maternal and foetal morbidity and mortality worldwide. The risk factors for pre-eclampsia are well established, and the traditional method of risk assessment (based on binary risk factors) allows counselling, enhanced monitoring, and commencement of aspirin prophylaxis in higher-risk individuals. This method has sensitivity of approximately 77% and specificity of 54% [12].

Jhee et al. constructed several models for the prediction of late-onset pre-eclampsia using different AI techniques. The best results were achieved with stochastic gradient boosting, which gave an accuracy of 97.3% and false positive of 0.9%, using inputs of maternal factors and commonly available antenatal laboratory data [13]. The prediction of early-onset pre-eclampsia has also been addressed by Maric et al., who considered 67 variables and used an elastic net algorithm, achieving an area under the curve of 0.89 with a true-positive rate of 72.3% and false-positive rate of 8.8% [14].

The clinical validation of these methods has the potential to transform the way in which women are risk assessed and counselled for this important condition.

25.4.3 Prediction of Gestational Diabetes Mellitus

Gestational diabetes mellitus (GDM) is an important diagnosis since it is associated with adverse perinatal outcomes, including stillbirth, and has long-term implications for maternal health such as increased risk of type 2 diabetes mellitus in later life. Screening for GDM, usually with a glucose tolerance test, is generally offered at approximately 24–28 weeks' gestation to those with the presence of binary risk factors, but AI may allow for earlier and more accurate diagnosis. For example, in a retrospective analysis of 588,622 pregnancies, Artzi et al. were able to use a machine learning approach to predict GDM with an area under the curve of 0.85. This was true even at the beginning of pregnancy, which could allow for much earlier intervention and may prove cost-effective by reducing the need for glucose tolerance tests in lower-risk groups [15].

25.4.4 Prediction of Preterm Birth

Preterm birth is an important cause of perinatal morbidity and mortality, and attempts have been made at its prediction using AI methodologies. For example, Gao et al. used electronic health record data from 25,689 deliveries and a recurrent neural network to predict preterm birth, achieving an area under the curve of 0.827. Further, using this model they were able to predict preterm birth up to eight weeks before it occurred [16]. Bahado-Singh et al. evaluated six different machine learning techniques, including deep learning, for prediction of preterm birth <24 weeks' gestation among asymptomatic women with cervical shortening (<15 mm). Their input data included proteomics, metabolomics, and ultrasound data, and they were able to achieve an area under the curve of 0.89 [17].

The application of models such as these to clinical practice has the potential to reduce preterm birth and its associated morbidity and mortality, since interventions such as progesterone supplementation and cervical cerclage have been shown to be effective.

25.4.5 Stillbirth Prediction

Prediction and prevention of stillbirth are core tenets of antenatal care, but research in this area is beset with challenges, such as relatively low event rates and the fact that datasets likely include live births that would have resulted in stillbirths were it not for timely delivery (the 'treatment paradox'). This is an area where AI methodologies have the potential to be particularly impactful, and some attempts have already been made.

For example, Malacova et al. used national birth data from Australia over a 35-year period to build several predictive models for stillbirth using machine learning techniques. The best-performing classifier (XGBoost) was able to predict 45% of stillbirths [18].

Koivu and Sairanen used almost 16 million observations to build their models, which included ANN and gradient-boosting decision tree techniques. They were able to achieve an area under the curve of 0.76 for early stillbirth and 0.63 for late stillbirth, and the authors suggest that the predictive power of these tools could be further improved by the inclusion of biochemical or biophysical markers [19].

25.5 Pregnancy Ultrasonography

Ultrasound examination of the foetus is a cornerstone of antenatal care: pregnancy dating, aneuploidy risk assessment, monitoring of foetal growth, and identification of foetal abnormalities are among its many uses. Skilled operators are required, and even with experienced sonographers there is often an element of subjectivity in the selection of an image or placement of callipers and so on. There are many ways in which AI could be applied to this field, from identification and quality control of image planes to construction of reference charts. Some examples are presented here.

25.5.1 Foetal and Placental Segmentation

Foetal segmentation, or the identification of foetal anatomical structures on ultrasound, is at best semi-automatic and often entirely manual. This is time-consuming, may be technically challenging, and there is often inter-observer variability. AI may provide a solution to these issues. For example, Namburete et al. were able to use a convoluted neural network to localize the foetal brain and segment anatomical structures from three-dimensional ultrasound images. Similar approaches have also been used to segment other anatomical planes [23]. There is also a growing body of work highlighting the potential significance of first-trimester placental volume and vascularity in the prediction of adverse outcomes [24]. For these parameters to have clinical utility, automation and reproducibility are key. There are several AI tools available to assist with assessment of the first-trimester placenta, such as the OxNNet convoluted neural network, which can perform fully automated real-time placental segmentation from three-dimensional images [25].

25.5.2 Identification of Foetal Abnormalities on Ultrasound

Xie et al. have shown that deep learning algorithms can be used not only for segmentation of the foetal brain, but also for the binary classification of brain ultrasound images as normal or abnormal. Using standard sonographic planes, they were able to achieve an overall accuracy of 96.3%. This lays the foundation for the identification of extra-cranial abnormalities using similar techniques [26].

25.5.3 Construction of Growth Charts

There are numerous references for foetal growth in use, and an ongoing debate about the relative merits and pitfalls of prescriptive, descriptive, or customized approaches. AI may represent an entirely new means of assessing foetal growth that might make these discussions redundant and, most importantly, improve prediction of adverse outcomes.

Naimi et al. used several different AI methodologies (including random forests, Bayesian additive regression trees, and generalized boosted models) to predict estimated foetal weight from data available at birth. They propose that this be used to recover missing estimated foetal weight information in population birth records, the lack of which is a problem in epidemiological research (particularly at early gestations). This raises the possibility of AI being used in future to construct antenatal growth charts themselves [27].

25.5.4 Gestational Age Estimation in Late Pregnancy

Accurate estimation of gestational age is essential to allow for appropriate antenatal care and timely intervention. Pregnancies are usually dated from measurement of the crown–rump length (CRL) in the first trimester, except in cases of in vitro fertilization where the date of embryo transfer is known. Where CRL has not been measured in the first trimester, gestational age can be estimated either from the date of the last menstrual period (if known), or from biometric measurements (such as head circumference) taken later in pregnancy. The former is sometimes unknown or uncertain, the latter problematic due to variations in growth later in pregnancy, which may lead to under- or over-estimation of gestational age. Papageorghiou et al. used a machine learning algorithm, the 'Genetic Algorithm', to assess >64,000 combinations of potential combinations of biometric parameters to create polynomial equations to predict gestational age – an approach that would not be feasible without AI. The most accurate predictions of gestational age were achieved using a novel equation incorporating second-trimester head circumference and femur length measurement [28].

25.6 Foetal Heart Rate Monitoring

Cardiotocography (CTG), the monitoring of variations in foetal heart rate, is a key test of foetal well-being used both antenatally and during labour. Despite the availability of several guidelines, the interpretation of CTG can sometimes be difficult. Failure to recognize abnormal patterns can have devastating consequences and has important medico-legal implications. Electronic tools have been developed to assist with CTG interpretation, such as the Dawes–Redman system, but the development of AI may further assist clinicians in the identification of cases at greater risk of adverse outcomes.

25.6.1 Antenatal Cardiotocography

Foetal growth restriction (FGR), the failure of a foetus to achieve its growth potential, is associated with stillbirth and other adverse perinatal outcomes. Antenatal diagnosis of FGR is essential in order to reduce the risk of such outcomes, and a consensus definition has been developed based on a constellation of ultrasound markers [29]. Targeted ultrasound assessment of pregnancies at greater risk of FGR is contentious, and better tools are needed to identify those at risk.

One possible solution is proposed by Signorini et al., who tested the performance of 15 machine learning techniques in the binary classification of foetuses as healthy or FGR, based on a single antenatal CTG recording. The best results were achieved using the random forests method, which gave a mean classification accuracy of 0.911. This raises the possibility that CTG could be used as a screening test to identify those pregnancies requiring further ultrasound assessment and surveillance [30].

25.6.2 Intrapartum Cardiotocography

AI methodology has also been applied to the interpretation of intrapartum CTG. For example, Warrick et al. used a database of healthy and pathological cases (those with arterial blood gas derangement or those with neurological deficit at birth) to train SVM classifiers. They were able to identify 50% of cases deemed pathological, with a false-positive rate of 7.5% [31].

Other groups have had greater success. For example, Fergus et al. used CTG data, maternal age, umbilical cord gas data, and Apgar scores to classify normal vaginal and caesarean section deliveries using several machine learning algorithms. The greatest sensitivity and specificity were achieved with a deep learning approach (94% and 91%, respectively, with area under the curve of 99%) [32]. However, a systematic review and meta-analysis compared visual CTG assessment with AI, including three randomized control trials and six cohort studies. AI was not shown to reduce the incidence of adverse perinatal outcomes compared with visual assessment, and inter-rater reliability was moderate, with Cohen's kappa of 0.49 (0.32–0.66) [33].

The K2 INFANT® system (K2 Medical Systems, Plymouth, UK) is one example of a commercially available CTG interpretation tool and is based on numerical algorithms involving a database of over 400 rules and a small ANN [34]. Although a large randomized control trial has not shown this system to improve clinical outcomes for mothers or babies [35], the continued development of AI in this area is of great academic, clinical, and commercial interest. It is probable that significant advances in the field of foetal heart rate monitoring will be seen in the near future.

25.7 Intrapartum Care

The ability to accurately predict intra-partum complications allows for advanced planning to facilitate safer birth and, in some cases, to offer early delivery or delivery by pre-labour caesarean section. These decisions can have profound implications, and so using AI to improve predictive accuracy is an attractive prospect.

25.7.1 Shoulder Dystocia

Shoulder dystocia can result in serious complications for babies, including brachial plexus injuries, fractures, hypoxic brain injury, and death. Appropriate prediction and counselling about mode and timing of birth therefore have important clinical and medico-legal implications.

Tsur et al. developed a machine learning model for prediction of shoulder dystocia based on foetal ultrasound biometry and maternal risk factors, with an area under the curve of 0.75. They showed this to be significantly better at predicting shoulder dystocia than the currently used risk factors of estimated foetal weight and the presence of maternal diabetes [20].

25.7.2 Post-partum Haemorrhage

Post-partum haemorrhage (PPH) is a major cause of maternal morbidity and mortality. Prediction of those at risk of PPH allows for preventative and precautionary measures to be taken, such as active management of the third stage of labour or cross-matching of blood in anticipation of blood transfusion being required.

Venkatesh et al. built several machine learning models to predict blood loss >1 L based on an input of 55 different risk factors and a dataset containing >150,000 births. The best prediction was achieved with an extreme gradient-boosting model that had a C-statistic of 0.93. This could form part of future risk assessment strategies and be used to inform the making of birth plans [21].

25.7.3 Prediction of Successful Vaginal Birth after Caesarean Section

Women who have had a previous caesarean section may opt for vaginal birth in future pregnancies. Attempting vaginal birth after caesarean section (VBAC) has a number of advantages, but may also confer a significant risk of adverse events such as emergency caesarean section or scar rupture. Lipscheutz et al. have shown that machine learning techniques can be used to create a personalized risk score for a successful VBAC, and such tools that can help with the prediction of adverse events may help empower women to make better-informed decisions [22].

25.8 Postnatal Care

The postnatal period is one of enormous physical and emotional adjustment for new mothers, during which time women remain at risk of a number of pregnancy-related complications such as pre-eclampsia, venous thromboembolism, and mental health disturbance. The application of AI to this aspect of women's health seems somewhat limited so far, despite its importance. However, one condition of particular interest where AI has been applied is postnatal depression (PND).

25.8.1 Postnatal Depression

Postnatal Depression (PND) is a relatively common health issue affecting women in the postnatal period. Most cases will recover if the right support and treatment are offered, but sadly maternal suicide remains a significant cause of maternal mortality, accounting for 17% of maternal deaths in the first year after a pregnancy (`https://www.npeu.ox.ac.uk/assets/downloads/mbrrace-uk/reports/maternal-report-2020/MBRRACE-UK_Maternal_Report_Dec_2020_v10_ONLINE_VERSION_1404.pdf`). In a retrospective cohort study, Shin et al. have used a machine learning approach to develop nine different predictive models for PND. The greatest success was achieved using a random forest technique, which gave an area under the ROC curve of 0.884, demonstrating that machine learning approaches may have utility in the prediction of PND, thereby facilitating targeted intervention [36].

25.9 Menopause

Menopause and the climacteric can have a significant physical and emotional impact, and AI has been employed to better understand and manage this transition. For example, Ryu et al. used five different machine learning models to analyse the factors associated with development of vasomotor symptoms, identifying several important contributors that might form part of a decision-support system [37]. Lee et al. used an intelligent data-mining model to analyse the relationship between hormone replacement therapy (HRT) and breast cancer, often a particular concern for those commencing HRT, and were able to identify particular phenotypes that may be at greater risk [38].

Compared with menstrual tracking and ovulation prediction, there are far fewer consumer apps to assist those going through menopause. One notable example though is the Caria app, which incorporates an AI chat assistant with which users can interact to access personalized health data, insights, and recommendations.

25.10 Gynaeoncology

Gynaecological malignancy remains an important cause of morbidity and mortality among women worldwide. In most cases, early diagnosis and prompt intervention are key to minimizing long-term sequelae, including mortality. There are many examples of AI applied to this field and only a small selection can be presented here.

There is also a significant body of work relating to the interpretation of ultrasound, computer tomography (CT), and magnetic resonance imaging (MRI) using AI, much of which has relevance to the diagnosis or staging of gynaecological malignancies [39–50]. However, in the interests of brevity, topics relating to radiology in the context of gynaecological malignancy are not discussed here in detail.

25.10.1 Cancer Screening

Cervical cytology (a 'Pap test' or 'smear test'), along with screening for human papillomavirus (HPV) infection, forms the basis of screening for cervical intraepithelial neoplasia (CIN), and this is the most widely employed screening strategy for any gynaecological malignancy. There are numerous reports of the use of AI to assist with cytological image analysis [51–53]. Machine learning has also been applied to HPV typing data, combined with various biomarkers, to predict CIN2 or greater with an accuracy of 81.4% [54].

AI may yet facilitate screening for other gynaecological cancers too. For example, Makris et al. have shown that it is possible to predict endometrial malignancy and hyperplasia from cytological analysis, with an accuracy of 90% using an automated system based on a deep learning model, and Troisi et al. used machine learning methods to assess the serum, with a diagnostic accuracy of 99% for the presence or absence of endometrial cancer [55, 56]. However, it is important to consider that there may be other practical barriers to the use of these methods for screening despite the promise of AI.

25.10.2 Further Investigation of Suspected Malignancy

25.10.2.1 Colposcopy

AI has been used to assist with colposcopic image analysis, an important step in the diagnosis of cervical malignancy. For example, Xue et al. used images from 19,435 cases to develop a deep learning–based system for diagnosis at colposcopy and to facilitate guided biopsy. The results of AI-guided biopsies were more accurate than those that were guided by the operator alone (82.2% vs 65.9%) [57].

25.10.2.2 Hysteroscopy

Hysteroscopic assessment of the endometrial cavity is used to assist in diagnosis of endometrial cancer and facilitate targeted biopsy, but visual assessment of the cavity may be subjective, and targeted biopsies are only useful if taken from the right areas. It may be possible to improve upon the diagnostic accuracy of hysteroscopy using AI. Takahashi et al. used deep learning to evaluate hysteroscopic images of cases with and without confirmed malignancy. Using conventional methods, they found that diagnostic accuracy was approximately 80%, and this improved to 90% with the use of AI [58].

25.10.3 Differentiating Benign and Malignant Ovarian Tumours

Benign ovarian cysts and adnexal masses are relatively common, and differentiating these from malignant disease is not always straightforward. Several attempts have been made to solve this problem using AI. For example, Akazawa and Hashimoto used five machine learning algorithms to analyse various demographic characteristics, haematological parameters, and tumour markers, as well as CT image features. A diagnostic accuracy of 80% was achieved using the XGBoost machine learning method. This might not be adequate to translate into clinical practice, but it serves as a proof of concept [59].

Serum CA 125 concentration is often used in combination with other clinical features as part of tools such as the risk of malignancy index to help risk assess and guide initial management of suspected ovarian malignancy. Tanabe et al. showed that evaluation of serum CA 125 and HE4 values using a deep learning model could achieve a diagnosis rate of 95%, which may represent an alternative to more traditional methods [60].

25.10.4 Prognostication

Accurate prognostication is important in counselling patients about their treatment options, and this is another area where AI may add value. For example, Obrzut et al. used a probabilistic neural network to predict 10-year overall survival in patients with cervical cancer after primary surgical treatment. Results compared favourably with logistic regression analysis and gave an area under the curve of 0.809 [61].

Metastasis to the lymph nodes is an important feature in the staging of endometrial cancer, as well as having a bearing on long-term outcomes. Being able to predict lymph node involvement therefore has important implications for patient counselling and surgical planning. Günakan et al. used a machine learning model based on a number of pathological features (tissue type, vascular invasion, tumour diameter, deep muscle invasion, cervical invasion, etc.) to predict lymph node involvement. The predictive accuracy of lymph node involvement was approximately 85% [62]. As predictive accuracy improves, it is likely that AI-based risk assessments will be used more and more in the assessment of such cases.

25.11 The Future of AI in Obstetrics and Gynaecology

The scope of use of AI within the field of obstetrics and gynaecology is truly enormous, and it is clear that some areas, such as reproductive medicine and gynaeoncology, are leading the way in terms of the size of the literature base. In order for the theoretical to be translated into the practical, prospective validation and regulatory approval of tools are necessary so that they can be adopted into clinical practice.

There is mounting evidence that AI, used as decision support, could help improve outcomes within women's health and reduce the risk of iatrogenic harm. If we accept that this is true, then there is a moral imperative to ensure that available tools are used, and that AI-based tools are developed where they do not currently exist. This is of particular importance in areas that so far have attracted less research interest, such as general benign gynaecology.

Where AI really has the potential to revolutionize care is in the development of entirely new models of assessment. For example, should we use AI to automate foetal growth scans, or might AI be used to develop better means of predicting adverse outcomes from other parameters such that growth scans eventually become redundant?

We must be meticulously wary of algorithmic bias to ensure that use of AI does not exacerbate existing health inequality, particularly along racial and socioeconomic lines. Caution is required when developing tools using datasets that were not created specifically for this purpose, and so the prospective collation of datasets with AI in mind should be encouraged, as should collaborative relationships between clinicians, data scientists, and engineers.

The next phase of AI implementation, eagerly anticipated, is likely to be the widespread demonstration of improved real-world outcomes using AI tools in clinical practice, although the timeframe for this relies on multiple factors, including the development of robust evidence, regulatory pathways, information governance and data security, systems interoperability, and acceptance by the clinical community.

KEY INSIGHTS

- **AI has been applied to some of the most topical challenges in women's health, from improving the diagnosis of gynaecological cancers to modelling the risk of stillbirth.**
- **In order for the theoretical to be translated into the practical, prospective validation and regulatory approval of tools are necessary so that they can be adopted into clinical practice.**
- **There is mounting evidence that AI, used as decision support, could help improve outcomes within women's health and reduce the risk of iatrogenic harm.**
- **The development of proprietary algorithms embedded within monetized consumer apps is an important driver of progress in this field. However, there is a risk that such technologies circumvent the conventional pathway of publication and peer review, which is arguably an important safety check.**
- **Although AI is of great interest across a broad range of areas within obstetrics and gynaecology, the development of AI-based tools for improved foetal heart rate monitoring is of particular clinical and commercial interest.**

Declarations of Interest

Lucy Mackillop is supported by the NIHR Oxford Biomedical Research Centre and is an employee of EMIS Group plc. Lucy Mackillop and Sam Mathewlynn both hold shares in Sensyne Health plc., which has not been referred in this chapter.

References

1. Cavalera F, Zanoni M, Merico V et al. A neural network-based identification of developmentally competent or incompetent mouse fully-grown oocytes. *Journal of Visualized Experiments* 2018(133):56668.
2. Goodson SG, White S, Stevans SM et al. CASAnova: a multiclass support vector machine model for the classification of human sperm motility patterns. *Biology of Reproduction* 2017;97(5):698–708.
3. Carrasco B, Arroyo G, Gil Y et al. Selecting embryos with the highest implantation potential using data mining and decision tree based on classical embryo morphology and morphokinetics. *Journal of Assisted Reproduction and Genetics* 2017;34(8):983–990.
4. Güvenir HA, Misirli G, Dilbaz S et al. Estimating the chance of success in IVF treatment using a ranking algorithm. *Medical & Biological Engineering & Computing* 2015;53(9):911–920.
5. https://flo.health.
6. www.miracare.com.
7. Pichon A, Jackman KB, Winkler IT, Bobel C, Elhadad N. The messiness of the menstruator: assessing personas and functionalities of menstrual tracking apps. *Journal of the American Medical Informatics Association* 2022;29(2):385–399.

For additional references and Further Reading please see www.wiley.com/go/byrne/aiinclinicalmedicine.

26

AI in Ophthalmology

Nima John Ghadiri

University of Liverpool, Liverpool University Hospitals NHS Foundation Trust, Liverpool, UK

Learning Objectives

▪ Understand the backstory and rationale for AI developments in ophthalmology.
▪ Explore how AI will impact diagnostics and therapeutics in ophthalmology.
▪ Review the challenges and pitfalls of these technologies in eye care.
▪ Explore exciting avenues for future progress.

26.1 Introduction

Ophthalmology is at the forefront of medical specialties galvanized by AI. With the rapid advancement of technologies and non-invasive diagnostic modalities in this field, ophthalmology has access to the Big Data needed for progression of AI in this area.

The rationale for using AI in ophthalmology came from the technological developments and capability to diagnose disease through the application of deep learning, as well as motivation to provide equitable healthcare while minimizing treatment delays in a field that has become one of the busiest of outpatient specialties [1]. Age-related eye diseases, such as age-related macular degeneration (AMD) and diabetic retinopathy (DR), are of particular significance as the incidence of these conditions continues to increase. This surge will likely be a burden felt the most in healthcare systems that have a shortage of trained ophthalmologists and lack economic infrastructure and human resources. Moreover, early detection and treatment are critical to preserve the vision in several ophthalmologic diseases. In these conditions, AI has the potential to be an integral tool in recognizing pathology early, and to ensure that patients with critical eye diseases are flagged for treatment earlier.

AI systems have already shown promising results when compared with human experts for detecting DR and AMD; however, caveats remain about generalizability and practical challenges such as access to imaging and economic viability.

AI in Clinical Medicine: A Practical Guide for Healthcare Professionals, First Edition. Edited by Michael F. Byrne, Nasim Parsa, Alexandra T. Greenhill, Daljeet Chahal, Omer Ahmad, and Ulas Bagci.
© 2023 John Wiley & Sons Ltd. Published 2023 by John Wiley & Sons Ltd.
Companion website: www.wiley.com/go/byrne/aiinclinicalmedicine

26.2 Looking into the Eye: A Historical Perspective

Since Herman von Helmholtz invented the direct ophthalmoscope (which he dubbed the Augenspiegel, or 'eye mirror') in 1851, it has become possible to examine the back of the eye, visualizing blood vessels and the optic nerve [2]. In 1886, William Thomas Jackman and J.D. Webster pioneered ophthalmic imaging by taking photos of the fundus with long-exposure cameras while using candles to provide the required illumination, as shown in Figure 26.1 [3].

The examination of the fundus was not readily possible until the development of the first commercially available fundus camera by Carl Zeiss in 1926 [4]. From 1950 onwards, advances in camera technology such as the electronic flash tube enabled a paradigm shift in the diagnosis of threatening conditions such as AMD, diabetic eye disease, retinal vascular diseases, and glaucoma [5]. The next evolution was the advent of digital fundus imaging, which enabled comparison of higher-quality images and storage of larger quantities of data [6]. The emergence of optical coherence tomography (OCT) in 1991 enabled a higher resolution with a swift and non-invasive method of examining a cross-section of the back of the eye in vivo, a technique that remains a cornerstone for the diagnosis of AMD, glaucoma, and DR [7]. OCT is an inexpensive imaging method with wide global uptake that has transformed the management of retinal and optic nerve disease. It has also provided the three-dimensional (3D) architecture and structural detail of the retina, something that was otherwise inaccessible via examination or conventional imaging.

(a)

(b)

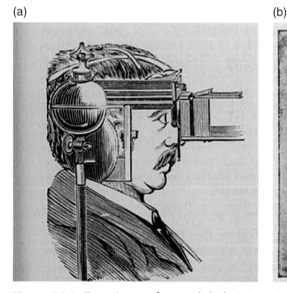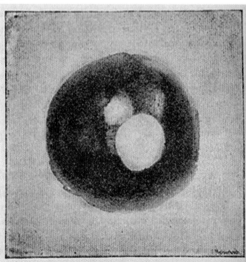

Figure 26.1: Two pictures from ophthalmic imaging history. (a) Photographing the eye of the living human retina. *Photographic News, England*, 7 May 1886. (b) On photographing the eye of the living human retina. The large circle represents an artifact, where the smaller circle at the top left shows the optic nerve. *Philadelphia Photographer*, 5 June 1886.

Source: [3].

26.3 Deep Learning and Ophthalmology

Early work in this field has mainly focused on more prevalent diseases with large imaging datasets. The ubiquity of colour fundus and OCT imaging in retina clinics and community optician practices ensures a large amount of data for training neural networks. Moreover, advances in modelling and cloud-based storage have accelerated this training. The cornerstone of deep learning in ophthalmology is convolutional neural networks (CNNs), which either classify or segment an image, for example a fundus photo or an OCT image, as shown in Figure 26.2. The convolutions generate feature maps from an image by employing a filter, and when split into various channels these represent different features of the input image.

From these foundations, to classify or segment aspects of the imaging, architectures are built for the algorithm to learn which features to select from the image, for example subretinal fluid [9], intra-retinal fluid cysts, haemorrhages, and exudates. Deep convolutional networks transcend conventional machine learning methods in their ability to segment anatomical boundaries; when taken as input, 3D OCT images provide further contextual information. This work prompted the exploration of a deep learning architecture called the DeepMind-Moorfields system, which allowed for a device-independent representation of tissue segmentation [10], as shown in Figure 26.3.

The architecture of this model comprised two neural networks. Firstly, a segmentation network was manually trained via 877 segmented images, the objective being to create a transitional representation of the image within which the pathological features have been delineated. This was subsequently fed into a classification network, and the output data was trained with 14,884 scans to provide quantifiable data and make a triage assessment (routine, semi-urgent, urgent) alongside a diagnosis. Ensemble methods then used a combination of learning algorithms to hone a better prediction for each scan, with an intermediate tissue representation in the segmentation network acting as an indispensable component to highlight and quantify the relevant retinal pathology for a clinician to review and highlight any

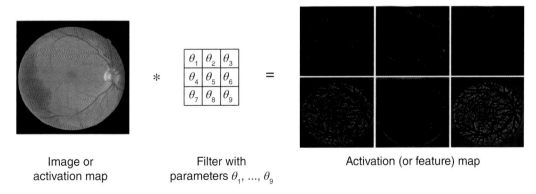

| Image or | Filter with | Activation (or feature) map |
| activation map | parameters $\theta_1, ..., \theta_9$ | |

Figure 26.2: Example of a convolution in which a filter convolves an image through learnable filters to produce a feature map that displays a different feature of the input image.
Source: [8].

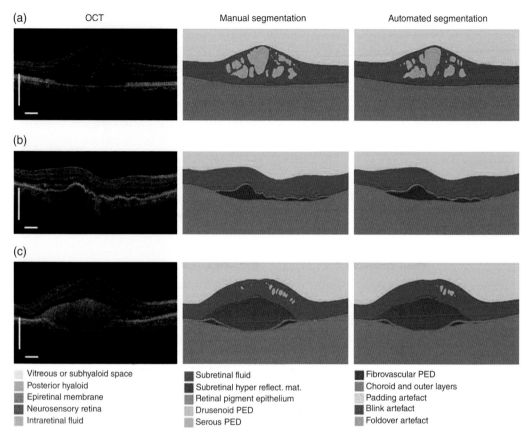

(a) OCT | Manual segmentation | Automated segmentation

(b)

(c)

- Vitreous or subhyaloid space
- Posterior hyaloid
- Epiretinal membrane
- Neurosensory retina
- Intraretinal fluid

- Subretinal fluid
- Subretinal hyper reflect. mat.
- Retinal pigment epithelium
- Drusenoid PED
- Serous PED

- Fibrovascular PED
- Choroid and outer layers
- Padding artefact
- Blink artefact
- Foldover artefact

Figure 26.3: Example of the segmentation of morphological features used in the DeepMind-Moorfields system, with a patient with diabetic macular oedema (a), a patient with choroidal neovascularization as a consequence of age-related macular degeneration (AMD) (b), and a patient with neovascular AMD (c).

Source: De Fauw et al. 2018 / with permission of Springer Nature.

borderline cases. Tested on 1000 new cases, the model asked the question 'Would you refer this patient?' and found that in more than 94% of cases, the referral recommendation made was correct (see Figure 26.4). Promisingly, this model was used to assess more than 50 different retinal diseases, and the AI system's performance reached or exceeded that of experts [10].

In ophthalmology, the eye is a window to systemic disease. Observational cohorts with large datasets, such as the UK Biobank (www.ukbiobank.ac.uk), EyePACS (www.eyepacs.com), and Messidor2 (https://www.adcis.net/en/third-party/messidor2/) databases, may be used to unlock the potential to identify ophthalmic features associated with health and disease. As an example, retinal features can be used to identify cardiovascular disease, including changes in vessel calibre, tortuosities, bifurcations, and microvascular changes [11]. Fascinatingly, these deep learning models predicted a person's age, body mass index, sex, and smoking status after validation on two independent datasets of 12,026 and 999 patients [12]. These are risk factors not previously considered quantifiable or even identifiable in images.

(a)   (b)

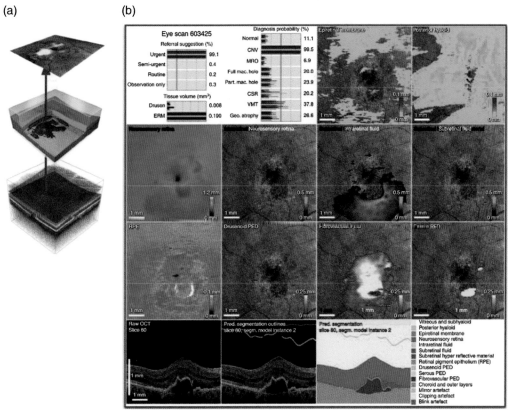

Figure 26.4: A visualization screenshot from the Moorfields-DeepMind deep learning system. (a) Average intensity projection of the optical coherence tomography (OCT) scan along with the frontal view of the eye, overlaid with a thickness map of a fibrovascular pigment epithelium detachment (PED). (b) A referral recommendation on the top left with highlighted bars corresponding to the segmented segmentation model. First–third rows, thickness maps of the 10 relevant tissue types from segmentation model instance. Displayed in a black-blue–green–brown–white colour map are two healthy tissue types (high-level retina and retinal pigment epithelium). Displayed as an overlay on a projection of the raw OCT scan are the pathological tissues (all others). The thin white line indicates the position of slice 80. Fourth row, slice 80 from the OCT scan and the segmentation map from the segmentation model instance.

Source: De Fauw et al. 2018 / with permission of Springer Nature.

Deep learning applied to these ocular biomarkers of systemic disease (the burgeoning field of *oculomics* [13]) can help researchers understand the complex relationships underlying diseases, opening new and unforeseen avenues for diagnosis and risk stratification. For example, a machine learning model that combined imaging, demographics, and other systemic data from the UK Biobank identified a correlation between glaucoma progression and lung function [14]. These developments open new possibilities as the imaging modalities used, primarily OCT, are widely available in community optician practices. Implemented in under-resourced settings, AI can be used to screen for eye disease and possibly even systemic disorders.

26.4 AI-Informed Diagnostics in the Eye Clinic

The prime focus of AI in ophthalmology has been to target common diseases via imaging modalities commonly used in eye clinics, with the aim of earlier detection and staging of sight-threatening disorders.

26.4.1 Age-Related Macular Degeneration

AMD is one of the leading causes of visual disturbance in the world, and is a multifaceted disease with several risk factors. It can be subdivided into early, intermediate, and late AMD, with an increasing prevalence worldwide due to a globally aging population. AMD is characterized by changes to the retinal pigment epithelium in the early stages of the condition that can subsequently progress into geographic atrophy and neovascularization. Deep learning systems have emerged using the AREDS dataset, with the objective to determine whether an image is referable or not. One automated grading model has shown a fair diagnostic accuracy of around 90% for referable AMD, and a further study using the same dataset showed a sensitivity of 84.2% for detecting any AMD, although these systems have not yet been externally validated [15,16]. An AI system was introduced to predict progression to exudative AMD (exAMD) in the fellow eye of patients who already have a diagnosis of exAMD in one eye [17]. This system, trained on scans of almost 2800 patients, predicted conversion to exAMD during a six-month period in which therapy with anti-vascular endothelial growth factor (anti-VEGF) drugs could make a difference to disease progression again. Further clinical validation is necessary.

Geographical atrophy is a vision-threatening manifestation of non-neovascular AMD, and thus far has no proven method for early detection. Composite deep learning models show considerable promise in both detecting and quantifying geographical atrophy from 984 OCT images, enabling ophthalmologists to identify and localize the early disease process (Figure 26.5) [18]. The algorithm tested favourably against ophthalmic specialists.

26.4.2 Diabetic Retinopathy

DR is a common complication of diabetes, and a leading cause of preventable blindness in adults worldwide [19]. DR is a microvascular consequence of diabetes characterized by microaneurysms, haemorrhages, and vascular abnormalities, and if untreated leads to irreversible blindness. Diabetic macular oedema (DMO) is an important complication that is characterized by the thickening of the macular region in the retina as a consequence of fluid build-up due to vascular leakage. Current treatments such as anti-VEGF drugs, intravitreal steroid injections, and laser photocoagulation are particularly important in the early stages of DMO and can prevent sight loss and stabilize vision. Figure 26.6 demonstrates the iDX-DR algorithm, an example of a deep learning system for DR screening [20].

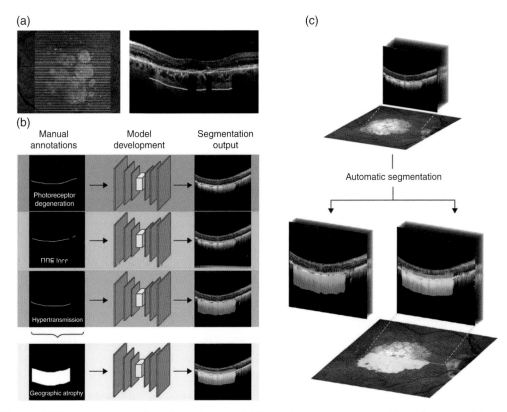

Figure 26.5: An example deep learning model for automatic segmentation of geographic atrophy and its constituent retinal features. (a) A B-scan with the manual demarcation of areas of damage to the retinal pigment epithelium. (b) An image analysis pipeline with models trained on segmentations of specific features of the input image. (c) The validation dataset with each scan automatically segmented.

Source: Zhang G et al. 2021 / with permission of Elsevier.

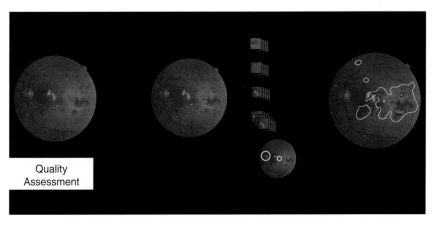

Figure 26.6: An example of a deep learning system for diabetic retinopathy (DR) screening – the iDx-DR algorithm. The first stage is a quality assessment that judges whether the image can be used for analysis. Secondly, a deep learning algorithm using convoluted neural networks screens the image for clinical biomarkers such as haemorrhages and microaneurysms. Thirdly, a disease assessment is made based on the clinical biomarker assessment and classified into no DR, moderate DR, or vision-threatening DR.

Source: [20].

DR screening can be performed by a variety of healthcare professionals, from ophthalmologists and optometrists to clinical photographers and technicians, and incorporates several methods from slit-lamp microscopy to retinal imaging and retinal telemedicine. The challenge of establishing DR screening programs worldwide has often focused on the necessary economic burden and human resources. AI can be essential in screening and staging DR using retinal images and OCT, and in assessing the disease severity by following the International Clinical Diabetic Retinopathy severity scale.

One system from Google AI Healthcare was developed using over 128,000 images graded for DR and DMO by a panel of 54 ophthalmologists, with an impressive diagnostic performance (area under the curve [AUC] above 0.99) [21]. Similar screening systems have been developed to detect referral-warranted DR [22], such as the EyeArt (https://www.eyenuk.com/en/products/eyeart) and EyeStar (https://eyestar.ai/en) systems. Promisingly, a CNN-based model achieved high sensitivity and specificity (0.97 and 0.92, respectively) for distinguishing referral-warranted macular oedema [23]. Other studies have explored AI to assess response to treatment with anti-VEGF injections [24]. These retrospective studies have not yet been tested in real-world screening programmes with heterogeneous populations. The system reported by Ting et al. used external datasets from six countries [25]. Many of these screening systems have been developed and validated on two-dimensional imaging, rendering the recognition of elevated lesions a challenge and signalling the importance of multimodal imaging for the future.

26.4.3 Glaucoma

Glaucoma is a disease of the optic nerve, precipitated by an increase in ocular pressure, and is a leading cause of blindness around the world. Characterized by optic nerve head cupping, which refers to erosion and excavation of the neuroretinal rim, glaucoma is a disease that is often asymptomatic in the initial stages, during which early treatment can delay progression. The value of AI therefore lies in facilitating community screening to ensure earlier diagnosis and referral to a glaucoma specialist, and earlier treatment before there is irreversible loss of sight. Could there be a role for AI in differentiating between optic nerve appearances that are equivocal, aiding the non-glaucoma specialist in their judgement call?

There is hope. In one single-centre study, a deep learning system rated 110 randomly sampled photographs, and outperformed five out of six ophthalmologists in diagnostic performance, though this was not statistically significant [26]. In another study, optic disc images from almost 4000 patients trained a model for referring glaucomatous optic neuropathy with a specificity of 0.980 and sensitivity of 0.956 [27]. More objective quantitative data come from OCT imaging than from disc photos. One study examining more than 32,820 pairs of optic disc photographs and

OCT images from 2312 eyes was able to discriminate eyes with glaucomatous field loss from healthy eyes, showing the potential for the assessment of progression and monitoring structural optic nerve changes over time [28].

Huge potential exists in implementing AI algorithms in visual fields, which are a keystone of glaucoma monitoring, based on spatial pattern analysis [29]. Thakur et al. developed an algorithm that appears to detect more slowly progressing and earlier glaucomatous field changes, highlighting the promise of better AI-augmented monitoring [30]. AI could also have a role in identifying disc appearances associated with specific visual field loss across a range of disc sizes.

The most exciting possibility for AI is in early glaucoma prediction, well before disease onset. Deep learning can potentially predict glaucoma one to three years before clinical signs manifest. Could deep learning deliver a tailor-made management plan and determine the risk of requiring surgery or experiencing vision loss, with or without treatment?

26.4.4 Other Eye Diseases

Retinopathy of prematurity (ROP) is a vaso-proliferative condition that affects premature infants, and is one of the leading causes of blindness in children globally. Adequate screening of low-birthweight children ensures that early treatment can be effective. AI screening is important in developing countries, as improved neonatal critical care means reduced mortality for premature babies. However, the lack of a national programme for screening infants translates to an increasing incidence of ROP.

There is considerable heterogeneity in the variability of disease severity assessment in ROP, and the implementation of AI, telemedicine, and retinal photography can ensure access to trained expertise for reviewing and classifying ROP. AI models have been successful in determining the presence and severity of ROP from fundus images, with a specificity of 0.969 and sensitivity of 0.849 [31]. A deep learning system that could diagnose plus disease (the most significant feature of severe ROP) has also shown promise [32], and the i-ROP DL system (https://i-rop.github.io) could produce a severity score that might allow monitoring for disease progression and response to treatment [33].

A plethora of other ophthalmic subspecialties have experienced early explorations in AI. These include the development of a protocol classifying eyelid melanomas as malignant or not [34], grading of the corneal keratoconus [35], and using slit-lamp images to grade pediatric cataracts [36], though the AI platform subsequently developed for diagnosing childhood cataracts exhibited less accurate performance in comparison with specialists [37]. AI systems trained on facial photographs to assess eight periorbital measurements used in the oculoplastic clinic have shown similar performance compared with human experts [38]. A deep learning model using 6465 corneal tomographic images has also demonstrated promising results in screening patients prior to refractive surgery [39].

26.5 Assistive Technology Applications of AI in Ophthalmology

The administration of medical therapies to the eye has long been a challenge due to the various anatomical barriers in the eye preventing a drug from reaching the target tissue. In recent years, drug-delivery devices and new formulations have been rapidly developed [40]. AI may have a pivotal role in our understanding of drug constituents and help inform new formulations and technologies that can lead to breakthroughs in ophthalmic therapeutics. The work of modelling the human proteome from DeepMind will open new gateways for more accurate structure-based drug design, enabling the optimization of small-molecule drugs [41].

As a supportive technology in the ophthalmic setting, AI will also play an important role for the visually impaired. The implementation of AI within image-recognition technology serves to open up the digital world. This has become increasingly pertinent as interactive media evolve from being primarily text based to integrating various other modalities. Examples of such technologies include screen readers, which interpret video, images, or text using image-recognition technology, and AI algorithms in smart glasses to detect features that can then be presented to the user either via audio or more easily readable text (see Figure 26.7).

26.6 Caveats and Challenges

The gulf is closing between eagerness for these new AI technologies and clinical validation. Recent reviews demonstrate that the diagnostic performance of deep learning models is equivalent to those of healthcare professionals in medical imaging in numerous specialties, including ophthalmology [42]; a caveat is that there was poor reporting and unreliable interpretation of the diagnostic accuracy in all but 14 studies. For many studies, a combination of limitations needs to be considered [43]. An understanding of the data used to train the algorithms is important so that results will be generalizable to the populations intended. Study design and data analysis must highlight clinical significance, as statistical significance has less consequence

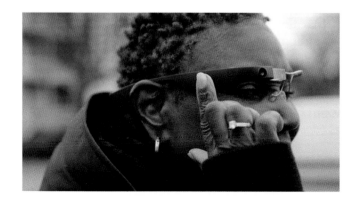

Figure 26.7: AI-assisted smart glasses can help the visually impaired using colour and object recognition.

Source: Envision.

when dealing with large amounts of data (since even minor differences may show statistical significance). Many studies fail to document the power calculation, which is critical for standardization and fine-tuning of the deep learning algorithms.

Validation of both Big Data and AI study results in independent study cohorts is crucial. In many cases, study outcomes focus on the comparison of AI systems to doctors' performances instead of measuring improvements in patient outcomes. The advent of more robust reporting standards will no doubt accelerate the uptake of these new technologies in the eye clinic setting, and increase acceptance by clinicians and patients alike.

The transition from studies to real-world settings for image-based AI systems, such as those used in ophthalmology, depends on good-quality input data. In an attempt to train AI systems, the data used may not meet quality standards, resulting in performance uncertainty. Deep learning integrated image filtering can be used to remove poor-quality images, thus ensuring that the subsequent 'selective eating' leads to a higher level of input data quality. This should help in the promised enhancement of performance of established AI diagnostic systems, as illustrated in a study of over 40,000 fundus images [44].

Over-reliance on technology is a pitfall in many fields, and ophthalmology is no exception. The excitement that accompanies AI can include the temptation to side-step important parts of the eye clinic evaluation. AI is an adjunctive tool rather than a clinical surrogate; there are many nuances to an ophthalmic examination that AI is unable to synthesize, particularly the social and psychological aspects.

Every paradigm shift in AI within ophthalmology needs to reflect an ethical standpoint. It is crucial to ensure transparency so that AI algorithms are not biased to ethnicity or gender. (For more information see Chapters 39 and 40). Researchers must test the algorithms on heterogeneous population groups. Newer models should seek to avoid data imbalance and domain generalization [45]. A human-centred evaluation of deep learning for detected DR underscores the value of ensuring that AI is generalizable and replicable [46]. Patient trust and acceptance in AI-based/ AI-augmented screening or monitoring systems are crucial if they are to be recognized and promoted. Economic evaluations also need to be considered, particularly where there is the need for the assembly of ophthalmic imaging technologies and processing infrastructure in healthcare systems that do not have this already [47].

There are many unpredictable factors when using AI in ophthalmic imaging, and these can be problematic when used on a large scale. For example, when interpreting the presence of additional human marking on images (annotations and measuring rulers are examples), neural networks may suggest that pathology is more likely to be present on an eye image. It is easy to fool these clever tools, and apprehension arises if practitioners ignore their better judgement and are affected by automation bias [48]. For AI to succeed, clinicians need adequate education and training.

Thus far, the diagnostic implementation of AI in ophthalmology has focused on common diseases, to the detriment of rarer entities. However, the combined morbidity from rare ophthalmic diseases is large [49]. Intraocular inflammation, a rare ophthalmic disease, causes 10% of blindness worldwide. Some common conditions, such as cataracts, are not routinely imaged in clinical practice, so the amount and quality of data available to train AI models are less in these diseases. It is important that future progress does not ignore these diseases, which are not as easily algorithmized or recorded.

26.7 The Future of Artificial Intelligence in Ophthalmology

Current ophthalmic AI research has concentrated on the detection and staging of diseases from retinal and OCT imaging. The goal is for these systems to be clinically validated and to be slowly integrated into practice to detect, stage, refer, and treat eye diseases earlier. AI can extract unanticipated features from various imaging modalities to potentially identify new biomarkers of the eye and systemic disease. Indeed, there are undiscovered realms of application for AI in ophthalmology, and the empowerment of scientists and clinicians in this field is crucial to its advancement. The hope, and indeed challenge, will be in integrating technologies and information streams. This spans new modalities of imaging to data from the spheres of the '-omics', including genomic, proteomic, and metabolomic information. The advent of home monitoring and patient-acquired sensor and smart app data, integrated with new wearable technologies, will add further sources of rich information, and expand the prospects for personalized medicine and more accurate diagnosis. Integrating this data in a real-world setting will be a challenge for AI to solve, in particular the integration of electronic health record (EHR) data with deep learning datasets. The history and examination findings and data such as visual acuities and intraocular pressures, which are key parts of the ophthalmic examination, are hindered by the variability between EHR platforms. There is tremendous promise and possibility for these technologies, but there needs to be global collaboration and sharing between the ophthalmic clinician, the vision scientist, and the data scientist communities. From the patient and clinician perspective, obtaining and interpreting integrated data increase the prospects for timely access to the right ophthalmic care. They also provide the opportunity for longer and richer consultations with patients, dealing with the subtleties and nuances in ophthalmic and systemic health that no machine can truly address.

The developing world has barriers to the implementation and uptake of AI, including infrastructure elements such as telecommunications and networking, but the arrival of cloud-based infrastructures may help with these barriers. The lack of digital data may present a challenge with the lack of datasets, or it may provide an opportunity for early-stage implementation of AI-integrated imaging and EHR systems. However, the over-riding aspiration is the potential for AI to improve the standard of care and provide optimum care to every patient in nations that have a shortage of eye specialists.

The most potent accelerator for progress is collaboration and sharing of ophthalmic datasets between departments, nationally and internationally, while safeguarding participant privacy and securing against data breaches. Developing flexibility is critical, whether by ensuring that neural networks can be retrained for various diagnostic devices or by safeguarding clinical validation that can span different environments and healthcare systems.

KEY INSIGHTS

- Early AI work in ophthalmology has concentrated on the diagnosis and screening of common diseases, employing the more abundant imaging modalities used in eye clinics.
- The accuracy of deep learning systems is encouraging when compared with human experts, but more rigour in reporting standards is needed.
- Further research and collaboration are important to evaluate the clinical efficacy, safety, and expense of deep learning and AI systems within ophthalmology.
- AI as an assistive instrument in eye clinics and community settings can revolutionize access to timely care, streamline clinical flow, and enhance patient outcomes.
- As more data sources and imaging modalities become available, AI's role will expand to integrating complex data streams and providing a multimodal decision-support tool to screen common eye conditions and uncover eye manifestations relating to systemic disorders.

References

1. NHS Digital. *Hospital Outpatient Activity, 2017–18*, 2018. https://digital.nhs.uk/data-and-information/publications/statistical/hospital-outpatient-activity/2017-18.
2. Helmholtz H. Correspondence. *Ophthalmic Review* 1865;1:312.
3. Jackman WT, Webster JD. On photographing the retina of the living eye. *Philadelphia Photographer* 1886;23:340–341.
4. Mann WA. Newer developments in photography of the eye. *American Journal of Ophthalmology* 1935;18(11):1039–1044.
5. Hansell P, Beeson EJG. Retinal photography in color. *British Journal of Ophthalmology* 1953;37:65–69.
6. Cideciyan A, Nagel J, Jacobson S. Modeling of high resolution digital retinal imaging. *Proceedings of the Annual International Conference of the IEEE Engineering in Medicine and Biology Society*, 1991;13:264–266.
7. Huang D, Swanson EA, Lin CP et al. Optical coherence tomography. *Science* 1991;254(5035):1178–1181.

For additional references and Further Reading please see www.wiley.com/go/byrne/aiinclinicalmedicine.

27

AI in Orthopaedic Surgery

David Burns[1], Aazad Abbas[2], Jay Toor[1], and Michael Hardisty[1,3]

[1] Division of Orthopaedic Surgery, Department of Surgery, University of Toronto, Toronto, Canada

[2] Temerty Faculty of Medicine, University of Toronto, Toronto, Canada

[3] Sunnybrook Research Institute, Toronto, Canada

Learning Objectives

- Developments in wearable technology and machine learning algorithms have provided a robust and accessible platform for accurate and objective tracking of patient physical activity.
- Digital outcomes and activity tracking with wearable devices yield novel insights in orthopaedic clinical research not typically captured with patient-reported outcome measures.
- Orthopaedic clinical prediction rules, based on numerical scores, trade simplicity and interpretability for accuracy and calibration.
- Automatic image segmentation with neural networks yields rapid bone models that can be used for templating, fracture risk analysis, pre-operative planning, and custom instrument and implant manufacture.
- AI and machine learning can amplify the effectiveness of business and operations management strategies in improving health systems efficiency.
- Artificial neural networks have yielded accurate predictions for post-operative length of stay and discharge disposition.

27.1 Activity Tracking and Digital Outcomes

27.1.1 Activity as a Clinical Outcome and Prognostic Variable

Modern AI algorithms have enabled robust video- and sensor-based human activity recognition and tracking applications that have begun to yield novel insights to clinical outcomes research in orthopaedic surgery, with potential for future application in routine clinical practice. Artificial neural networks offer substantial improvement in processing both video data and wearable sensor data over classical non-neural algorithms, enabling accurate automated tracking, quantification and

AI in Clinical Medicine: A Practical Guide for Healthcare Professionals, First Edition. Edited by Michael F. Byrne, Nasim Parsa, Alexandra T. Greenhill, Daljeet Chahal, Omer Ahmad, and Ulas Bagci.
© 2023 John Wiley & Sons Ltd. Published 2023 by John Wiley & Sons Ltd.
Companion website: www.wiley.com/go/byrne/aiinclinicalmedicine

analysis of basic activities (e.g. walking, cycling, jogging, resting, etc.), or assessment of more complex activities such as weight training, physiotherapy exercise, gait, and sleep quality. Advances in wearable technology (e.g. smart watches) and their increasing adoption have allowed these devices to serve as a robust and accessible platform for data collection in orthopaedic patients.

The impact of disease states and orthopaedic treatments on activity and function are of prime interest in orthopaedic research, and questions related to activity status are universal within orthopaedic patient-reported outcome measures (PROMs). However, PROMs suffer from a number of significant limitations in attempting to quantify activity: they are subject to a number of different patient biases (e.g. recall bias), typically have low granularity that limits sensitivity in outcomes assessment, and often are collected intermittently, thus yielding a sparse view on the recovery process.

Digital outcome measures, which are defined broadly as outcome measures collected using a digital health technology tool such as a mobile phone app or smart watch, can include accurate and objective measures of activity as well as subjective patient perspectives collected continuously or very frequently throughout treatment and recovery. These measures are being increasingly used and accepted to supplement PROMs in orthopaedic outcomes research in diverse applications.

Patient physical activity levels may also be considered of prognostic value, and may guide clinical decisions in patient pre-operative assessment, and in ongoing treatment. For instance, patient home shoulder physiotherapy exercise can be tracked using artificial neural networks to process inertial sensor (accelerometer and gyroscope) data recorded on a smart watch (Figure 27.1), and this technology has been

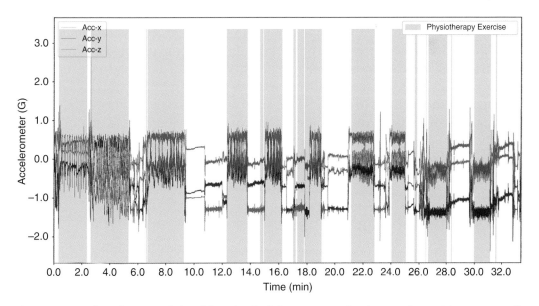

Figure 27.1: Classification of shoulder physical therapy exercise by a patient with rotator cuff pathology. A sliding window segmentation and fully convolutional neural network were used to detect the exercises.

Source: Burns et al. [1] / CC BY-SA 4.0.

used to demonstrate and quantify the link between physiotherapy adherence and recovery in patients with rotator cuff pathology [1]. There may also be an opportunity to leverage such technology in an interventional fashion to promote better physical therapy adherence, or inform clinical decision-making in the rehabilitation process. Digital outcome measures have been used to guide return-to-sport decisions in patients following anterior cruciate ligament surgery, concussion, and others.

27.1.2 Machine Learning Methods for Activity Tracking

Inertial sensors embedded in wearable devices measure the device acceleration and rotational velocity, and with repeated sampling produce a multivariate time series that can be processed in a machine learning pipeline to infer the type of activity being performed by the wearer of the device. The first step in the pipeline is to break the time series into segments of fixed length (usually 2–10 seconds), in a process called sliding window segmentation. The segments are then processed by a machine learning classifier to determine which activity is being performed during that segment of time. Historically, non-neural classifiers such as random forest or support vector machine were used. However, these required the inertial data first to be transformed into a feature representation consisting of various heuristics such as mean, variance, zero crossings, and so on. The modern approach uses an artificial neural network, typically a convolutional neural network (CNN), which classifies the segments directly and in theory learns an optimal feature representation during training. Figure 27.2 depicts an example of a neural network architecture for inertial activity tracking.

Both neural and non-neural models for inertial activity recognition are typically quite compact, relative to their counterparts in the image processing domain, due to the lower dimensionality of the time-series data; in comparison to an image with potentially millions of pixels, a typical segment of inertial data may have only 2400 sensor samples based on the number of sensors (6), the sampling rate (50 Hz), and the length of the segment (8 seconds). As a result, it is feasible to process the inertial data and classify activity in real time, either through a cloud-based model deployment or with edge computing (on-device) architecture. The latter approach has the benefit of reducing the required network bandwidth, which is substantial in the setting of continuous activity tracking.

27.1.3 Limitations and Challenges

There are a number of important limitations to these activity recognition techniques in clinical applications. Firstly, orthopaedic patient activity performance can differ significantly from healthy controls, can vary between individuals, and can change over time as patients recover. This presents a significant challenge to models trained on healthy subjects, where model accuracy can be substantially degraded for even simple tasks such as step counting in the context of disease or post-surgical states. It is important that the algorithms employed in clinical contexts are validated on

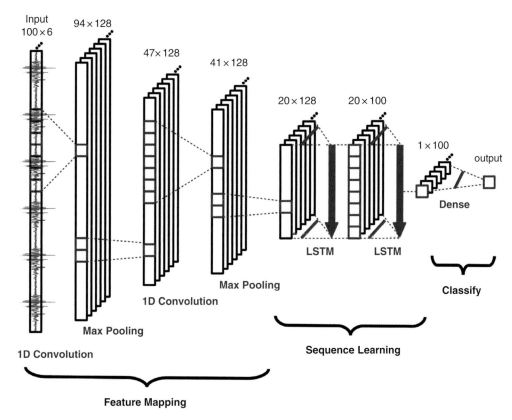

Input
100×6

94×128

47×128

41×128

20×128 20×100

1×100

output

Dense

LSTM   LSTM

Classify

Max Pooling

1D Convolution

Sequence Learning

Max Pooling

1D Convolution

Feature Mapping

Figure 27.2: Example of a convolutional recurrent neural network architecture for classifying activity from inertial time-series data. In this case, the input to the network is a 'segment' of 100 samples of six-axis inertial data (three-axis accelerometer, three-axis gyroscope). The segments are generated from the inertial time series using a sliding window segmentation. LSTM, long short-term memory.

the intended population prior to implementation. In cases where machine learning models trained on healthy subjects have poor performance in patients with musculoskeletal pathology, it can be challenging, expensive, and time-consuming to acquire sufficient patient data to train or retrain a robust model that can account for a large degree of heterogeneity in performance. In this context, we have used a patient-specific approach to activity classification that leverages patient-specific data to improve model performance and generalizability.

Out-of-distribution (OOD) detection refers to a machine learning classifier's ability to identify instances where a new class (one not in the training set) is encountered. OOD detection is a significant challenge for activity classification algorithms, and specifically problematic for neural network classifiers. For example, it would be unsurprising if a neural network for physiotherapy tracking misclassified tooth brushing as physiotherapy, if it had not been specifically trained on tooth-brushing data. This issue stems from an overconfidence bias that is typical of most neural network implementations. There are various approaches to improving OOD performance and overconfidence [2], but this remains an open problem for activity recognition and it is important to be cognizant of this issue, as these algorithms can easily have a high false-positive rate when deployed in practice.

The ethical and health policy considerations around patient activity tracking, and in general surveillance of patient self-management strategies, such as physical therapy and rehabilitation, is a complex and challenging topic. Use of this technology in consenting adults within research protocols approved by institutional research ethics boards is well accepted. However, the implications of broader deployments of such technology must be carefully assessed. There are important considerations around how collection, interpretation, and sharing of activity tracking data might negatively impact care access or influence clinical decisions for some patients, and how these risks may be mitigated. A multidisciplinary approach with the involvement of bioethicists, health policy experts, and patient advocates is important in developing and deploying ethically conscious system designs that will hopefully benefit both patients and health systems.

> **KEY INSIGHTS**
>
> ◼ **Digital outcomes measures incorporating objective metrics of activity can supplement PROMs to better characterize the natural history and treatment response in a wide variety of orthopaedic applications.**
> ◼ **Tracking of patient health self-management strategies, such as physical therapy participation, requires careful consideration of data usage and sharing policy to ensure ethically conscious system designs.**

27.2 Image Processing and Analysis

AI has revolutionized image processing and analysis techniques and capabilities across many domains, including medicine, and in particular orthopaedics. Medical image data is very well suited for the application of machine learning because of the structure of the data and because routine clinical practice produces large databases of images. This section will focus on specific advances with impacts on the orthopaedic field.

27.2.1 Image Analysis with AI

The dominant machine learning framework for image processing and analysis uses pixel (2D) or voxel (3D) arrays from images as inputs for training and prediction. First, image features are extracted from the pixel/voxel arrays (examples of features include edges, or mean intensity). Secondly, algorithms including classifiers – a type of algorithm that predicts categorical variables (i.e. Fracture yes/no) – and

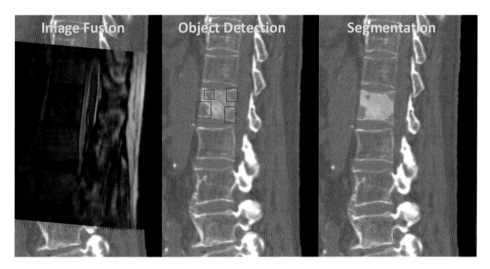

Figure 27.3: AI image analysis. Examples of tasks that are commonly performed with AI algorithms in image processing and analysis. The example depicts a metastatically involved spine. The example tasks are image fusion of magnetic resonance T2 imaging with computed tomography, object detection applied to lytic tumour detection, and segmentation of lytic (green) and blastic (yellow) tumour within the vertebral body.

regressors – a type of algorithm that predicts continuous variables (i.e. length of hospital stay) – can combine extracted features with patient information (age, sex, PROMS, etc.) to derive models that address a wide variety of clinical needs (i.e. identify fractures, make predictions of outcomes, and quantify disease). Common image processing tasks that are good candidates for AI algorithms are image fusion, tumour/bone/implant detection, and image segmentation (Figure 27.3).

27.2.2 Feature Extraction

27.2.2.1 Image-Derived Machine Learning Engineered Features for Predicting Musculoskeletal Cancer Outcomes

Engineered image features are related to the intensity (i.e. colour), texture, and shape of whatever is imaged. A good example of using image features to solve an image analysis problem in orthopaedics is the use of computed tomography (CT)-derived radiomic features in the diagnosis, segmentation, and prediction of metastatic tumours, osteosarcoma, chondrosarcomas, and cartilaginous tumours [3]. Here the disease affects tissue quality, which shows up in CT imaging as changes in both the intensity and texture of bone. These changes get quantified as a difference in texture and intensity mathematically by calculating radiomic features. In this way, the images are transformed into a common set of established radiomic features and turned into data that can then be combined with other clinical data and used for bioinformatics. Engineered features can be combined with statistical and machine learning techniques for regression and classification problems. For instance, in the case of chondrosarcoma, five radiomic-based features are combined with a logitboost classifier for disease classification. Logitboost is a classifier that 'boosts' performance by overweighting misclassified points during training, and uses a weighted sum of simple classifiers to make predictions.

27.2.2.2 Deep Learning–Based Segmentation for Analysing Frailty and Sarcopenia from Imaging

Measures of frailty and sarcopenia have been shown to be related to orthopaedic surgical outcomes, predicting length of hospital stay, mortality, and complications leading to reoperation. Deep learning for medical image segmentation, CNNs, and fully connected networks (FCNs) present a solution to automated sarcopenia and frailty quantification from routine clinical CT. The CNN allows features to be learnt at a variety of spatial levels and combines the information from the different spatial levels. It is by combining information from multiple levels that CNNs can incorporate intensity, texture, and shape differences to make excellent predictions and characterize images. With deep learning methods, instead of calculating known features, the network learns how to calculate features and how to combine the features and make predictions, all from the training data. In this way, it is a more data-driven approach. These methods have enabled rapid and automated quantification of measures of musculoskeletal (MSK) health that can be combined with other patient factors, and used to improve surgical outcome predictions and affect clinical decision-making. Deep learning models have become dominant in most image analysis problems, having state-of-the-art performance in multiple image analysis tasks in orthopaedics, including detection of abnormality in X-rays, hip fracture prediction from X-ray, spine model segmentation, fracture detection, bone age estimation, and tumour identification.

27.2.3 Opportunities

Treatment planning and navigation present great opportunities for AI algorithms to have an impact on orthopaedic surgery. Custom implant designs and locations based on the analysis of diagnostic medical imaging have the potential to create powerful tools for planning and simulating surgical cases prior to surgical interventions. Patient simulation is a natural extension of image segmentation, where voxels within medical imaging volumes are labelled, allowing for patient-specific geometry of many tissues to be visualized and interacted with. Personalized implants are another area where deep learning is well suited to generate implant geometry from AI-enabled medical image analysis. The approach involves training a network to generate implant geometry from medical images by providing examples of implant geometry and matched patient imaging. This technique is more developed for bone craniofacial implant designs. Implant geometries are generated by training algorithms with synthetic defects created from healthy skulls. Predicting ideal implant placement is another area that could have large impacts on orthopaedics. Currently methods exist to detect and localize implants within medical imaging volumes. These data could be used to help guide AI-enabled implant placement algorithms for computer-assisted or robotic surgery.

27.2.4 Limitations and Challenges

Similar to other areas of AI, large, well-labelled datasets, with adequate variation, are crucial for training AI-enabled image processing and analysis algorithms. This is particularly challenging with image processing and analysis because, while relatively large volumes of imaging are produced, most are not labelled. Natural language processing applied to electronic medical records and tied to medical imaging records presents a possible solution. Furthermore, there are many initiatives to create large high-quality, well-labelled and open imaging datasets (i.c. Medical Image Computing and Computer Assisted Intervention [MICCAI] challenge datasets, Cancer Imaging Archive, University of California Irvine Machine Learning Repository). Open imaging datasets are repositories of imaging data that are accessible to the public and researchers. The datasets are organized and maintained to aid in scientific discovery and technology development. Greater data availability brought about by open data initiatives will accelerate the development and adoption of AI medical imaging processing algorithms, allowing the creation of robust and generalizable methods.

KEY INSIGHTS

- ■ **AI has revolutionized image processing and analysis, creating methods that are fast, robust, and accurate.**
- ■ **Common image processing tasks that are amenable to AI algorithms are fracture detection, bone and tumour segmentation, and sarcopenia assessment.**
- ■ **AI image processing algorithms have benefited from large open datasets, and new initiatives will lead to even more advances.**

27.3 Clinical Outcome Prediction and Decision Support

27.3.1 Predictive Scores in Orthopaedic Surgery

Clinical outcome prediction scores and models have been utilized in the orthopaedic field for decades to aid in clinical decision-making and guide treatment. Some notable examples include the Kocher criteria for predicting paediatric hip septic arthritis [4], Mirels criteria for predicting pathological fracture in metastatic bone disease [5], and the Instability Severity Index Score [6], which predicts recurrent shoulder instability after arthroscopic stabilization. These predictive tools, and others like them, employ categorical or dichotomized clinical variables that are assigned integer weights and summed to produce an easily calculated predictive score. While simple for surgeons to use in clinical practice, this type of scoring tool often has poor predictive performance. There is a substantial opportunity to employ modern machine learning models and methods to better assist clinical decision-making.

These prototypical orthopaedic predictive scores are derived from retrospective data, and they are in essence linear machine learning models. The choice of a score-based linear model sacrifices accuracy and model expressivity to derive a tool that is both easy to calculate and also easily interpretable. However, in many cases rigorous methods have not been used to dichotomize/categorize numerical variables, derive optimal variable weights such as with logistic regression, and conduct internal and external validation. For instance, the Mirels score (Table 27.1) assigns an integer value of 1, 2, or 3 to four clinical variables and sums them [5]. Although each of the clinical variables is important in predicting pathological fracture, the weights assigned in each variable category are identical to optimize score simplicity, and do not necessarily have an optimal calibration given the data. The categorization of continuous data (e.g. lesion size) also reduces model performance in favour of simplicity. In a well-calibrated model, the actual risk increases proportionally to the score, and different combinations of variables yielding the same score should have approximately equal risk.

Revisiting these scoring tools with more complex models and rigorous machine learning methods for model development and validation in an effort to improve accuracy and calibration is an attractive idea, but can also have significant challenges.

27.3.2 Challenges

One major challenge occurs when the predicted outcome has become more rare due to clinical practice changes. For instance, revising the Mirels score could be challenging for this reason. Prophylactic stabilizations performed for patients predicted to have bone tumours at risk of fracture reduce the number of observed

Table 27.1: Mirels score for predicting risk of pathological fracture [5]. A score of 1–3 is given for each of the four criteria and then summed. The authors suggest that patients with a score greater than 8 may benefit from prophylactic internal fixation prior to radiation.

Criteria	Score		
	1	2	3
Site	Upper limb	Lower limb	Peritrochanteric
Pain	Mild	Moderate	Functional
Lesion	Blastic	Mixed	Lytic
Size	$<1/3$	$1/3–2/3$	$>2/3$

Source: Adapted from Mirels, Hilton (1989).

pathological fractures, and also create bias in the population of observed new cases, complicating derivation of new predictive models. The same challenge might exist for revisiting the Instability Severity Index Score, as many patients with large bone defects (an element of the score) are offered the Latarjet procedure instead of arthroscopic stabilization, which would be predicted to have a high likelihood of failure. Ultimately, in order to revise a predictive score with new data, it is necessary to observe sufficient numbers of both positive and negative outcomes of the prediction.

Another challenge with more complex machine learning models is interpretability, which is the degree to which a human can understand the cause of the model decision. It may be acceptable to use an app or website to calculate a complex prediction, but it is generally less acceptable if it is unclear how the model is making that prediction. There are multiple examples in the literature highlighting the risk of undesirable features that can be learnt from the data, and hidden within a non-interpretable model. A notable, but non-orthopaedic, example is provided by Caruana et al. [7], where a rule-based method they used to predict pneumonia mortality erroneously learnt that patients with asthma were at lower risk. This counter-intuitive result stemmed from the more aggressive clinical management and practice of routine hospital admission used for this patient group that is generally known to be at higher risk from pneumonia. Since the purpose of the tool is to assess the need for admission, it is clearly an undesirable result. However, the rule-based method used is readily interpretable, and so this issue with asthmatics was apparent in the model itself, allowing the issue to be detected and corrected by the researchers. Had they used a non-interpretable model, such as a neural network or random forest, it is likely that this undesirable characteristic for asthmatics would be learnt from the data but hidden within the black box of the model and be very challenging to identify.

27.3.3 Interpretable Models

For the majority of risk prediction applications involving categorical and numerical data, a logistic regression model with rigorous methods applied to model development, variable selection, and then validation serves as an excellent baseline for achieving a well-calibrated model that is easily interpretable. Aside from needing a calculator or app to compute the score, the chief downside of logistic regression is that it models each independent predictor variable with a linear effect, which in some cases does not match reality (e.g. risk from radiation exposure). Interaction effects between two variables are also sometimes very important in risk modelling or outcome prediction. However, interaction terms are typically not used in logistic regression, chiefly because doing so makes the model weights difficult to interpret.

There are a few choices when it comes to easily interpretable models for risk prediction, and these include logistic regression, naive Bayes, decision trees and their variants, and general additive models. The latter two are capable of modelling interaction effects in an interpretable way. K-nearest neighbour can also arguably be considered an interpretable model, as it derives its predictions from the outcomes of k other patients from the training set that are most similar to the predicted case. Although the reason for the decision is understandable by humans, it does not reveal any insights into the importance or effect of the individual clinical variables.

27.3.4 Opportunities

A major advance in orthopaedic clinical outcome prediction enabled by modern machine learning methods is the ability to model more complex data sources with artificial neural networks (ANN). For instance, ANNs can directly model 2D or 3D image data, multivariate time-series data (e.g. a 12-lead electrocardiogram [ECG] tracing), and natural language, which was largely impractical with non-neural machine learning models. This advance presents novel opportunities to leverage these additional data sources in predicting clinical outcomes. For example, good results have been achieved using a CNN to predict risk of pathological fracture directly from an X-ray of the proximal femur [8].

The application of modern machine learning methods to outcome prediction in orthopaedic surgery is a rapidly evolving area, still in its infancy. A recent systematic review identified 59 such studies, most of them published in the last few years [9]. Of note is that the most commonly used models were non-interpretable (neural network, random forest). Many studies also performed only limited validation, with calibration reported in just 26 (34%) studies. Ultimately, deployment of non-interpretable models with incomplete validation should be approached with trepidation. There are excellent guidelines for developing and appraising clinical prediction models such as the CHARMS checklist, and these should be considered when appraising prediction rules regardless of the underlying model.

KEY INSIGHTS

- Familiar orthopaedic scores such as the Kocher criteria and Mirels score are machine learning models that sacrifice prediction accuracy and calibration for simplicity of use.
- While it is tempting to apply complex machine learning models (e.g. neural networks) to risk prediction, interpretable models such as multivariate logistic regression are safer because human beings can understand the formula for the model's prediction.
- Neural networks allow complex data sources such as text, 2D and 3D image data, and time series to be effectively modelled.

27.4 Health Systems Efficiency and Optimization

The delivery of orthopaedic care entails the management of a high volume of patients, with each episode of care typically associated with considerable financial impact. Expenses are often correlated with operating room (OR) surgical duration, inpatient length of stay (LOS), and instrumentation costs.

Most cost containment efforts in public health systems have focused on regulating the use of hospital resources through approaches such as surgical case prioritization, inpatient LOS reduction, and purchasing and procurement strategies. These fundamental cost-containment techniques are steps in the right direction, but may have consequences such as increasing patient wait times for surgery, decrements in clinical outcomes, and declining provider satisfaction. Notably, cost containment is less of a concern in private-payer systems. More sophisticated efforts aimed at increasing efficiency rather than constraining expenditure have also been made, such as dedicated trauma room time, staff on-call float pooling, and scheduling optimization. These operational optimization techniques, derived from the business world, are beneficial to both public and private health systems.

27.4.1 Currently Implemented Optimization Techniques

Many hospitals attempt to divert cases away from expensive after-hours operating room (OR) time via daytime dedicated orthopaedic trauma rooms. However, there is some hesitation associated with this scheduling practice, as orthopaedic trauma presentation is temporally variable. This may lead to unused OR time that would have otherwise been used for elective surgery.

Another solution to improve efficiency is to optimize the scheduling of surgical procedures based on expected duration of surgery (DOS) and LOS. However, optimization often relies on the accuracy of these predictions, and currently employed methods lack sophistication. Not only do most institutions still use ad hoc scheduling mainly led by surgeons, but even leading centres in this regard are also limited to rudimentary methods such as historical scheduling and moving averages for DOS and LOS predictions.

Other optimization techniques involve adjusting the number of hospital staff during periods of high demand. For example, many hospitals annually add an extra inpatient hospitalist medicine team during the flu season. As alluded to earlier, this may be challenging in orthopaedics due to the high variability of trauma presentation. Figure 27.4 demonstrates the variability of average daily demand on the orthopaedic service at a level I trauma centre throughout the year. In addition, staffing availability itself can be inherently variable due to unplanned absences. Common strategies entail overtime pay to incentivize staff, as well as the use of on-call float pools of staff to be called if needed. However, these strategies can be financially and operationally burdensome.

27.4.2 Opportunities Presented by AI

Many of these techniques have been analogously applied in the field of business and operations management. For example, retail stores often face the same challenge of over- or under-stocking inventory to meet customer demand, which is highly variable. However, the retail industry has been a much earlier adopter of machine learning techniques, which they have utilized to predict their short- and long-term demand and optimize their inventory accordingly. In the same fashion, machine learning may

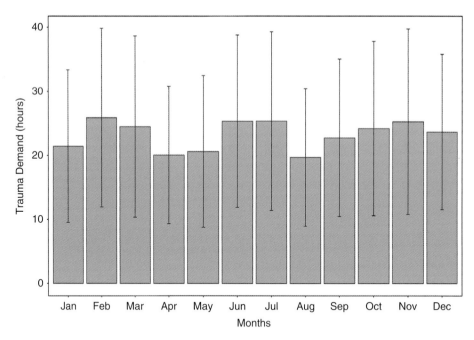

Figure 27.4: Average daily demand on the orthopaedic service stratified by month at a level I trauma centre in North America over an eight-year period (2012–2019). This demonstrates the variation in demand throughout the year.

be leveraged to both predict trauma volume and elective care resource consumption to optimize scheduling. Despite work in this area being in its infancy, ANNs may prove to be highly amenable to these predictions due to their ability to reproducibly model time-series data and non-linear relationships. Useful inputs into these networks related to trauma volume include seasonality, day of week, weather, and traffic patterns. Preliminary work in using these factors to predict orthopaedic trauma volumes at a level I trauma centre in North America is shown in Figure 27.5. These predictions may be used as part of optimization frameworks, allowing for the ideal scheduling of trauma cases, allocation of hospital resources, and staffing assignment.

Aside from predicting orthopaedic trauma volumes, there is also the challenge of determining case-level resource utilization for both trauma and scheduled elective care. Accordingly, there has been substantial traction in using clinical and operational factors to predict key markers of resource utilization such as DOS, LOS, and discharge disposition. Work by Ramkumar et al. has proven ANNs to be useful in generating both LOS and discharge disposition predictions, with factors such as patient demographics, comorbidity status, admission type, illness severity, mortality risk, income quartile, and operational factors such as hospital type and admission date proving essential to these models [10]. Such methods of resource utilization prediction can be integrated with staffing absence pattern predictions to generate ideal staffing assignments.

Despite the reported accuracy of these models ranging from 75% to 80%, a limitation is that they are often not superior to using the statistical mode (i.e. the value

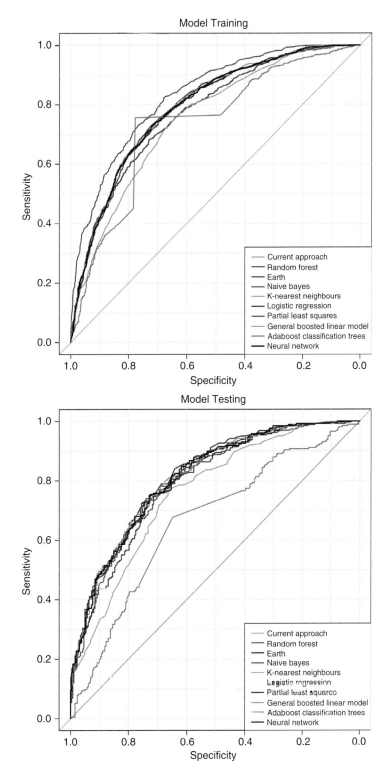

Figure 27.5: Prediction of orthopaedic trauma volumes at a level I trauma centre in North America. Multiple models were used to predict the trauma volumes. Reproduced by permission from Jay Toor and Aazad Abbas.

that appears most often in the dataset), which suggests potential for over-estimation of their utility. Future work should incorporate the statistical mode as a benchmark for such models to ensure their utility. In addition, the majority of the work has yet to integrate variability of LOS and readmission over time, as a large body of the current work is predicated on randomly stratifying the training and testing data. Incorporating the temporal difference in these outcomes is necessary for real-world application of these models.

27.4.3 Future Directions

Notably, generalizable predictions of DOS using AI have not yet been demonstrated, most likely due to the highly variable and multifactorial nature of DOS. Efforts using traditional statistical analysis have demonstrated the dependence of DOS on factors such as surgeon, procedure type, and surgical team composition [11]. These factors are hospital and institution specific, which implies that it may not be possible to generate generalizable predictions of DOS for any one particular institution solely based on large databases. However, a strength of ANNs is they may be trained on large datasets and subsequently adapted to a particular setting by updating the model weights with training a smaller corpus of institution-specific data. This technique of transfer learning may allow institutions to generate reliably accurate predictions of their DOS, allowing for optimization of their surgical scheduling. In addition, a challenge in applying machine learning for the purposes of operational optimization is that a successful model will alter operational practice, and may subsequently neutralize the benefits of the machine learning model itself. Adaptive modeling provides a solution to this as well, as it allows continuous updating of the model based on subsequent improvements.

Effectively integrating established business and operations management tools into orthopaedic surgery can generate tremendous benefits to health systems striving to minimize expenses by maximizing efficiency. Although attempts have been made to apply such techniques, AI and machine learning can offer improved model performance to help overcome the barriers hampering broader adoption.

KEY INSIGHTS

- **While many cost-reduction strategies are orientated around constraining OR time and inpatient capacity, some more sophisticated business-style strategies include dedicated daytime trauma room time, daily schedule optimization, and staff assignment optimization.**
- **The efficiency savings of these techniques are curtailed by the high variability within health systems, and in particular orthopaedics. Machine learning and AI therefore have significant potential to overcome this barrier, amplifying the effectiveness of these techniques and facilitating widespread adoption.**

Conflicts of Interests

David Burns is a Founder at Halterix and has received grant support from the Workplace Safety and Insurance Board. Aazad Abbas is an Associate at Primus Healthcare Solutions and has received grant support from CONMED Corporation. Jay Toor is a Founder at Primus Healthcare Solutions and has received grant support from CONMED Corporation. Michael Hardisty holds shares in Halterix and has received grant support from Synaptive Medical, Varian Medical Systems, and Altis Labs.

References

1. Burns D, Boyer P, Razmjou H, Richards R, Whyne C. Adherence patterns and dose response of physiotherapy for rotator cuff pathology: longitudinal cohort study. *JMIR Rehabilitation and Assistive Technologies* 2021;8(1):e21374. https://doi.org/10.2196/21374.
2. Boyer P, Burns D, Whyne C. Out-of-distribution detection of human activity recognition with smartwatch inertial sensors. Sensors 2021;21:1669. https://doi.org/10.3390/s21051669.
3. Gitto S, Cuocolo R, Annovazzi A, et al. CT radiomics-based machine learning classification of atypical cartilaginous tumours and appendicular chondrosarcomas. *EBioMedicine* 2021;68:103407. https://doi.org/10.1016/j.ebiom.2021.103407.
4. Kocher MS, Zurakowski D, Kasser JR. Differentiating between septic arthritis and transient synovitis of the hip in children: an evidence-based clinical prediction algorithm. *Journal of Bone & Joint Surgery* 1999;81(12):1662–1670. https://doi.org/10.2106/00004623-199912000-00002.
5. Mirels H. Metastatic disease in long bones. A proposed scoring system for diagnosing impending pathologic fractures. *Clinical Orthopaedics and Related Research* 1989;249:256–264.
6. Balg F, Boileau P. The instability severity index score. A simple pre-operative score to select patients for arthroscopic or open shoulder stabilisation. *Journal of Bone and Joint Surgery* 2007;89(11):1470–1477. https://doi.org/10.1302/0301-620X.89B11.18962.
7. Caruana R, Lou Y, Gehrke J et al. Intelligible models for healthcare: predicting pneumonia risk and hospital 30-day readmission. *Proceedings of the 21st ACM SIGKDD International Conference on Knowledge Discovery and Data Mining.* New York: Association for Computing Machinery; 2015, 1721–1730. https://doi.org/10.1145/2783258.2788613.

For additional references and Further Reading please see www.wiley.com/go/byrne/aiinclinicalmedicine.

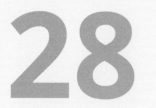

28
AI in Surgery

Jesutofunmi A. Omiye, Akshay Swaminathan, and Elsie G. Ross

Stanford University School of Medicine, Stanford, CA, USA

Learning Objectives

▪ Be able to describe current cutting-edge applications of AI in surgery with relevant use cases.
▪ Be able to outline the unique challenges of surgical AI and potential ways to overcome them.
▪ Identify future directions for research and development.

28.1 Introduction

Modern surgical practice has come a long way from its roots formed in the 1700s when the concepts of 'scientific surgery' were first cemented, and surgery was performed in homes and theatres by those who had been trained through non-standard apprenticeships, and when surgical techniques were still primitive [1]. Today, the pace of surgery is fast and dynamic, the systems in which patients are treated are much more complex, and the tools for treatment are ever more sophisticated. It is in the backdrop of this growing complexity that machine learning and AI can be applied to enable more precise, timely, and effective surgical practice. From just-in-time data-driven clinical decision support, to automated intra-operative assistance technology populating operating rooms (ORs) of the future (Figure 28.1), to enhanced post-operative recovery, AI is poised to usher in the next era of advanced surgical care. In this chapter we will discuss the promises and challenges of AI in surgery using a framework that focuses on the pre-, intra-, and post-operative periods, alongside the opportunity to leverage AI for surgical education.

28.2 Pre-operative Care

The pre-operative period hinges upon obtaining the appropriate diagnosis to ensure that an adequate and effective treatment plan can be enacted. In addition to this, there are a myriad of questions, including whether a patient is an adequate surgical

AI in Clinical Medicine: A Practical Guide for Healthcare Professionals, First Edition. Edited by Michael F. Byrne, Nasim Parsa, Alexandra T. Greenhill, Daljeet Chahal, Omer Ahmad, and Ulas Bagci.
© 2023 John Wiley & Sons Ltd. Published 2023 by John Wiley & Sons Ltd.
Companion website: www.wiley.com/go/byrne/aiinclinicalmedicine

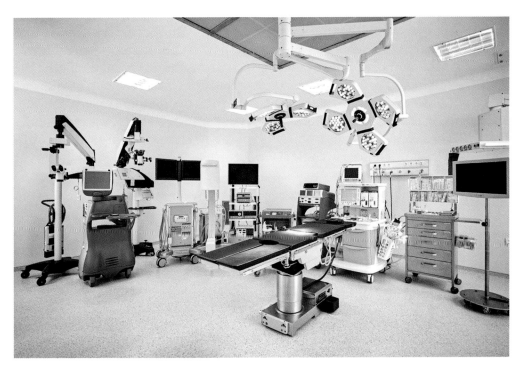

Figure 28.1: The operating room of the future. Various AI technologies are synchronized to provide real-time information and aid surgical intervention during the intraoperative phase of surgical care.

Source: Maier-Hein et al. 2017 / Springer Nature.

candidate, if and to what extent patient-specific factors can be optimized before surgical intervention, and what surgical approach can maximize the chances of a good outcome and minimize harm. Current AI technologies aim to assist with timely diagnosis, more precise risk stratification, and surgical planning.

28.2.1 AI-Assisted Diagnosis

CLINICAL VIGNETTE

Jake is involved in a minor motor vehicle accident and is brought to the emergency department (ED) with vague complaints of generalized body aches, but no visible signs of injury, and vital signs are within normal limits. He quickly undergoes a trauma survey, including a series of imaging studies, per protocol, to rule out any underlying fractures or related problems. The ED is busy, and because Jake's injuries appear to be minor the clinical team start to prioritize other patients who are flooding the ED. The radiologist on call is also dealing with interpreting an onslaught of studies. The hospital has recently implemented an AI system that quickly evaluates all the images in the radiology queue, provides a plausible diagnosis, and triages them. Images that indicate that surgical intervention may be needed are prioritized for the radiologist to read. The AI model identifies that Jake has a pneumothorax on his chest X-ray, which was initially so small it was missed by the trauma team. The radiologist confirms the finding and calls the ED physician taking care of Jake. The ED physician goes back to attend to Jake just as Jake begins desaturating on the monitor – the pneumothorax has worsened, and Jake is on the brink of cardiopulmonary collapse. A chest tube is expediently inserted and Jake's vital signs stabilize. Had the AI system not prioritized Jake's chest X-ray, a worse outcome could have occurred.

A recent focus of surgical AI platforms has been developing ways to improve time to detection of urgent surgical diagnoses. In partnership with an academic institution, General Electric (GE; Boston, MA, USA), for example, developed AI models to identify pneumothoraces on chest X-rays [2]. Once a pneumothorax is identified, the diagnosis is automatically communicated to the technologist, and the image is prioritized in the queue for review and confirmation by the on-call radiologist. This model was US Food and Drug Administration (FDA) approved in 2019 and integrated with GE X-ray devices [3].

A similar platform was developed by Aidoc (Tel Aviv, Israel), a health technology firm with FDA-approved AI imaging technologies. Its AI platform leverages advanced deep learning to classify and interpret a wide array of images, and can detect spinal fractures, pulmonary embolism, and intracranial bleeding. Similar to the GE system, Aidoc triages images based on acuity for further evaluation by the radiologist. Some healthcare systems in Europe and the USA have implemented Aidoc, and through this platform clinicians can diagnose emergent surgical conditions faster, potentially improving surgical outcomes [4]. Aidoc algorithms, importantly, have been validated and found to be highly accurate, with one research team finding that Aidoc's intracranial haemorrhage models have an overall accuracy of 98% when using non contrast head computed tomography (CT) scans [5]. Other companies that offer similar capabilities include Icometrix (Leuven, Belgium), Arterys (San Francisco, CA, USA), and Imagen (New York, USA). Each company offers FDA-approved technologies that can automatically interpret brain magnetic resonance imaging (MRI) scans, detect lung cancer, and detect wrist fractures, respectively. Through use of these AI software platforms, patients can be diagnosed early, encouraging prompt surgical intervention when required [6].

28.2.2 AI-Assisted Risk Prediction Model

While the aforementioned companies focus nearly exclusively on imaging data, there is a smaller number of companies that aim to leverage another large data source in modern healthcare – electronic health records (EHRs). With the explosion of EHR data, machine learning methods can be deployed to comb through massive amounts of sparse data for the early identification of patients suffering from surgical diseases and provide more accurate risk stratification for expected post-operative outcomes.

Traditional risk scores are well known in the surgical field, with the most notable ones being the American Society of Anesthesiologists (ASA) risk score and the American College of Surgeons National Surgical Quality Improvement Program (ACS-NSQIP) risk calculator [7]. These established scores enable assessment of the likelihood of post-operative morbidity and mortality for those undergoing major surgery, primarily using an assessment of the severity of patient comorbidities. However, these risk scores have traditionally assumed a linear relationship between variables, and used a small number of risk factors. In addition, evaluating the severity of patient risk factors can be subjective [7]. Bertsimas and colleagues sought to build a machine learning–based risk calculator for surgical morbidity and mortality risks for emergency surgery (ES) patients [7]. The goal of this calculator was to apply novel machine learning techniques to produce an interactive and holistic risk score for patients. Using data from over 300,000 ES patients in the ACS-NSQIP database, they built what is known as a Predictive OpTimal Trees Emergency Surgery Risk (POTTER) calculator to assess the risk of post-operative morbidity and mortality, alongside specific 30-day post-operative complications like surgical site infection, pneumonia, and sepsis [7]. An optimal classification trees algorithm was used, and the risk calculator produced superior results compared to the traditional ACS-NSQIP risk score and the standard Emergency Surgery Score. Specifically, the morbidity C-statistic for the machine learning–based approach was 0.84, and the mortality C-statistic was 0.92 compared to ASA's 0.87 [7]. To fast-track deployment, the authors built a freely available visual interface for surgeons to interact with the risk calculator (Figure 28.2) [8], and their models have been validated in a wider array of patient populations [9].

One company that aims to utilize large amounts of clinical data to deploy surgical AI solutions is KelaHealth (San Francisco, CA, USA). KelaHealth uses registry data from NSQIP to train models that can be deployed within different EHR systems. One published application for its platform addresses surgical site infection (SSI) [10]. In vascular surgery, the older patient distribution and the comorbid status of patients significantly increase the risk of SSI [11]. SSI also contributes to an estimated increase in health costs of $10,149 per incidence [10]. KelaHealth developed a deep learning prediction model for SSI using 72,435 cases from the NSQIP dataset. The authors then applied the model to a retrospective cohort of patients who underwent major vascular surgery at a single institution to see who the model would have flagged as high risk for wound infection. These high-risk patients could theoretically have been treated with more aggressive measures, including the use of closed-incision negative-pressure therapy. Thus, prospective use of an SSI model can help surgeons pre-operatively decide on wound management plans. Applied to institutional data, KelaHealth's model achieved an area under the curve (AUC) of 0.68, a sensitivity of 0.83, and a negative predictive value of 0.91 [10]. In total, the authors estimated that use of the deep learning model could have decreased SSI by 40% by better matching of patients to their high and low infection risk categories, potentially saving $231–458 per patient [10].

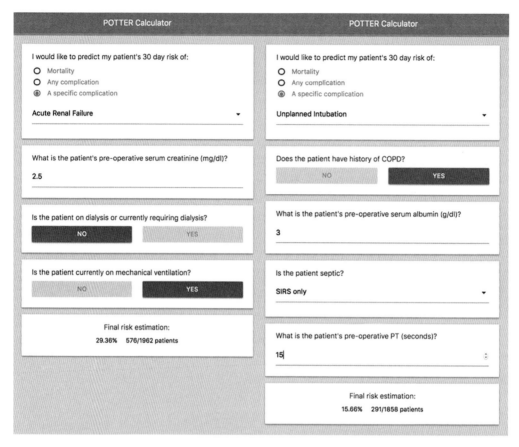

Figure 28.2: A snapshot of the interactive AI-based POTTER risk calculator. Here, the model predicts the 30-day risk of acute renal failure and unplanned intubation for a patient scheduled for surgery.

Source: Bertsimas et al, 2018 / with permission of Wolters Kluwer Health Inc.

While KelaHealth and the POTTER systems are examples of helpful AI-based platforms for pre-operative risk prediction, it should be noted that their currently described models are built on large-registry data. This has pros and cons. On the one hand, using large-registry data enables patient sampling from a wide variety of patients, potentially making models more generalizable. However, this generalizability can come at the cost of higher accuracy. Future model iterations can benefit from two approaches: (i) utilizing the full breadth of data within the EHR to further train and validate model performance; and (ii) retraining models for local environments. EHR data has been found to be useful in a wide number of tasks, including predicting future major adverse cardiovascular events [12], time to wound healing [13], and heart failure readmission [14]. Complete EHR data, including unstructured clinical text combined with time-sequence data, can improve model performance in some important ways, especially given that nearly 80% of data in healthcare are unstructured [15]. Lastly, each health system treats a subsample of larger populations, and thus retrained models can better capture unique local patient characteristics and practice patterns, ultimately improving model accuracy.

28.2.3 AI-Assisted Surgical Planning

In addition to pre-operative risk assessment, surgical planning based on imaging is of utmost importance in all surgical fields. The needs of each field are often unique, and thus each specialty uses particular tools that can augment imaging to improve surgical planning such as the Proprio system (Seattle, WA, USA) in neurosurgery [16] and TeraRecon (Durham, NC, USA) for cardiovascular surgical planning [17]. These platforms leverage different degrees of AI to assist in the planning process. For example, TeraRecon leverages AI to provide measurements such as enhanced coronary calcium scoring for CT coronary angiograms, and automates the detection and segmentation of different body structures to decrease the time required to plan endovascular interventions. Looking towards the future, Ceevra Health (San Francisco, CA, USA), an AI-augmented imaging start-up, aims to build interactive AI-based 3D models from radiological imaging [18]. As an illustration of the potential impact of its interactive platform, Ceevra conducted a single-blind randomized clinical trial of its 3D models for robotic nephrectomy cases, and found that a surgeon's use of its platform led to decreased operative time, blood loss, clamp time, and patient length of stay [19].

28.3 Intra-operative Care

The intra-operative phase of surgical care represents one of the most high-stakes, high-cost periods of the patient journey through the health system. During this time, the surgeon works with teams of other clinicians, nurses, and technologists to perform a series of tasks that are currently still too complex to be neatly summarized or executed by computer modelling or robotics alone. However, there are many promising surgical AI technologies that aim to enhance the abilities of those in the OR.

28.3.1 Multi-modal Operating Room Solutions

Modern ORs include a panoply of technology, such as multiparameter monitors that provide live feeds of patient vital signs, high-definition surgical cameras, 3D imaging panels, and interconnected devices that work together to aid the surgical team in providing safe, effective care [20]. Despite this, the traditional OR is often considered inefficient and cluttered [20,21]. The opportunity for AI to transform intra-operative care has been steered by advances in computer vision over the past decade.

Computer vision algorithms can be trained on hundreds of surgery videos obtained across different procedures and provides insights into important patterns. For example, Khalid and colleagues developed a model using labelled data of 103 surgery videos from eight surgeons from the Johns Hopkins University Intuitive

Surgical Gesture and Skill Assessment dataset that included surgeons performing specific tasks like suturing and needle passing [22].The goal for the machine learning model was to accurately detect the type of surgical task being done, and estimate surgical competence by assessing the technical skills performed. The model achieved a precision of 1.00 for suturing and 0.91 for needle passing. It also estimated scores that ranged from 0.85 to categorize a surgical task as novice level to 0.80 for expert-level categorization [22]. The success of this model showed that AI models can identify associations in surgical videos and potentially provide immediate feedback during a surgical procedure by identifying the specific task conducted. A similar model described by Khalid et al. was implemented by Surgical Safety Technologies (Toronto, Canada) to develop the OR BlackBox® [22,23], which leverages multi-modal data including audio, video, imaging, and patient vitals, to provide insights for surgical analytics and quality improvement [23]. The OR BlackBox has already been adopted in some hospitals in the USA, Canada, and Europe to improve surgery safety. It does this by capturing intra-operative data and providing AI-based insights on the safety checklist use, OR efficiency, communication, and other important metrics [23].

28.3.2 Intraoperative Imaging Guidance

The field of vascular surgery has seen a rise in the complexity of minimally invasive aortic aneurysm repair. With the development of sophisticated aortic endografts with multiple side branches to vital organs, surgeons can benefit from AI-augmented tools that help guide complex intraoperative endovascular repair. Cydar Medical (Cambridge, UK) applies computer vision analytics and 3D fusion imaging to intraoperative aortic angiograms for precision stenting during complex endovascular aortic aneurysm repair. Maurel and colleagues showed that the use of Cydar's platform was associated with a 30% reduction in radiation dose to patients and surgeons [24].

28.3.3 Reducing Surgical Errors

AI can play a large role in reducing intra-operative errors in the future. Medical errors account for about 210,000–400,000 deaths in hospitalized patients [25], and adverse safety events related to surgery have been estimated to cost about $1.5 billion in the USA per annum [26]. Madani and colleagues set out to use machine learning techniques to minimize intra-operative errors. They developed a GoNoGoNet model that identifies dangerous and safe zones of dissection during laparoscopic cholecystectomy (Figure 28.3) [27]. The model was trained on 290 cholecystectomy videos from 37 countries and 153 surgeons worldwide. The Intersection-Over-Union (IOU) metric that evaluates the overlap between model prediction and reality was the primary outcome for the model and revealed 0.53 for the safe zones and 0.71 for the non-safe zones [27]. Accuracy was 0.94 for the safe zones and 0.95 for the dangerous resection zones. The specificity of the model was equally high at 0.94 and 0.98 for safe and dangerous zones, respectively, even though a lower sensitivity of 0.69 for

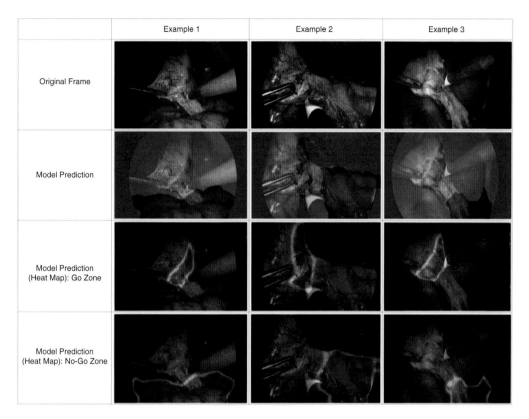

	Example 1	Example 2	Example 3
Original Frame			
Model Prediction			
Model Prediction (Heat Map): Go Zone			
Model Prediction (Heat Map): No-Go Zone			

Figure 28.3: GoNoGoNet model prediction showing safe (green overlay) and dangerous (red overlay) zones, developed by Madani and colleagues.

Source: Madani et al. 2020 / Wolters Kluwer Health Inc.

the safe and 0.80 for the dangerous zones was achieved [27]. While this was a preliminary study that demonstrates a proof of concept, the authors provide valuable lessons on designing AI models for intra-operative surgical safety that can one day be deployed in every OR.

28.3.4 AI-Augmented Robotics Surgery

Robotics have become more common in surgical practice since the FDA approval of the da Vinci system developed by Intuitive Surgical (Sunnyvale, CA, USA) [28]. Since adoption, over 10 million robot-assisted surgical procedures have been performed in more than 67 countries [28,29]. Robotic surgery is increasingly used for uro-oncological, general surgery, and gynaecological procedures [30]. However, most robotic surgery technologies follow the 'master–slave' principle, where a surgeon controls the robot remotely to perform specific surgical tasks [30]. This is the traditional robotic surgery approach, and AI can revolutionize this process by utilizing multi-modal data. For example, AI embedded in robotic systems can be used for skill assessment, warn of dangerous surgical zones, provide haptic feedback to surgeons, and even fine-tune movements [30].

Preliminary work towards AI-augmented robotic surgery was conducted by Hwang and colleagues, who developed a machine learning model to automate a peg transfer task, a common training procedure in robotic surgery [31]. Using the da Vinci surgical robot, Hwang and colleagues' machine learning model achieved 99.4% accuracy for the peg transfer task, which also requires depth sensing to achieve high accuracy [31]. Using machine learning for this task showed that AI in robotic surgery can enable robots to rapidly execute smooth and more accurate motions in the OR. This finding has huge implications for what AI-assisted robotic surgery can look like in the future. There is the potential to automate robotic-assisted surgery to enhance the surgeon's capabilities in the OR, increase accuracy, and reduce or compensate for fatigue. Furthermore, an upcoming robotic system known as Microsure (Eindhoven, Netherlands), a novel robot system for microsurgery, aims to integrate machine learning and data from patient-related features to improve the precision of their robotic tools [32,33].

28.4 Postoperative Care and Long-Term Management

Post-operative care and long-term management of the surgical patient provide opportunities for reinvention. The current focus of AI technologies in the post-operative aspects of care includes effective tracking of acute post-operative recovery, prognostication, and long-term rehabilitation.

28.4.1 Surgical AI in the Acute Post-operative Phase

Similar to pre-operative risk assessments, post-operative care can be guided by risk scores. For example, surgeons can estimate risk of post-operative complications specific to their surgeries, and/or general complications such as likelihood of deep venous thrombosis or myocardial infarction. While these risk scores can aid clinical decision-making, current scoring metrics are often based on a small number of pre-defined criteria with limited precision. Machine learning algorithms applied to large datasets can improve this aspect of surgical care. An example of this is the machine learning–based post-operative risk score developed by Han and colleagues using data from the Samsung Medical Center in South Korea [34]. The risk score was built to stratify patients for risk of developing a post-operative pancreatic fistula from a pancreatoduodenectomy, with the goal of early intervention to mitigate morbidity [34]. Investigators retrieved data on patients' sociodemographic and clinico-pathological characteristics, surgical technique (including the type of anastomotic method) used in the OR, as well as peri-operative management on 1769 patients from the medical database of their institution. They used neural network algorithms to develop a model, resulting in an AUC of 0.74. This was better than other standard risk scores, and the developers of this model made it freely available to the general public [35]. This use case highlights an important aspect of developing AI models.

The most useful models are likely to be ones that focus on a specific surgical case with well-defined actionable steps to improve outcomes.

For patients transferred to the intensive care unit (ICU) for recovery after surgery, it is important to reduce the number of days spent in intensive care, as this has been correlated with improved surgical outcomes [36]. Beyond this, active mobilization of critically ill patients can reduce complications like pneumonia and bedsores, and increase survival [37]. Yeung and colleagues developed technology, using computer vision algorithms, that can automate detection of mobility in the ICU. The study used prospectively collected data on 563 instances of mobility activities and 98,801 frames of video from the Intermountain LDS Hospital ICU to train and test these models. The data were collected using depth-sensing cameras installed in the ICU, and could also identify the number of personnel associated with each activity. Their models achieved an average AUC of 0.938, with mean sensitivity and specificity of 87.2% and 89.2%, respectively, for activities including 'getting out of bed', 'getting in bed', 'getting out of chair' and 'getting in chair' [38]. In addition to patient-specific benefits, models generated from this work have the potential to improve operational capabilities such as aiding in staff planning and personalization of mobility protocols in the ICU. These models are already implemented at Stanford Healthcare, with research ongoing as to the effect of such technology on patient outcomes [39].

28.4.2 Surgical AI for Disease Recurrence Prediction

In the field of surgical oncology, recurrence prognosis is of great importance. Historically, data on post-surgical recurrence rates have used epidemiological methods that identify only those risk factors for which large effect sizes are seen on a population level [40,41]. While epidemiological studies provide insights into broad risk factors, it can be difficult to extrapolate data to provide individual patients with a precise prediction of recurrence rates [42,43]. Given the growing importance of personalized medicine in surgical oncology [44], machine learning techniques have been utilized for prognostication, leveraging multi-modal data by integrating clinical and genomic data points [45]. For example, a study by Lou and colleagues demonstrated that a neural network model was superior in predicting the 10-year recurrence rate of breast cancer after surgical resection with an AUC of 0.99 [46]. Another example includes machine learning models developed for predicting hepatocellular carcinoma recurrence after surgical resection. In addition to clinical data, the investigators incorporated radiomics analysis (a technique that utilizes extracted features from imaging) of CT imaging, resulting in near perfect prediction of disease recurrence [47]. This study was conducted on 470 patients with external validation on a subset of 153 patients. Clinical validation of the model successfully stratified patients into various recurrence groups, demonstrating clinical relevance. The model showed superior prognostic performance compared to other staging systems [47]. When such models are integrated into clinical decision-support tools, they will enhance education and communication between patients and surgeons, and help produce more tailored post-operative surveillance and treatment plans.

28.4.3 AI for Post-operative Rehabilitation and Recovery

AI is also being integrated into surgical workflows through enhancement of remote patient rehabilitation protocols. In a small cohort of 25 patients who underwent total knee arthroplasty (TKA), patients were monitored using a smart orthotic device with sensors that collected movement data [48]. This was paired with a mobile application to document post-surgery recovery exercises, and a dashboard for surgeons and the health team to accurately track patients' recovery in real time. Patients could also document their pain scores, opioid usage, and functional activities [49]. In their assessment of the feasibility of a machine learning–based remote monitoring system, Ramkumar and colleagues analysed multi-modal data from patients, including steps, opioid use, and patient-reported outcome measures. The machine learning component provided real-time feedback on progress to patients and providers. Primary outcomes were patient compliance, which was 88%, and mean mobility post-TKA, which was found to return to baseline within six weeks. All patients surveyed at the completion of the study enjoyed interacting with the interface, in part due to the automated feedback provided [50]. Similar technology has been built by FocusMotion (Santa Monica, CA, USA) to provide AI-augmented solutions that remotely track, assess, and report post-operative recovery progress to the surgical team [49]. This niche area has enormous space for growth. Wearable sensors can create unique digital signatures that can further personalize the recovery process for post-operative patients, and even predict recovery time based on machine learning–driven insights.

28.5 Surgical Training

Poor technical skills are associated with an increased risk of readmission and complications after surgery [48,51]. In addition, several studies show that direct feedback to surgical trainees is associated with improved surgical skills, increased motivation, and trainee satisfaction [52,53]. Advances in computer vision and other emerging technologies like augmented reality (AR) and virtual reality (VR) are providing solutions to enhance surgical skills and usher in a new era in the training of surgery residents.

A Canadian team of clinicians and engineers developed a virtual operative assistant (VOA) that uses AI to provide automated feedback on surgical metric performance to users, based on an expert performance benchmark. The machine learning model used to develop the VOA tool was built on a small dataset of 50 individuals who participated in 250 brain tumour resections [54], and was then validated on 28 neurosurgery attendings and trainees, alongside 22 novice participants in the early stages of residency training [55]. The VOA demonstrated an accuracy of 92% and a sensitivity of 100% in classifying the surgical skills of participants [55]. Although this system was tested on a relatively small group of surgeons, there is the potential for this technology to be introduced into surgical training to deliver real-time assessments to trainees learning a particular procedure, alongside keeping track of proficiency improvements over time.

Some startups are integrating AI and computer vision technologies into surgical videos to aid in training and skill improvement for professionals. Theator (Tel Aviv, Israel), has built a surgical AI-powered platform that assists surgeons in automatically annotating key portions of laparoscopic surgery to enable focused review, and the platform also performs automated analysis of operative performance. These capabilities enable learners and experienced surgeons to identify areas for improvement in their surgical practice. The potential is made possible by near-accurate surgical skill classification based on hand movements. The model used by this company demonstrated an accuracy of over 90% in detecting surgical phases for laparoscopic cholecystectomy, for example, thereby providing an important benchmark for the deployment of related models for surgical training [56].

28.6 Challenges and Opportunities

The key challenges in the adoption of AI in surgery can be described under three broad headings:

- Lack of robust data sources.
- Uncertainty regarding adoption of surgical AI technologies.
- Difficulty in implementation.

28.6.1 Lack of Robust Data Sources

Surgery is one of the least penetrated fields in healthcare when it comes to AI, particularly compared to specialties like radiology, pathology, and dermatology. One of the reasons for this discrepancy is likely the amount of routine data collection. For example, fields like radiology and pathology that generate and store immense amounts of image data each day lend themselves well to developing AI models that leverage computer vision and image recognition [6]. In contrast, large amounts of data collected in the OR have not been routinely formatted in ways to enable model building and training on as large a scale as imaging slides in pathology or digital imaging and communications in medicine (DICOM) images in radiology.

Recently, some institutions have established surgical AI centres, with the goal of labelling already available data and acquiring more data from videos and installation of cameras/sensors [57]. The introduction of these tools is an important step in generating large, high-quality datasets that can be used to train surgical AI models. To date, most published use cases of AI in surgery have been small-scale proofs of concept validated on small datasets [58]. As more ORs are outfitted with data-capture technology, the amount of data available to train and validate AI models will grow.

Investments in data mining, accurate labelling of data, and making data widely available for AI in surgery research will go a long way in achieving the potential of AI in surgery. Specifically, open-source surgical datasets can accelerate surgical AI research and development. For instance, the Stanford Center for Artificial

Intelligence in Medical Imaging (AIMI) has teamed up with Microsoft's AI for Health to make the large repository of de-identified imaging datasets freely available to the general public for AI research purposes [59]. Similar efforts have accelerated the adoption of AI in other medical fields, such as the publicly available imaging dataset developed by the American College of Radiology [60] and a recently launched open-source dataset referred to as Nightingale Open Science [61]. These efforts underscore the opportunity for industry, academia, providers, and payers to collaboratively develop large datasets to drive research and development in surgical AI. Multi-institutional datasets sponsored by professional surgical societies can also play a defining role in actualizing AI in surgery and mitigating the current lack of adequate data.

28.6.2 Uncertainty in Adoption of Surgical AI Technologies

Some surgical innovations have caught on like wildfire. Since the introduction of laparoscopic surgery for gallbladder removal was introduced in the 1980s, it took only three years for 75% of cholecystectomies to be done this way [62]. Even so, the pace of innovation adoption is not distributed equally across surgical procedures and specialties [62,63]. Charles Wilson, the pioneering neurosurgeon, outlined multiple factors that affect the rate of adoption of surgical technology [64]. While patient demand is one common theme, other prevailing themes include compatibility with current practice, simplicity of the new technology, the learning curve for said technology, and perceived benefit from different stakeholders [64]. Given these factors, it is difficult to say a priori what AI technologies will be major successes, but one can surmise that successful technologies will be built around fully understanding the pain points that face surgeons and their teams, and ensuring that AI solutions do not overly complicate existing practices, but integrate well within existing systems and provide large benefits to important stakeholders that include surgeons, patients, payers, and other health providers. While there is always room for disruptive technology, such use cases will likely need to provide outsized benefits to multiple involved parties to reach successful adoption. Furthermore, technologists will need to focus on generating appropriate evidence to support the use of AI technology, as evidence-based medicine still stands as the ideal standard for surgical practice.

28.6.3 Difficulty in Implementation

Practical implementation challenges are often overlooked in the research and development of medical AI tools [65]. Important questions that must be answered include: How will an AI solution impact the workflow and dynamics of the surgical team? Who on the team needs to review the data provided by AI technologies? Who will act on these data? And what specific action will they take? How much capacity does anyone on the team have to take action on insights provided and what are the associated costs? Thinking about deployment early in the design of surgical AI solutions can help mitigate implementation challenges, and partnerships with the surgical team can provide better results than building tools in silos without consultation with the intended user [65]. Furthermore, given the multiple AI platforms in development, how will teams and health systems prioritize and/or integrate AI solutions from different vendors? Surgical AI implementation is an emerging topic with a lot of opportunities for both academia and industry, bridging disciplines such as surgical practice, process design, business, and organizational behaviour and culture change.

Another challenge in implementation has to do with physician versus AI technology liability. Many of the systems we describe do not aim to *replace* clinicians in the quest to improve patient care. The reasons for this, while multifactorial, are likely due to two major issues. First, helping clinicians, rather than replacing them, can increase technology utilization given our current healthcare paradigm [64]. One can imagine that a technology that plans to replace a clinician would receive hostility from the medical community. Another important point is that AI platforms in healthcare have generally avoided being liable for making final decisions about diagnoses or care recommendations. In doing so, medical AI companies may avoid significant liability and larger consequences associated with missed diagnoses or incorrect recommendations. Moving forward, an emerging question arises: as AI models become more accurate and are trained on larger bodies of real-world data, will there ever be a point where clinicians are disintermediated in a way that reduces liability risk? The answer to this question is likely to evolve iteratively with changing technological and regulatory environments.

28.7 Caveats for AI in Surgery

While we have described a broad array of important use cases for surgical AI, it is important to remember some caveats. No AI system to date can boast 100% accuracy in the task at hand, especially when used in different settings. Mistakes generated from automated surgical AI systems can be costly on multiple fronts. Thus, tools that provide enhancement of human capabilities where there is still appropriate human oversight can mitigate the problem of 'machines run amok'. The potential for bias in AI systems is also a concern. Many AI models, even those trained exclusively on imaging data, use data from a small subset of the population [66]. This can cause prediction accuracy to break down when applied to the larger population. Worse yet, predictions may adversely affect certain groups whose data are not well represented in training datasets. Increasing data availability and paying attention to the diversity (or lack thereof) of the data used to develop AI technology are of paramount importance. Another important caveat is that conflicts of interest must be evaluated when AI technologies are being developed in conjunction with industry. Misaligned incentives can lead to speedy development of technology that is at best not helpful, and at worst harmful. While industry–academia partnerships should be encouraged, the principles of 'do no harm' should sit at the forefront of these partnerships.

28.8 Conclusion

Machine learning and the AI applications generated are set to transform the world, with research estimating the market to be worth $13 trillion in the coming decades [67]. Though healthcare, in general, is known for slow technology adoption, the unique aspects of surgical practice that embrace technology and innovation, as well as current inefficiencies in diagnosis, risk stratification, education, and OR logistics, make the field ripe for improvement via the adoption of AI technology. While AI can augment surgical care in incredible ways, roadblocks to achieving maximum success include lack of robust data sources and difficulty in addressing implementation challenges, to name just a couple. Removing these barriers will accelerate research, development, and adoption of surgical AI solutions.

KEY INSIGHTS

- The focus of surgical AI to date has been on diagnosis of acute surgical diseases, pre- and post-operative risk stratification, and some proof-of-concept use cases related to prognostication and real-time surgical safety during certain procedures. Other exciting use cases that are being developed and deployed include improving the pre-operative planning capabilities through AI-based 3D modeling, AI-assisted robotic surgery, and enhancement of post-operative recovery.
- Key challenges cover data availability for technology development, implementation constraints, and uncertainty regarding surgeon interest in, and adoption of, AI tools.
- Key opportunity areas include development of large, representative surgery-specific datasets, working together with surgical teams to identify key pain points and solutions that best fit into the surgical workflow, and prospectively studying the impact of surgical AI technologies to form a sound evidence base for technology adoption.
- Future issues to be addressed include how health systems and providers will prioritize and/or integrate AI systems built by disparate teams and companies for different use cases, as well as how increasingly accurate systems may affect our interest or ability to remove clinicians from certain medical decisions or tasks.

References

1. Kapp KA, Talboy GE, Kapp K. *John Hunter, the Father of Scientific Surgery.* CC2017 Poster Competition. Chicago, IL: American College of Surgeons; 2017, 34–41.
2. Taylor AG, Mielke C, Mongan J. Automated detection of moderate and large pneumothorax on frontal chest X-rays using deep convolutional neural networks: a retrospective study. *PLoS Medicine* 2018;15(11):e1002697.

3. Bai N. Artificial intelligence that reads chest x-rays is approved by FDA. *UCSF Research*, 12 September 2019. https://www.ucsf.edu/news/2019/09/415406/artificial-intelligence-reads-chest-x-rays-approved-fda.

4. Ginat D. Implementation of machine learning software on the radiology worklist decreases scan view delay for the detection of intracranial hemorrhage on CT. *Brain Science* 2021;11(7):832.

5. Ojeda P, Zawaideh M, Mossa-Basha M, Haynor D. The utility of deep learning: evaluation of a convolutional neural network for detection of intracranial bleeds on non-contrast head computed tomography studies. *Proceedings Medical Imaging 2019: Image Processing*. Bellingham, WA: SPIE; 2019, 899–906. https://www.spiedigitallibrary.org/conference-proceedings-of-spie/10949/109493J/The-utility-of-deep-learning--evaluation-of-a-convolutional/10.1117/12.2513167.full.

6. Topol EJ. High-performance medicine: the convergence of human and artificial intelligence. *Nature Medicine* 2019;25(1):44–56.

7. Bertsimas D, Dunn J, Velmahos GC, Kaafarani HMA. Surgical risk is not linear: derivation and validation of a novel, user-friendly, and machine-learning-based Predictive OpTimal Trees in Emergency Surgery Risk (POTTER) calculator. *Annals of Surgery* 2018;268(4):574–583.

For additional references and Further Reading please see www.wiley.com/go/byrne/aiinclinicalmedicine.

29

AI in Urological Oncology: Prostate Cancer Diagnosis with Magnetic Resonance Imaging

Sherif Mehralivand and Baris Turkbey

Molecular Imaging Branch, National Institutes of Health, Bethesda, MD, USA

Learning Objectives

- Understand the importance of multiparametric magnetic resonance imaging (MRI) in prostate cancer detection.
- Review the value of AI algorithms in prostate lesion detection.
- Understand current scientific achievements in AI-assisted prostate lesion detection.
- Gain knowledge of the future prospects and value of AI algorithms in multiparametric prostate MRI.

29.1 Introduction

AI in prostate cancer diagnostics is a relatively new domain. Historically, prostate cancer was not diagnosed using diagnostic imaging. Before the introduction of prostate cancer screening programmes, prostate cancer was mainly diagnosed in the late metastatic stages or incidentally in pathological specimens after transurethral resection of the prostate for benign prostatic hyperplasia.

The discovery of the prostate-specific antigen (PSA) in serum enabled its use as a cancer biomarker and eventually as a screening tool. In the late 1980s and early 1990s, widespread population-based screening programmes were introduced to advance the early detection of prostate cancer, and therefore improve oncological outcomes by early treatment of localized disease and prevention of metastatic disease [1]. However, prostate cancer lesions are not visible on transrectal ultrasound (TRUS), meaning that prostate biopsy specimens had to be obtained systematically by targeting pre-defined areas within the organ according to a standardized biopsy template. Although this approach significantly reduced the proportion of metastatic prostate cancer diagnoses and led to a decrease in disease-specific mortality, over-diagnosis and over-treatment of early clinically insignificant disease remain among the main challenges in prostate cancer management. However, there are still high numbers of prostate cancer patients who die from the disease [2].

AI in Clinical Medicine: A Practical Guide for Healthcare Professionals, First Edition. Edited by Michael F. Byrne, Nasim Parsa, Alexandra T. Greenhill, Daljeet Chahal, Omer Ahmad, and Ulas Bagci.
© 2023 John Wiley & Sons Ltd. Published 2023 by John Wiley & Sons Ltd.
Companion website: www.wiley.com/go/byrne/aiinclinicalmedicine

29.1.1 Imaging Diagnostics

Over the last decade, advancements in magnetic resonance imaging (MRI) have led to improvement in detection of prostate cancer [3]. Multiparametric MRI (mp-MRI) combines anatomical and functional MRI sequences to enable the detection and localization of prostate cancer lesions, and promotes the visualization of prostate cancer lesions on medical imaging. As a consequence, a more targeted prostate biopsy approach was developed, and we can now obtain biopsy samples directly from prostate cancer lesions made visible on mp-MRI [4].

However, like all medical imaging modalities, inter-reader reproducibility is a significant challenge, and success is dependent on reader expertise and experience. This is particularly challenging in mp-MRI imaging due to the complexity of integrating anatomical and functional MRI sequences into a whole assessment [5]. AI-based solutions can aid radiologists during the reading process by offering objective assistance. This is shown to be especially beneficial for less experienced radiologists. However, due to the special characteristics of mp-MRI, data preparation and annotation must adhere to certain standards and techniques.

29.1.2 Imaging AI for Prostate Cancer Detection

The first attempts to develop AI detection systems for prostate cancer lesions using mp-MRI were mainly based on 'classical' machine learning techniques [6]. These algorithms were trained on small institutional datasets using well-established machine learning classifiers like support vector machines, random forest, or logistic regression. Significant data preparation and pre-processing are required before algorithm training. Imaging features (handcrafted) must be extracted and pre-tested, and standardization and transformation procedures are applied before final model training is performed. As a tremendous amount of hand-crafting is required, a process that is both tedious and time-consuming, this results in only small datasets available for model training.

29.1.3 Data-Related Challenges

A key challenge is that institution-based overfitting can introduce human bias into the training data, resulting in poor performance in clinical practice. We refer to overfitting in the context of machine learning based on imaging features and patient characteristics inherent to an institution. In our experience, this effect is particularly visible in AI algorithms trained on mp-MRI datasets, as MRI images can differ significantly between vendors. The MRI signal can vary based on the construction of the MRI scanner, for instance scanner length or aperture. More importantly, the post-processing of the raw MRI signal is calculation intensive and heavily dependent on the vendor's scanner software. This is in contrast to computed tomography (CT), where scanner engineering and software are much more standardized among vendors. We see from our experience that AI algorithms trained on CT images are less prone to institution-based overfitting, and demonstrate more consistent performance on images from different vendors compared to MRI scans.

Magnet field strength (B_0) is another factor influencing the signal-to-noise ratio (SNR) that directly translates into image resolution. Theoretically, B_0 is linearly proportional to SNR. Newer scanners with $B_0 = 3$ Tesla (T) can therefore double the resolution compared to older 1.5 T machines, and include additional advantages such as fewer motion artifacts and shorter scanning time. However, many older 1.5 T scanners are still in use, and differing image resolution is a significant challenge for AI model training and external validity. In addition, there are other differences inherent to the multiparametric technique.

29.1.4 Multiparametric MRI Imaging for Prostate Cancer

As previously mentioned, mp-MRI combines different anatomical and functional sequences for prostate cancer lesion detection and characterization. T2-weighted imaging is the backbone of anatomical imaging, while diffusion-weighted imaging (DWI) and dynamic contrast-enhanced (DCE) imaging are functional sequences. These MRI sequences demonstrate higher signal intensities in areas of high cellularity or vascularity. Cancer lesions tend to have higher contrast, and are therefore more visible than the surrounding benign tissue.

DCE imaging has come under increased scrutiny recently [7]. While proponents praise its value in improving detection sensitivity, especially for smaller and less visible lesions, opponents question its risk–benefit ratio with regard to the long-term negative effects of gadolinium contrast application as compared to subtle detection improvements.

DWI is the main functional sequence in multiparametric prostate MRI. The b-value determines the degree of diffusion weighting, and usually lies between 0 and 1000 s/mm². The higher the b-value, the higher the contrast between prostate cancer lesions and the background, which is represented by healthy prostate tissue and other benign forms of prostate lesions. Thus, the 'high b-value' sequence has become an integral part of multiparametric MRI protocols [8]. Although not clearly defined, current guidelines recommend b-values between 1500 and 2000 s/mm². Higher tissue contrast comes at the cost of resolution and anatomical detail, which is the main reason for combining T2-weighted and DWI. Furthermore, higher b-values result in greater susceptibility to motion artifacts caused by rectal peristalsis during the scanning process.

Different approaches have been proposed to mitigate the effects of rectal peristalsis, ranging from administering peristalsis-inhibiting medication to applying rectal enemas prior to scanning the patient. The application of an endorectal coil is another variable affecting prostate MRI resolution and quality [9]. An endorectal coil can improve the resolution of prostate MRI images up to fourfold due to its anatomical proximity to the rectum. While there is an increasing agreement that 1.5 T scanners should use endorectal coils to guarantee sufficient image resolution for prostate cancer lesion detection and classification, widespread consensus about the necessity of endorectal coil use in 3 T machines does not exist. Proponents praise the improved detection rate due to higher image resolution, while opponents criticize the additional inconvenience to patients with no or only subtle clinical benefit.

29.1.5 AI Overcomes Inter-Reader Variability

Like all medical imaging techniques, mp-MRI for prostate is subject to inter-reader variability, in relation to detected lesions and classification. Because the reading process is highly complex and MRI images lack objective quantitative information, the subjective interpretation by readers with varying experience and expertise leads to different results and outcomes [10,11].

AI-based solutions have tremendous potential in assisting less experienced readers in this highly specialized and complex field of genitourinary radiology by offering objective assistance based on algorithms that were trained on large clinical datasets. Empirical data from our institution and others demonstrate that AI provides improved outcomes with regard to prostate cancer lesion detection, particularly for readers with low to intermediate levels of experience.

Greer et al. published the results of a large international multicentre reader study of an AI-based computer-aided diagnosis (CADx) system in 2018 [12]. Nine radiologists with different backgrounds in mp-MRI were involved in the study (equally split between low, intermediate, and significant experience). A total of 163 patients were included: 110 patients had undergone robotic-assisted radical prostatectomy, and 53 patients had negative MRIs and no cancer pathology on biopsy. The AI model was based on a random decision forest classifier trained by tumour contours and targeted biopsy histopathology as labels. Its outputs were cancer probability maps highlighting areas of increased prostate cancer risk (Figure 29.1).

In the first arm of the study, readers were presented with MRI exams alone, and were asked to detect and classify cancer-suspicious lesions. After a washout period of five weeks, readers were tasked to evaluate the same MRI scans (in a different random order) using AI assistance. Overall, detection sensitivity showed a statistically significant improvement – 98% with AI assistance compared to 92.7% without AI assistance (p = 0.002).

The results were very different among readers who had different levels of evaluation experience. AI assistance demonstrated a statistically significant improvement in detection sensitivity among moderately experienced readers (98.2% sensitivity with AI assistance compared to 91.5% without AI assistance, p = 0.015). Although high- and low-experience readers also demonstrated improvements in detection sensitivity, this difference was not statistically significant. These results are essentially consistent with other AI models from other institutions, which demonstrated that highly experienced readers do not benefit from AI assistance while low to moderately experienced readers can gain significantly benefit, depending on their skills and training. AI assistance also significantly decreased specificity among all reader

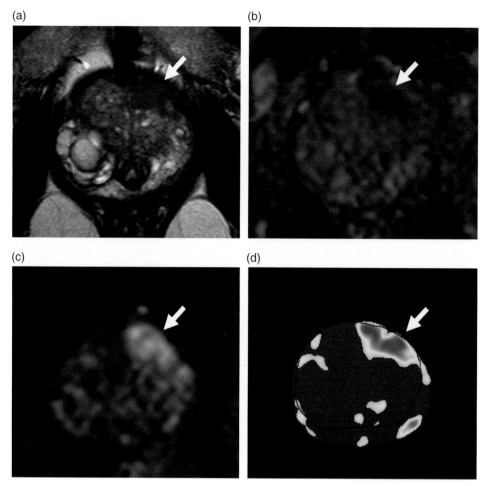

Figure 29.1: Imaging to identify areas of increased prostate cancer risk in a 70 year old male with a serum prostate-specific antigen (PSA) of 10.45 ng/mL. The arrow shows the location of a left apical anterior transition zone lesion by (a) axial T2-weighted magnetic resonance imaging (MRI); (b) apparent diffusion coefficient (ADC) map; (c) b1500 diffusion-weighted MRI; (d) AI algorithm probability map highlighting area of increase prostate cancer risk. Targeted biopsy of this lesion revealed Gleason 3+4 prostate adenocarcinoma.

Source: NIH, National Cancer Institute / U.S. Department of Health and Human Services / Public domain.

groups from 54.2% to 16% (p < 0.001). This is a common trend among many AI tools, and is caused by an increased false-positive rate in lesion presentation by the algorithm. In our experience, the majority of these false-positive lesions occur in the transition zone of the prostate, where benign prostatic hyperplasia (BPH) is commonly found in elderly men [13]. This disease is caused by hyperplasia of smooth muscle cells, which can lead to obstruction and micturition problems. Although it is a benign disease with no association with prostate cancer, it has similar prop erties in multiparametric MRI, and these can be challenging to differentiate with the human eye and AI alike.

BACKGROUND ON DEEP LEARNING IN MEDICAL IMAGING

The last decade was shaped by tremendous progress in deep learning technology. Deep learning is a sub-branch of machine learning using deep neural networks. These neural networks use deep hidden layers; that is, many serial layers that can solve much more complex tasks compared to 'shallow' neural networks. Although they are not a new concept, deep neural networks have re-emerged over the last decade due to several simultaneous advancements [14].

Firstly, there have been improvements in algorithm theory, like fast implementation of convolutional neural networks (CNN) and recurrent neural networks (RNN). The use of Graphics Processing Unit (GPU) implementations of backpropagation training has accelerated the training process, and enabled the use of much more complex networks. Furthermore, GPU computational power has steadily increased over the past several years.

Deep learning mainly benefits from the use of large amount of well curated data; that is, large labelled datasets that are representative of the population of interest. These data have become much more available with the rise of the internet, smart phones, and social media. Deep learning has several advantages compared to machine learning. A common issue with conventional machine learning–based approaches for medical imaging is the need for feature engineering (i.e., hand-crafted feature modeling and extraction). This method is prone to overfitting, since image features are selected and generated by hand, leading to increased human interference during the training process. Deep learning methods like CNNs theoretically reduce this interference, since the filters – that is, the kernels – are not manually generated, but trained by large datasets using backpropagation.

However, deep learning can also be prone to overfitting, especially when using small datasets for training. This is still an issue, especially in medicine, where large datasets are relatively unavailable compared to industry and social media. There are two main reasons for that. First, there are more patient privacy-related restrictions in relation to data availability and sharing. Larger patient datasets are often part of a clinical trial or protocol, which significantly impedes data sharing and accessibility. Second, data labelling, which is essential for deep learning algorithm training, is more tedious and expensive since highly specialized experts, such as genitourinary radiologists, need to dedicate a significant amount of their workforce to evaluate, contour, and label data on medical imaging examinations.

Nevertheless, we believe that deep learning is the future of AI-based applications in medical imaging due to its advantages. Its shortcomings can be overcome by multi-institutional and international collaborations to ensure that large representative well-curated datasets are available for model training and validation. It must be emphasized that large datasets alone will not suffice. Deep learning models trained on large datasets from a single institution are prone to institution-based overfitting. For instance, as already mentioned, mp-MRI images can differ significantly among institutions due to differences between scanner vendors, software, patient preparation, and patient demographics. As a consequence, an algorithm trained on a single-institution dataset might perform well in validation and testing cohorts on patients from this same institution, but its performance will significantly drop when used on patients from other institutions or geographical regions, limiting external validity.

29.2 Deep Learning Algorithms for Prostate Cancer Diagnosis

To train a deep learning model for the prediction of prostate cancer on multiparametric MRI, we started an initiative in 2019 to gather large, labelled datasets for multiparametric prostate MRI, adhering to the highest reading standards available. A dedicated top expert in the field with more than 15 years of experience and more than 1500 reads per year was engaged to start labelling scans from our institution. MRI scans were retrospectively evaluated, and lesions were contoured using in-house segmentation software. Lesions were then compared to MRI-TRUS fusion-guided prostate biopsy results, and lesions were labelled as positive in cases of proven prostate cancer.

We blended our dataset with a publicly available dataset, called PROSTATEx, created for an AI challenge (which concluded in 2017 and it has since been made available for public use). This resulted in a total of 525 patient scans, which were used for model training, validation, and testing.

Two different deep learning algorithms were used in this study, the U-Net and the recently proposed AH Net. This network architecture enables the training of detection and segmentation algorithms for medical imaging tasks. U-Net and AH-Net were both trained using 3D masks of prostate cancer lesions on multiparametric MRI. To optimize training, a prostate segmentation algorithm (based on a similar previous algorithm [15]) first highlighted the borders of the prostate. The predicted organ boundaries were then used to crop out the prostate from the rest of the MRI scan in order to improve algorithm performance. Detection sensitivity was 72.8% for the U-Net and 63% for the AH-Net in the test set. This came at the cost of a mean of 1.9 false-positive lesions per patient for the U-Net and a mean of 1.4 false-positive lesions per patient for the AH-Net.

Both models demonstrated higher detection sensitivities compared to previous AI algorithms not based on deep learning. However, direct comparison of detection performance is only valid through comparative studies. We are currently working on solutions to deploy this new deep learning algorithm in our picture archiving and communication system to make it available to radiologists at our institution. We can therefore apply this infrastructure in future studies.

29.3 Future of AI in Prostate Cancer Diagnosis

We believe that deep learning will superscde conventional machine learning approaches in medical imaging classification and detection tasks for prostate cancer. There are a large number of studies reporting the development and performance of AI models that aim to detect prostate cancer automatically at MRI. A meta-analysis conducted in 2019 by Cuocolo et al. included 12 studies that aim to detect clinically significant prostate cancer using machine learning or deep learning AI models [16]. The overall pooled area under the receiver operating characteristic for AI models in clinically significant prostate cancer detection was 0.86 (95% confidence interval [CI] 0.81–0.91). The results of this meta-analysis indicate that AI models yielded a comparable performance in prostate cancer detection compared to human readers. However, these results should be interpreted with caution, since these AI models were not trained on large-scale or diverse datasets, and were not sufficiently tested in multicentre study designs with direct comparison to radiologists [16].

The availability of larger multicentre clinical data will benefit AI-based approaches, as has been demonstrated in other domains. While the AI approach for cancer detection is mainly still at the research phase and is not yet ready for widespread clinical adoption, there are currently some AI solutions that aim to assist the prostate MRI reading process by providing automated prostate segmentation for PSA density calculation and biopsy guidance [17–22]. With access to more large-scale, diverse, multicentre training datasets with a more reliable ground truth for model training purposes, we expect that more robust prostate MRI AI algorithms will be commercially available to assists radiologists and urologists in their clinical workflow.

Although some of the first experiences with deep learning are promising, the true value of these algorithms can only be determined by direct comparison to the gold standard: namely, expert human evaluation. In medical imaging, said experts are radiologists with specialized training in their respective fields. Due to inter-reader variability and differences in training and expertise, multi-reader studies are often employed to compare outcomes. Despite their promise, AI algorithms are still subject to false negatives as well as a significant number of false-positive lesions. Therefore, a standalone AI application to detect prostate cancer is still not feasible.

We believe that the focus should be on developing AI tools that work in conjunction with radiologists during the reading process, and can be used for both clinical and teaching applications. Preliminary data have shown significant improvements in reading outcomes, especially among readers with low to intermediate experience. Multi-reader studies comparing prostate lesion detection outcomes on mp-MRI for radiologists with different levels of experience, with and without AI assistance, are planned. Other areas of improvement include algorithm optimization through the use of larger and more diverse MRI datasets, as well as testing new network architectures.

KEY INSIGHTS

- Deep learning is gaining ground in medical imaging-related tasks.
- Large and diverse medical datasets improve algorithm performance and generalizability.
- In prostate cancer lesion detection, false negatives and especially false positives are still very high, precluding standalone application.
- Currently, AI tools will mainly serve as adjunct assistance tools during prostate MRI reading.
- Comparative multi-reader studies are needed to determine the true value of AI assistance in clinical practice.

References

1. Schroder FH, Hugosson J, Roobol MJ et al. Screening and prostate cancer mortality: results of the European Randomised Study of Screening for Prostate Cancer (ERSPC) at 13 years of follow-up. *Lancet* 2014;384:2027–2035.
2. Siegel RL, Miller KD, Jemal A. Cancer statistics, 2020. *CA: A Cancer Journal for Clinicians* 2020;70(1):7–30.
3. Turkbey B, Pinto PA, Mani H et al. Prostate cancer: value of multiparametric MR imaging at 3 T for detection—histopathologic correlation. *Radiology* 2010;255:89–99.
4. Ahdoot M, Wilbur AR, Reese SE et al. MRI-targeted, systematic, and combined biopsy for prostate cancer diagnosis. *New England Journal of Medicine* 2020;382(10):917–928.
5. Rosenkrantz AB, Ginocchio LA, Cornfeld D et al. Interobserver reproducibility of the PI-RADS version 2 lexicon: a multicenter study of six experienced prostate radiologists. *Radiology* 2016;280:793–804.
6. Wang S, Burtt K, Turkbey B, Choyke P, Summers RM. Computer aided-diagnosis of prostate cancer on multiparametric MRI: a technical review of current research. *BioMed Research International* 2014;2014:789561.
7. Turkbey B, Rosenkrantz AB, Haider MA et al. Prostate Imaging Reporting and Data System Version 2.1: 2019 Update of Prostate Imaging Reporting and Data System Version 2. *European Urology* 2019;76(3):340–351.

For additional references and Further Reading please see www.wiley.com/go/byrne/aiinclinicalmedicine.

AI in Pathology

Stephanie Harmon and Kevin Ma

National Cancer Institute, National Institutes of Health, Bethesda, MD, USA

30

Learning Objectives

- Learn how digital pathology is transforming clinical care.
- Understand areas of digital pathology where AI can make an impact.
- Recognize the challenges in data collection and annotation specific to digital pathology.
- Review successful components of AI studies for clinical validation.
- Discuss limitations and solutions for AI applications in resource-limited settings.

30.1 Digital Pathology: Beginning of a New Era

Pathological evaluation is an essential part of diagnostic and treatment decision pathways in modern medicine. For several years, tissue specimens were reviewed only with the microscope. In the past few years, advances in technology have enabled the routine scanning and digital assessment of pathology specimens, which is shown to be comparable to traditional microscopic assessment. The clinical benefits of digital assessment include improved quality, efficiency, and access to high-quality healthcare. Pathologist interpretation and reporting are often limited to providing a qualitative assessment of diagnosis and grading. With the recent US Food and Drug Administration (FDA) approval of whole slide imaging (WSI) systems, opportunities for the clinical deployment of AI systems in this area have increased substantially. AI has the potential to drastically speed up time-consuming evaluation by the pathologist while improving the inter-observer variability. Currently, there is only one FDA-approved AI algorithm for the diagnosis of prostate cancer on digital pathology images from biopsy samples (https://www.fda.gov/news-events/press-announcements/fda-authorizes-software-can-help-identify-prostate-cancer). However, several algorithms that have undergone successful training and robust validation for potential clinical translation will be discussed in this chapter. Compared to similar work in radiology, digital pathology presents a unique challenge to the annotation, development, and deployment of image-based

AI in Clinical Medicine: A Practical Guide for Healthcare Professionals, First Edition. Edited by Michael F. Byrne, Nasim Parsa, Alexandra T. Greenhill, Daljeet Chahal, Omer Ahmad, and Ulas Bagci.
© 2023 John Wiley & Sons Ltd. Published 2023 by John Wiley & Sons Ltd.
Companion website: www.wiley.com/go/byrne/aiinclinicalmedicine

AI algorithms due to the large image size and scale. Diagnostic pathology includes standard anatomical review, using haematoxylin and eosin (H&E) staining, and increasingly more immunohistochemical (IHC) molecular markers. Digitization and automation in both areas will be important for the successful translation of AI into routine clinical care.

30.2 Successful Applications of Clinical Pathology AI: The Basics

There are several potential areas for the application of AI in digital pathology, such as cellular segmentation, cancer detection, cancer diagnosis, cancer grading, and prognostic prediction. A large proportion of clinically relevant AI research in this field is in the cancer domain.

The application of AI in digital pathology ranges from microscopic (individual cells in the order of several micrometres) to macroscopic (tumour grading in the order of several millimetres) evaluation. Images are often several gigabytes per slide, and scanners can achieve resolution up to 40× magnification, presenting a challenge for dataset aggregation and annotation. For these reasons, AI algorithms learn on small patches of data extracted at specific sizes and magnification. Additional post-processing is often necessary to determine a slide-level or patient-level diagnosis. An example of patches extracted at different magnifications is shown in Figure 30.1.

The first critical component to a successful AI algorithm is dataset selection and annotation. Different medical centres have different methods for tissue fixation and processing that can affect the generalizability of trained AI models. Without

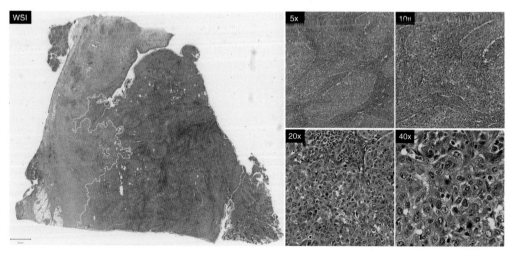

Figure 30.1: Whole slide imaging of bladder cancer specimen from TCGA-BLCA collection (https://portal.gdc.cancer.gov) with tumour regions outlined in yellow. Representative image tiles reflecting histology architecture to nuclear features are shown ranging from 5× to 40×, representing resolution of 2 μm/pixel and 0.25 μm/pixel, respectively.

Source: Stephanie Harmon and Kevin Ma.

millions of WSIs representing all known disease entities for training, AI algorithms can only achieve the highest predictive performance by training on a high-quality dataset that accurately represents a discase entity.

Once the algorithm is trained, researchers perform rigorous validation on an independent testing set to evaluate the performance within the clinical context. This step is essential to demonstrate how easy it is to integrate that particular AI algorithm into clinical practice without negatively impacting the workflow of the pathologist. Given the known inter-observer variability, the performance metrics of AI tools should be evaluated against several expert readers to gauge the reliability of these tools in comparison to the current clinical standard.

30.2.1 Application Use Case: Grading in Prostate Cancer

The development of automated detection and grading for prostate cancer is a highly challenging task frequently studied in recent literature. Clinically, the Gleason grading system is used for treatment decision-making and determining the risk of recurrent cancer after definitive treatment for localized prostate cancer. This scoring system is, however, prone to inter-observer variability. The system combines the most prevalent and the second most prevalent entities present in a specimen to determine the final grade. Therefore, AI systems developed to support this grading system must detect and classify each morphological entity with high accuracy to produce an accurate slide-level prediction. Successful AI algorithms have used cascaded approaches, such as multi-step algorithms, to solve this problem. Recently, a large study from Sweden trained a diagnostic-quality algorithm on core needle biopsies from >900 patients to achieve expert-level agreement concordance between AI and pathologists [1]. They trained a set of AI classification algorithms to determine the probability of cancer and tumour grade in patches corresponding to ~0.5 mm dimensions at 10× magnification. Probabilities from all patches were then fed into an additional algorithm to determine slide-level tumour grade. Success in this study was enabled by consistent and detailed annotations, use of an independent test set, and clinical benchmark comparison to 23 independent pathologists. In the independent test set, the AI algorithm achieved a mean pairwise kappa of 0.62 with the 23 independent pathologists. *Importantly, this concordance is similar to the pairwise kappas when comparing one pathologist against another pathologist (mean 0.60), showing that AI has a similar level of agreement with pathologists as they do among themselves.* The final algorithm provides twofold clinical benefits: streamlining the diagnostic workflow by identifying benign cores with high accuracy, and standardizing grading with expert-level performance concordance.

30.2.2 Application Use Case: Staging in Breast Cancer

Beyond cancer detection and grading of localized disease, a critical task for pathologists is the identification of tumour seeding outside the primary organ. For localized breast cancer, nodal staging is an essential step in the selection of treatment regimens. The clinical task of identifying cancer cells in these lymph nodes is time-consuming and error prone due to the 'needle in a haystack' nature of the task. The sensitivity of pathologists for correctly identifying cancer-containing lymph nodes is <50% using H&E slides alone. AI can play a critical role in this area, given the challenging nature of searching through the entire image to be able to find these small cancer cell deposits. An algorithm created by Google AI Healthcare recently underwent rigorous clinical validation, and demonstrated that an AI-assisted work-flow can improve the sensitivity for detection beyond 90% [2]. The classification algorithm was trained using a large publicly available dataset (CAMELYON16) and predicts the likelihood (probability) that a given 32 × 32 μm area contains cancer. This classification algorithm was then applied to WSIs to produce a probability heatmap for identifying local areas of cancer. Success in this study was enabled by the design and use of AI assistance for diagnostic review by the pathologists, and by evaluating the algorithm's clinical performance against six pathologists using two external patient cohorts.

The results demonstrate that a combination of AI and pathologist interpretation was more accurate than either alone, and the time needed for pathologists to review images was nearly halved. The sensitivity of micro-metastasis detection improved from a mean of 83% to a mean of 91% with AI assistance, with 5 of 6 pathologists showing individual improvement in sensitivity when using AI assistance. Attention-based systems such as these have the potential to streamline the diagnostic workflow by quickly highlighting suspicious areas with high sensitivity, and giving pathologists more time to review difficult cases. It is worth noting that the patch size for this application is ~100× smaller than the previous prostate cancer example, underscoring the task-specific nature and domain knowledge needed to identify clinically relevant datasets for algorithm training.

30.2.3 Application Use Case: Prognosis in Colorectal Cancer

The previous two examples have focused on achieving high performance within currently accepted pathology standards; that is, routine clinical definitions. Most often, these pathology standards and definitions are driven by the need for reproducible morphology patterns that validate the correlation with disease severity or outcome. In some clinical settings, tumour stage and grade by standard pathological assessment do not completely stratify patients at high risk for poor clinical outcomes.

To evaluate the potential for AI to improve prognostic prediction, many researchers have focused on predicting outcomes from the images themselves. A critical component to the success of these algorithms is the collection of non-biased patient cohorts. Skrede et al. proposed a deep learning solution to discover and develop biomarkers from WSI for colorectal cancer prognosis [3] Four different patient cohorts, consisting of resectable non-synchronous colorectal cancer patients from stages I to III, were included in model training and testing. Images categorized as distinct 'good' or 'poor' outcomes were used in the training cohort, while images with non-distinct outcomes were used for tuning. One convolutional neural network (CNN) model was used to automatically segment cancerous tissues, and a second CNN model provided prognosis categories. The classification model consisted of five separate networks, each providing a prognostic score. The overall prognostic score was aggregated from the five networks. Overall, the trained classifier of the new biomarker was a significant predictor of survival in stage II and stage III (p = 0.01 and <0.0001, respectively).

The outcome of this multivariable classifier showed the potential for identifying new biomarkers to consider in risk assessment in clinical environments. A strong correlation of biomarkers and outcome may inform discussion with patients with stage II and III colorectal cancer regarding treatment options. In this setting, AI provides additional information to existing clinical workflows at no cost to the pathologist.

30.3 AI for Streamlined Clinical Workflow

The previous examples have all detailed successful use cases for AI in challenging clinical, diagnostic, and prognostic settings. AI has other applications that can increase efficiency and accuracy for general yet time-consuming tasks. One of the most commonly researched areas is the segmentation of nuclei on digital histological imaging.

Nuclei segmentation and classification are used in both the H&E and IHC assessment of many cancers, including the segmentation of mitotic figures in breast cancer specimens and the automated cellular counting of expression markers like programmed death ligand-1 (PD-L1) or nuclear protein Ki-67. For each of these entities, it is desirable to have a quantitative assessment of the number and distribution within a given specimen. Another area for streamlined histopathological assessment is screening, where cytology or histology samples are quickly reviewed for abnormalities that then trigger a further diagnostic work-up. We have provided further reading suggestions (see the end of this chapter).

30.3.1 Tumour-Infiltrating Lymphocytes

The presence of tumour-infiltrating lymphocytes (TIL) is an important biomarker for predicting invasive breast cancer outcomes and evaluating treatment response, especially with the emergence of immunotherapy. Several research groups have published on the development of patch-based TIL detection algorithms and the correlation to clinical outcomes [4,5]. Here, high-resolution patches are often classified as high versus low/no TIL infiltration, and the spatial distribution within a tumour sample is characterized (Figure 30.2).

A key example where higher TIL concentration levels are predictors of survival is in certain types of breast cancers, such as human epidermal growth factor receptor 2 positive (HER2+) or triple-negative subtypes. Current practice requires pathologists to manually segment and evaluate TIL concentration

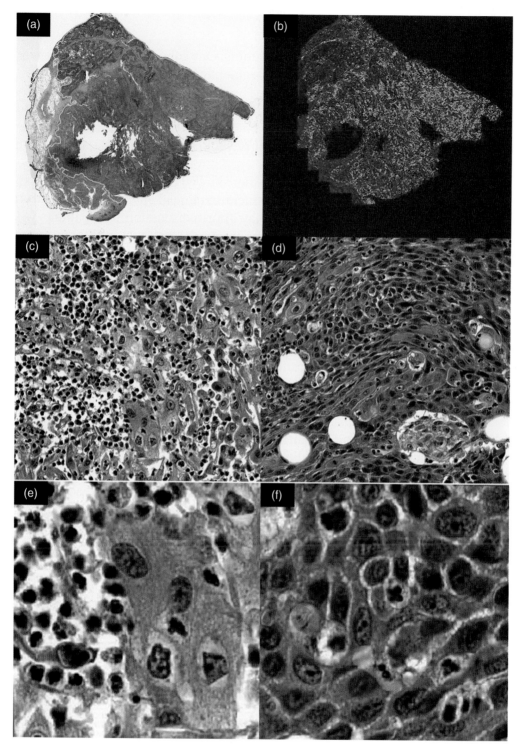

Figure 30.2: Example tumour-infiltrating lymphocyte (TIL) detection map for whole slide imaging (WSI). (a) Bladder cancer WSI with tumour regions outlined in yellow. (b) AI-based TIL detection probability map using an algorithm initially published by Saltz et al. [4] and modified for use by Harmon et al. [5]. Probabilities range from 0 (dark blue) to 1 (dark red). Representative regions within the same tumour demonstrate high (c) and low (d) infiltration. High-power regions of high (e) and low (f) infiltration representing ~100 × 100 μm at 40×.

Source: Stephanie Harmon and Kevin Ma.

within a tumour, which is intrinsically qualitative and time-consuming. Le et al. proposed a deep learning model that automates the detection of breast cancer regions in large-scale datasets of WSIs [6]. In this study, researchers validated their AI algorithm against pathologist assessment and correlated it with clinical outcomes. In the first analysis, three pathologists rated 500 patches as having low, medium, or high TIL content in comparison to AI-based assessment in the same patches. The results showed high correlation between pathologist scoring and AI output (>0.75 inter-rater concordance), representing a modest improvement to inter-pathologist correlation (0.72 concordance). Next, the AI-based TIL prediction results were correlated with overall survival using the TIL infiltration score, a continuous variable calculated as a fraction of the predicted tumour area containing lymphocytes. The mean of the TIL infiltration score, 6.4%, served as a threshold to separate the low infiltration group (n = 695) and the high infiltration group (n = 281). After correcting for other survival predictors such as stage (I, II, III, and IV) and gene expression subtype (LumA, LumB, PAM50 Basal, HER2), the binarized TIL infiltration fraction was predictive of survival with p < 0.05. The analysis results showed the accuracy of AI in detecting and quantifying TIL concentration and spatial distribution in tumours, the reproducibility of prediction results agreeing with expert pathologists, and the clinical relevance in survival prediction for invasive breast cancer.

30.3.2 Screening Populations

Worldwide, the use of population screening via cervical tissue cytology analysis reduces the burden of patients diagnosed with cervical cancer. In cytology, screening experts review cellular morphology under the microscope to detect abnormal cells, which, if present, trigger further diagnostic testing. In screening applications, it is crucial to evaluate both the sensitivity and the specificity of a given test, as the pre-test probability of each entity is massively imbalanced (containing more negative samples than positive samples). This contrasts with other diagnostic settings where clinical symptoms or testing have already indicated a suspicious finding and resulted in a sample biopsy.

A recent study in a large screening cohort demonstrated that AI-assisted cytology had high concordance with expert cytologists, and could improve the sensitivity of various histologically confirmed cervical lesions by 4.5–6.8% while maintaining a <0.5% decrease in specificity [7]. This system worked by first detecting individual cells in the sample and then classifying them according to normal, abnormal, and inadequate criteria. The final score produces a probability of severity (abnormality). The system then sorts slides needing further attention: those with a high likelihood of abnormality versus those that only need a rapid review due to a low likelihood of abnormal findings. Algorithms such as these could have a particularly important application in resource-limited settings by improving equity of care without overburdening smaller or rural healthcare systems.

30.4 Major Challenges

Several major roadblocks challenge the development of AI algorithms in current clinical practice, including:

- Availability and quality of digital WSI.
- Infrastructure for storage, and clinical systems for reviewing digital WSI.

Advances in whole slide scanners in digital pathology have provided high-definition, high-contrast images for diagnostic, educational, and research purposes. Investment in a scanner is not the only consideration: the infrastructure needed for a fully operational digital department requires a large amount of storage, and an electronic health IT system to handle digital review and sign-out by pathologists.

Digital pathology images are often very large, representing a challenge both for storage and dataset curation for AI purposes. Pixel-wise annotations in pathology, often needed in developing deep learning solutions in radiological images, are very time-consuming, presenting a unique challenge in AI research. Images are often several gigabytes per slide, and scanners can achieve resolution up to 40× magnification. Therefore, the time it takes to complete retrospective annotation of existing pathology archives at large centres is prohibitive. Furthermore, there are currently only a limited number of publicly available datasets for research use.

These limitations often mean that AI models are developed on small, potentially biased datasets for training. Training under such conditions can limit the generalizability and successful deployment of algorithms. Specifically, such algorithms may be prone to bias from a specific scanner, tissue fixation and staining characteristics of a certain centre, and overfitting to the training population. Evaluating model robustness to factors such as scanning and staining appearance should be completed during the validation phases of AI development. Furthermore, performing failure analysis with expert review and interpretability analysis of the AI output can provide researchers with key insights for evaluating model confidence and successful clinical adoption.

In addition to dataset considerations, it is important to evaluate the impact of scanner quality on AI algorithms. While most modern scanners provide autofocus and sharpening functionalities, these WSIs can still suffer from artifacts such as out-of-focus/blurry areas and variance in contrast/hue, which decrease diagnostic value and affect the outcome of the computerized image analysis system. These artifacts are identified on images by visual inspection, a time-consuming task. Problem areas on the images must be rescanned, disrupting the clinical or image processing workflow.

One of the aims in developing AI-based systems was to provide solutions to these image quality issues. One such system, DeepFocus, was developed to automatically detect and segment blurry areas in WSIs [8]. In the study by Senaras et al., a CNN was used to develop the DeepFocus program. The training data included four digital slides with different stains (H&E, Ki67, CD21, and CD10) from four different patients. Images were divided into 6 mm^2 patches (with a pixel size of 0.2461 μm × 0.2461 μm) as regions of interest (ROI), and each ROI was manually fine-tuned to ensure that autofocus features were correctly aligned. The focus of each region was then adjusted by a fixed offset value, such that each ROI contained a set of images with different focal planes.

An image was identified as in focus if its focal plane was within the margin of error. To identify if an ROI was in focus or blurry, the CNN learnt from the training data. When compared with a state-of-the-art detection algorithm, DeepFocus is on average 23.8% more accurate (93.2% vs 69.4%), with lower variability. Evaluated with test data from a different scanner, the algorithm's overall detection accuracy was generally equal or higher across images with different stains. Its advantages include higher accuracy among multiple stain types and tests using multiple scanners with different patients/diseases, as well as a higher speed of processing by allowing GPU implementation.

30.5 Future Potential

The development of AI algorithms that are robust and generalizable enough for clinical pathology deployment is still in its early days. AI's immediate impact in pathology is for quality assurance in clinical care, including the improved concordance of pathologists in the assessment of subjective grading and quantification tasks. Digital pathology and AI algorithms can improve the efficiency of telepathology practices for consulting, slide archiving, and diagnostic workflow in general. Storage of digital data in cloud-based platforms allows for equal access by pathologists and algorithms alike. An active area of research is the use of AI for difficult and rare diseases. Algorithms that can predict the site of origin for indeterminate cancers [9] or algorithms that can produce search engine–like results based on the histological appearance on digital imaging can aid pathologists in the most challenging of settings, and serve as a digital consultant.

30.5.1 On the Microscope

The applications discussed in this chapter are limited to AI applications on digital pathology images. The adoption of digitization is ongoing, and currently, for the most part, limited to large academic centres due to the investment and infrastructure needed for scanning, storage, and digital reading platforms. It is therefore critical to acknowledge the research and development of AI algorithms that can be integrated onto a conventional microscope.

A recent study from researchers in China demonstrated that the adoption of AI algorithms in a standard microscope via augmented reality could improve reproducibility and agreement in Ki-67 IHC scoring for breast cancer specimens [10]. To achieve this, 30 pathologists of varying experience for scoring slides with and without AI augmentation were recruited. In this setting, while AI assistance increased accuracy and agreement, it also increased reading time for the pathologist as they adjusted to the augmented reality view (an average of 12 seconds longer per slide). Nonetheless, including AI in the standard clinical workflow is an attractive option in resource-limited settings where digitization is not feasible. This exciting application has the potential to expand the reach of AI algorithms in the field.

30.5.2 The Prospect of Personalized Medicine

Subjective pathology standards used in clinical medicine today highlight the need for reproducible morphology patterns detected by the human eye. In the growing landscape of treatments targeting specific biological properties of cancer, it is difficult for clinicians to decide which treatments are most likely to benefit their patients. The development of additional AI algorithms beyond the current pathological grading criteria could provide companion diagnostics that would help link patients and treatments for truly personalized medicine. This active area of research includes the development of algorithms that predict a patient's prognosis, in addition to algorithms that predict a patient's response to treatment.

It is challenging for pathologists to 'discover' new, important features in this space, given the complexity and heterogeneity of cancer within and across patient samples. AI has the potential to fully exhaust the features within an image set to identify novel and important signatures for treatment prediction. AI research directed at the discovery of human-interpretable features that are relevant for treatment selection, response, and prognosis prediction is likely to be transformative in the coming decades.

30.6 Conclusions

As institutions around the globe move to digital scanning and review of pathology specimens, the deployment of AI algorithms has the potential to impact all points of clinical care, from quality assurance to diagnosis and review. In this chapter we have reviewed several case studies of successful AI applications in pathology. Each case has demonstrated the essential components required for successful clinical integration: clinical feasibility, AI validation compared to human readers, and the value of AI-assisted readouts. While outside the scope of this chapter, future digital pathology research with other data, such as serum biomarkers or genomic panels, has the potential to further enhance personalized medicine initiatives and improve algorithm accuracy in patient care settings.

KEY INSIGHTS

- **Clinical benefits of digital assessment include improved quality, efficiency, and potential to improve health-related outcomes.**
- **Digital pathology presents a unique challenge to the annotation, development, and deployment of image-based AI algorithms due to large image sizes and scale.**

- AI algorithms for automated quality control of digital pathology images are critical for clinical review and downstream AI applications.
- AI algorithms have shown the ability to improve pathologist agreement and reduce review time for detection and grading of various cancer types.
- Not all centres have the resources to support digital pathology, and advancements in microscope technology enable AI incorporation within the standard workflow.

References

1. Ström P, Kartasalo K, Olsson H et al. Artificial intelligence for diagnosis and grading of prostate cancer in biopsies: a population-based, diagnostic study. *Lancet Oncology* 2020;21(2):222–232.
2. Steiner DF, MacDonald R, Liu Y et al. Impact of deep learning assistance on the histopathologic review of lymph nodes for metastatic breast cancer. *American Journal of Surgical Pathology* 2018;42(12):1636–1646.
3. Skrede O-J, De Raedt S, Kleppe A et al. Deep learning for prediction of colorectal cancer outcome: a discovery and validation study. *Lancet* 2020;395(10221):350–360.
4. Saltz J, Gupta R, Hou L et al. Spatial organization and molecular correlation of tumor-infiltrating lymphocytes using deep learning on pathology images. *Cell Reports* 2018;23(1):181–193.e187.
5. Harmon SA, Sanford TH, Brown GT et al. Multiresolution application of artificial intelligence in digital pathology for prediction of positive lymph nodes from primary tumors in bladder cancer. *JCO Clinical Cancer Informatics* 2020;4:367–382.
6. Le H, Gupta R, Hou L et al. Utilizing automated breast cancer detection to identify spatial distributions of tumor-infiltrating lymphocytes in invasive breast cancer. *American Journal of Pathology* 2020;190(7):1491–1504.
7. Bao H, Sun X, Zhang Y et al. The artificial intelligence-assisted cytology diagnostic system in large-scale cervical cancer screening: a population-based cohort study of 0.7 million women. *Cancer Medicine* 2020;9(18):6896–6906.

For additional references and Further Reading please see www.wiley.com/go/byrne/aiinclinicalmedicine.

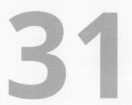

31

Introduction to AI in Radiology

Shu Min Yu and Amarpreet Mahil

Department of Radiology, Vancouver General Hospital, Vancouver, BC, Canada

31.1 Introduction

Radiology is naturally primed for the implementation of AI, as the practice already holds a readily available database of digitized images. As such, AI and computer assistance are not novel to the field of radiology. In 1998, computer-assisted detection for screening mammography, plain chest radiography, and computed tomography (CT) chest imaging received US Food and Drug Administration (FDA) approval [1]. This form of AI was used to identify and highlight areas of suspicion for review based on pattern recognition. However, recent advancements in the field of deep learning and machine learning have significantly expanded the use case of AI in radiology, from detection to prognosis, to workflow optimization, to quality control, and more. Therefore, overall reviews of the many applications and potential applications for AI in radiology are presented in Chapters 32–35.

31.2 AI in Diagnostic Imaging

In Chapter 32, we describe the applications of AI in diagnostic imaging, and the incorporation of AI in assisting the radiologist to detect and identify abnormalities in an imaging study. The radiologist's interpretation can be subjective at times. In contrast, AI excels at highlighting complicated patterns in imaging data, and can deliver an automatic quantitative judgement. AI can also analyse the full series of images in the study protocol, and provide quantitative metrics and segmented volumes that would otherwise be far too laborious and time-consuming for the radiologist to produce during their workflow.

There is a wide range of use for AI within diagnostic Imaging. However, the implementation of AI in healthcare has not always been simple. For example, training an algorithm to detect a certain disease necessitates a vast dataset of imaging studies from several institutions. This has proven difficult due to the siloed structure of

AI in Clinical Medicine: A Practical Guide for Healthcare Professionals, First Edition. Edited by Michael F. Byrne, Nasim Parsa, Alexandra T. Greenhill, Daljeet Chahal, Omer Ahmad, and Ulas Bagci.
© 2023 John Wiley & Sons Ltd. Published 2023 by John Wiley & Sons Ltd.
Companion website: www.wiley.com/go/byrne/aiinclinicalmedicine

data storage, privacy issues, and regulatory limitations [2]. With the acceleration of AI research and development, academic and health institutions must evolve their data management practices to provide solutions that can support such data-intensive research.

31.3 Enhancement of Radiology Workflow

Chapter 33 explores the ability of AI to improve the current radiology workflow by influencing numerous key points along the patient pathway. The radiologist benefits from AI by the automation of repetitive activities, removing human fatigue. As a result, the radiologist may read pictures with greater sensitivity and specificity in a shorter amount of time. It is also critical to reduce the turnaround time for completed imaging examinations in order to improve workflow [3]. A common target for workflow optimization is study prioritization and a triage system in the reading worklist. Targeted diagnoses and treatments in medicine are now possible thanks to algorithms that can deliver automatic suggestions based on multi-input data. Natural language processing is also used to flag studies for follow-up, organize requisitions for patient booking, and generate actionable items from the radiologist's report directly to the clinician.

31.4 Medical Imaging Processing – Powered by AI

AI has also been leveraged to enhance existing medical imaging hardware, and to improve image processing, resulting in better image quality, greater radiation safety, and lower costs for accessibility. In Chapter 34, the main technique discussed is convolutional neural networks, a subset of deep learning, for image reconstruction. Here, the main concept is that traditional algorithms for image reconstruction are based on physics and statistical image correction techniques, and do not utilize all the information contained within the digital image. By pairing raw data received by device sensors with the ideal 'output' or generated image, a reconstruction network can be trained to reconstruct images from any type of sensor input. This is known as a sensor domain–based AI solution. When sensor data are not available, an image domain–based solution is implemented where suboptimal images are paired with optimal-quality images for training. These techniques have been used to improve the quality of image reconstructions, resulting in lower image acquisition times and reduced exposure to radiation. These techniques also allow the reconstruction of high-quality images from cheaper and energy-efficient scanners, which in turn leads to the reduction of barriers preventing access to medical imaging.

31.5 Future Outlook and Obstacles

Finally, in Chapter 35 we conclude with a discussion on the trajectory of AI in radiology and where it is headed. The current gap between the demand and supply of radiology services is exacerbated by the shortage of radiologists and radiology support staff, as well as the backlog of cases and long wait times resulting from the COVID-19 pandemic. Due to this, there is generally a high motivation to adopt AI in order to improve productivity, increase operational efficiency, and reduce the workload and burnout experienced by radiology staff. With these driving factors, it is likely that we will face a future where AI takes on a more expansive role in radiology, from managing many of the tasks of a radiologist to automating scheduling, billings, and other administrative tasks.

When discussing the future of AI in radiology, it is also necessary to discuss the obstacles in the pathway of AI development and adoption. Ethical considerations include concerns over data ownership and privacy – will patients be consenting to the use of their archived data, and who will own the derived data used for AI training? Healthcare authorities must also consider exposure to liability – who is responsible when the AI algorithm makes a mistake, the radiologist or the vendor? Finally, as we strive towards a future where AI informs clinical decision-making and influences the treatment plan, it is important that we avoid a 'black-box' algorithm, and instead provide a transparent framework that is communicable to both the physician and the patient. This will support transparent reporting and the identification of errors in the AI output in the field of radiology.

References

1. Lee, LIT, Kanthasamy S, Ayyalaraju RS, Ganatra R. The current state of artificial intelligence in medical imaging and nuclear medicine. *BJR Open* 2019;1(1):20190037.
2. Tollinsky N. AI improves diagnostic imaging at Canadian hospitals. *Canadian Healthcare Technology*, 30 March 2020. https://www.canhealth.com/2020/03/30/ai-improves-diagnostic-imaging-at-canadian-hospitals.
3. Dikici E, Bigelow M, Prevedello LM, White RD, Erdal BS. Integrating AI into radiology workflow: levels of research, production, and feedback maturity. *Journal of Medical Imaging* 2020;7(1):1. https://doi.org/10.1117/1.jmi.7.1.016502.

32

Clinical Applications of AI in Diagnostic Imaging

Mohammed F. Mohammed[1], Savvas Nicolaou[2,3], and Adnan Sheikh[2,3]

[1] *Department of Radiology, King Faisal Specialist Hospital & Research Center, Riyadh, Saudi Arabia*

[2] *Department of Radiology, Vancouver General Hospital, Vancouver, BC, Canada*

[3] *University of British Columbia, Vancouver, BC, Canada*

Learning Objectives

- Discover the current radiology AI market and available solutions.
- Understand the impact of current radiology AI solutions in different radiological specialties.
- Illustrate tools for objective assessment and appraisal of AI systems.
- Identify hidden costs of AI in healthcare and radiology.

32.1 Introduction

The growth of the AI industry over the last decade has been staggering. AI technology has been implemented in some form or another in nearly all aspects of our lives, from intelligent assistants on our wrists, to semi-autonomous driving, to the ads we see while checking out our AI-recommended shopping basket. As of 2018, 154,000 AI patents had been filed, a majority of which were by Microsoft [1]. The AI market is expected to reach $62 billion in 2022 [2] and hit $360 billion by 2030 [3]. Medical imaging is poised to have a significant share of that market, with a predicted value of $1.2 billion by 2025, representing a compound annual growth rate of nearly 36% [4]. This is not surprising given that in 2020 there were only 21 US Food and Drug Administration (FDA)-approved imaging-based AI products related to radiology, whereas at the time of writing this chapter there are 160 FDA-approved AI products for radiology [5]. Clearly, radiology is an appealing area for AI companies to concentrate their efforts, as it is somewhat standardized with an expected number of acquisitions, views, or techniques for any given clinical scenario.

Despite this explosion in AI solutions, radiology remains a thriving medical specialty with a record number of applicants to the field worldwide. This has been associated with a notable shift from 'AI versus human' narratives to research that

AI in Clinical Medicine: A Practical Guide for Healthcare Professionals, First Edition. Edited by Michael F. Byrne, Nasim Parsa, Alexandra T. Greenhill, Daljeet Chahal, Omer Ahmad, and Ulas Bagci.
© 2023 John Wiley & Sons Ltd. Published 2023 by John Wiley & Sons Ltd.
Companion website: www.wiley.com/go/byrne/aiinclinicalmedicine

embraces AI augmentation of radiologist capabilities to enhance and elevate patient care. The AI market reflects this shift as well, with the industry realigning priorities to focus on its main consumer, the radiologist [6–9].

In this chapter we will discuss the current state of clinical, image-based AI solutions that are available on the market, as well as potentially impactful AI tools that are currently in the research stage. We will discuss the tools and metrics that can be used to assess and evaluate AI solutions prior to clinical implementation, and some hidden costs of implementing AI solutions. We will conclude with a summary of the relevant points discussed, and possible ways in which radiology practice may evolve in the near future as a result of the widespread adoption of AI.

32.2 Clinical AI Solutions in Radiology

32.2.1 Current State of the Radiology AI Market

The AI showcase at the 2021 Radiological Society of North America (RSNA) annual meeting featured 95 exhibitors and vendors demonstrating the gamut of AI solutions. This number was down from the 2019 RSNA Annual Meeting, likely owing to multiple mergers in the industry and consolidation of services. There has also been growth in the number of AI orchestration and distribution platforms that essentially act as 'app stores', providing users with multiple tools that can be used to meet specific needs in a single interface. Examples of such platforms include deepc's deepcOS (www.deepc.ai), Arterys (www.arterys.com), and Terarecon's Eureka Clinical AI Platform (https://www.terarecon.com/artificial-intelligence), all of which offer access to several products and tools from a variety of vendors that can be integrated into the clinical workflow.

The American College of Radiology (ACR) maintains a list of FDA-approved image-based radiology solutions as part of the ACR Data Science Institute's (DSI) AI Central (https://aicentral.acrdsi.org), which can be accessed by anyone who wants to learn about these solutions and view a product description page and data sheet curated by the editors of AI Central (Figure 32.1). The products are divided into computer-aided detection (CADe) solutions, computer-aided diagnosis (CADx) solutions, computer-aided detection and diagnosis (CADe/x) solutions, computer-aided triage (CADt) solutions, and image processing/quantification solutions. A brief definition of these terms and use case examples are presented in Table 32.1. Users may also search by radiology subspecialty, body area, the interrogated finding, and the modality on which the solutions function.

Another approach to classifying image-based AI algorithms was described by Tadavarthi et al. [10], dividing solutions into four major groups by the tasks they are meant to accomplish: repetitive, quantitative, explorative, and diagnostic. This division is fairly similar to the one adopted by the ACR-DSI with the exception of *explorative tasks*, which Tadavarthi et al. define as 'are designed to allow a radiologist to select an area of interest with a pathology they may not be familiar with (for example, fibrotic lung disease), and return similar-appearing regions from other

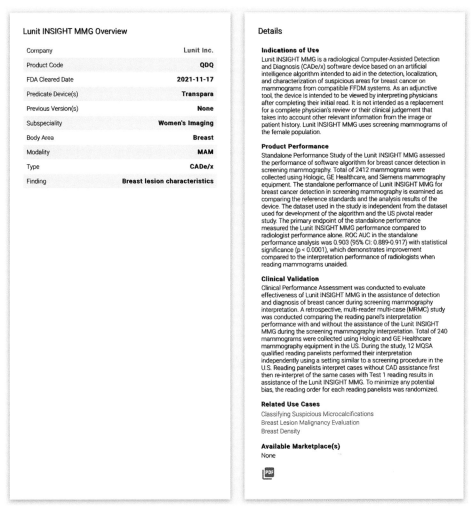

Figure 32.1: Product description page and data sheet curated by the editors of AI Central.
Source: Lunit INSIGHT MMG (n.d.) / American College of Radiology / CC BY-4.0.

scans in a database with associated diagnoses'. Currently, there are no FDA-approved algorithms capable of performing explorative tasks, even though this is a high-value, high-impact area for image-based AI development.

Despite having many solutions and algorithms that are FDA or Conformité Européenne (CE)-approved on the market, up to two-thirds may not have undergone any clinical validation in a peer-reviewed manner. Van Leeuwen and colleagues showed that out of 100 radiology AI solutions that had FDA or CE approval, only 36 had any peer-reviewed publications describing accuracy or real-world impact [11]. A database similar to the ACR-DSI database – AI for Radiology (`https://grand-challenge.org/aiforradiology`) – was used, and it includes information on CE approval as well.

These findings highlight the importance of radiologists learning the skills needed to evaluate AI tools and validate vendor claims in order to select solutions that perform as required by the radiologist.

Table 32.1: Definition of Terminology Used to Describe Commercial Ai Solution Types By The American College of Radiology Data Science Institute (Acr-Dsi) Based on Food and Drug Administration Categorization of These Tools.

Solution type	Definition	Use case example
Computer-aided detection (CADe)	Aids in localizing/marking regions that may reveal specific abnormalities	Detection of pulmonary nodules without risk stratification
Computer-aided diagnosis (CADx)	Aids in characterizing/assessing disease, disease type, severity, stage, progression	Stratifying a pulmonary nodule into benign or malignant
Computer-aided detection and diagnosis (CADe/x)	Aids in localizing and characterizing conditions	Detection of an abnormality on a mammogram and assigning a BI-RADS category to it
Computer-aided triage (CADt)	Aids in prioritizing/triaging time-sensitive patient detection and diagnosis	Alerting the radiologist and interventionist to a large vessel occlusion on a head CTA by prioritizing the study on a worklist or generating an automated alert
Image processing/ quantification	Aids in acquisition or optimization of images, or performs measurements, segmentations, or quantitative functions on images	Providing 'super-resolution' on MRI brain images Segmenting a tumour and providing the volume Quantifying hepatic steatosis

BI-RADS, Breast Imaging–Reporting and Data System; CTA, computed tomography angiogram; MRI, magnetic resonance imaging.

32.2.2 An Introduction to Available AI Solutions

AI in radiology has the advantage of a large number of commercially available solutions that work with the medical imaging infrastructure and are able to integrate into practice to varying degrees, as opposed to research-only or locally developed algorithms in other clinical healthcare areas. Due to that fact, we will focus on these commercial products, while highlighting non-commercial or research-only tools when relevant. Both the ACR-DSI and AI for Radiology demonstrate a similar number of radiology AI offerings (160 and 191, respectively). Focusing on the ACR-DSI list shows that neuroradiology, chest imaging, and breast imaging have the largest number of available solutions by far. We will divide the solutions by radiological subspecialty, and discuss the most notable products and algorithms currently on offer in these respective areas.

32.2.2.1 Neuroradiology

Neuroradiology also represents one of the first areas demonstrating the clinical success of AI in healthcare. Neuroradiology AI solutions make up the bulk of commercially available AI software, representing nearly a third of the FDA-approved solutions, and overtaking chest imaging in the last two years.

In 2018, Viz.ai introduced its ContaCT AI algorithm (since renamed Viz LVO), which detects large vessel occlusions on head computed tomography (CT) angiograms, and sends an alert to all specialists involved in managing stroke, accelerating access to care, and potentially reducing the time to the delivery of specialized care in established stroke centres. In 2020, Viz LVO became the first AI software to be granted reimbursement in the USA by the Centers for Medicare & Medicaid Services through the New Technology Add-on Payment pathway (which incentivized hospitals to use new products during the initial 2–3-year period of product market entry) of up to $1040 per use, which was recently renewed through to 2022 [12]. This was following demonstration of portability and result consistency [13], as well as clear benefits on access to care [14] and on patient outcomes [15].

Since then, other similar solutions such as RapidAI (Figure 32.2), AIdoc, and Avicenna were granted reimbursement through the incentivization pathway

(a)

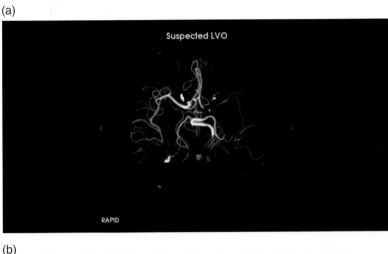

(b)

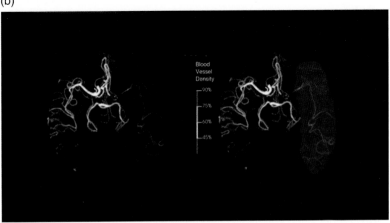

Figure 32.2: Automated alert and image postprocessing of a suspected large vessel occlusion by iSchemiaView's Rapid AI, demonstrating the area of occlusion (a), as well as quantifying collateral vessel density (b), to help with treatment planning.

Source: Automated alert and image postprocessing of a suspected large vessel occlusion by iSchemiaView's Rapid AI. (n.d.). Photograph by RapidAI.

(New Technology Add-on Payment) as well [12]. These can mainly be categorized as CADt solutions, as the primary task of the algorithm is to enable accurate triage of high-priority cases, alerting the radiologist, interventionalist, and other care team members of a potentially impactful finding on a scan. In this way, a scan can then be reviewed and confirmed by a human reader, and a clinical decision on optimum treatment can be made. There are 18 such FDA-approved neuroradiology AI algorithms listed by the ACR-DSI.

The majority of neuroradiology AI algorithms, however, focus on image processing or quantification tasks on CT, magnetic resonance imaging (MRI), or positron emission tomography (PET), such as segmentation of tumours or multiple sclerosis plaques, brain structure segmentation and volumetry, or measurement of volumes of infarcted tissue or intracranial haematomas. These tools can potentially improve the efficiency of radiologists, and reduce the burden of repetitive tasks that do not require a high level of cognitive engagement.

Some tools in this space focus on whole-brain volumetry for the purposes of dementia classification and monitoring of disease progression, despite the lack of concrete clinical evidence that such measurements provide any benefit or can offer any planned intervention that may improve outcomes. This highlights an issue with image-based AI, where algorithms can be developed and marketed without the input of key clinical stakeholders or end-users, driven by unverified claims. Should such algorithms become widespread, the risk of increasing 'noise' over 'signal' in an already hype-filled market could lead to delayed development and adoption of truly impactful solutions.

32.2.2.2 Chest Imaging

One of the earliest applications of image-based AI in healthcare was on chest X-rays [16]. Since then there has been sustained growth in the chest imaging market, with a current offering of 36 FDA-approved solutions listed on AI Central. A portion of chest algorithms focus on detection (CADe) of pulmonary nodules on chest CTs, highlighting suspected nodules and presenting them to the radiologist for verification. One pulmonary nodule algorithm, the Optellum Virtual Nodule Clinic, allows users to define a region of interest over a nodule and outputs a score that differentiates benign from malignant nodules (Figure 32.3). Baldwin and colleagues assessed the tool on 1397 patients from three cities across the UK, demonstrating a receiver operating characteristic (ROC)–area under the curve (AUC) of 89.6, and sensitivity and specificity of 99.57% and 28.03%, respectively, to exclude a malignant nodule when a threshold score of 1.28 was used [17]. Within the studied sample, there was only a single false-negative case, but there were 837 false-positive cases. Algorithms such as this, although valuable in excluding a disease, may result in an increase in downstream testing or investigation, and these impacts should always be considered when implementing in practice.

Other chest imaging AI solutions focus on automated lines and tubes labelling, segmentation of airways or emphysema calculations, or triage (CADt) of studies based on urgent findings such as pneumothorax, pneumoperitoneum, pleural

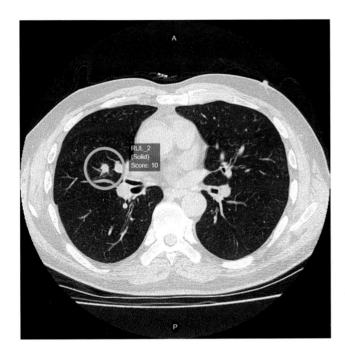

Figure 32.3: LCP score as seen in Optellum's Virtual Nodule Clinic. A score of 10 is almost certainly a malignancy. Courtesy of Optellum and Oxford University Hospitals NHS Foundation Trust.

effusion, or pulmonary embolism. A few solutions allow the labelling, automated measurement, and longitudinal tracking of lung pathology.

There are 22 chest AI algorithms that are CT-based algorithms compared to 11 X-ray–based algorithms, despite chest X-rays having jump-started image-based AI interest.

32.2.2.3 Cardiac Imaging

Cardiac AI applications have also seen steady growth in the last few years, with 21 cardiac applications currently on the market compared to 1 FDA-approved solution in 2020. These applications mainly focus on cardiac structure segmentation, volumetry, and image analysis. There are 7 ultrasound-based solutions on the market as well, mainly performing automated segmentation and calculation of ejection fractions.

HeartFlow remains the sole provider of FDA-approved CT based fractional flow reserve. Negative fractional flow reserve results have been shown to predict lower adverse outcomes and coronary events in patients with stable coronary artery disease [18].

32.2.2.4 Breast Imaging

Breast imaging remains a high-interest area due to the value of early detection of breast cancer by screening mammography. A number of mammography-based solutions focus on disease detection and risk stratification by providing a score for the findings (CADe/x; Figure 32.4). Other solutions focus on breast density measurements and automated result generation based on the ACR BI-RADS Atlas [19]. Since 2020, there has been an increase in algorithms capable of tomosynthesis

(a)   (b)

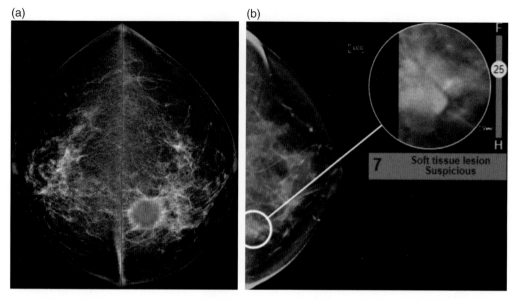

Figure 32.4: Examples of computer-aided detection and diagnosis (CADe/x) solutions highlighting suspicious findings using heatmaps (a), or region of interest and labels (b), from Lunit Inc. and Therapixel, respectively.

Source: Lunit Inc. (n.d.). Lunit Inc. Retrieved March 11, 2022, from https://www.lunit.io/en/company).

(three-dimensional mammography) analysis, with 11 tomosynthesis-capable FDA-approved algorithms currently on the market. There is a single MRI-based offering, focusing on lesion segmentation and analysis.

Breast imagers are very familiar with augmented workflows, having adopted CAD tools since the early 2000s when their use was encouraged by an increase in reimbursement by the Centers for Medicare & Medicaid Services. However, these tools did not improve upon patient outcomes or accuracy, and may have had a negative impact on performance, as demonstrated by Lehman et al. [20]. Lessons learnt could potentially improve how AI tools enhance performance, such as better integration of AI tools into the workflow instead of disrupting clinical readouts by using a separate system or additional screen, and by linking incentives to improving patient outcomes rather than to utilization [21].

32.2.2.5 Abdominal Imaging

There are currently 17 FDA-approved algorithms listed by ACR-DSI, nearly all of which perform image processing, segmentation, or quantification. There is a notable increase in prostate-related AI algorithms (Figure 32.5), in keeping with the market's interest in improving the performance and efficiency of repetitive tasks and screening programmes. However, no clinical validation of these claims is available.

Liver AI algorithms focus mainly on automated quantification of iron, fat, or fibrosis. A few tools aid in segmentation and pre-surgical planning. A single CADt algorithm is currently on the market for triaging cases with pneumoperitoneum on abdominopelvic CTs.

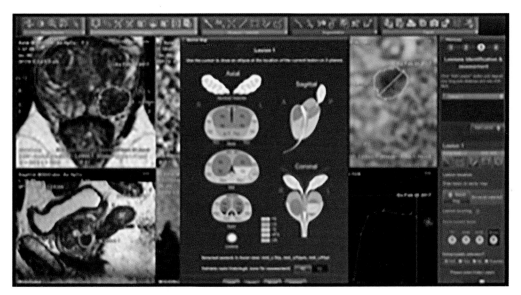

Figure 32.5: Example of GE Healthcare's automated prostate workflow PROView demonstrating lesion segmentation and automated visual report generation.

32.2.2.6 Musculoskeletal Imaging

There is a paucity of FDA-approved musculoskeletal AI solutions despite early research concentrating on fracture detection and diagnosis. Current offerings include detection of wrist or spine fractures, osteoarthritis grading, image segmentation, and automated spine display.

32.2.2.7 Paediatrics and Nuclear Medicine

The development in the paediatrics space has been extremely limited, despite the need for technologies that can improve detection and speed up examinations in this population. Currently, the only application is an ultrasound-based automated hip dysplasia measurement tool. Other ultrasound-based measurements such as pyloric measurements and hydronephrosis grading, as well as image-acquisition acceleration, dose-lowering algorithms, and motion-correction algorithms, are all potential areas of development with potentially impactful results.

Nuclear medicine offerings remain limited to image-quality improvement on PET/CT. There are no quantitative or automated tracking tools on offer. There are no general nuclear medicine algorithms currently on the market.

32.2.3 Radiomics

Radiomics is an area where AI can potentially have notable impact. Radiomics is the application of AI and machine learning principles to extract a large number of quantitative and textural features from medical images. These features demonstrate disease characteristics that are difficult to identify by human vision alone, but may have direct impact on decision-making in regard to disease processes or findings.

Examples include algorithms that could detect triple-negative breast cancer based on mammographic features or predict lung cancer response to immunotherapy. Currently there are no advanced radiomics products on the market; however, there are a few companies with products in the pipeline that have undergone clinical validation. SUNDIAL-chemorad by Radiomics (`https://radiomics.bio`), for example, is currently undergoing prospective validation for predicting survival in patients with non-small cell lung cancer treated with chemoradiotherapy based on baseline CT imaging.

32.2.4 Opportunistic Screening and Multi-Organ Algorithms

Opportunistic screening – where patients are screened for diseases unrelated to the reason for presentation – is an exciting area for AI application. Consider that on a single abdominopelvic CT scan, the lumbar spine and femoral necks could be used to screen for osteoporosis and fracture risk [22,23], the aortic calcium score could screen for risk of a cardiac event [24], visceral fat could be used to screen for metabolic syndrome [25,26], the bulk of the muscles for sarcopenia [25], the liver surface for chronic liver disease, and the hepatic parenchyma for hepatic steatosis [27,28]. There is even potential to take this further by screening an unprepared bowel for colon cancer or high-risk polyps, the kidneys for chronic kidney disease, and the pancreas for pre-diabetes or undiagnosed diabetes. A large number of these algorithms have been validated, and work is underway to create a viable tool for use in clinical practice (Figure 32.6) [29]. In the current AI marketplace these algorithms would work separately, requiring separate tools, payment models, and infrastructure. However, if these algorithms were to function as a single tool, either through the creation of an efficient multi-organ assessment algorithm or by being integrated seamlessly on a single platform and presented in a unified visual style, this would greatly improve the user experience and user adoption.

An example of a multi-organ algorithm that works on abdominopelvic CT scans was recently published, and demonstrates good accuracy for a range of common pathologies, including kidney stones, gallstones, hepatic lesions, pulmonary nodules, and another 11 common findings [30]. If algorithms like this can provide high true-negative results with a fair number of false positives, then these tools can be extremely valuable in clinical practice for rapid triage and swift clearance of negative studies that do not require immediate expert attention.

32.3 Evaluation of AI Tools for Clinical Implementation

As mentioned earlier, a large proportion of AI tools and algorithms that are commercially available have not undergone rigorous clinical validation or prospective assessment in a clinical trial [11]. As such, the onus for assessing an algorithm for appropriateness, acceptable performance, and clinical utility will likely fall upon the radiologist. Understanding what metrics and tools are available for interpreting an algorithm's performance is essential.

(a)

CT scan images from original screening study

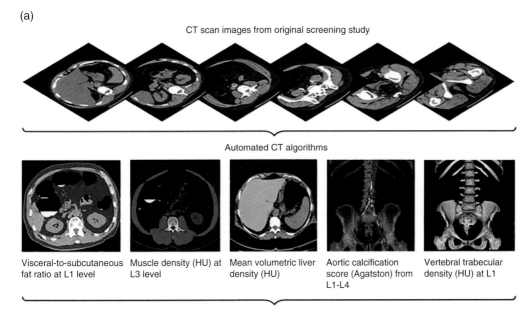

Automated CT algorithms

Visceral-to-subcutaneous fat ratio at L1 level

Muscle density (HU) at L3 level

Mean volumetric liver density (HU)

Aortic calcification score (Agatston) from L1–L4

Vertebral trabecular density (HU) at L1

Longitudinal follow-up for adverse clinical outcomes

(b)

CT scan 12 years after original study

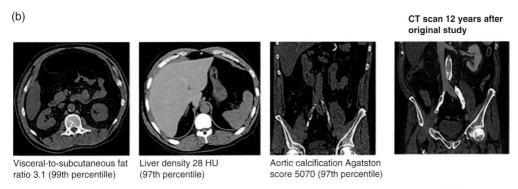

Visceral-to-subcutaneous fat ratio 3.1 (99th percentille)

Liver density 28 HU (97th percentile)

Aortic calcification Agatston score 5070 (97th percentile)

Figure 32.6: Automated computed tomography (CT)-based cardiometabolic tools for assessment of (second row of images, left to right) bone, aortic calcium, visceral to subcutaneous fat ratio, muscle attenuation, and liver attenuation biomarkers from original abdominal CT data. In practice, a visual correlate allows for quality assurance for the automated segmentation results in individual patients. The specific CT biomarkers shown have all been validated in prior works.

Source: Daniel C. Elton.

32.3.1 Essential Performance Evaluation Statistical Tools

Most AI tools used in medical imaging perform either classification tasks or segmentation tasks. For classification tasks, the binary contingency table can be one of the most valuable sources of information. The table highlights true-positive, true-negative, false-positive, and false-negative results. In an excellent example highlighted by England and Cheng [31], an algorithm for detecting a disease that has a prevalence of 1 in 1000 would have an accuracy of 99.9% if it labelled every examination as negative. This algorithm would, on paper, look like an incredible tool, while not fulfilling its main objective of detecting said disease. A contingency table of the algorithm's performance on 2000 studies would show that it had 0 true positives, 1998 true negatives, 2 false negatives, and 0 false positives. The evaluator would be able to tell that this algorithm is incapable of detecting the disease when present and is unsuitable for that task. It always important to place diagnostic performance parameters such as sensitivity, specificity, positive predictive value, and negative predictive value within the appropriate context to be able to assess performance in a meaningful way.

Other commonly used metrics in algorithm performance reporting are the $F1$ score, the Youden J index, and the ROC–AUC. The $F1$ score provides a single value that summarizes the binary contingency table, assuming that true negatives are unimportant and that false-positive and false-negative results are equally undesirable. The Youden J index is similar to the $F1$ score in assuming that false-positive and false-negative results are equally undesirable; however, it accounts for true-negative results as well as true positives.

The ROC–AUC is useful when a numerical value can be used to assign a threshold for a binary classifier; for example, if a lesion has an algorithm score of less than 2, it is almost certainly benign. In this case, the ROC–AUC is useful at providing information across the whole operating range of the algorithm, and an optimum threshold can be selected based on the desired sensitivity and specificity.

For segmentation algorithms, the most commonly described metrics are the Dice similarity coefficient and the Hausdorff distance. These can be used in conjunction, as the Dice similarity coefficient describes the overlap between a prediction and the ground truth (1 = perfect overlap, 0 = no overlap), while the Hausdorff distance describes the distance between the edge of ground truth and prediction in two dimensions [32].

32.3.2 Checklists and Data Cards

Recently, several checklists have been introduced that can be utilized by stakeholders to make an informed decision on an AI algorithm by assessing several crucial areas such as methodology, study design, patient population or test population, demographics, technical methodology and test methods, end-points, and evaluation metrics and results. The Checklist for AI in Medical Imaging (CLAIM) is an excellent checklist that requests vendors or authors to submit information on algorithm details in 42 questions separated into 6 major domains [33]. Since then, several other checklists have become available, such as the SPIRIT-AI (Standard Protocol Items: Recommendations for Interventional Trials – Artificial Intelligence) [34] and CONSORT-AI (Consolidated Standards of Reporting Trials – Artificial Intelligence) [35]. (See Chapter 42 for more detailed discussion.)

Given how lengthy these tools are, some authors have created abbreviated assessment questions, datasheets, or model labels, which still cover the essential information required for informed decision-making in regard to an algorithm [36,37]. Another useful tool that is gaining support is the concept of a dataset nutrition label that distils key information into a label similar to the dietary nutrition labels on food items [38].

32.3.3 Acceptance Testing and Monitoring

There are no standardized practices for user acceptance of an AI algorithm. The application of tools and checklists such as those mentioned allows for the assessment of these algorithms objectively based on reported performance. It is equally important that users considering implementation of such tools in practice demand external validation on local data and compare them to reported performance or desired performance metrics. In case there are wide discrepancies between reported performance and real-world performance, retraining of the algorithm on local data to achieve the desired performance is recommended.

There is also lack of guidance on how algorithms should be tested for any drop in performance over time. Suggestions include the creation of 'virtual phantom studies', which could be synthetic images generated for the purpose of testing the algorithm over time. Another potential solution would be to reserve a small percentage of local studies (say, 5–10%) that do not undergo interrogation by the algorithm, and instead utilize them for annual or biannual testing.

32.4 The Hidden Costs of Implementing AI in Practice

The development and execution of complex AI algorithms require an immense amount of energy, and in turn have a large impact on the environment. Radiology, as it is, is a significant producer of greenhouse gases [39,40], possibly responsible for up to 1% of global emissions. Developing and running AI require significantly larger amounts of energy and produce much larger amounts of waste. By some estimates, the training of a single advanced natural language processing algorithm may require as much energy as a trans-American flight. A single complex algorithm could end up producing the waste equivalent of five passenger vehicles over their entire lifespan [41,42]. With the growing complexity of algorithms, the desire of academic centres to set up large-scale AI labs, and the growing climate crisis, it is imperative that we are conscious of the consequences of developing, deploying, and utilizing these technologies. It is reasonable to favour algorithms that prioritize efficiency and large gains in patient outcomes over those that result in marginal improvements in accuracy without overall impact on patient care.

Additionally, there is concern that AI could propagate health inequities due to encoded biases at the time of algorithm development and training. Although this may seem like an abstract concept, a team of international radiology AI researchers were able to demonstrate that AI algorithms could detect a patient's self-identified race with an astounding degree of accuracy [43] – an AUC of up to 0.99, meaning near-perfect classification on algorithms designed for entirely unrelated clinical tasks such as lung pathology detection on X-ray and CT. What was even more surprising was the fact that the researchers could not demonstrate how the algorithms were able to detect race with such accuracy, as there are no image-based findings that may suggest race. The algorithms continued to perform well after the introduction of low-pass and high-pass filters, essentially rendering the images uninterpretable by human readers. This raises two major concerns. Firstly, it highlights that an algorithm may behave in ways that the developers could never anticipate or account for, and as such they would not be able to eliminate or correct an undesirable behaviour such as this. Secondly, the COVID-19 pandemic has highlighted the severe disparities in healthcare delivery based on socioeconomic status and race in many parts of the world and the USA in particular [44–48]. If AI tools propagate these entrenched biases, they could further increase disparities in healthcare delivery for minorities and vulnerable peoples. We must ensure that algorithms include a diverse population that is representative of the intended area of deployment, and that outcomes are reported in relation to the patient demographics so that any adverse outcomes may be detected early.

32.5 Conclusion

The image-based radiology market continues to mature at an impressive rate, with FDA-approved solutions growing nearly eightfold in two years. However, the offerings continue to be piecemeal solutions dedicated to niche tasks rather than solutions working together to analyse multiple aspects of an examination and provide true support to the radiologist. The introduction of AI platforms that offer multiple solutions working in conjunction to present information in a unified visual language and within an integrated space for radiologists aims to alleviate those concerns to a certain extent, and to allow for multi-organ assessment. As these systems become more ubiquitous, radiologists will have to become familiar with tools and metrics used to assess and vet AI algorithms to ensure safe deployment within their practices. This must be balanced with the potential negative environmental and socioeconomical impacts of AI, and steps should be taken to minimize those effects when possible.

As radiology AI systems mature and a greater number of repetitive, low-yield, and low-impact tasks can be automated, radiologists will be free to engage in high-impact activities such as focusing on complex cases, dedicating greater time to interventional procedures in their subspecialty domains, and engaging with patients and clinicians in integrated care clinics or screening clinics.

KEY INSIGHTS

■ **The narrative of AI in radiology has shifted from 'AI versus radiologists' to the artificial augmentation of the radiologist's capabilities by AI to enhance and elevate the radiology services and patient care provided; radiologists have become the radiology AI market's main consumer.**

- Most AI solutions offered are concentrated in neuroradiology, cardiothoracic, and breast imaging subspecialties, and are divided into computer-aided detection, computer-aided diagnosis, computer-aided detection and diagnosis, computer-aided triage, and image processing/quantification solutions.
- Examples of clinical application include accurate triage of high-priority cases to alert the radiologist for prioritization, automated segmentation and volumetry, and classification and labelling of imaging features.
- Some tools for the evaluation of AI performance include contingency tables for binary classifiers and diagnostic performance parameters (sensitivity, specificity, positive predictive value, negative predictive value), the *F*1 score, Youden *J* index, ROC–AUC for binary classification or numerical values based on a threshold, and the Dice similarity coefficient and Hausdorff distance for segmentation metrics.
- Before implementing AI algorithms into clinical practice, they must be assessed by the methodology of the performance evaluation, patient population, test population, demographics, metrics, and results.
- As algorithms are trained on human-labelled data, and humans are subject to bias, measures must be taken to ensure that algorithms do not propagate these biases, and this means training and validating algorithms on a diverse dataset that is representative of the intended location of deployment; this may mean that an algorithm approved for clinical implementation still requires optimization to and validation on a local dataset before it is deployed to ensure it is accurate for the local population.

References

1. Columbus L. Microsoft leads the AI patent race going into 2019. *Forbes*, 6 January 2019. https://www.forbes.com/sites/louiscolumbus/2019/01/06/microsoft-leads-the-ai-patent-race-going-into-2019/?sh=3bca1db744de.
2. Gartner. Gartner forecasts worldwide artificial intelligence software market to reach $62 billion in 2022. Press release, 22 November 2021. https://www.gartner.com/en/newsroom/press-releases/2021-11-22-gartner-forecasts-worldwide-artificial-intelligence-software-market-to-reach-62-billion-in-2022.
3. Fortune Business Insights. Artificial intelligence (AI) market to hit USD 360.36 billion by 2028; surging innovation in artificial Internet of Things to augment growth. *Global Newswire*, 16 September 2021. https://www.globenewswire.com/news-release/2021/09/16/2298078/0/en/Artificial-Intelligence-AI-Market-to-Hit-USD-360-36-Billion-by-2028-Surging-Innovation-in-

Artificial-Internet-of-Things-AIoT-to-Augment-Growth-Fortune-Business-Insights.html.
4. Allied Market Research. *AI in Healthcare Market*, 2021. https://www.alliedmarket research.com/artificial-intelligence-in-healthcare-market.
5. AI Central. https://aicentral.acrdsi.org.
6. Ridley EL. IBM to sell Watson Health assets to private equity firm. AuntMinnie.com, 21 January 2022. https://www.auntminnie.com/index.aspx?sec=sup&sub=aic&pag=dis&itemId=134788.
7. Ridley EL. AI market churn continues as Sirona buys AI assets from Nines. Aunt Minnie.com, 18 February 2022. https://www.auntminnie.com/index.aspx?sec=sup&sub=aic&pag=dis&itemId=135039.

For additional references and Further Reading please see www.wiley.com/go/byrne/aiinclinicalmedicine.

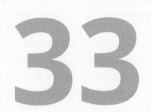

33

AI for Workflow Enhancement in Radiology

Sabeena Jalal[1], Jason Yao[2], Savvas Nicolaou[3], and Adnan Sheikh[3]

[1] Department of Radiology, Vancouver General Hospital, Vancouver, BC, Canada

[2] McMaster University, Hamilton, ON, Canada

[3] University of British Columbia, Vancouver, BC, Canada

Learning Objectives

- Understand AI's role in supplementing the imaging workflow.
- Describe the benefits of using AI in protocolling.
- Understand the importance of quality assurance and peer review, and how AI-based methods can augment retrospective and prospective second-reader applications.
- Highlight the challenges involved in developing AI in radiology.

33.1 Introduction to Imaging Workflow

As a result of the ever-expanding body of literature, it can be challenging to keep up with the latest trends in AI research. Increasing processing power of computers has allowed for tools to enhance decision-making and improve access to up-to-date medical information, augmenting efficiency and allowing more time for tasks that actually need a physician's attention. Over 135 million imaging examinations were performed in a selection of seven US healthcare networks and Ontario, Canada, between the years 2000 and 2016 [1]. Now imagine how high the number for North America as a whole would be. This sheer volume has significantly increased the radiologist's workload [2]. Radiology is essential for many time-sensitive applications such as trauma, stroke, and fractures, making it indispensable for medical decision-making and developing a treatment plan, so any improvements to workflow will be very welcome (Figure 33.1).

Radiology information systems (RIS) gather imaging data, resulting in the creation of extensive datasets that could be used for AI training. AI can be integrated into many aspects of the radiology workflow, including voice recognition software, picture archiving and communication systems (PACS), and clinical decision-making [3].

AI in Clinical Medicine: A Practical Guide for Healthcare Professionals, First Edition. Edited by Michael F. Byrne, Nasim Parsa, Alexandra T. Greenhill, Daljeet Chahal, Omer Ahmad, and Ulas Bagci.
© 2023 John Wiley & Sons Ltd. Published 2023 by John Wiley & Sons Ltd.
Companion website: www.wiley.com/go/byrne/aiinclinicalmedicine

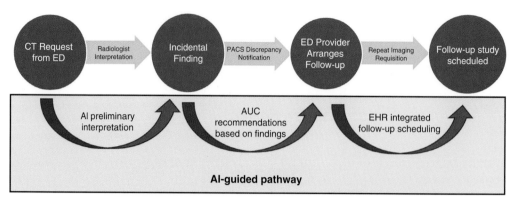

Figure 33.1: Proposed AI-guided clinical decision-support model. In this example, the traditional emergency department (ED) model for addressing incidental computed tomography (CT) findings involves the radiologist reporting the results in the dictated report. In most cases, it is up to the ordering clinician to arrange for both imaging and clinical follow-up. AI can integrate into this pathway at several stages: (i) providing a preliminary interpretation of incidental findings so they can be flagged for the radiologist and clinician; (ii) providing automated recommendations for follow-up based on appropriate use criteria (AUC); and (iii) automatically arranging for follow-up based on the imaging findings, reducing lag time and referral error.

These solutions can play a fundamental role, not just in a patient's imaging workflow but also in providing support to clinicians, such as in deciding whether an imaged patient requires medical care, surgical care, or can be safely discharged [3].

This chapter aims to explore applications of AI-guided imaging workflow systems within a radiology department.

33.2 Image Display Protocols

Workflow efficiency in the reading room is a critical factor in a fast-moving radiology department. PACS have allowed for a revolution in efficiency, enabling departments to keep up with ever-increasing imaging demands. While diagnostic applications of AI are well known, applications of AI as a tool to assist radiologists in their day-to-day workflow have also been proposed.

Digital hanging protocols are algorithms that display images from the examination along with relevant prior studies. Depending on the study and imaging modality, they can be useful for the interpreting radiologist to view relevant series, and to make comparisons to prior studies regarding interval changes. A previous survey of radiologists has shown that they perceive hanging protocols as the most impactful task on productivity, with an estimated 9% of time on a study spent on modifying image layout [4]. With more advanced imaging modalities and sequences, such as those seen in magnetic resonance imaging (MRI), hanging protocols are also becoming increasingly complex due to the volume of information from different pulse sequences and planes. Therefore, these protocols are one of the most common non-diagnostic applications of AI for radiology workflow enhancement.

Historically, hanging protocols have relied on Digital Imaging and Communications in Medicine (DICOM) sequences that contain metadata coding specific anatomical data, the Primary Anatomic Structure Sequence (PASS), to categorize exams based on image structure. However, hard-coded metadata may contain false tags and lack nuance (for example, basal lung fields may be present in a computed tomography [CT] scan of the abdomen), which can result in fetching and display errors. Methods of optimizing hanging protocols have included user-level algorithms, which consider the radiologist's preferences, and use performance metrics to analyse efficiency and recommend potential optimal protocols, as well as image-level algorithms that use pixel data to identify relevant image features and display them based on anatomy and sequences most relevant to the task. Commercially, these algorithms have already started to be integrated into PACS, with vendors developing proprietary smart imaging informatics systems that use contextual learning to provide workflow assistance [5].

Research into the use of image segmentation and classification models for workflow optimization is currently ongoing, with significant overlap in the core technologies underlying diagnostic and non-diagnostic applications. Groups have shown applications of combined classification and segmentation networks for identifying relevant regional anatomy on CT, with one group achieving 96.2% accuracy on identifying chest, abdomen, and pelvis anatomy on a pan-CT [6]. Proposed future applications will build on these core frameworks.

Beyond hanging protocols, other applications that have been proposed include automated spatial linking between studies to facilitate parallel scrolling, and intelligent cache-management systems to facilitate automated pre-fetching of archived studies.

Spatial linking in multi-planar imaging is currently achieved by manually or automatically matching two images of the region of interest in corresponding studies, so that anatomical slices align and can be scrolled in parallel. This is typically used to compare the study of interest to a previous study for interval change, oncology monitoring being a common application. While this approach works relatively well for images acquired using the same equipment and protocol, linking issues can occur when comparing images acquired from different machines, different hospitals, or different modalities (such as MRI and CT). While most PACS have mechanisms to correct for differences in slice thickness and protocol, these systems are not dynamic and may still encounter errors. AI has been proposed as a potential solution, using anatomical landmarks to dynamically link studies. While several groups have shown promise in AI-guided acquisition, patient positioning, and plane prescription [7], there have been few attempts at characterizing the clinical use of localization strategies post-acquisition.

Cache management is also an active area of research in radiology workflow optimization. Given the volume and storage requirements for imaging data, most PACS architectures are based on a hybrid model of local and off-site storage, such that recently acquired or accessed images are available immediately from on-premises servers, and more remote images are archived in the secure cloud. However, this introduces the problem of latency when accessing off-site records, as large image files must be retrieved and downloaded onto local servers – a time-consuming process, as studies can be hundreds of megabytes each. Most PACS have pre-fetch protocols for anticipating studies that are likely to be accessed. However, these are typically based on static scenarios (for instance, fetching previous CT chest studies in lung cancer surveillance). With increasing use of multi-institutional PACS, greater heterogeneity in imaging data may require more dynamic solutions for cache management. AI-based solutions have been proposed, such as dynamic pattern-recognition algorithms that learn from usage patterns [8]. Described approaches have used multilayer perceptron and decision trees to model user behaviour. In conjunction with these algorithms, image-level analysis with deep learning may be used for image tagging at the time of acquisition [7], to categorize relevant images, and to facilitate identification and retrieval.

33.3 Quality Assurance and Peer Review: 'Second Reader' Applications

Peer review is a method used by radiology departments to maintain high imaging standards and to provide quantifiable metrics for performance. Most departments have some form of peer review process, typically involving a double read of a random subset of studies. Quantifiable scales for reviewer concordance with the original report have been developed, most notably RADPEER™ from the American College of Radiology (ACR). In this system, cases are assigned a grade of 1–4 depending on the presence of discrepancy and difficulty of the case (scores 3–4 representing a significant discrepancy with the expected interpretation). However, these tools have been found to have low intra-reader reliability [8], and require radiologist time that could otherwise be used to report on new studies. AI has been proposed as a tool to improve the peer review process, using algorithms for second reads to assess for concordance in both prospective and retrospective applications.

Many of these algorithms have overlapping functionality with computer-assisted diagnosis models, which have been shown in applications for improving reader accuracy and efficiency at time of reporting. Computer-aided diagnosis (CAD) applications for image interpretation are discussed in further detail elsewhere in this book; we will focus on applications as they pertain to imaging workflow and quality assurance. At the time of publication, no study has directly assessed the use of AI for quality assurance, although several retrospective applications have shown high AI sensitivity in second-reader applications, including for chest radiographs [9] and trauma CT [10]. In second-reader applications, AI has been proposed as a tool for flagging high-risk studies that were reported as normal, based on neural network image analysis of common radiological findings. Prospective applications of this have been demonstrated, including in intracranial haemorrhage (ICH), a 'can't miss' diagnosis often requiring immediate medical intervention [3,8]. Using an AI-based model for ICH detection, Seyam et al. demonstrated that AI assistance reduced communication time for critical findings and demonstrated high overall ICH detection rates [11], a finding that has been supported by other publications in the literature [12,13].

AI has also been demonstrated for peer review in non-interpretative contexts, including targeted case sampling and knowledge-based peer learning. For instance, AICloudQA (Real Time Medical, Ontario, Canada) is a QA platform that provides both prospective and retrospective peer-review solutions, based on historical user data. It proposes intelligent case sampling using analysis of previous user discrepancies, addressing a limitation of traditional random peer-review methods that have been found to have low yield for identifying discrepancies. Additionally, it proposes user-specific learning recommendations based on performance, presenting a potential opportunity for trainee education. Combined with image-based networks, these applications have the potential to both improve clinical detection and department quality assurance methods [13].

33.4 Clinical Decision Support

AI-powered clinical decision-support systems have been an aspirational target for AI researchers since the inception of the technology. A 'black-box' algorithm that can provide automated recommendations based on multi-input data introduces the possibility for targeted diagnostics and interventions in medicine. Radiomics and AI-assisted diagnostics, discussed in Chapter 32, are just one element of how AI can be used to assist in radiology decisions. Beyond the reading room, AI can also integrate into clinical workflows, and assist radiologists and patient-facing clinicians in making decisions regarding patient management based on radiographical findings.

In most institutions, there is limited streamlined workflow once the radiologist's report is sent to the ordering provider; while urgent findings may be called in, it is typically up to the primary care team to follow up on findings or order additional imaging if needed. This introduces the potential for latency and missed findings based on communication errors during transfer of care. One study found that 47.6% of errors occurred with relation to communication of imaging results – the single most common stage for communication errors to occur in the overall workflow. The impact of these errors ranged from unnecessary imaging follow-up to delays in diagnosis of malignant or emergent findings. A commonly encountered case is a patient who has a CT abdomen in the emergency department (ED) to rule out an acute process, but has an incidental adrenal nodule noted on imaging requiring radiographic follow-up. While these incidental findings are reported by the radiologist, it is up to the emergency physician to note the discrepancy and to plan for follow-up, typically with the patient's family physician. With a workflow going through three providers, errors are common. AI, automated booking, and electronic health record (EHR) direct patient-flow tracking are solutions that can help ensure that patients receive appropriate follow-up care, and also provide additional guidance to clinicians.

Clinical decision-support frameworks have historically relied on knowledge-based frameworks, using pre-determined rules based on best evidence guidelines. The computer-assisted reporting and decision support (CAR/DS) framework is an example of this, introduced by the ACR to incorporate evidence- and consensus-based guidelines into radiology workflows [14]. In the previous example of an incidental adrenal adenoma, CAR/DS can provide a structured reporting framework based on nodule features (size, history of malignancy, interval change) and make recommendations for follow-up care. Using CAR/DS, ordering providers were found to be twice as likely to order follow-up imaging and hormonal screening for incidental adrenal nodules [15].

AI-based clinical decision-support frameworks have the potential to go beyond knowledge-based approaches, using image-level and textual features to automatically identify findings and make care suggestions. In a fully automated setting, AI-CDS could identify abnormalities using image-level neural networks or natural language processing (NLP) text parsing of radiology reports, suggest recommended follow-up based on appropriate use criteria and previous provider behaviour, and schedule additional investigations or imaging based on a priority queue. While this level of automation does not yet exist, several AI-based CDS models have been introduced commercially, such as CareSelect® (Change Healthcare, Nashville, TN, USA), which integrates into existing EHR workflows to suggest appropriate imaging indications based on patient data, provider, and care setting. Of course, provider preference must be taken into consideration with any framework, meaning that increasingly advanced semi-automated AI-CDS systems like CareSelect will likely be the direction for future applications of this algorithm class.

33.5 Natural Language Processing

NLP is a growing class of AI designed to process human language and speech. Consumer applications of NLP have been at the forefront in recent years, with examples of voice-recognition and text-processing algorithms powering everyday applications such as smart assistants, search engines, and chatbots.

In radiology, NLP has been applied in both imaging and clinical-facing applications. One of the most common uses of NLP is in report dictation. Historically, the process of reporting a radiology study involved the radiologist creating an audio report that was transcribed into text by a transcriptionist. However, this introduced delays in report processing, and required the radiologist to review transcriptions for accuracy prior to finalization. The advent of speech recognition introduced live transcription, allowing the radiologist to dictate and finalize the report during interpretation, and giving clinicians near-instant access to imaging results. Specialty transcription algorithms have been developed for use in radiology, based on similar algorithms to those seen in consumer-facing applications but optimized for common medical terminology. Earlier studies of the technology have shown that speech recognition has reduced report turnaround time by 81% [16], a number that has likely further increased with greater radiologist familiarity with the workflow and algorithm optimizations.

NLP models can also play a role in radiology research and education. Models may be combined with image interpretation networks to extract clinical variables from previously dictated reports, automating data mining that would have previously required significant human resources to achieve. As most radiology reports consist of unstructured text, NLP models are well equipped to identify key in-text phrases that can label relevant images and code clinical variables into a structured format. Models have been developed for applications such as assessing treatment response in oncology [17] and in a variety of quantitative applications. One example is in myocardial perfusion imaging, where quantitative/ semi-quantitative variables such as perfusion and flow reserve can be trended to assess treatment response. Compared to human reviewers, NLP algorithms have been found to have similar sensitivity and specificity for identifying these abnormalities in unstructured text reports [18], saving time and standardizing the review process. Several systematic reviews of NLP applications have been published [19], with applications in diverse subspecialties including musculoskeletal, breast, and chest radiology.

33.6 Medical Image Protocolling

In radiology there are tasks that are often repeated, such as protocolling of medical imaging requests. Protocolling is tedious and time-consuming, as imaging studies are multi-modal – ultrasound, X-ray, CT, MRI, and nuclear medicine – each requiring that parameters be adjusted, such as phasing, contrast, and perfusion. In the literature, radiology trainees have acknowledged protocolling as a cause for exhaustion and burnout, a factor that not only affects the physician's level of satisfaction with the work they do, but also adversely affects the quality of patient care [20]. Reducing disparities and discrepancies is imperative in the process, so that the radiology technologist can do the correct task [21,22]. It has been noted that inaccuracies in protocolling could range between 3% and 5% in large hospitals, potentially resulting in misdiagnosis, unnecessary investigations, tardy patient care, and consequently poor outcomes [22].

There have been efforts towards developing AI systems and neural networks that would essentially mechanize the method of protocolling medical imaging requests [23,24]. This would improve the efficiency of the radiologist. Triage strategies vary by modality – for example in CT, where volumes are higher and scan time is fast, the priority may be to expedite urgent scans based on clinical presentation [23]. However, in MRI, which has longer acquisition times, more focus may be placed on modifying MRI protocols and their sequence selection according to the clinical question and also the radiological image request. Electronic order-entry systems have been designed to incorporate machine learning models that can perform some elements of triage and pre-screening based on the requested study [24]. Artificial intelligence systems that automate the process of protocolling of medical imaging requests have the ability to allow the radiologist to focus their time and energy on reaching an accurate diagnosis rather than investing their time on repetitive tasks [25].

33.7 Image Acquisition and AI support

Developments in the field of radiology have led to improvements in image quality, at the level of both the scanner and post-processing. Image-reconstruction algorithms are a broad class of algorithms that have been enhanced by technological advancement in AI. A full discussion of these algorithms can be found in Chapter 32. Here, we will briefly focus the discussion as it pertains to workflow. For example, iterative reconstruction algorithms have substituted filtered back projection [26]. These algorithms have not only increased the image quality attained by the CT scans, but have also resulted in a decrease in the quantity of the dose of radiation that is required to carry out the test [27].

The integration of the radiology technologist's workflow with electronic order-entry systems has also been proven to be beneficial. Once a request for imaging is approved and protocolled by the radiologist, the radiology technologist can access the information using an import function, which mechanically adjusts the scanner for the particular patient's clinical scenario. This improves the technologist's workflow, which in turn streamlines the department's workflow and reduces time delays. All these stages of workflow could be further enhanced by AI support. This enhances the radiologist's efficiency in attaining precise diagnoses in a reduced amount of time, and consequently reduces the overall time taken to reach a decision pertaining to the patient's treatment plan [28].

33.8 Imaging Pathway in an Emergency and Trauma Radiology Department

At any hospital, the department of emergency and trauma radiology plays an important role in ensuring that quality healthcare is provided to patients who come to an ED [29,30]. Emergency and trauma radiologists work hard to meet the amplified imaging volume load, to achieve a low discrepancy rate, to generate accurate reports, and to provide a rapid turnaround time of finalized imaging reports. The demand for improved efficiency in delivering quality care to acute patients has led to the proposed applications of AI in emergency radiology [31], in order to help the radiologist in dealing with an increasing imaging volume and workload (Table 33.1) [32].

AI applications have the potential to enhance the existing workflow at several essential points along the typical patient pathway. At the centre of Figure 33.2 is the emergency and trauma radiologist. AI assists the radiologist by facilitating repetitive tasks, addressing the human element of tedium and fatigue, and enabling the radiologist to read images with a higher sensitivity and specificity in a smaller period of time. This is desirable, as shortening the turnaround time for finalized imaging studies enhances workflow and improves outcomes [33].

A patient's journey through the emergency and trauma radiology department commences prior to their arrival at the hospital's ED. Paramedics who bring the

Table 33.1: Applications of AI for radiology workflow enhancement.

Clinical decision support

- Order entry
- Appropriate use criteria screening

Study protocolling

- Study/sequence selection
- Safety assessment (renal function, allergies, metal, device compatibility)

Study triage

- Worklist prioritization
- Preliminary interpretation
- EHR clinical correlation

Image acquisition

- Image optimization
- Scan time reduction
- Sequence prescription

Image display

- Hanging protocols
- Cache management
- Worklist distribution

Quality assurance

- Second-reader applications
- Peer review/learning
- Department metric analytics

Natural language processing

- Study dictation/pre-dictation
- Report interpretation
- Clinical variable extraction

patient to the ED communicate relevant patient history and findings from physical examination to the triage physicians [34]. For trauma and stroke patients, the emergency radiology department is alerted of the possible requirement for imaging before the patient arrives at the ED [34,35]. Neural network models, when incorporated at this point in emergency radiology, could automatically compute the acuity scores in the ED. This could be done with enhanced precision compared to standardized systems, such as the Emergency Severity Index [35]. This triage information could in turn be made available to the emergency and trauma radiologist and assist with the prioritization of the worklist. There has also been a recent trend showing an increase in the use of portable CT scanners – when the patient is on the way to the ED – which utilize integrated AI software to support triage and patient placement [36]. These portable scanners that have in-built decision-support software may enhance patient transport metrics, and consequently decrease time to treatment and reduce delays in care.

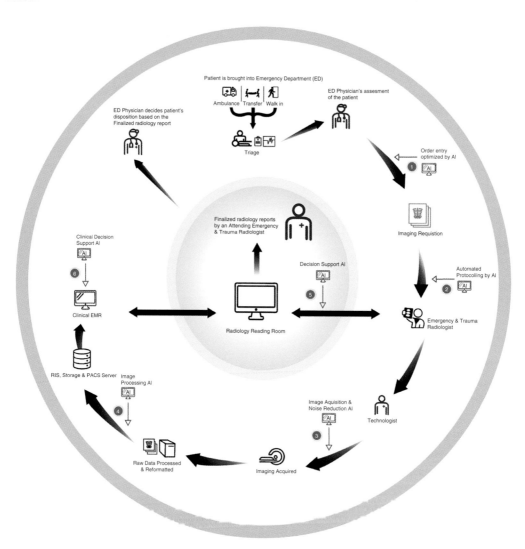

Figure 33.2: AI supported workflow in an emergency and trauma radiology department. A graphical representation of an imaging pathway. Implementing AI and integrating it into the workflow of the emergency and trauma radiology department would assist the radiologist.

Source: Jalal S et al. 2021 / with permission of Sage Publications.

AI can also be used to reduce unwarranted imaging studies. The ACR and the Canadian Association of Radiology have published several checklists and scoring systems to define appropriateness criteria [37]. ED doctors rely on electronic order-entry systems to request imaging studies from the department of radiology [21]. The process of order entry for radiological studies is not always straightforward. These checklists and scoring systems aim to streamline the process, and reduce irrelevant and unnecessary imaging. Electronic ordering systems may be used to automatically incorporate appropriateness criteria into imaging workflows using AI, with data automatically captured from the patient's medical record.

These AI-reinforced techniques could considerably enhance both the emergency radiology and emergency medicine department's workflow and efficiency [38].

33.9 Challenges Related to AI Use

There are several challenges associated with AI use for imaging workflow: lack of properly annotated patient data, high-dimensionality feature vectors, complex and interdependent patient features, and complex relationships between patient features and final diagnosis. Additionally, from an adoption perspective, the deployment of AI has to overcome numerous barriers, including acceptance of AI applications, knowledge and education regarding the technology, availability of appropriate data, and, most importantly, the ethics involved [19].

While there may be stigma surrounding AI in the radiology community given the narrative that these tools will work to replace radiologists, it is important to note that most applications of AI have been designed to enhance radiologist workflow, rather than act as the primary interpreter.

As AI itself cannot process unforeseen insights and conjure disease diagnosis based on diverse scenarios, workflow-enhancement tools are poised to remain the foremost clinically relevant applications in radiology in the short term. For greater acceptance of the technology, more knowledge-translation activities need to be undertaken in order to explain this narrative to the medical community. Another issue when training AI algorithms is data governance. Medical data are personal, and access to them can pose challenges for AI research. Promoting a data-centric view that sees value in integrating and sharing data is crucial. A final challenge relates to resource and personnel requirements – when a radiologist wants to design an algorithm for a task, this requires a lot of resources. A holistic team including personnel with diverse expertise is required, and this team may need to work on optimizing algorithms for a significant period of time. This translates into an ongoing drain on financial resources, and highlights the importance of greater interdisciplinary collaboration between radiologists, AI scientists, and computer engineers [19].

A radiologist interested in developing AI applications needs appropriately annotated data, suitable hardware infrastructure, precise labels, and health outcomes data. Accumulating a suitable dataset is vital for AI training, validation, and eventually testing of the algorithm. In designing a network, there are several issues to consider, such as which covariates need to be added to the training dataset (different scanners, illnesses, body parts, and modalities). All of this adds to the intricacies related to acquisition of patient data and algorithm validation. The more varied the combinations, the more difficult it is to address all the dimensions. Clinical heterogeneity might render the process even more arduous owing to the heterogeneity of patient populations, distinctive features and characteristics of the disease, and variation in patient geographical location. Algorithms may often fail to generalize, meaning they may work in one hospital setting with a high accuracy, but fail in another hospital setting [19]. Consequently, setting realistic goals is crucial at the beginning of an AI development project in radiology.

33.10 Conclusion

The application of AI technology in the field of radiology undoubtedly assists a radiologist. All stages of the radiology workflow – protocolling a radiology exam, image order placement, and communication of finalized imaging reports – can be carried out in a more efficient manner by the integration of AI techniques. Radiologists are in a privileged position to train, utilize, and assimilate AI technology into patient care as they have access to an enormous amount of data. This offers an opportunity to improve patient outcomes, and to add value to the healthcare industry.

KEY INSIGHTS

- **AI technology supplements imaging workflow – reduces discrepancies, decreases finalized report-turnaround time, and assists in repetitive tasks.**
- **AI technology increases the efficiency and effectiveness of a radiologist.**
- **The automation of tasks can prevent burnout among staff and trainees, providing an opportunity to focus on diagnosis and decision-making.**
- **The incorporation of AI into radiology can promote quality patient care.**

References

1. Smith Bindman R, Kwan ML, Marlow EC et al. Trends in use of medical imaging in US health care systems and in Ontario, Canada, 2000–2016. *JAMA* 2019;322(9):843–856. https://doi.org/10.1001/jama.2019.11456.
2. Mendoza D, Bertino FJ. Why radiology residents experience burnout and how to fix it. *Academic Radiology* 2019;26(4):555–558.
3. Tang A, Tam R, Cadrin Chênevert A et al. Canadian Association of Radiologists white paper on artificial intelligence in radiology. *Canadian Association of Radiologists Journal* 2018;69(2):120–135.
4. Padole A, Ali Khawaja RD, Kalra MK, Singh S. CT radiation dose and iterative reconstruction techniques. *American Journal of Roentgenology* 2015;204(4):W384–W392.
5. Lynch M. Intelligent tools for a productive radiologist workflow: how machine learning enriches hanging protocols. *Silo.Tips*, 18 June 2017. https://silo.tips/download/intelligent-tools-for-a-productive-radiologist-workflow-how-machine-learning-enr.
6. Philips. Philips is first to bring adaptive intelligence to radiology, delivering a new approach to how radiologists see, seek and share patient information. Press release

27 November 2016. https://www.philips.com/a-w/about/news/archive/standard/news/press/2016/20161127-philips-is-first-to-bring-adaptive-intelligence-to-radiology.html.

7. Filice RW, Stein A, Pan I, Shih G. Federated deep learning to more reliably detect body part for hanging protocols, relevant priors, and workflow optimization. *Journal of Digital Imaging* 2022;35(2):335–339. https://doi.org/10.1007/s10278-021-00547-x.

For additional references and Further Reading please see www.wiley.com/go/byrne/aiinclinicalmedicine.

34

AI for Medical Image Processing: Improving Quality, Accessibility, and Safety

Leonid L. Chepelev[1], Savvas Nicolaou[2], and Adnan Sheikh[2]

[1] University of Toronto, ON, Canada

[2] University of British Columbia, Vancouver, BC, Canada

Learning Objectives

- Understand some of the challenges of medical image acquisition in radiology and the practical impact of those challenges on everyday patient care.
- Understand some of the potential applications of AI in addressing image quality challenges.
- Develop appreciation of the measures taken for risk mitigation with radiation and contrast dose reduction, and how AI-based techniques can further assist in these areas.
- Explore some of the potential investigational solutions for the use of AI-based image processing beyond image quality improvement.
- Explore the uses of AI in assisting image-guided procedures and interventions.

34.1 Introduction

More than a decade has now passed since the demonstration of AlexNet by the team of Krizhevsky, Sutskever, and Hinton at the University of Toronto [1], which was a tremendous scientific achievement that transformed the field of machine learning. This triumph was closely followed by boundless optimism and assertions that no new radiologists should be trained, as the newly demonstrated convolutional neural networks (CNNs) would be capable of completely supplanting radiologists. The basis for this claim was the impressive accuracy of CNNs in image classification, and the widespread availability of computational hardware to carry out CNN training and deployment. While initial success in simple classification tasks with a finite differential space and well-behaved imaging inputs produced early successes in tasks such as pneumonia detection [2] and bone age characterization [3], an increasing

AI in Clinical Medicine: A Practical Guide for Healthcare Professionals, First Edition. Edited by Michael F. Byrne, Nasim Parsa, Alexandra T. Greenhill, Daljeet Chahal, Omer Ahmad, and Ulas Bagci.
© 2023 John Wiley & Sons Ltd. Published 2023 by John Wiley & Sons Ltd.
Companion website: www.wiley.com/go/byrne/aiinclinicalmedicine

realization of the nuances of practical implementation and the significant caveats to frontline clinical deployment of AI-based solutions [4,5] have facilitated a more mature outlook on the role of AI in medical imaging in the years following the CNN breakthrough. A decade after AlexNet, the adversarial sentiment towards the role of human experts has been recanted and significantly revised, with the current contention being that of a mutually beneficial relationship between radiology and AI where AI augments rather than replaces the radiologist [6]. Certainly, as noted elsewhere in this book, a wide array of daily tasks that typically limit productivity in medical imaging could potentially benefit from the introduction of clinically validated AI-based solutions. In some cases, rather than limiting the role of radiologists, novel AI-based solutions are already expanding the potential spectrum of applications of medical imaging, the value of medical imaging in patient care, as well as the affordability, accessibility, and safety of medical imaging.

In this chapter, we will first provide a very brief background overview of several medical imaging technologies to set the stage for the discussion of AI-mediated solutions. We will introduce some of the basic imaging terms and concepts in medical image acquisition and reconstruction. Using these concepts, we will then discuss some of the major applications of AI-based solutions in computed tomography (CT), magnetic resonance imaging (MRI), and fluoroscopy-guided interventions. We will focus primarily on the application of CNNs in medical image acquisition and processing, and on how AI-based techniques deployed in this context facilitate improvements in the value of radiology. We will then extend the discussion to potential novel developments in imaging hardware, and novel applications of the techniques described, to expand the value and role of medical imaging in patient care.

34.2 Basic Introduction to Medical Image Processing Concepts

Before embarking on an informed discussion of the applications of AI-based solutions in medical imaging, an introduction of the basic medical imaging concepts is imperative to ground this discussion. A complete examination of medical imaging physics is far beyond the scope of this chapter and could be found elsewhere [7]. This introduction is followed by a brief and simplified overview of some of the greatest ongoing challenges in medical imaging and the role of AI-based image processing techniques in addressing these challenges. Subsequent sections will then lay out the specific examples of some of the applications of AI-based image processing techniques available in the peer-reviewed literature.

34.2.1 Basic Medical Imaging Concepts

While numerous medical imaging technologies exist, the most frequently performed imaging procedures include roentgenography (also known as X-ray or fluoroscopy where time-resolved X-ray images are obtained), CT, ultrasound, and MRI.

In roentgenography, object shadows are formed by exposing an object to high-energy photons in the X-ray spectrum and reading the image from a detector plate. Higher-density objects such as bones allow fewer photons to pass through and form darker shadows than lower-density objects, therefore allowing distinct visualization of bones, for example. While shadows are dark on a bright background when one uses for instance a flashlight, in radiology the convention is to invert the colours of the shadows such that the shadows are bright while the background is dark. Therefore, the brighter structures are actually the denser ones and block photons more effectively (Figure 34.1).

The high-energy photons needed to adequately visualize anatomical detail to enable medical diagnosis are termed *ionizing radiation*, since the amount of energy carried by these photons renders them capable of enabling electrons to leave their orbits, therefore causing molecular damage. When this damage involves DNA, it may result in errors in gene sequences that can then increase the risk of significant mutations and carcinogenesis.

CT is simply the application of the same X-ray photons using a circular array of photon sources and detectors rotating around the patient at high speeds (Figure 34.2).

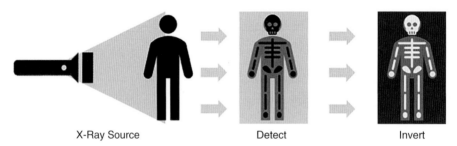

X-Ray Source   Detect   Invert

Figure 34.1: Image formation in radiography. An X-ray source is used to shine powerful photons at a patient, and the detector positioned on the opposite side of the source detects the intensity of photons reaching it and thus forming an image. This image is inverted by convention. Fluoroscopy is an imaging technique that acquires many radiographs in a rapid succession of several frames per second to track movement of instruments and contrast to help guide procedures and inform diagnosis, for example in examining coronary arteries.

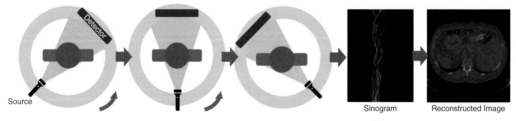

Figure 34.2: Basic operation of a computed tomography scanner. The patient (viewed from the top here) is placed inside a cylinder containing a source of X-rays and a detector. By taking images as the detector rotates around the patient, an intermediate image called a sinogram is generated. This sinogram is then reconstructed into an anatomical image of a patient's cross-section, called an axial image, as the table moves on in the craniocaudal axis. A stack of such images is generated to visualize a 3D region of the patient's body.

Generally, the more thorough is the anatomical coverage in a scan and the higher the photon dose, the better is the scan quality as measured by the signal-to-noise ratio (SNR), but the higher is the cancer risk. Minimizing cancer risk while optimizing image quality for diagnostic purposes is one of the key concerns in radiological safety. Furthermore, since blood has similar density to soft tissues – that is, a similar ability to block transmission of X-ray photons – it can be difficult to distinguish between the different soft tissues and adjacent vessels. To improve this distinction, iodine-containing contrast agents are injected into venous circulation. Iodine absorbs photons effectively and therefore appears as bright on CT images. Differential uptake of iodine by different tissues and the timing of imaging since contrast injection help differentiate the various soft tissue structures and types of blood vessels (arteries or veins), based on how much dense contrast is present. Unfortunately, contrast cannot be given to people who are allergic to it and to people who have poor renal function. For such patients, other techniques such as dual-energy CT or MRI must be considered.

In MRI, no ionizing radiation is used (Figure 34.3). Instead, MRI uses the principle where some atomic nuclei (in medical imaging, most often ^{1}H nuclei) have a non-zero spin that can exist in two states, up or down. Practically, such nuclei are in a constant precession about their axis and have a weak magnetic dipole. When an external magnetic field is applied, the spin axes of these atoms align with the external field axis, with the total nucleus population splitting into two spin states: low- and high-energy states based on the direction of alignment with the external magnetic field. Since the energy difference associated with these states is miniscule, the populations of the two spin states are similar. The stronger the

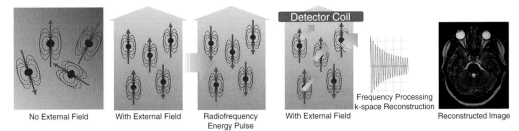

No External Field   With External Field   Radiofrequency Energy Pulse   With External Field   Frequency Processing k-space Reconstruction   Reconstructed Image

Figure 34.3: Basic principles of magnetic resonance imaging application. Some atoms, like hydrogen atoms, have a spin property and are in constant precession around their axis, with an associated magnetic dipole formed. When an external field is applied, it becomes slightly more energetically favourable for the protons to align with the field than against it, creating a net difference in the number of atoms aligned with and against the external field, and thus a net dipole. When external energy is provided using radiofrequency pulses, some of the low-energy atoms aligned with the field flip against the field using the extra energy supplied. Once this extra energy is removed, the atoms flip back to their low-energy alignment, emitting radiofrequency waves that are detected and analysed to first reconstruct a k-space image, which is an inverse representation of the real space image, and then the real space image of patient anatomy.

external field applied is, the larger the energy difference grows, and the greater is the difference in the numbers of nuclei between the two states. When an external boost of energy is applied using radio frequency waves, some atoms in the low-energy state have enough energy to jump in alignment against the field. When the radio frequency energy is removed, the two populations equilibrate back to the original distribution. As this equilibration occurs, the MRI scanner collects signals that correspond to the energy released by the atoms that jumped to the higher-energy state as they return to the lower-energy state, in the form of electromagnetic radiation.

Advanced processing of these data allows the scanners to populate an inverse space of the real Euclidean space, known as the k-space. In the k-space, each data-point contains information regarding the entirety of the image in the real space. The more datapoints are added to the k-space, the easier it is to reconstruct the images of the real space; however, doing so prolongs the scan times. Different combinations of radio frequency pulses allow different ways of visualizing tissues, highlighting ^1H atoms in different circumstances, for example separating those atoms that are found in fat from those that are found in water or those atoms that are moving (e.g. fluid and cells in vessels) from those that are stationary. Generally, the more times the radio frequency pulses are repeated, the more points can be obtained in the k-space and the better is the SNR, but the longer is the scan. Additionally, the higher is the external magnetic field, the greater is the difference in the two populations of ^1H nuclei, and the better is the SNR, but the more expensive is the MRI machine. Similar to CT, different gadolinium-based contrast agents administered intravenously help better delineate different soft tissues, organs, and types of lesions in order to support diagnosis.

In CT, the principal goal in optimizing imaging is to find the minimum amount of radiation dose and contrast dose necessary to obtain diagnostic images with optimal SNR, contrast-to-noise ratio (CNR), and spatial resolution. In MRI, the goal is to find the technique that provides the best spatial resolution, SNR, and CNR, best tissue differentiation, lowest contrast dose, shortest acquisition time, and lowest external magnetic field. In X-ray and fluoroscopy, the principal goal is to expose the patient to the least possible radiation in as little time as possible. All of these techniques are subject to possible introduction of image artifact, as further discussed in what follows.

34.3 Basic AI-Based Image Quality Improvement Approaches

Before embarking on the discussion of general problems in improving medical image quality and the specific examples of solutions provided in peer-reviewed literature, a discussion of some of the basic AI-based image reconstruction approaches is necessary. Here, we arbitrarily divide such solutions into sensor domain–based solutions and image domain–based solutions (Figure 34.4).

(a)

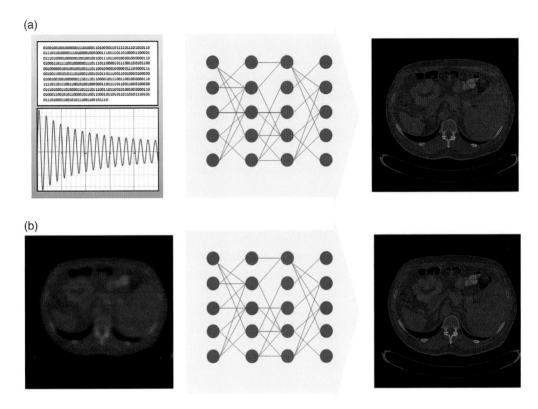

(b)

Figure 34.4: Sensor and image domain–based solutions. (a) In sensor domain–based solutions, the raw data from device sensors are obtained in order to generate an image directly. To train the reconstruction network in this case, pairs of inputs (sensor signals) and outputs (ideal images) are provided. The network then is able to reconstruct an image from any sensor input. (b) In image domain–based solutions, suboptimal images from low-quality instruments or images with artifact paired with optimal versions of these images are used to train reconstruction networks, which then can be applied to arbitrary suboptimal low-quality images to create high-quality images.

34.3.1 Sensor Domain–Based Solutions

In sensor domain AI image reconstruction solutions, the principal assumption is that traditional physics-based image reconstruction algorithms and statistical image correction techniques do not utilize all of the imaging data to the full potential, and that replacement of the physics-based mapping of the data from the sensor domain to the image domain can provide a better basis for image reconstruction. In order to train such techniques, one starts with a pairing of the ideal-quality 'perfect' images with suboptimal sensor data. Within the sensor data, one may introduce perturbations that either increase overall noise, emulate the results of decreasing radiation dose for CT imaging, emulate the results of limited k-space characterization by shorter image acquisition times in MRI, or emulate image artifacts in any technique. The combination of the imperfect sensor data and the paired perfect image sets is used to train an intermediary CNN that maps the two, and is subsequently capable of reproducibly accounting for the arbitrary sensor limitations. One of the earliest and best known of such applications in MRI is AUTOMAP, which is essentially a modified denoising autoencoder [8]. Because arbitrary perturbations can be achieved for the sensor data, similar approaches are not specific for a specific artifact type. While traditional physics-based image reconstructions must necessarily fall back on the theoretical underpinnings of image formation and derivation of statistical methods that are specific to each artifact type, image reconstruction through a CNN generally relies on only minimally perturbed approaches for training, ensuring that image sensor data would be maximally leveraged regardless of imaging artifact type.

34.3.2　Image Domain–Based Solutions

Where sensor data are not immediately available to train a neural network mapping, encoder–decoder architectures can be used to train networks capable of image optimization based on paired examples of suboptimal- and optimal-quality images. Since raw sensor data occupy a large amount of space on disk, medical scanners typically maintain these data for 24–48 hours, after which additional image reconstructions from raw data are not available. This means that unless explicitly used for the highest possible quality reconstruction (e.g. with the thinnest axial image slice), some data will be lost after the limited time window following image acquisition, and in some cases this may result in repeating the studies to ensure optimal visualization. To bypass this limitation, a number of approaches using a set of suboptimal or limited images paired with optimal images have been demonstrated, typically using an encoder–decoder framework or generative adversarial networks. The solutions demonstrated could be based on techniques utilizing two-dimensional images or complete three-dimensional imaging volumes. For example, such approaches have been used to improve image resolution in cardiac imaging [9], and to boost reduced-dose contrast signal [10], or create synthetic contrast-enhanced images bypassing contrast administration altogether [11], as well as predicting the appearance of lesions on entirely different modalities. In principle, any pair of images may be used for training and subsequent prediction. For example, imagine training an image domain–based network by pairing pre-chemotherapy and post-chemotherapy images on a range of patients including those for whom chemotherapy worked well and those in whom it was less effective, and then using this network to help predict whether specific chemotherapy regimens would be likely to succeed in a specific patient, and using this information to help target therapy.

34.4　Specific Problems and AI-Based Solutions

34.4.1　Denoising and Artifact Reduction

Medical images are often subject to image noise and imaging artifact. Noise may result from a number of sources, including, for example, photon scatter in CT and plain films, and endogenous patient radiofrequency emissions combined with accumulated instrument errors in MRI. Imaging artifact refers to systematic errors. For example, a single detector broken on a CT scanner will produce a 'ring artifact' that will create a ring of abnormal signal in a specific position on every single image. Introducing radio frequency signal interference inside an MRI scanner, such as by leaving the door to the scanner room open and thus disrupting the scanner Faraday cage, produces a characteristic radiofrequency interference artifact. Similarly, systematic distortions to the homogeneity of the intrinsic magnetic field within an MRI scanner by physical alterations of internal physical shimming hardware would result in systematic image distortion [7].

Traditionally, in order to decrease the amount of image noise, one must either increase the amount of time that the images are acquired for during MRI – which decreases patient throughput and thus increases cost while restricting access to vital imaging – or increase the amount of energy of the photons used in CT, thus increasing the radiation dose. Numerous computational techniques have been developed to harness various statistical and physical principles to address noise and artifact problems prior to the advent of CNN-based solutions. Unfortunately, physics-based solutions are limited by the quality of the inputs and physics-based constraints, as well as computational tractability.

AI-based approaches have been developed to significantly reduce arbitrary image noise, both using the unprocessed or processed sensor domain data directly and based on already reconstructed image data directly [8]. Similar approaches have been deployed by others, including, for example, to accelerate knee MRI [12], with the aim of bringing down the MRI acquisition time to the point where other traditional methods such as radiographs would no longer be the recommended entry point of imaging workups due to improved MRI costs. Additional important recent developments have been made in enabling cheap, energy-efficient, low magnetic field MRI instruments to generate diagnostic images on a par with the much more expensive and much less portable machines used conventionally. This could improve instrument affordability with limited compromises to image quality [13], representing just one example of AI-enabled novel imaging instrument development. The low magnetic field MRI could potentially represent a major breakthrough in changing global healthcare by fundamentally altering imaging affordability and accessibility of MRI to wider populations and clinical settings.

34.4.2 Image Resolution

In some instances, the image resolution available on already existing images is insufficient for the purposes of complete diagnosis or patient-specific treatment planning. For example, a patient entering the emergency department at a local hospital with a vague complaint of pain would, if appropriate, receive CT imaging that is routinely optimized for immediate diagnosis of a wide variety of conditions while minimizing the necessary radiation dose, and images reconstructed would typically be widely spaced (low axial resolution). If it is discovered that this patient has a tumour that lies in close proximity to a vital anatomical structure, more closely spaced images would be required. Invariably, a repeat CT or MRI study is performed specifically for treatment planning, which exposes the patient to additional risks, and increases care costs and care delays.

AI-assisted super-resolution algorithms have recently entered the mainstream with products such as NVIDIA's Deep Learning Super Sampling (DLSS), and have been made popular by widespread implementation in film and video game processing hardware. These techniques allow less powerful graphics cards to leverage CNNs to improve the resolution of images on the fly, and to improve the temporal resolution of video streams, upgrading a 30 frame per second (FPS) image stream to 60 FPS, for example. Thus, the original image generated at lower resolution and reduced cost would be upscaled to much higher resolutions not previously achievable by the installed hardware through explicit graphical calculations.

These super-resolution algorithms could be directly utilized in improving image quality, reconstructing missing images within a CT [14], or improving the quality of MRI [15] scans, and enhancing the temporal resolution, such as imaging of the heart throughout the cardiac cycle, as will be exemplified later in the chapter [9]. A solution that can be imagined here as an exercise is to dramatically reduce the radiation dose using the FPS boosting functions to improve fluoroscopic examinations. For example, in interventional percutaneous coronary angiograms, one can envision using the existing video frame rate-boosting techniques to improve the visualization of blood flow through the coronary arteries using less radiation and with fewer actual radiation pulses taken to help support more accurate diagnosis. For example, a 2 FPS examination could potentially be boosted to 3 FPS or 4 FPS through post-processing.

34.4.3 Reducing Time and Radiation Dose Requirements of Imaging

The problem of decreasing the minimum data requirements for reconstruction of diagnostically viable images is a direct corollary of the problems of denoising and artifact reduction discussed earlier. Any imaging technique capable of deriving more information from existing sensor data would be capable of directly reducing the necessary radiation doses in CT. For example, a currently commercially available deep learning–assisted image reconstruction algorithm deployed on a clinical scanner was compared to more traditional CT image reconstruction algorithms, and was found to be superior in quality in comparison to traditional reconstruction techniques, while significantly reducing radiation dose [16].

In the case of MRI, this approach would result in decreased scan times, as fewer points would need to be acquired in the k-space to populate the image adequately. Both of these measures would improve the accessibility and safety of medical imaging directly. For example, in paediatric cardiac MRI, reducing the time necessary for image acquisition is of tremendous importance, as younger children are generally unable to reliably comply with instructions to remain still and hold their breath, and may consequently require anaesthesia for some imaging procedures. Deep learning image reconstruction has been recently validated in children and young adults, significantly accelerating image reconstruction, and thus dropping the acquisition time and requirement for controlled breath holds during image acquisition [17]. The application of AI-based image reconstruction techniques in this context holds the promise of maximizing the utilization of sensor data and already reconstructed image data. It may be argued that in the future, AI assistance in targeting and directing the imaging protocols has the potential to eliminate unnecessary imaging, while more specifically tailoring and taking pre-emptive steps for improving image quality where the need for precise planning is detected during a scan.

Numerous AI-based solutions have been deployed to facilitate image acquisition and planning. More generally, in cardiac MRI where adequate visualization of the heart is crucial to diagnostic accuracy, AI-based solutions can help accelerate image planning by proposing optimal imaging planes [10], and easily identifying key diagnostic tissue parameters from limited data [18] to help boost the productivity of radiologists and technologists. In the future, such algorithms may eventually be involved in automated quality evaluation as part of a semi-automated workflow to alert the technologists and radiologists to potential alterations in imaging protocols [19]. Furthermore, a side product of accelerated MRI is the improved accessibility of this imaging modality through dramatically increased throughput, as discussed earlier.

These benefits in technique are not only limited to CT and MRI. Fluoroscopic procedures can be significantly improved from the standpoint of radiation dose administered by the use of AI-assisted image optimization methods, and this was validated on fluoroscopy-guided endoscopic procedures, resulting in decreased radiation exposure to the patient and medical personnel by half in comparison to procedures not assisted by AI [20].

34.4.4 Intravenous Contrast Dose Reduction

Where possible, minimization of additional administration of any substance as part of the diagnostic workup is encouraged. While modern CT iodinated contrast agents and MRI gadolinium-based agents have excellent safety profiles, they are not completely without risk, including the direct risk of anaphylactic reaction. Acute kidney injury is another feared complication of iodinated contrast administration, and iodinated contrast is avoided in patients with decreased or dropping renal function who are not already on dialysis. For gadolinium-based contrast agents, nephrogenic systemic fibrosis is a rare but feared complication of contrast administration, resulting in avoidance of contrast administration in patients with reduced renal function. From the point of view of patient safety, while reduction in the dose of contrast does not reduce the risk of true anaphylaxis, some reactions and the extent of kidney injury may be mitigated by administering lower amounts of contrast, while lowering scan costs due to decreased consumption of contrast agents. Algorithms aimed at boosting the signal associated specifically with intravenous contrast are therefore of potential tremendous utility.

For example, a generative adversarial network-based image domain reconstruction algorithm was used to boost the contrast signal, allowing reduction in administered contrast by half without compromising diagnostic accuracy [21]. In MRI, techniques aimed at significantly reducing the contrast are in constant development, including, for example, a recent study validating the use of 10% of the typical intravenous contrast dose for brain imaging [22], as well as ongoing commercial developments poised to create synthetic contrast-enhanced images without any intravenous contrast.

34.4.5 Cross-Modality Alignment and Information Redundancy

In some cases, adequate visualization of pathology requires the use of complementary imaging techniques. For example, for a Pancoast lung tumour that invades the adjacent ribs and neurovascular bundles, CT provides excellent visualization of the degree of bone involvement while MRI can detail the precise neurovascular structures involved. The combination of the two scans provides a comprehensively accurate depiction of anatomy to enable patient-specific preoperative planning. Unfortunately, the repositioning of the patient on the CT table and subsequent transfer to the MRI scanner results in patient motion and anatomical deformation between the scans, thus complicating the alignment of CT and MRI images. Automated image alignment is therefore highly useful in mitigating issues with image co-registration. Additionally, the ability to bypass one of the modalities or, in the case of MRI, one of the sequences altogether would be tremendously valuable in accelerating patient care. Cutting out additional time-consuming MRI sequences by using existing data to reconstruct these sequences, or cutting out the CT examination by predicting CT images from the MRI data or alternative MRI sequences from existing MRI sequences, would be tremendously useful in such settings [23].

34.5 Potential Pitfalls

While impressive and encouraging for medical imaging, AI-based solutions must be carefully understood and considered within the specific clinical setting for which they are optimized. In this section, we will discuss the importance of validating any AI-based image quality-improvement technique and considering its ongoing utility in the setting of additional concurrent software solutions and ongoing data drift.

34.5.1 The Importance of Quality Assurance and Validation

To place the need for algorithm quality assurance and validation in perspective, in one large-scale analysis of breast cancer screening, 94% of the 36 tested AI systems were found to be inferior and of no added value in comparison to an unassisted radiologist [24]. In another study, all assessed algorithms touted as capable of detecting/prognosticating for COVID-19 were found inadmissible due to method-ological flaws and biases [5].

For successful implementation, it is important to understand that practical and clinically meaningful implementation of AI-based image quality-improvement solutions are potentially open to an equally wide array of limitations. Solutions that are published are not necessarily available for clinical use [5], and where they are available for use, significant practical deployment barriers may exist. If deployment challenges are overcome, solutions must first be validated in a specific clinical setting and on specific imaging hardware. Furthermore, it must be ascertained that any AI-based solution is capable of failing safely, which necessitates adequate unit testing. Only then can such solutions begin to improve perceptions of their value and become sufficiently trusted to participate in direct patient care [25]. The precise mechanisms of evaluating and implementing AI-based software are beyond the space constraints of this chapter, and in-depth evaluations of this topic exist elsewhere [26].

34.5.2 Algorithm Orchestration and Provenance

In the story of the tower of Babel, humans begin the construction of a tower that reaches the heavens, only to have their arrogance punished by the curse of different languages, resulting in a lack of mutual understanding of humankind and the abandonment of the construction project. Where active software development by multiple entities occurs, resultant software frequently runs into the *computational tower of Babel* problem with a lack of software compatibility, interoperability, and seamless integration. Above all, this manifests in a lack of mutual awareness and records of the different software solutions working within a single pipeline. To illustrate, consider a computational pipeline where an AI-assisted image reconstruction algorithm is used in conjunction with another algorithm that emulates intravenous contrast, as well as a third algorithm that alerts radiologists to potential critical findings. If each algorithm was only validated on unprocessed images obtained directly from the scanner, a situation where these algorithms are deployed in sequence (e.g. contrast enhancement > denoising > prioritization) would not be sufficiently validated. Furthermore, the interchange of the order in which the different algorithms are deployed, or the version of a specific algorithm, can further potentially substantially alter the final result, with real impact on patient care. Therefore, algorithm version number, any additional steps taken to train/optimize/modify the algorithm, and the order in which any image processing was performed would likely need to be stored as part of the medical record in the future.

The number of medical AI companies with unique solutions has seen explosive growth, which further propagates and complicates the tower of Babel problem as well as the storage of the relevant provenance information. A vendor-neutral computational fabric that allows uniform algorithm deployment and orchestration supported by common ontologies such as RadLex [27] and Digital Imaging and Communications in Medicine (DICOM) workgroup standards would be indispensable in supporting seamless AI integration. Alternatively, various PACS or instrument vendors could develop a collection of 'app marketplaces' to provide an environment for algorithm deployment.

34.5.3 Ongoing Quality Assurance and Drift

The quality assurance/quality improvement initiatives are unlikely to succeed unless they are carried out on an ongoing basis. The reason for this is drift, which includes population drift, algorithm drift, instrument drift, and imaging technique drift, among others. For example, algorithms validated for a specific population may not be resistant to demographic changes or directly transferable to an area where socioeconomic or ethnic subgroups with unique challenges and healthcare needs were not fairly represented in the initial training data. The potential magnitude and clinical significance of fair population distribution in training and validation sets are reflected in the capability of CNNs to accurately identify patient race from chest radiographs [28]. Additional considerations, including changes in local disease prevalence, changes in imaging hardware, and changes in personnel and practices, can likely provide an equally considerable effect on the quality of the AI-based image processing results, as observed on networks with performance degradation over time [29].

34.6 Looking Ahead: Beyond Image Acquisition

The range of AI-assisted applications in medical imaging is virtually limitless. Beyond image acquisition, AI-based applications have been instrumental in supporting nascent developments in medical imaging. For example, one of the recent momentous developments has been the widespread introduction of 3D printing and advanced visualization. Image post processing with precise segmentation is key to supporting these precision medicine applications in a wide range of clinical scenarios [30]. Since segmentation is extremely time-consuming, architectures such as nnU-Net have been successfully employed in these tasks, achieving excellent accuracy [31] to significantly facilitate this process and enable on-the-fly, accurate segmentation. The resultant medical 3D-printed models can be used in hyperrealistic simulations where encoder–decoder frameworks can dynamically generate augmented reality video streams based on an input video stream of 3D-printed model manipulations, thus facilitating physician training and procedure planning [32].

Aside from tremendously facilitating a wide range of menial tasks in lung cancer screening, and supporting advanced secondary image analysis including cardiac strain analysis, similar techniques to those described here could be used in entirely novel ways. For example, paired images of patients with cancer before and after treatment can be used in frameworks that are nearly identical to the noise-reduction frameworks to predict disease evolution over time or in response to specific therapy, with the aim of more precisely tailoring treatment plans. Similar approaches can be used in a range of pathologies, for example predicting stroke evolution and helping support decision-making on the fly. Combined with AI-based solutions that may enable 'digital biopsy' through radiomic evaluation of disease to more accurately establish malignant potential based on imaging alone [33], AI can dramatically alter the role of medical imaging.

34.7 Conclusions

The introduction of CNNs has presented a wide range of tremendous opportunities for medical imaging. Far from replacing radiologists, AI-based solutions stand poised to expand the role of medical imaging and significantly facilitate patient safety, the accessibility of medical imaging, and the cost of medical imaging and post-processing. Radiologists of the future would have to maintain an enriched skillset rendering them capable of centralizing all aspects of medical imaging within a single transcendent imaging department in order to support further positive transformation of the scope, accessibility, and throughput of radiology. This transformation, however, will have to be carried out with careful attention to justice, quality, and safety considerations.

KEY INSIGHTS

- **The process of machine learning–mediated image reconstruction allows imaging hardware to harness sensor data to a more complete extent than previously enabled by traditional physics-based reconstructions and image improvement techniques.**
- **The two main approaches for the implementation of AI in medical imaging include reconstruction of images from sensor data and image reconstruction from previously reconstructed suboptimal image data, using convolutional neural networks (CNNs) to map sensor data or suboptimal image data to high-quality image reconstructions. Both approaches include mechanisms for built-in image quality improvement at no additional cost.**
- **AI-based image reconstruction must be implemented properly in order to be effective, and requires vigilance in the form of ongoing quality assurance and customized, validated deployments with careful attention paid to implementation details.**
- **Reductions in the amount of data necessary to reconstruct diagnostic images, and improvements of image acquisitions enabled by AI, directly translate into decreased radiation dose requirements for CT, decreased image time requirements for MRI, lower permissible doses of intravenous contrast, and therefore decreased risks associated with imaging and improved cost and accessibility.**

- **AI-based image reconstruction enables novel low-cost imaging instruments such as low-field MRI, which could be used in urgent settings and could be affordable enough for use in developing countries.**
- **The techniques used in AI-based image reconstruction can be extended beyond image quality, and can help improve prognostic performance and clinical decision-making.**

References

1. Krizhevsky A, Sutskever I, Hinton GE. ImageNet classification with deep convolutional neural networks. In: Pereira F, Burges CJC, Bottou L, Weinberger KQ (eds), *Advances in Neural Information Processing Systems 25*. Redhook, NY: Curran Associates; 2012, 1097–1105.
2. Pan I, Cadrin-Chênevert A, Cheng PM. Tackling the Radiological Society of North America pneumonia detection challenge. *American Journal of Roentgenology* 2019;213(3):568–574.
3. Pan I, Thodberg HH, Halabi SS, Kalpathy-Cramer J, Larson DB. Improving automated pediatric bone age estimation using ensembles of models from the 2017 RSNA machine learning challenge. *Radiology: Artificial Intelligence* 2019;1(6):e190053.
4. Tang A, Tam R, Cadrin-Chênevert A; Canadian Association of Radiologists (CAR) Artificial Intelligence Working Group. Canadian Association of Radiologists white paper on artificial intelligence in radiology. *Canadian Association of Radiology Journal* 2018;69(2):120–135.
5. Roberts M, Driggs D, Thorpe M et al. Common pitfalls and recommendations for using machine learning to detect and prognosticate for COVID-19 using chest radiographs and CT scans. *Nature Machine Intelligence* 2021;3(3):199–217.
6. Reardon S. Rise of robot radiologists. *Nature* 2019,576(7787):S54–S58.
7. Huda W. *Review of Radiologic Physics*, 4th edn. Philadelphia, PA: Lippincott Williams & Wilkins; 2016.

For additional references and Further Reading please see www.wiley.com/go/byrne/aiinclinicalmedicine.

35

Future Developments and Assimilation of AI in Radiology

Aakanksha Agarwal[1] and Timothy É. Murray[2,3]

[1] *Department of Radiology, University of British Columbia, Vancouver, BC, Canada*

[2] *Department of Radiology, St. Paul's Hospital, Vancouver, BC, Canada*

[3] *Department of Radiology, University of British Columbia, Vancouver, BC, Canada*

Learning Objectives

- Project forward from known AI trends, both specific to medical imaging and generalizable to all sectors.
- Understand the challenges in adapting to fast-paced changes in AI in medical imaging.
- Understand the benefits of incorporating AI in medical imaging.
- Highlight the challenges with the ethical development and incorporation of AI, and in developing a reasonable path forward.
- Understand legal and payment model complexities that will shape the future implementation of AI in medical imaging.

35.1 Introduction

Radiology and medical imaging were among the first healthcare fields to adopt digitization. The shift from hard copy to digital processing, storage, analysis, and dissemination was driven by multiple parallel factors: namely, lowering costs and complexity, enabling after-the-fact image processing, and expediting turn-around times. This digitalization created enormous amounts of data that facilitated downstream advances in analytics, machine learning, and AI. These have ensured that radiology is at the forefront of AI in clinical medicine, with a longer lead-time and a greater depth of experience than many less data-intensive domains of medicine.

In looking to the radiology department of the future, it is worth defining the typical links of the value chain covered within a typical radiology department or clinic. These include:

- Request receipt
- Request protocolling
- Study scheduling

AI in Clinical Medicine: A Practical Guide for Healthcare Professionals, First Edition. Edited by Michael F. Byrne, Nasim Parsa, Alexandra T. Greenhill, Daljeet Chahal, Omer Ahmad, and Ulas Bagci.
© 2023 John Wiley & Sons Ltd. Published 2023 by John Wiley & Sons Ltd.
Companion website: www.wiley.com/go/byrne/aiinclinicalmedicine

- Study performance
- Study interpretation
- Study reporting
- Report dissemination and follow-up
- Quality assurance (of all aspects of the process)
- Teaching (of radiology doctors, non-radiology doctors, technologists, and all levels of non-medical staff)
- Billing and finance
- Compliance
- Radiation safety

The extent to which these tasks have been at least partly automated varies, and takes into account complex local factors including patient needs and expectations, legislation, and culture. Although the core function of radiology is well suited to generating large amounts of data that can be analysed, many of the related functions of any radiology department rely on labour-intensive processes. The pace of adoption of AI has demonstrated that in almost any arena, AI can improve productivity or replace human input. There is little reason to think that the radiology department of the future will be spared from the AI-spearheaded drive for productivity, led today by private industry.

Many imaging studies are conducted in large hospital-based academic departments or private clinics which combine multiple image modalities. This is typically conducted with the support of technologists, clerical staff, and a variety of support staff on-site. A main driver for centralization has been the need to manage human resources, and to concentrate expertise. However, in a future where almost all aspects of a study are automated, the need for centralization for staffing purposes will presumably diminish. As with fully automated vending-machine stores now seen in airports and malls (often representing a satellite of a big box retailer), a fully autonomous computed tomography (CT) or magnetic resonance imaging (MRI) machine in similar settings would seem likely in the future. The potential use of AI and automation across the entire spectrum of a radiology practice is clearly enormous, and offers limitless scope for disruption.

35.2 Future of Radiology Reporting

A broad base of research supports the current shift from narrative reports to a structured reporting format. This makes the reports more readable and reduces errors. Machine learning in AI can be employed to automatically generate report impressions, and can be customized to the reporting radiologist's preference. AI can detect diagnoses suggested in the report, and automatically suggest consensus guideline recommendations. Additionally, it can facilitate billing by ensuring that the correct language is entered in the reports. Deep learning software can aid in automatically suggesting grades or classifications available in the literature, depending upon the imaging findings. For example, AI can automatically classify fractures or assist in deciding the correct Reporting and Data System (RADS) classification. This may improve efficiency, and maintain consistency and accuracy in reporting. AI software can 'learn' incidental findings, and add them instantly to the report along with consensus guidelines, thus greatly reducing the cognitive load upon the radiologist.

With voice recognition software, differences in a radiologist's voice can make the identification of certain erroneous words. AI software can use algorithms to proofread reports to ensure that such context errors are not transmitted, and thus reduce the need for creating addenda [1]. AI software can be used for computer-aided detection of lesions, for example in chest X-rays and CT scans. The radiologist can then categorize the lesions.

For follow-up imaging, measurements are of utmost importance, particularly when applying the RECIST (Response Evaluation Criteria in Solid Tumours) criteria or following up tumoral pathologies. Standardization is possible using AI-automated tools for measurement of dimensions and volume of a lesion [2].

Machine learning software can be developed to mine critical information pertaining to the imaging diagnosis from patients' electronic medical records. For example, AI can look into a patient's records for relevant history of any known personal or family history of malignancy, history of autoimmune disease, and so on. This can alter the significance of an imaging finding, and change appropriate workup recommendations. This will save the reporting radiologist's time, improve efficiency, and provide a more clinically useful report.

A radiology report typically includes a diagnosis, and often a suggestion or recommendation regarding further investigation or management. It is not possible for any one person to keep track of all such recommendations, incorporating the latest research or society guidelines. AI can assist in ensuring that the recommendations are scientifically sound, and then also manage a follow-up on all signed reports. This may also permit report recommendations to be retrospectively updated in the future, should future guidelines change current management. Where several competing classification systems exist, clinicians may also indicate their preference for a particular classification system. The variety of current and predicted future capabilities illustrates the potential of AI to improve all aspects of a radiologist's report.

35.3 Beyond the Radiologist

Radiology is an information-dense speciality. A multitude of studies have demonstrated the ability of AI to detect subtleties and textures beyond the expert reader. Quantitative image analysis can provide extractable data for mathematical analysis, a field described as radiomics (Figure 35.1). Deep learning and other machine learning software can be employed to use imaging data to calculate and predict in-hospital mortality, readmission, length of stay, and discharge diagnoses better than currently used clinical models [3–5]. The ability of AI to keep 'learning' will allow AI to integrate new research as it becomes available [6].

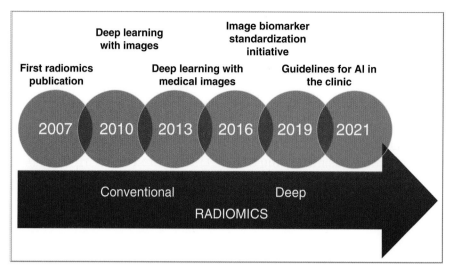

Figure 35.1: Timeline of progress in radiomics. The evolution of radiomics from the first publication in 2007 to full clinical integration today.

Source: Aakanksha Agarwal and Timothy É. Murray.

The current radiology department is radiologist centred, with the radiologist occupying a reporting station, while performing or delegating a series of tasks including administrating, protocolling, and performing studies. There are few roles within a department that cannot be in part, or even fully, automated with software and hardware solutions. In 50 years from now, a department where a patient meets no human staff while attending for an imaging study is entirely feasible, as is one where the data acquired is reviewed and processed by a set of algorithms only. Once an algorithm has been shown to outperform (and undercut) the best-in-field human, the benefit of paying for an objectively worse human interpretation will surely be questioned by payers.

35.4 Future for Patients

AI has been embraced as a tool to improve all aspects of the customer experience, and medical imaging will undoubtedly provide similar opportunities. AI-backed innovation and improvement have the potential to impact every aspect of the patient's interaction, from scheduling to the completion of safety questionnaires, to patient information dissemination, to scan performance, to follow-up. A combination of rules-based AI-augmented scheduling software and chatbots will back-end ('everything the user of a website does not see') the websites that link the patient's portal to their medical imaging encounter. AI-backed software can propose answers to a patient safety questionnaire based on their electronic medical records or prior imaging (presence of any metal devices, calculating renal volume, and so on). The patient can simply confirm the AI-suggested answers to save time and reduce error.

The performance of medical imaging in concentrated centres or large multi-unit outpatient centres in current practice may also change to better suit the patient, as barriers to decentralization will fall with the replacement by AI of roles currently undertaken by people. Competing providers will offer medical imaging studies as close to the consumer as possible. Remotely monitored imaging pods dispersed throughout the community will enhance patient access to medical imaging.

The impact that AI will have on cost is uncertain at this time. AI clearly offers major efficiencies in terms of reducing human input for a variety of tasks, and reducing scan time (thus increasing throughput on fixed assets, driving down fixed costs). There may, however, be legislative or cultural hurdles to such shifts. Furthermore, the many benefits of AI in image interpretation and reporting are often predicated on less human input (and thus less overhead), but the relationship between the two is unlikely to simply represent an inverse correlation. Until clearer trends emerge clarifying who is paying for clinical AI tools, it is challenging to predict the effect this will have on payer prices in the future.

35.5 Future for Administrative Staff

AI-based interactive platforms can be employed to answer telephone calls and stratify them; those from physicians requiring urgent direct communication with the radiologist can be directly transferred, while calls from patients enquiring about services can be handled by the software itself. This will provide the administrative staff with more time to strategize workflow more productively. Automated messages can be sent to patients regarding pre-arrival requirements for routine, recurring, and straightforward investigations. AI can facilitate placing reminders in patients' electronic calendars for their upcoming appointment, and provide a 'click to confirm appointment' interface. This will reduce human administrative requirements, and allow the patient to respond at a moment of their choosing, while also improving the departments' efficiency and financial performance.

35.6 Ethical Considerations in Radiology

35.6.1 Data Related

If medical data are well used, they can lead us to an era of personalized medicine. Conversely, misuse of data can cause harm, and needs to be regulated [7].

35.6.2 Data Ownership and Privacy

All AI-based algorithms need access to data for training, testing, and validation. Ethics related to data handling are fundamental to the incorporation of AI in radiology. They reflect trust in data acquisition, management, and assessment, and include informed consent, patient privacy, data protection, genuine ownership,

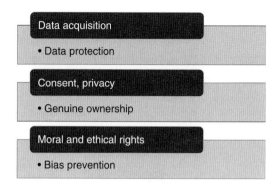

Figure 35.2: Challenges in data protection. With increasing cyber-crimes, the need for data protection is paramount while trying to integrate AI into routine practice.

Source: Aakanksha Agarwal and Timothy É. Murray.

transparency, and ensuring that access rights are moral and meaningful (Figure 35.2) [8]. The radiologist's prerogative is to use the available data to further medical research for the common good, while ensuring that it does not cause undue harm to the patient in any manner. Well-labelled datasets, linked to reports or other outcomes, are in great demand for development, training, and validation of AI software and machine learning. Unethical capitalization of data can lead to harm. Vigilance in the creation or capitalization of such datasets is required to prevent legal suits and costly mistakes (see Chapter 37) [9].

35.6.3 Algorithm-Related Ethics

It is inevitable that ethical issues will retrospectively be discovered as AI expands its scope and prevalence in medical imaging. To prepare for the inevitable retrospective scrutiny that this is sure to invite, a robust system of checks and balances should be considered. Ultimately, although AI-derived/supported outcomes will likely be superior in most areas of radiology with sufficient time, there will inevitably be failures. These will be held to account in human terms, requiring explanation to the courts, to the public, to shareholders, and to healthcare users. Retreating into the details of the algorithm for a mathematical explanation is unlikely to suffice in addressing the various stakeholders' concerns. Software providers must be able to explain to the public how a decision was made in a comprehensive fashion [10,11].

35.6.4 Practical Ethics

The field of AI in radiology is a complex ecosystem (Figure 35.3). Deciding the correct path on moral grounds can be, at times, intellectually challenging. The bias of automation hovers over practical ethics. Humans may develop a tendency to trust AI-derived decisions and disregard conflicting opinions from other humans or data. They may fail to recognize a failure of AI, resulting in an omission bias, and consciously and erroneously accept an incorrect AI decision in the presence of contradictory evidence, resulting in commission bias [9].

Research is needed to prevent clinical data, as well as social, environmental, and ethical factors, from creating significant bias, as such bias will impair the

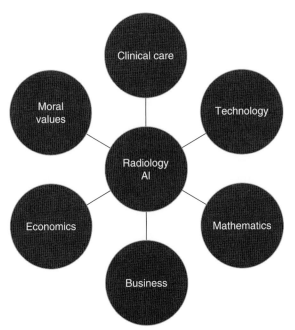

Figure 35.3: Radiology AI ecosystem. The radiology ecosystem is complex, and consolidates elements of clinical care, technology, mathematics, business, economics, and moral values.

Source: Aakanksha Agarwal and Timothy É. Murray.

productivity and reliability of AI software. Provocative questions may arise. If a particular radiomic pattern of brain texture is linked to a diagnosis of homicidal ideation, should this prompt referral to law enforcement or psychiatry? If so, does this create a potential risk of profiling people of a particular ethnic group in whom this finding may be more common? Or does this create a liability towards future homicide victims if this finding was not reported? The scope for troubling radiomic or imaging associations is limitless and profound. It needs to be determined how much a practising physician is willing to risk when trusting AI-made decisions that may turn out to be erroneous. The exact nature of physician liability has to be ascertained as AI expands itself in the field of radiology (Figure 35.4).

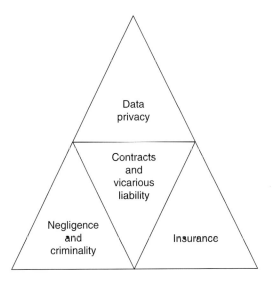

Figure 35.4: Sources of liability. The pyramid of liability is multi-pronged, and needs consideration of various contributory sources to ultimately ascertain the physician liability.

Source: Aakanksha Agarwal and Timothy É. Murray.

35.7 Legal and Ethical Challenges in Radiology

The liability for errors on the part of AI systems currently predominantly falls on the radiologist, who is responsible for the content of the report. As the role of AI encroaches on the role of the human reader, this may shift. Who will be responsible for any individual patient harm in clinical use, or unethical results arising out of data sharing, or AI software malfunction? The domain of individual medicolegal responsibility has ample legal precedent and well-established trends, but exactly how nascent AI liability will evolve is unclear.

AI software incorporation will require financial input, as well as provision of technology and infrastructure. This may further increase disparities between developed and developing nations in radiology practice. Conversely, should AI reduce the need for human capital, this may reduce costs, which would disproportionately benefit lower-income countries where even marginal cost reductions can increase access. It remains to be seen if future AI in medical imaging will ultimately represent a democratizing tool capable of reducing health inequalities, or if it will increase cost along with quality (which may result in gross negative outcomes within developing nations).

35.8 Differential Role of AI across Imaging Modalities

The scope for AI augmentation is perhaps greatest in volumetric imaging modalities, which provide greater volumes of data for analysis and interpretation. As MRI field strengths increase, MRI technology becomes more accessible, and as AI-backed abbreviated sequences and virtual sequences develop, MRI is poised to become a rapid imaging modality with unrivalled tissue characterization properties. Radiography and CT have inherent physical limitations in terms of tissue characterization, and require commensurate radiation. These unparalleled advantages of MRI may drive MRI to become the workhorse modality, with multiple MRI scanners performing rapid study acquisitions, thus anchoring the radiology department. Radiation-dependent modalities and ultrasound may be relegated to supporting roles and for procedural guidance.

35.9 Using Future Predictions to Guide Current Planning

Reducing MRI scan times from 30 minutes to 10 minutes (as has been described to be possible for a number of body parts) will dramatically reduce the relative share of a fixed cost borne by each patient. This favourable change in the value proposition of MRI relative to other modalities will doubtless increase the role of MRI within a radiology department. This has far-reaching implications, in terms of requirements for technologist and radiologist training, in addition to floor-space assignment and up-front capital investment requirements.

Additional changes to the structure of a department include the requirements for on-site servers and storage. There are a variety of models in use, ranging from AI that is entirely self-enclosed within the host's radiology department, to fully cloud-based solutions where the information is stored and analysed off-site. Many departments currently have considerable on-site storage and server demands; how these evolve with the coming of AI-backed software remains to be seen. In the longer term, the human-centric design of every aspect of the radiology department (where hardware is often centred in an adjacent control room) may change as AI incorporates a greater share of human-performed technologist activities.

Given the multiple vendors with AI solutions, how these will make it to the workstation is uncertain. Several picture archiving and communications system (PACS) platforms sell own-brand AI solutions as discrete purchasable add-ons. Several other PACS platforms have internal marketplaces where third-party AI functions can be purchased and incorporated. Other standalone software can work independently, or with limited integration into separate PACS software. In more mature software markets, companies who design specific operating systems occupy dominant positions in internal application marketplaces. The PACS landscape is currently more fragmented than computer operating system markets (with multiple vendors, none of whom occupies a dominant market position). This suggests that we are unlikely to see dominant 'app stores'. While many PACS offer substantially overlapping features, it is likely that any PACS software that facilitates a range of third-party in-program clinical AI applications, while permitting ease of billing for these additional services, will have a competitive advantage over PACS that does not incorporate third-party AI. This will likely be a key driver of change in the PACS market in the future. Until such time, the radiology department looking to the future may wish to lean towards vendor-neutral solutions or solutions that integrate third-party applications, to avoid being contracted to a PACS solution that prohibits effective AI integration and ultimately impacts competitiveness.

35.10 Determining Who Pays

AI for medical imaging has attracted considerable investment from a spectrum of established players in the medical imaging space, as well as information technology conglomerates and unaffiliated investment firms. The premise underwriting this inward investment has been the development of a product or service capable of generating profit exceeding investment at a point in the future. While many applications of AI have proven useful in research, and increasingly in a clinical setting, the payment model is heterogeneous. In general terms, while all parties desire the benefits of AI, there is less enthusiasm for paying. Ultimately, payment will be derived from the patient or payer. Should the additional fee for AI input be added to current fee structures, or should it come from the radiologist fee? To cloud things further, the AI function may have a subscription model, a per-use model, or a per-finding model. Thus, even itemized billings of patients will likely prove challenging. The ability of an AI tool to demonstrably reduce the requirement for radiologist input, or improve output in a measurable and cost-reducing manner, and thus financially justify incorporation into current business models, would seem like the easy pathway to payment in the near term. Alternative payment models, such as government funding or freeware, may have a role in the future (see Chapter 45).

35.11 Conclusion

AI was feared as an antagonist to the radiologist, a competitor threatening the current business model, and potentially undercutting investment in high levels of education and training. Much of this fear has been converted into hope that AI will represent a virtual assistant that can reduce missed diagnoses, automate the mundane aspects of reporting, and increase the value of AI-assisted reports. To quote Dr Curtis Langlotz, 'AI won't replace radiologists, but radiologists who use AI will replace radiologists who don't' [12]. Synergistic functioning between AI and radiologists in harmony is a likely path forward, at least in the short term. The entire lifecycle of an imaging exam – starting from the decision to place an order to acting on the subsequent report – can be rendered more efficient at all points using AI. Advanced information analysis, radiomics, result preparation, provision of clinically relevant data to the radiologist at the time of reporting, and prognostication remain aspirational goals of AI. For the radiologist, incorporation of AI will enhance efficiency. AI must be applied in an ethical manner, promoting improved health outcomes while minimizing harm. Data protection is of utmost importance, and any AI tool should be thoroughly vetted by a regulatory board before being introduced in practice. Striving to developing a code of ethics and regulations for AI to best serve the community will be a continuous and iterative process.

The radiology department of the future is likely to see many shifts, primarily driven by AI-derived enhancements to image acquisition and interpretation, but also including other elements of the value chain from order placement to follow-up. The relationship between patients, healthcare workers, software, and hardware is set to evolve in line with these AI-derived enhancements as they take aim at the three domains underpinning all aspects of any service industry: namely cost, quality, and turnaround time.

KEY INSIGHTS

- **Medical imaging has already seen the adoption of AI into clinical practice, and the scope of AI is certain to encroach into all aspects of the medical imaging value chain.**

- The relationship between patients, healthcare workers, software, and hardware is set to evolve in line with these AI-derived enhancements as they take aim at the three domains underpinning all aspects of any service industry: namely, cost, quality, and turnaround time.
- AI-driven automation has permitted other industries relying on blended hardware–software products (such as vending machine kiosk-type automated stores in airports) to deliver autonomous units closer to the consumer; this would seem broadly applicable to medical imaging, where fully autonomous medical imaging units could be placed beyond the geographical limits of a physical department or clinic.
- Future AI research in medical imaging offers limitless scope for innovation and improved patient outcomes; it poses significant ethical questions, however, and requires vigilance to prevent bias and confounding of racial/socioeconomic disparities.
- Accelerated scan times permitted by AI stand to disproportionately benefit MRI; a commensurate reduction in the relative fixed cost of MRI studies may change the value proposition of MRI, and increase its share in the department of the future relative to other modalities.
- A patchwork of varied payment models currently exists. The optimal model for payment (and who should pay) remains to be determined.
- Future planning for any radiology department should favour PACS software that integrates with third-party AI software, rather than vendors who restrict integration to self-designed software.

References

1. Rad AI. *The Future of AI in Radiology.* https://www.radai.com/webinars/www.radai.com/webinars/the-future-of-ai-in-radiology.
2. Syed AB, Zoga AC. Artificial intelligence in radiology: current technology and future directions. *Seminars in Musculoskeletal Radiology* 2018;22(5):540–545.
3. Kassner A, Thornhill RE. Texture analysis: a review of neurologic MR imaging applications. *American Journal of Neuroradiology* 2010;31(5):809.
4. Rajkomar A, Oren E, Chen K et al. Scalable and accurate deep learning with electronic health records. *NPJ Digital Medicine* 2018;1:18.
5. Syeda-Mahmood T. Role of big data and machine learning in diagnostic decision support in radiology. *Journal of the American College of Radiology* 2018;15(3 Pt B): 569–576.

6. Gupta A, Raja AS, Khorasani R. Examining clinical decision support integrity: is clinician self-reported data entry accurate? *Journal of the American Medical Informatics Association* 2014;21(1):23–26.

7. Brady AP, Neri E. Artificial intelligence in radiology—ethical considerations. *Diagnostics* 2020;10(4):231.

For additional references and Further Reading please see www.wiley.com/go/ byrne/aiinclinicalmedicine.

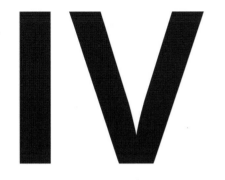

IV Policy Issues, Practical Implementation, and Future Perspectives in Medical AI

Design and Implementation

The Way Forward

36

Medical Device AI Regulatory Expectations

Vesna Janic[1], Helen Simons[2], and Taimoor Khan[3]

[1] *Satisfai Health, Vancouver, BC, Canada*

[2] *StarFish Medical, Victoria, BC, Canada*

[3] *StarFish Medical, Toronto, ON, Canada*

Learning Objectives

- Describe the European Union (EU), Food and Drug Administration (FDA), and Health Canada regulatory requirements for devices, including software and AI in particular.
- Review the EU, FDA, and Health Canada Medical device classification for software.
- Identify the FDA Medical device classification for software.
- Describe the breakdown on specific guidance relating to software submissions.
- Understand the relation to IEC 62304 and comparison between new FDA draft guidance and current guidance.
- Provide a summary of AI/machine learning in Software as a Medical Device (SaMD).
- Expand on the current action plan proposed by the FDA.

36.1 Introduction

This chapter focuses on the current guidance, regulatory requirements, and relevant classification rules for medical devices that include software in the EU, Canada, and the USA. It also provides a summary of the FDA's action plan and best practice guidelines for AI/machine learning–based SaMD.

This chapter is designed to guide physicians and developers who intend to develop AI/machine learning devices as applied to medicine. Regulatory strategy, including risk classification determination, is a key initial task in medical device development, as the pathway selected will influence the development of the product. This chapter lays out specific areas to consider.

AI in Clinical Medicine: A Practical Guide for Healthcare Professionals, First Edition. Edited by Michael F. Byrne, Nasim Parsa, Alexandra T. Greenhill, Daljeet Chahal, Omer Ahmad, and Ulas Bagci.
Companion website: www.wiley.com/go/byrne/aiinclinicalmedicine

36.2 EU Regulatory Requirements for Medical Devices, Including Software and AI

To be able to market a medical product in the EU, you are required to show compliance with either the Medical Device Regulations (MDR) [1] or the In Vitro Diagnostic Regulations (IVDR) [2]. The EU identifies four levels of medical device class: Class I, Class IIa, Class IIb, and Class III, where Class I is the lowest risk and Class III is the highest. There is an equivalent grading of in vitro diagnostics, but the identifiers are A, B, C, and D. The relevant classification is determined by reviewing the rules laid out in Annex VIII of the regulations.

Class I/A products can be self-declared, whereas higher-class devices require a notified body to be involved in the approval process. All devices are required to build a technical file and comply with the General Performance and Safety Requirements listed in Annex I. For any device including software, the EU has published guidance, MDCG 2019-11 Qualification and Classification of Software [3], to help with the classification process, as shown in Table 36.1.

Both the EU guidance and the equivalent Health Canada guidance refer back to the International Medical Device Regulators Forum (IMDRF), 'Software as a Medical Device': Possible Framework for Risk Categorization and Corresponding Considerations [4].

In addition to medical-specific expectations, in April 2021 the EU published a proposal for an AI regulation (COM/2021/206) [5] that would be applicable to all AI products. The general approach appears to be aligned with processes already required for medical devices, but this will need to be confirmed when the final version of this regulation is enacted.

Table 36.1: MDCG 2019-11 Qualification and Classification of Software. This table provides a risk classification based on the state of healthcare situation or patient condition.

		Significance of information provided by the software to a healthcare situation related to diagnosis/therapy		
		High Treat or diagnose	**Medium** Drives clinical management	**Low** Informs clinical management
State of healthcare situation or patient condition	**Critical** situation or patient condition	Class III	Class IIb	Class IIa
	Serious situation or patient condition	Class IIb	Class IIa	Class IIa
	Non-serious situation or patient condition	Class IIa	Class IIa	Class IIa

Source: [3] / European Union / CC BY-4.0.

36.3 Health Canada Regulatory Requirements for Medical Devices Including Software

To be able to market a device in Canada, you need to comply with the Canadian Medical Device Regulations (cMDR) [6]. Health Canada identifies four levels of device class, Class I, Class II, Class III, and Class IV, where Class I is the lowest risk and Class IV is the highest.

Similarly to the EU, Health Canada uses a rule-based system to classify devices, and provides two guidance documents for classifying devices: Guidance Document: Guidance for the Risk-based Classification System for In Vitro Diagnostic Devices (IVDDs) [7] and Guidance Document – Guidance on the Risk-based Classification System for Non-In Vitro Diagnostic Devices (non-IVDDs) [8].

Class I devices only require a Medical Device Establishment Licence to register the company making the product, whereas higher classifications are required to gain a product-specific Medical Device Licence and provide a submission to Health Canada to gain this. The expectations of the content of the submission are laid out in the cMDR [6].

For SaMD, they also refer back to the IMDRF guidance [4], and summarise the classes as shown in Table 36.2.

To distinguish between Class II or III, it is III if an erroneous result could lead to immediate danger. To distinguish between Class I or II, it is II if the software is intended to image or monitor a physiological process or condition.

It is interesting to note the similarities in approach but different outcomes between the EU and Health Canada's risk profiling.

Table 36.2: Health Canada's Canadian Medical Device Regulations (cMDR). This table provides a risk classification based on the state of healthcare situation or patient condition and is based on the International Medical Device Regulators Forum system.

		Significance of information provided by the software to a healthcare situation related to diagnosis/therapy		
		High Treat or diagnose	**Medium** Drives clinical management	**Low** Informs clinical management
State of healthcare situation or patient condition	**Critical** situation or patient condition	Class III	Class III	Class I or II
	Serious situation or patient condition	Class II or III	Class II or III	Class I or II
	Non-serious situation or patient condition	Class I or II	Class I or II	Class I or II

Source: Adapted from [6].

36.4 FDA Regulatory Requirements for Medical Devices Including Software

36.4.1 Device Classification and Regulatory Pathways

The FDA identifies three levels of device classes, Class I, Class II, and Class III, where Class I is the lowest risk and Class III is the highest risk.

The class that a given product falls into is determined on the basis of what class previous products of a similar type were classified as. Hence, the first step in determining the regulatory pathway for new medical software products is to research if there is a product that could be considered a predicate, with the same intended use and similar technological solutions.

If a predicate can be identified, then the FDA databases can be consulted to determine the class of the predicate device. Class 1 devices are usually exempt from requiring a pre-market submission, Class 2 devices may require a pre-market submission but can often choose the 510(k) pathway, which is based upon providing evidence of substantial equivalence to the predicate approved device. All Class III devices are required to have a pre-market application (PMA).

At this time, only a few AI/machine learning–based products have been approved, so it may be difficult to find a suitable predicate. If this is the case, it is possible to leverage a De Novo process where a submission is made, and the FDA agrees that it is a novel product, but falls into the lower-risk classifications.

36.4.2 Specific Guidance for Software Content in Submissions

Once a regulatory pathway and device classification have been selected for a product, product development can begin. This is where technical standards and FDA guidance documents need to be addressed. For any product including software, whether it is AI/machine learning or not, they need to address the requirements of the FDA's Guidance for the Content of Premarket Submissions for Software Contained in Medical Devices [9]. In November 2021, the FDA issued a new draft version of this guidance, which among other changes renamed it Content of Premarket Submissions for Device Software Functions [10]. This draft guidance is intended to replace the previous guidance on the subject from May 2005.

36.4.3 Background

The original guidance, over 15 years old, is well used and understood by industry. Because of the existing industry acceptance, the changes in this new version will require significant shifts in mindset and process about how to carry out and document software development. *While draft guidance documents are intended to be drafts for comment, there is an understanding that they are the latest thinking from the FDA and should be considered when developing medical devices.*

This draft guidance document is intended to provide information regarding recommended documentation that should be included in pre-market submissions for the FDA's evaluation of the safety and effectiveness of device software functions. It applies to the following types of submissions:

- Premarket Notification (510(k)).
- De Novo Classification Request.
- Premarket Approval Application (PMA).
- Investigational Device Exemption (IDE).
- Humanitarian Device Exemption (HDE).
- Biologics License Application (BLA).

This list has been expanded to reflect the submission types that are now available compared to those in 2005. Additional documentation may also be required for post-market activities relating to software. This guidance specifically looks at documentation needed for submission. It also clarifies that it applies to both Software in a Medical Device (SiMD) and Software as a Medical Device (SaMD), but it does not apply to automated manufacturing and quality system software or software that is not a device. This is a helpful delineation of scope.

36.4.4 Changes from Previous Version of This Guidance

The guidance from 2005 categorized software into three risk classifications or levels of concern: Minor, Moderate, Major. These levels were somewhat aligned with the relevant process standard IEC 62304:2015 Medical Device Software – Software life cycle processes [11], which had classes A, B, and C. At the very least, they had the same number of levels.

The new guidance now defines the documentation level. The recommended documentation for a pre-market submission depends on the device's risk to a patient, a user of a device, or others in the environment of use:

- *Basic documentation* should be provided for any pre-market submission that includes device software functions where enhanced documentation does not apply.
- *Enhanced documentation* should be provided for any pre-market submission that includes device software functions, which include any of the four subsequently stated risk factors in the next section.

The new guidance reduces the software documentation categories from three to two, which raises the question of how the previous classifications relate to the new classifications.

36.4.5 Determination of Risk Compared to Previous Guidance

Firstly, let us look at what triggers the higher-level, enhanced documentation. If the software exhibits any of the following **Risk Factors**, then it requires the enhanced documentation:

1. The device is a constituent part of a combination product.
2. The device (a) is intended to test blood donations for transfusion-transmitted infections; or (b) is used to determine donor and recipient compatibility; or (c) is a Blood Establishment Computer Software.
3. The device is classified as class III.
4. A failure or latent flaw of the device software function(s) could present a probable risk of death or serious injury, either to a patient, user of the device, or others in the environment of use. These risk(s) should be assessed prior to implementation of risk control measures. The risk(s) should be considered in the context of the device's intended use; the direct and indirect impacts to safety, treatment, and/or diagnosis; and other relevant considerations. ['Probable' is intended to capture reasonably foreseeable software and hardware risks associated with the device.]

In comparison, the previous guidance required a determination of Level of Concern through answering the following questions:

- If the answer to any one question below is Yes, the Level of Concern for the Software Device is likely to be **Major**.
    1. Does the Software Device qualify as Blood Establishment Computer Software?
    2. Is the Software Device intended to be used in combination with a drug or biologic?
    3. Is the Software Device an accessory to a medical device that has a Major Level of Concern?
    4. Prior to mitigation of hazards, could a failure of the Software Device result in death or serious injury, either to a patient or to a user of the device? Examples of this include the following:
        a. Does the Software Device control a life supporting or life sustaining function?
        b. Does the Software Device control the delivery of potentially harmful energy that could result in death or serious injury, such as radiation treatment systems, defibrillators, and ablation generators?
        c. Does the Software Device control the delivery of treatment or therapy such that an error or malfunction could result in death or serious injury?

    d. Does the Software Device provide diagnostic information that directly drives a decision regarding treatment or therapy, such that if misapplied it could result in serious injury or death?

    e. Does the Software Device provide vital signs monitoring and alarms for potentially life-threatening situations in which medical intervention is necessary?

■ If the Software Device is not Major Level of Concern and the answer to any one question below is Yes, the Level of Concern is likely to be **Moderate**.

    1. Is the Software Device an accessory to a medical device that has a Moderate Level of Concern?

    2. Prior to mitigation of hazards, could a failure of the Software Device result in Minor Injury, either to a patient or to a user of the device?

    3. Could a malfunction of, or a latent design flaw in, the Software Device lead to an erroneous diagnosis or a delay in delivery of appropriate medical care that would likely lead to Minor Injury?

■ If the answers to all of the questions above are No, the Level of Concern is **Minor**.

Immediately one can see the correlation with Risk Factors 1 and 2 from the new guidance, with questions 1 and 2 under Major Level of Concern in the old guidance.

Risk Factor 3, in the new guidance, has some alignment with the sub-questions under question 4 of Major Level of Concern in the old guidance, and the generalization that all class III devices including software will require enhanced documentation is understandable, as these high-risk devices will be expected to provide more detailed and extensive documentation throughout the submission and not just for software.

It is interesting that the questions about accessories to a medical device are no longer explicitly stated, but it is inferred that this is being covered by the risk assessment.

Finally, Risk Factor 4 in the new guidance has been worded more generically to cover all the remaining considerations from Major and Moderate questions in the previous guidance from 2005.

36.4.6 Assessment of Risk Compared to IEC 62304

Risk Factor 4 is the first conflict with IEC 62304 [11], as in the guidance it specifically states 'these risk(s) should be assessed *prior* to implementation of risk control measures', whereas the assessment flow chart from IEC 62304 (Figure 36.1) shows an expectation that the classification is determined *after* risk controls are applied. This could lead to different risk profiles being defined for the same software, leading to different documentation expectations. This is in addition to the difference between the two levels in the guidance and the three levels in IEC 62304.

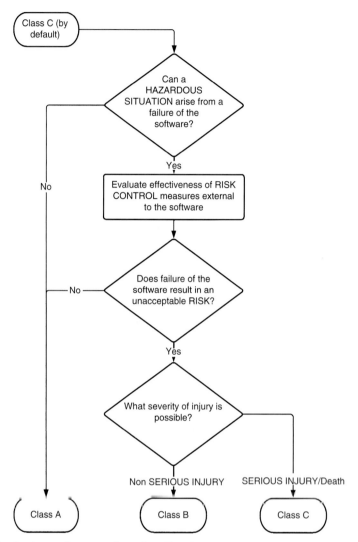

Figure 36.1: Assigning software safety classification.
Source: IEC 62304: 2015 [11].

In a departure from previous guidance, the recent document sets an expectation that software will be developed in accordance with IEC 62304, and states under the category of 'Software Development and Maintenance Practices' that a Declaration of Conformity to IEC 62304 can be provided.

36.4.7 Documentation Required by the Guidance

When looking at what documentation is required, both the previous and new versions of the guidance provide a helpful table of what is expected for classification of software and offer further details on the content of those documents. The Documentation Requirements comparison in Table 36.3 is only a summary and

Table 36.3: Documentation requirements comparison between 2005 and 2021 guidance documents.

Software document elements	Previous (2005) guidance [9]			New (2021) guidance [10]	
	Minor concern	**Moderate concern**	**Major concern**	**Basic level**	**Enhanced level**
Level of Concern/ Documentation Level Evaluation	A statement indicating the Level of Concern and a description of the rationale for that level			A statement indicating the appropriate Documentation Level and a description of the rationale for that level	
Software Description	A summary overview of the features and software operating environment			Software description, including overview of operationally significant software features, analyses, inputs, and outputs	
Device Hazard Analysis/Risk Management File	Tabular description of identified hardware and software hazards, including severity assessment and mitigations			Risk management plan, risk assessment demonstrating that risks have been appropriately mitigated, and risk management report	
Software Requirements Specification (SRS)	Summary of functional requirements from SRS	The complete SRS document		The complete documentation, describing the needs or expectations for a system or software, presented in an organized format and with sufficient information to understand the traceability of the information with respect to the other software documentation elements (e.g. risk management file, software design specification, system and software architecture design chart, software testing as part of verification and validation)	
Architecture Design Chart/System and Software Architecture Design Chart	No documentation is necessary in the submission	Detailed depiction of functional units and software modules. May include state diagrams as well as flow charts		Detailed diagrams of the modules, layers, and interfaces that comprise the device, their relationships, the data inputs/ outputs and flow of data, and how users or external products (including IT infrastructure and peripherals) interact with the system and software	

(Continued)

Table 36.3: (Continued)

Software document elements	Previous (2005) guidance [9]			New (2021) guidance [10]	
	Minor concern	Moderate concern	Major concern	Basic level	Enhanced level
Software Design Specification (SDS)	No documentation is necessary in the submission	Software design specification document	Software design specification	None	The complete documentation, including sufficient information that would allow the FDA to understand the technical design details of how the software functions, how the software design completely and correctly implements all the requirements of the SRS, and how the software design traces to the SRS in terms of intended use, functionality, safety, and effectiveness
Traceability Analysis	Traceability among requirements, specifications, identified hazards and mitigations, and Verification and Validation (V&V) testing			See SRS	
Software Development Environment Description/Software Development and Maintenance Practices	No documentation is necessary in the submission	Summary of software life cycle development plan, including a summary of the configuration management and maintenance activities	Summary of software life cycle development plan. Annotated list of control documents generated during development process. Include the configuration management and maintenance plan documents	A Declaration of Conformity to IEC 62304 **OR** a summary of the life cycle development plan and a summary of configuration management and maintenance activities	A Declaration of Conformity to IEC 62304 **OR** **Basic Documentation Level PLUS** complete configuration management and maintenance plan document(s)

Verification and Validation Documentation/Software Testing as Part of Verification and Validation	Software functional test plan, pass/fail criteria, and results	Description of V&V activities at the unit, integration, and system levels. System-level test protocol, including pass/fail criteria, and tests results	Description of V&V activities at the unit, integration, and system levels. Unit-, integration-, and system-level test protocols, including pass/fail criteria, test report, summary, and tests results	A summary description of the testing activities at the unit, integration, and system levels. System-level test protocol including expected results, observed results, pass/fail determination, and system-level test report	**Basic Documentation Level PLUS** unit and integration level test protocols including expected results, observed results, pass/fail determination, and unit- and integration-level test reports
Revision Level History	Revision history log, including release version number and date			Revision history tabulating the major changes to the software during the development cycle, including date, version number, a brief description of the changes relative to the previous version, and indication of the version on which testing was performed	
Unresolved Anomalies (Bugs or Defects)	No documentation is necessary in the submission	List of remaining software anomalies, annotated with an explanation of the impact on safety or effectiveness, including operator usage and human factors		List of remaining software anomalies (e.g. bugs, defects) annotated with an explanation of the impact on safety or effectiveness, including operator usage and human factors, workarounds, and timeframe for correction	

Source: Adapted from [9,10].

does not contain full details. See the detailed past and current guidance for more information [9,10].

Highlights from Table 36.3 include the following:

- The elements of the submission between the guidance documents remain similar, with the exception of traceability analysis, which was previously called out as its own item, but now is integrated into the Software Requirements Specification (SRS).
- The 'Device Hazard Analysis' element is now indicated as the 'Risk Management File', and describes a set of documents rather than the individual document. However, these documents would normally be included in a submission and are not an additional burden.
- The Major/Moderate expectations have been combined into the enhanced level of documentation, and the basic level has added in some of the Moderate-level descriptive aspects to the previous Minor-level requirements.
- Additional detail is being provided about the content of each element.

In summary, the impact of the changes between the two versions of the guidance is described in Table 36.4.

36.4.8 Alignment with IEC 62304

But how does the new FDA draft guidance [10] compare with the expectations of documentation and development activities from IEC 62304 [11]?

Enhanced-level documentation approximately aligns with Class B/C. Basic would be equivalent to Class A. However, due to the differences in assessing the risks associated with the software, a Class B from IEC 62304 that has a non-serious harm (prior and post-risk controls) could exist, which would then only need the basic-level documentation for submission.

A comparison of the documentation requirements between the new draft guidance [10] and IEC 62304 [11] is shown in Table 36.5.

Table 36.4: Summary of changes in guidance requirements.

Categories	Change
Was Minor, now basic	Additional descriptive documents required
Was Moderate, now enhanced	Additional descriptive documents required
	Additional Verification and Validation detailed protocols and reports
Was Major, now enhanced	No significant change

Table 36.5: Comparison of documentation between Guidance and IEC 62304.

Document type	Basic	Class A	Enhanced	Class B/C
Software Development Plan*		x		x
Documentation Level Evaluation (formerly Risk Classification)	x	x	x	x
Software Description**	x		x	
Software Architecture	x		x	x
Risk Management File	x	x	x	Specific Software Risk
Software Requirements	x	x	x	x
Software Design Specification		x	x	x
Software Development and Maintenance Practices	x	x	x	x
Software testing as Part of Verification and Validation	System	System	System, Unit, Integration	System, Unit, Integration
Revision Level History	x	x	x	x
Unresolved Anomalies	x	x	x	x

* Specific to IEC 62304.
** Specific to software submissions in accordance with FDA guidance.
Source: Adapted from [10,11].

For most items, the draft guidance and IEC 62304 are reasonably aligned, but discrepancies exist in the expectations for:

■ Software architecture – basic/Class A.
■ Software design specification – basic/Class A.

36.5 FDA's Action Plans for AI/Machine Learning in SaMD

AI and machine learning technologies have huge potential to change the way we look at our current healthcare practices. AI and machine learning enable new insights derived from the huge amount of data that is collected every day in the healthcare sector. Software algorithms can be used to learn from real-world applications to improve a product's performance. However, they present a set of new considerations due to the complexity in their development and the data that is collected.

In January 2021 the FDA released an action plan titled FDA Artificial Intelligence/Machine Learning (AI/ML)-Based Software as a Medical Device (SaMD) Action Plan [12]. This plan was developed in direct response to feedback from stakeholders to provide practical oversight and future considerations the FDA will make for AI/machine learning–based medical devices. The FDA's traditional model of medical device regulation was not designed for adaptive AI and machine learning technologies. Under its current approach to software modifications, the FDA anticipates that many of these AI/machine learning changes to a device may need a pre-market review.

As part of the action plan, the FDA highlights five key considerations that manufacturers should have when developing AI/machine learning–based SaMD:

- The principle of pre-determined change control plan – the FDA requests information about what aspects the manufacturer intends to change through learning; and the algorithm change protocol – how the algorithm will learn and change while remaining safe and effective.
- A proactive patient-centred approach to development and utilization that considers issues including usability, equity, trust, and accountability. One way in which the FDA is addressing these issues is through the promotion of the transparency of these devices to users and patients, which mostly pertains to the devices' functionality.
- Labelling for AI/machine learning–based devices, and the need for manufacturers to clearly describe the data used to train the algorithm, the relevance of its inputs, the logic it uses (if possible), the role intended to be served by its output, and evidence of the device's performance.
- Accounting for bias and generalizability. This is not an issue exclusive to AI/machine learning–based devices. Because AI/machine learning systems are developed and trained using data from historical datasets, they are vulnerable to bias, and AI/machine learning is prone to mirroring biases present in the data. Healthcare delivery is known to vary by factors such as race, ethnicity, and socioeconomic status. Therefore, it is possible that biases currently present in a healthcare system may be inadvertently introduced into the algorithms.
- The FDA believes that it is important for medical devices to be well suited to a racially and ethnically diverse intended patient population. This includes the need for improved methodologies for identification and improvement of machine learning algorithms.
- The FDA would like manufacturers to consider gathering real-world performance (RWP) data. Gathering performance data on the real-world use of the SaMD can allow manufacturers to understand how their products are being used, identify opportunities for improvements, and respond proactively to safety or usability concerns. Real-world data collection and monitoring can be used by manufacturers to leverage or mitigate the risk involved with AI/machine learning–based software modifications.

In October 2021, the FDA together with Health Canada and the UK's Medicines and Healthcare products Regulatory Agency (MHRA) jointly identified 10 guiding principles that can inform the development of Good Machine Learning Practices (GMLP) to describe a set of AI/machine learning best practices. More information on this list can be found in the guiding principles document itself [13].

Ten Guiding Principles That Can Inform the Development of GMLP to Describe AI/Machine Learning Best Practices

1. Multi-disciplinary expertise leveraged throughout the total product life cycle.
2. Good software engineering and security practices are implemented.
3. Clinical study participants and datasets are representative of the intended patient population.
4. Training datasets are independent of test sets.
5. Selected reference datasets are based upon best available methods.
6. Model design is tailored to the available data, and reflects the intended use of the device.
7. Focus is placed on the performance of the human–AI team.
8. Testing demonstrates device performance during clinically relevant conditions.
9. Users are provided with clear, essential information.
10. Deployed models are monitored for performance, and retraining risks are managed.

The FDA has provided a list of AI/machine learning–enabled medical devices marketed in the USA as a resource to the public [14].

36.6 Conclusion

This chapter has provided an overview of the current guidance and regulatory requirements for AI/machine learning–based medical devices and software in devices, as presented by the FDA, Health Canada, and the EU MDR. It also provides an overview of the current guidelines and relevant classification rules for medical devices that include software. By following these requirements and keeping up with updates for AI/machine learning as they are presented by regulatory bodies, medical device manufacturers can position themselves to understand and embrace the new regulations, and avoid mistakes or a last-minute rush to achieve compliance by implementing for these compliance requirements early on in their product life cycle.

KEY INSIGHTS

- Regulatory requirements in the EU, Canada, and the USA for devices including software and AI are important, and should be considered early in the development of any product.
- A comparison of the requirements of IEC 62304 and new FDA guidance Content of Premarket Submissions for Device Software Functions identifies changes in upcoming regulations.
- Insight into classifications of SaMD in the EU, Canada, and USA shows the similarities and differences between jurisdictions.

References

1. European Commission. Medical Device Regulations (2017/745). REGULATION (EU) 2017/745 OF THE EUROPEAN PARLIAMENT AND OF THE COUNCIL of 5 April 2017 on medical devices, amending Directive 2001/83/EC, Regulation (EC) No 178/2002 and Regulation (EC) No 1223/2009 and repealing Council Directives 90/385/EEC and 93/42/EEC. https://eur-lex.europa.eu/legal-content/EN/TXT/PDF/?uri=CELEX:32017R0745.

2. European Commission. In Vitro Diagnostic Regulations (2017/746). REGULATION (EU) 2017/746 OF THE EUROPEAN PARLIAMENT AND OF THE COUNCIL of 5 April 2017 on in vitro diagnostic medical devices and repealing Directive 98/79/EC and Commission Decision2010/227/EU. https://eur-lex.europa.eu/legal-content/EN/TXT/PDF/?uri=CELEX:32017R0746.

3. European Commission. MDCG 2019-11 Guidance on Qualification and Classification of Software in Regulation (EU) 2017/745 – MDR and Regulation (EU) 2017/746 – IVDR October 2019. https://ec.europa.eu/health/system/files/2020-09/md_mdcg_2019_11_guidance_en_0.pdf.

4. International Medical Device Regulators Forum (IMDRF). 'Software as a Medical Device': Possible framework for risk categorization and corresponding considerations, 18 September 2014. https://www.imdrf.org/sites/default/files/docs/imdrf/final/technical/imdrf-tech-140918-samd-framework-risk-categorization-141013.docx.

5. European Commission. Proposal for a Regulation of the European Parliament and of the Council laying down harmonized rules on artificial intelligence (Artificial Intelligence Act) and amending certain union legislative acts (COM/2021/206 final). https://eur-lex.europa.eu/legal-content/EN/TXT/?uri=CELEX%3A52021PC0206.

6. Government of Canada. Medical Devices Regulations SOR/98-282 FOOD AND DRUGS ACT Registration 1998-05-07. https://laws-lois.justice.gc.ca/eng/regulations/sor-98-282/fulltext.html.

7. Health Canada. Canadian Medical Device Regulations: Guidance for the risk-based classification system for in vitro diagnostic devices (IVDDs) 2016-10-07. https://www.canada.ca/en/health-canada/services/drugs-health-products/medical-devices/application-information/guidance-documents/guidance-document-guidance-risk-based-classification-system-vitro.html.

For additional references please see www.wiley.com/go/byrne/aiinclinicalmedicine.

37

Privacy Laws in the USA, Europe, and South Africa

Sara Gerke

Penn State Dickinson Law, Carlisle, PA, USA

Learning Objectives

- Learn about privacy laws in the USA, Europe, and South Africa.
- Understand some similarities and differences between the US HIPAA, the EU GDPR, and South Africa's POPI Act.
- Become aware that AI/machine learning in clinical medicine involves large amounts of health and non-health data that are likely to require compliance with privacy laws in order to be processed.

37.1 Introduction

AI is being implemented in clinical medicine in many countries across the world at a swift pace. For example, the US Food and Drug Administration has already cleared more than 500 AI and machine learning–enabled medical devices [1]. Examples include a diabetic retinopathy detection device [2], radiological computer-assisted triage and notification software [3], and coronary vascular physiological simulation software [4]. The hope is that AI will help improve clinical medicine in different meaningful ways, ranging from assisting physicians in making clinical decisions [5] to diagnostic tools [6] to optimizing the workflow in hospitals and relieving clinicians from administrative burdens such as clinical documentation [7].

AI/machine learning is unique because it can only realize its potential in clinical medicine with Big Data. AI/machine learning models are generally trained, tested, and validated on large datasets [8]. In addition, adaptive AI/machine learning algorithms (in contrast to so-called locked algorithms) can continuously learn from new real-world data [9]. Thus, it is not surprising that data has been named the 'new oil'; that is, the world's most valuable resource [10].

The fact that AI/machine learning relies on large amounts of data also brings ethical, legal, and practical challenges when implementing such tools in clinical medicine. One major challenge raised by AI/machine learning in clinical medicine is

AI in Clinical Medicine: A Practical Guide for Healthcare Professionals, First Edition. Edited by Michael F. Byrne, Nasim Parsa, Alexandra T. Greenhill, Daljeet Chahal, Omer Ahmad, and Ulas Bagci.
© 2023 John Wiley & Sons Ltd. Published 2023 by John Wiley & Sons Ltd.
Companion website: www.wiley.com/go/byrne/aiinclinicalmedicine

the adequate protection of patients' privacy. Patient data can be collected, used, and shared for different purposes, such as training the particular AI/machine learning model, providing an individual treatment recommendation, or providing access to data to industry for financial gain. With all of these applications, there is a real risk of compromising patient privacy.

Many countries worldwide have recognized the importance of data protection for individuals in the Big Data world and have passed new privacy legislation in recent years. This chapter will, for the first time, jointly discuss privacy laws in the USA, Europe, and South Africa in greater detail. It will first explore the US Health Insurance, Portability, and Accountability Act of 1996 (HIPAA) [11], and recent privacy legislation and initiatives at US state level. It will then look at Europe and provide an overview of the EU General Data Protection Regulation (GDPR) [12]. Subsequently, it will analyse the new Protection of Personal Information Act (POPI Act) [13] in South Africa. This will be followed by discussing some similarities and differences between these laws.

37.2 United States of America

The USA currently has a hotchpotch of privacy laws, making it hard for AI/machine learning companies and healthcare entities, such as hospitals, to keep track of the applicable provisions. At federal level, the Health Insurance, Portability, and Accountability Act of 1996 [11], more precisely its Privacy Rule, is the most relevant law for the protection of a patient's 'individually identifiable health information' ('protected health information' [PHI] under 45 C.F.R. § 160.103). HIPAA's scope is restricted to regulating the use and disclosure of PHI created by 'covered entities' – that is, healthcare clearinghouses, health plans, and most healthcare providers; or 'business associates' – that is, usually persons or organizations that provide particular services (e.g. data aggregation, consulting, or management services) to, or perform specific activities or functions (e.g. claims processing, quality assurance, data analysis) on behalf of, a covered entity that include the use or disclosure of PHI (45 C.F.R. § 160.103) [5,14].

This means that HIPAA mainly covers 'traditional', individually identifiable health information that is made part of a patient's medical record. It does not usually cover identifiable health information collected outside of the clinical context [5,15], such as by start-ups or companies manufacturing wearable health technology or health app developers. An exception applies if such information is transferred to the clinics, or more specifically if these organizations are business associates of the HIPAA-covered entity with regard to the patient's individually identifiable health information collected through wearables or apps.

Hospitals are also increasingly sharing health information with AI/machine learning companies these days. They typically share this information in 'de-identified' form most commonly involving the removal of 18 identifiers, including the patient's name, telephone number and so on – because HIPAA does not consider de-identified data as PHI, and thus their use and disclosure are possible without

HIPAA's constraints (45 C.F.R. §§ 164.502(d)(2), 164.514(a) and (b)) [14]. However, many scholars have criticized HIPAA's de-identification standard [5,15,16,17]. In the world of Big Data, even de-identified data do not guarantee that patients' privacy is secured. In particular, AI/machine learning companies may have other data at hand to effectively re-identify the data received from a HIPAA-covered entity [18]. Thus, it is important to establish safeguards – such as through contracts between the parties – to prevent the re-identification risk of de-identified data.

At state level, there have been many developments in recent years. California, Virginia, Colorado, Utah, and Connecticut have all passed new comprehensive privacy laws. The laws of these states all have in common that they aim to strengthen consumers' rights to have control over their own personal information/data. The California Consumer Privacy Act of 2018 has been effective since 1 January 2020. Some of its provisions have recently been amended by the California Privacy Rights Act of 2020 (Proposition 24), which has been fully operative since 1 January 2023, and further expands California consumers' privacy rights. The Virginia Consumer Data Protection Act (SB 1392) also became effective on 1 January 2023. In addition, the Colorado Privacy Act (SB 190) and the Connecticut Data Privacy Act (SB 6) will generally become effective on 1 July 2023, and the Utah Consumer Privacy Act (SB 227) on 31 December 2023. These state privacy laws aim to grant data rights to Virginia/Colorado/Connecticut/Utah consumers. Several other states, such as Michigan and Pennsylvania, also have active privacy bills that may be passed soon [19].

37.3 Europe

Europe is one of the leaders in data protection. The EU General Data Protection Regulation [12] applies to all EU Member States as well as Iceland, Liechtenstein, and Norway. It establishes 'rules relating to the protection of natural persons with regard to the processing of personal data and rules relating to the free movement of personal data' (Art. 1(1)). The term 'personal data' is interpreted as 'any information relating to an identified or identifiable natural person ("data subject")' (Art. 4(1)). Processing is broadly understood, and includes, for example, the collection, use, transmission, storage, disclosure, and destruction of personal data (Art. 4(2)).

The GDPR has an incredibly wide scope. Materially, it generally 'applies to the processing of personal data wholly or partly by automated means and to the processing other than by automated means of personal data which form part of a filing system or are intended to form part of a filing system' (Art. 2(1)). Thus, anonymous information that is, 'information which does not relate to an identified or identifiable natural person or to personal data rendered anonymous in such a manner that the data subject is not or no longer identifiable' – falls outside of the GDPR's purview (Recital 26). However, the GDPR does apply to personal data that have undergone 'pseudonymization' – that is, 'the processing of personal data in such a manner that the personal data can no longer be attributed to a specific data subject without the use of additional information, provided that such additional information is kept separately and is subject to technical and organisational measures to ensure that the personal data are not attributed to an identified or identifiable natural person' (Recital 26, Art. 4(5)).

Territorially, the GDPR 'applies to the processing of personal data in the context of the activities of an establishment of a controller or a processor in the Union, regardless of whether the processing takes place in the Union or not' (Art. 3(1)). Controllers and processors can be legal or natural persons, agencies, public authorities, or other bodies (Art. 4(7), (8)). The difference between the two is that controllers determine the means and purposes of the processing of personal data, and processors process personal data on the controllers' behalf (Art. 4(7), (8)). In addition, the GDPR 'applies to the processing of personal data of data subjects who are in the Union by a controller or processor not established in the Union' under the following two alternative conditions: first, 'where the processing activities are related to (. . .) the offering of goods or services, irrespective of whether a payment of the data subject is required, to such data subjects in the Union'; and second, 'where the processing activities are related to (. . .) the monitoring of their behaviour as far as their behaviour takes place within the Union' (Art. 3(2)). The GDPR also 'applies to the processing of personal data by a controller not established in the Union, but in a place where Member State law applies by virtue of public international law' (Art. 3(3)). Consequently, the GDPR applies not only to an EU establishment of a processor or controller, but also a non-EU establishment under certain circumstances. For example, an AI company established in the USA may be subject to the GDPR in cases where the company deliberately monitors the health behaviour of data subjects through smart devices in the EU [20].

If the GDPR applies, it provides, among other things, data subjects with multiple rights against controllers, such as the right of access (Art. 15), the right to erasure (Art. 17), and the right to data portability (Art. 20). In particular, the right to erasure (also called the 'right to be forgotten') is relevant in the context of AI/machine learning. Under Art. 17(1) of the GDPR, the data subject has the right against the controller to obtain 'the erasure of personal data concerning him or her without undue delay'. The controller is obliged 'to erase personal data without undue delay' so long as one of the grounds listed in Art. 17(1) of the GDPR applies, such as that 'the personal data are no longer necessary in relation to the purposes for which they were collected or otherwise processed' (a) or that 'the data subject withdraws consent on which the processing is based (. . .), and where there is no other legal ground for the processing' (b). Thus, the right to erasure may pose issues for AI/machine learning. For example, suppose personal data have already been used to train an algorithm, and one or more data subjects now have changed their minds and withdrawn their consent, on which the processing is based. A controller's obligation to erase data subjects' personal data may have implications for the AI/machine learning model and may require its retraining (e.g. also to mitigate potential biases). Solutions need to be explored on how best to address these 'right to erasure' requests in the AI/machine learning context. In some cases, a potential option may be to anonymize such data [21] and thus operate outside of the GDPR's purview. However, it should also be noted that the right to erasure under the GDPR is not absolute. Art. 17(3) of the GDPR lists five specific exceptions to this right, such as in cases where processing is necessary 'for exercising the right of freedom of expression and information' (a), 'for reasons of public interest in the area of public health' (c), or 'for archiving purposes in the public interest, scientific or historical research purposes or statistical purposes in accordance with Article 89(1) in so far as the right (. . .) is likely to render impossible or seriously impair the achievement of the objectives of that processing' (d).

In general, there are still some uncertainties about the application of the GDPR to AI/machine learning development. This can also be shown, for example, in the scholarly debate as to whether the GDPR contains a 'right to explanation' of automated decision-making and, if so, what this right entails [5]. Art. 22(1) of the GDPR states that '[t]he data subject shall have the right not to be subject to a decision based solely on automated processing, including profiling, which produces legal effects concerning him or her or similarly significantly affects him or her'. The term 'profiling' is defined as 'any form of automated processing of personal data consisting of the use of personal data to evaluate certain personal aspects relating to a natural person, in particular to analyse or predict aspects concerning that natural person's performance at work, economic situation, health, personal preferences, interests, reliability, behaviour, location or movements' (Art. 4(4)). Art. 22(2) of the GDPR also contains three exceptions to this right, such as if the decision 'is based on the data subject's explicit consent' (c). These exceptions are further restricted in cases where the decisions are based on 'special categories' of personal data (see later discussion and Art. 22(4)). The issue is that Art. 22 of the GDPR does not explicitly mention a data subject's 'right to explanation' of specific automated decisions. Only Recital 71 of the GDPR mentions such a right ('the right (. . .) to obtain an explanation of the decision reached after such assessment'), but Recitals are considered legally non-binding [5,22]. However, even if such a right to explanation does not exist under the GDPR, in cases 'of automated decision-making, including profiling, referred to in Article 22(1) and (4)', the data subject clearly has at least a right to obtain from the controller 'meaningful information about the logic involved, as well as the significance and the envisaged consequences of such processing for the data subject' (Art. 13(2)(f), Art. 14(2)(g), Art. 15(1)(h)) [5,22].

The GDPR also contains several principles concerning the processing of personal data (Chapter 2). In particular, Art. 9 of the GDPR regulates the processing of so-called special categories of personal data, such as personal data revealing ethnic or racial origin, data concerning health, and philosophical or religious beliefs. In the context of AI in clinical medicine, the term 'data concerning health' is especially pertinent, defined broadly as 'personal data related to the physical or mental health of a natural person, including the provision of health care services, which reveal information about his or her health status' (Art. 4(15)). The principle is that the processing of such data is prohibited (Art. 9(1)). However, Art. 9(2) of the GDPR contains ten exceptions, in which the processing of special categories of personal data is allowed, such as generally when 'the data subject has given explicit consent to the processing of those personal data for one or more specified purposes' (a). Consent is understood as 'any freely given, specific, informed and unambiguous indication of the data subject's wishes by which he or she, by a statement or by a clear affirmative action, signifies agreement to the processing of personal data relating to him or her' (Art. 4(11)). Other exceptions include cases where the 'processing is necessary for reasons of substantial public interest' (Art. 9(2)(g)) or where 'processing is necessary for archiving purposes in the public interest, scientific or historical research purposes or statistical purposes (. . .) which shall be proportionate to the aim pursued, respect the essence of the right to data protection and provide for suitable and specific measures to safeguard the fundamental rights and the interests of the data subject' (Art. 9(2)(j)). Member States can also introduce further constraints concerning the processing of certain special categories of personal data, such as data concerning health (Art. 9(4)).

37.4 South Africa

The Protection of Personal Information Act can be said to be South Africa's equivalent to the EU GDPR. The provisions in the POPI Act had different commencement days, but most of them came into effect on 1 July 2020, with an additional year to ensure compliance (i.e. 1 July 2021). The POPI Act has four main aims: (i) to 'give effect to the constitutional right to privacy, by safeguarding personal information when processed by a responsible party'; (ii) to establish 'minimum threshold requirements for the lawful processing of personal information'; (iii) to 'provide persons with rights and remedies to protect their personal information from processing that is not in accordance with this Act'; and (iv) to 'establish voluntary and compulsory measures, including the establishment of an Information Regulator, to ensure respect for and to promote, enforce and fulfil the rights protected by this Act' (§ 2).

The term 'personal information' is understood as 'information relating to an identifiable, living, natural person, and where it is applicable, an identifiable, existing juristic person' (§ 1). Examples include 'information relating to the race, gender, sex, pregnancy, marital status, national, ethnic or social origin, colour, sexual orientation, age, physical or mental health, well-being, disability, religion, conscience, belief, culture, language and birth of the person' (§ 1). Processing includes any kind of operations regarding personal information, such as collection, storage, use, alterations, or dissemination by means of transmission (§ 1). The responsible party is 'a public or private body or any other person which, alone or in conjunction with others, determines the purpose of and means for processing personal information' (§ 1). Data subjects are persons to whom personal information relates (§ 1). A 'person' can be a 'natural person or a juristic person' (§ 1). Operators are persons who process 'personal information for a responsible party in terms of a contract or mandate, without coming under the direct authority of that party' (§ 1).

The POPI Act has a broad scope. It 'applies to the processing of personal information (. . .) entered in a record by or for a responsible party by making use of automated or non-automated means: Provided that when the recorded personal information is processed by non-automated means, it forms part of a filing system or is intended to form part thereof' (§ 3(1)(a)). In addition, territorially, the responsible party must be domiciled in South Africa, but even in cases where the responsible person is *not* domiciled in South Africa, that person will fall under the POPI Act's scope if she or he 'makes use of automated or non-automated means in the Republic, unless those means are used only to forward personal information through the Republic' (§ 3(1)(b)).

It is important to note that the POPI Act, among other things, does *not* apply to 'personal information (. . .) that has been de-identified to the extent that it cannot be re-identified again' (§ 6). In the context of a data subject's personal information, 'de-identify' is interpreted as 'to delete any information that—(a) identifies the data subject; (b) can be used or manipulated by a reasonably foreseeable method to identify the data subject; or (c) can be linked by a reasonably foreseeable method to other information that identifies the data subject' (§ 1). In contrast, the term 're-identify' is defined in relation to a data subject's personal information as 'to resurrect any information that has been de-identified, that—(a) identifies the data subject; (b) can be used or manipulated by a reasonably foreseeable method to identify the data subject; or (c) can be linked by a reasonably foreseeable method to other information that identifies the data subject' (§ 1).

The POPI Act contains eight requirements for the lawful processing of personal information, ranging from accountability to information quality to security safeguards (§ 4). It also gives data subjects several rights such as to be notified that personal information about them is being collected, or to request, where necessary, the destruction, correction, or deletion of their personal information (§ 5). In the context of AI in clinical medicine, 'special' personal information, a subcategory of personal information, is relevant. Special personal information includes sensitive information, such as race or ethnic origins, health or sex life, or philosophical or religious beliefs (§ 26). The POPI Act clarifies that the processing of special personal information is generally prohibited (§ 26). However, it also contains some exceptions to this general ban. For example, the prohibition of processing of special personal information does not apply in cases where the data subject has given consent (§ 27(1)(a)) or for 'research purposes to the extent that (. . .) the purpose serves a public interest and the processing is necessary for the purpose concerned; or (. . .) it appears to be impossible or would involve a disproportionate effort to ask for consent, and sufficient guarantees are provided for to ensure that the processing does not adversely affect the individual privacy of the data subject to a disproportionate extent' (§ 27(1)(d)). Consent is understood as 'any voluntary, specific and informed expression of will in terms of which permission is given for the processing of personal information' (§ 1). In addition, the POPI Act contains specific exceptions for the processing of personal information regarding data subjects' health (§ 32). For instance, if a medical professional wants to process the personal information regarding a data subject's health, and 'such processing is necessary for the proper treatment and care of the data subject, or for the administration of the institution or professional practice concerned', then such processing is not prohibited under the Act (§ 32(1)(a)).

37.5 Similarities and Differences between HIPAA, GDPR, and the POPI Act

It will be important for AI companies and healthcare providers to be aware of the privacy laws in the USA, Europe, and South Africa and understand their similarities and differences. This knowledge will help them, for example, make clever investment decisions and comply with the applicable frameworks. In the following section, some of the similarities and differences between HIPAA, the GDPR, and the POPI Act will be revealed and analysed.

37.5.1 Limited versus Wide-Ranging Scope

While HIPAA is a key federal privacy law that exclusively applies to certain individually identifiable health information (i.e. PHI generated by covered entities or business associates), Europe and South Africa passed more wide-ranging privacy legislation. Both the GDPR and the POPI Act are much broader in their scope than HIPAA, and generally apply to the processing of personal data/information, including concerning data subjects' health. However, while the 'data subject' can be a natural or juristic person under the POPI Act (§ 1), the GDPR limits this term to a natural person only (Art. 4(1)). Territorially, the GDPR does not only apply to EU establishments of processors and controllers, but may also apply, under certain circumstances, to non-EU establishments, such as AI companies established in the USA (Art. 3). Even though the POPI Act's territorial scope seems to be narrower than that of the GDPR, it does apply to responsible parties domiciled in the entire Republic and, under certain conditions, even to those domiciled outside of South Africa (§ 3(1)(b)). While the GDPR uses the terms 'controller' (Art. 4(7)) and 'processor' (Art. 4(8)), the POPI Act's role players are called 'responsible party' and 'operator' (§ 1). Ultimately, however, a responsible party under the POPI Act is similar to a controller under the GDPR, and an operator under the POPI Act is similar to a processor under the GDPR.

As has been seen, HIPAA's limited scope leads to the unfortunate situation that it does not usually cover individually identifiable health information collected outside of hospitals, such as through health apps or wearables [5,15]. HIPAA also does not cover non-health information, even if it may provide indications about a patient's health, such as purchasing a pregnancy test on CVS.com [5,15]. Therefore, it is not surprising that US states have been getting active at the state level to close at least some of HIPAA's existing gaps. California, Virginia, Colorado, Utah, and Connecticut are the first five states that have recently passed new privacy laws to better protect consumers, and other states will likely follow them in the near future [19]. This mishmash of privacy laws in the USA, however, makes it particularly challenging for AI/machine learning companies to comply with the applicable provisions [17]. Although the GDPR and the POPI Act are certainly not easy waters to navigate, they have the advantage over the current US approach of being more comprehensive with a wide-ranging material and territorial scope. A comprehensive federal US law similar to the GDPR and the POPI Act would likely improve data protection across the country [17,23], and facilitate AI innovation by creating more legal clarity and transparency.

37.5.2 Anonymization, Pseudonymization, De-identification, and Re-identification

As discussed, HIPAA relies on de-identification as a privacy strategy [5,15,16]. De-identification can usually be achieved by stripping out 18 identifiers (45 C.F.R. § 164.514(b)). Once PHI has been de-identified, such information can be used and shared without limits [14]. However, such a strategy is weak because of the twenty-first-century risk of re-identification [18].

In contrast, as already noted, the GDPR does not use the term 'de-identification' but instead distinguishes between 'anonymous information' and personal data that have undergone 'pseudonymization' (Recital 26, Art. 4(5)). Only anonymous information falls outside of the GDPR's purview, but the term anonymous information is very narrowly interpreted as 'information which does not relate to an identified or identifiable natural person or to personal data rendered anonymous in such a manner that the data subject is not or no longer identifiable' (Recital 26). Thus, de-identified health information under HIPAA with its re-identification risk is usually insufficient to be considered anonymous information under the GDPR and thus is – similar to personal data that have undergone 'pseudonymization' – covered by the GDPR.

Similar to HIPAA, the POPI Act uses the term 'de-identify'. However, it seems that the laws differ in how they interpret this term. For example, in contrast to HIPAA, the POPI Act does not rely on the 'Safe Harbor' de-identification method; that is, removing 18 identifiers. Instead, the POPI Act's definition of the term 'de-identify' seems stricter, requiring the need 'to delete any information that—(a) identifies the data subject; (b) can be used or manipulated by a reasonably foreseeable method to identify the data subject; or (c) can be linked by a reasonably foreseeable method to other information that identifies the data subject' (§ 1). An objective standard is used to determine what constitutes a 'reasonably foreseeable method' [24].

Moreover, as discussed, the POPI Act also only excludes 'personal information (. . .) that has been de-identified to the extent *that it cannot be re-identified again*' (emphasis added, § 6). Thus, it seems that the POPI Act applies to de-identified health information that may *potentially* be re-identified. In comparison, under HIPAA, for a successful de-identification of PHI, it is sufficient that 'the covered entity *does not have actual knowledge* that the information could be used alone or in combination with other information to identify an individual who is a subject of the information' (45 C.F.R. § 164.514(b)(2)(ii)). Consequently, de-identified health information according to HIPAA may not always be enough to escape the POPI Act's scope (provided, of course, that the other requirements of its material and territorial scope are fulfilled).

When comparing the GDPR and the POPI Act, 'anonymous information' according to the GDPR also falls outside of the POPI Act's purview. However, personal data that have undergone 'pseudonymization' under the GDPR can technically be re-identified with the use of additional information (Art. 4(5)). Thus, the POPI Act would likewise cover such information (see the wording 'it cannot be re-identified *again*', emphasis added, § 6). In other words, the POPI Act's exclusion phrase in § 6 ('This Act does not apply to the processing of personal information (. . .) that has been de-identified to the extent that it cannot be re-identified again') is very close to the GDPR's term 'anonymous information' [24].

37.5.3 Protected Health Information, 'Special Categories' of Personal Data, and 'Special' Personal Information

In the context of AI in clinical medicine, the processing of individually identifiable health information is relevant. As seen, HIPAA regulates the use and disclosure of individually identifiable health information (called PHI) created by covered entities or business associates (45 C.F.R. § 160.103). In contrast, the GDPR and the POPI Act are much broader and generally apply to all personal data/information.

However, both the GDPR and the POPI Act have heightened requirements for 'special categories' of personal data under the GDPR, and 'special' personal information under the POPI Act. In particular, both laws are similar insofar as these subcategories of personal data/information refer to sensitive data/information, including 'data concerning health' (according to the term used under the GDPR, see Arts. 9(1), Art. 4(15)) or 'health' (according to the term used under the POPI Act, see § 26). Moreover, according to both laws, the processing of special categories of personal data or special personal information is principally banned (Art. 9(1) GDPR and § 26 POPI Act). However, the GDPR and the POPI Act both include particular exceptions where the processing of such sensitive data/information is allowed (Art. 9(2) GDPR and § 27 POPI Act). The POPI Act even contains exceptions specifically for processing personal information regarding data subjects' health (§ 32).

For example, the GDPR and the POPI Act both contain exceptions for the processing of special categories of personal data or special personal information in cases where the data subject has given (explicit) consent (Art. 9(2)(a) GDPR and § 27(1)(a) POPI Act). They also include exceptions from the processing ban for 'scientific or historical research purposes' or 'research purposes', respectively (Art. 9(2)(j) GDPR and § 27(1)(d) POPI Act). However, the POPI Act seems to rely more on informed consent as the primary legitimation for processing special personal information for research purposes when compared to the GDPR. This can be seen in the phrasing of the POPI Act's exception, which requires, among other things, as one alternative condition that 'it appears to be impossible or would involve a disproportionate effort to ask for consent' (§ 27(1)(d)).

37.6 Conclusion

Large amounts of data are needed to realize the potential of AI in clinical medicine, such as to train algorithms on diverse datasets and provide treatment recommendations. However, the need to process health and non-health information – from its collection to its use, storage, and sharing with third parties – requires stakeholders, such as AI/machine learning companies and healthcare providers, to be aware of the applicable privacy laws in order to be able to comply with their requirements.

This chapter has tried to shed some light on the complex privacy landscape around the world. To my knowledge, this is the first chapter of its kind that has jointly discussed the privacy laws in the USA, Europe, and South Africa in great detail, including comparing them and revealing some of the similarities and differences of the US HIPAA, the EU GDPR, and South Africa's POPI Act. Stakeholders in the health AI field will hopefully find this chapter useful as a starting point to understand what privacy laws exist in the USA, Europe, and South Africa, what these laws regulate, and whether the processing of (health) data/information that they are planning may fall within the scope of these privacy laws.

KEY INSIGHTS

- ■ **This chapter highlights that AI/machine learning in clinical medicine involves large amounts of health and non-health data that are likely to require compliance with privacy laws to be processed.**
- ■ **The chapter provides an overview of privacy laws in the USA, Europe, and South Africa.**
- ■ **It compares the US HIPAA, the EU GDPR, and South Africa's POPI Act and reveals similarities and differences.**

Acknowledgments

S.G. reports grants from the European Union (Grant Agreement no. 101057321 and no. 101057099), the National Institute of Biomedical Imaging and Bioengineering (NIBIB) of the National Institutes of Health (Grant Agreement no. 3R01EB027650-03S1), and the Rock Ethics Institute at Penn State University.

References

1. FDA. *Artificial Intelligence and Machine Learning (AI/ML)-Enabled Medical Devices*, 2021. https://www.fda.gov/medical-devices/software-medical-device-samd/artificial-intelligence-and-machine-learning-aiml-enabled-medical-devices.

2. Letter from the FDA to Digital Diagnostics Inc., 10 June 2021. K203629. https://www.accessdata.fda.gov/cdrh_docs/pdf20/K203629.pdf.

3. Letter from the FDA to Viz.ai, Inc., 18 March 2020. K193658. https://www.accessdata.fda.gov/cdrh_docs/pdf19/K193658.pdf.

4. Letter from the FDA to HeartFlow, Inc., 15 August 2019. K190925. https://www.accessdata.fda.gov/cdrh_docs/pdf19/K190925.pdf.

5. Gerke S, Minssen T, Cohen IG. Ethical and legal challenges of artificial intelligence-driven healthcare. In: Bohr A, Memarzadeh K (eds), *Artificial Intelligence in Healthcare*. London: Elsevier; 2020, 295–336. https://doi.org/10.1016/B978-0-12-818438-7.00012-5.

6. Babic B, Gerke S, Evgeniou T, Cohen IG. Direct-to-consumer medical machine learning and artificial intelligence applications. *Nature Machine Intelligence* 2021;3:283–287. https://doi.org/10.1038/s42256-021-00331-0.

7. Forbes. The future of voice AI In patient care, 11 February 2019. https://www.forbes.com/sites/insights-intelai/2019/02/11/the-future-of-voice-ai-in-patient-care/?sh=1ea63e33309c.

For additional references and Further Reading please see www.wiley.com/go/byrne/aiinclinicalmedicine

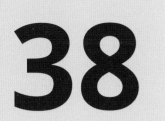

38 AI-Enabled Consumer-Facing Health Technology

Alexandra T. Greenhill

Department of Family Medicine, University of British Columbia, Vancouver, Canada; Careteam Technologies, Vancouver, Canada

Learning Objectives

- Explore trends and different types of AI-enabled consumer-facing or direct-to-consumer (DTC) health technology, which includes software and hardware.
- Review common issues and pitfalls as well as emerging regulation efforts for AI-enabled consumer-facing health technology.
- Recognize best practices for physician involvement with the creation and validation of AI-enabled consumer-facing health technology.
- Learn best practices of how to recommend and how to respond to patient-generated inquiries about AI-enabled consumer-facing health technology.
- Identify future directions for AI-enabled consumer-facing health technology.

38.1 Introduction

People interested in accessing health and wellness technology have choices that did not exist a decade ago: as of the time of writing, there are thousands of devices, over 370,000 apps in the app stores, and millions of various web-based solutions, and all those options are increasing year over year. While AI was initially a rarity, it is rapidly becoming a common component. In addition to health technology use that is managed through their healthcare providers, patients are increasingly independently accessing software (websites, computer applications, and mobile apps) and devices in what is now known collectively as a new category: consumer-facing or direct-to-consumer (DTC) health technology. Digital therapeutics (DTx) and Software as a Medical Device (SaMD) can be physician prescribed, but also increasingly be delivered directly to patients using evidence-based, clinically evaluated software and devices. Therefore, this chapter will include consumer-facing DTx and SaMD as a subset of consumer-facing AI-enabled health technologies.

All of these new, exciting technological offerings have good intentions and great potential benefits such as addressing unmet healthcare needs, as well as

AI in Clinical Medicine: A Practical Guide for Healthcare Professionals, First Edition. Edited by Michael F. Byrne, Nasim Parsa, Alexandra T. Greenhill, Daljeet Chahal, Omer Ahmad, and Ulas Bagci.
© 2023 John Wiley & Sons Ltd. Published 2023 by John Wiley & Sons Ltd.
Companion website: www.wiley.com/go/byrne/aiinclinicalmedicine

improving patient access and empowerment. They also have several significant issues related to execution, and respect of safeguards that must be identified and addressed. The hype surrounding AI in the public media includes exaggeration of both the benefits and the perils. As this is an emerging domain, unlike many other medical products and services, digital health and wellness technologies are currently often given or sold directly to individual patient consumers, without the safeguards established for food, supplements and over-the-counter (OTC) treatments, in terms of claims of both what they can achieve and that they are safe to use. In the next decade, there will be a tremendous effort from experts, regulators, and technology creators to fulfil the promise of AI in this area. It is imperative for physicians to understand the opportunities and issues, as there are important differences that exist amongst consumer-facing technologies, and given the fact that patients' use of such technologies could impact their medical care and health negatively [1].

Much of the discussion applies to digital health technology and to AI overall, with consumer-facing AI as an emerging and differentiated subset of policies, standards, regulations, and research. As that specific content is covered in more detail in other chapters of the book, this chapter will concentrate on the consumer-facing and AI dimensions in particular.

38.2 Trends and Patient Receptivity to AI-Enabled Consumer-Facing Health Technology

Four massive trends converge to explain this rapid proliferation of consumer-facing AI-enabled technology for healthcare. These are illustrated in Figure 38.1:

- *Production – easier, faster, and cheaper to create.* The barriers for creating such solutions have dramatically decreased, especially for software, but also for hardware. While there are a number of serious efforts, it is now possible

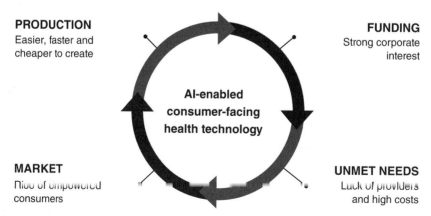

PRODUCTION
Easier, faster and cheaper to create

FUNDING
Strong corporate interest

AI-enabled consumer-facing health technology

MARKET
Rise of empowered consumers

UNMET NEEDS
Lack of providers and high costs

Figure 38.1: Trends fuelling the rise of AI-enabled consumer-facing health technology.

with a relatively small investment of time and money to create a product that appears to be a polished solution, and to add claims that often do not have to be substantiated. This can occur because there are still no specific regulations, accreditations, or standards to guarantee quality and mitigate risks for consumer-facing solutions. Conversely, while in the past there was usually a great difference in precision and quality between medical grade and consumer-facing technologies, some consumer-facing technologies are now sometimes on a par or even remarkably better than those made available to physicians.

- *Funding – strong corporate interest.* This approach attracts companies because the consumer-facing part of healthcare offers a large customer base, few regulatory barriers to entry, and no need to obtain the difficult-to-get buy-in from physicians and health systems. From 2011 to 2019, 21% of all health tech companies pursued the DTC route exclusively, with an investment of over $7 billion [2]. This already rapidly increasing trend has seen a massive jump due to the increased demand for consumer-facing health technology during the COVID-19 pandemic.

- *Market – rise of the empowered consumers.* With banking, ecommerce, and other services being offered online and via mobile apps, patients are now seeking these same conveniences when it comes to their health. Patients are demanding more flexibility and access to their health information, and more ways to improve their health and well-being. As of 2021, an estimated four in five US residents use a smart phone daily, three in five have downloaded at least one health app, and one in five owns a smart wearable device. These numbers are similar across all developed countries [3]. All these percentages are rapidly increasing as the declining costs of technology make it more accessible to a greater portion of the population. In addition, the increase in use for non-healthcare reasons makes more users of all ages and socioeconomic levels more comfortable using technology for health purposes as well.

- *Unmet needs – lack of providers and high costs.* There are significant numbers of people who cannot access healthcare due to lack of providers and/or challenges paying for services. When the health system does not have options to offer, consumers turn to self-directed approach to find solutions. In addition, organizations such as the US National Institute of Mental Health (NIMH), the UK National Health Service (NHS), health disease groups, payers, insurers, employers, and even retailers (such as pharmacies, grocery, and electronic stores) have all started to recommend apps and devices to address the substantial gaps in accessing healthcare – especially for preventative care, obesity, and mental health. This trend is even more powerful in developing nations that are unlikely to be able to meet sustainable human development goals in healthcare without the assistance of technology [4].

When exploring consumer attitudes towards AI-enabled health technologies, one of the challenges is that very often consumers are simply not even aware that there is AI in the application or device they are using, whether for health or non-health use. Experts are calling for greater informed consent in the healthcare context [2].

In this nascent domain, there is no clarity regarding consumer preferences. Many consumer surveys in the mainstream media and industry publications report that patients are overall increasingly open to new technologies in healthcare, including AI. However, in published medical articles, such as that from Yakar et al., the findings are that the general population's view on AI in medicine is leaning more towards a higher level of distrust, which is the opposite of positive publications in the mainstream media [5].

Interestingly, in a mixed-methods systematic review of studies on patient and general public attitudes towards clinical AI [6], only 26% of 23 studies assessed currently available or soon to be available AI tools. The remaining 74% of these studies assessed only hypothetical or broadly defined AI. This is significant if consideration is given to the substantial differences that exist in what patients say on surveys and focus groups, and what they actually do in real-world environments.

Patients have a generally positive attitude towards increased self-management through apps and devices. This is especially true if the patients are well educated and of higher socioeconomic status, leading to the perception that most of the users are the 'wealthy, worried, and well', and raising concerns regarding equity. This is, however, changing as the costs are decreasing, and while many patients can independently select and purchase health apps and devices, many receive them for free from governments, health disease groups, payers, insurers, employers, and even retailers (such as pharmacies, groceries, and electronic stores).

In surveys, consumers indicate a mix of excitement and distrust towards AI in health [5,7]. Some of the biggest reasons for consumer resistance to AI are technological (performance and communication), ethical (trust factors), and regulatory concerns [8], as well as 'uniqueness neglect', a concern that AI is less able than humans to account for consumers' unique characteristics and circumstances [9].

Even if the consumer-facing AI-enabled health technology performs well, the patient can afford it, and has the know-how to use it, the biggest challenges are low initial adoption and even lower ongoing use. Although patients may choose to purchase an app or a device, they most often do not start or continue to use it. Overall, 95% of apps that are downloaded are never looked at or are used only once, and the same trend applies to health technology. Considering the two dimensions of users' assessment of the technology and its capabilities (user experience), and their persistence at their health goals (intent), an emerging framework illustrates the four decisions that users might make after initial interaction: abandon use, limit use, switch, and continue use [10]. Findings to date suggest that a significant part of the low adoption and persistent use of consumer-facing AI-enabled health technology is due to perceptions of lack of trust around privacy, the current lack of evidence of their safety and effectiveness, and the limited usefulness of these technologies in their current state of performance [11].

38.3 Different Types of AI-Enabled Consumer-Facing Health Technology

AI-enabled consumer-facing health technologies lie along the full spectrum of healthcare, from promotion of wellness to identification of symptoms to treatment support to research. Compared to their non-AI counterparts, they offer a number of potential advantages such as passive collection of data, greater personalization and contextualization of care, and faster optimal insights from ever larger amounts of data [12].

Increasingly it is impossible to simply classify these technologies as software and hardware, as many solutions are offered online, on mobile, or by text messaging, and many devices come with a software component (web-based or app). In addition, it is often difficult to know the degree of automation, as some of these solutions are fully automated technologies while others are what is known as technology-enabled services, where humans use a given technology solution to provide the service.

This section will cover some broad categories, with illustrative examples, noting that widely adopted approach to such a classification does not yet exist. Most of the solutions that are in use remain to be proven to be safe and effective (as will be discussed in the next section about common issues). Of course, some solutions combine several of these categories, as illustrated in Figure 38.2:

- *Intended for encouraging or maintaining health and wellness.* These technologies allow consumers to actively monitor vital signs, weight, activity, and exercise; provide personalized daily motivational tips and automated coaching to reduce stress; or work on better eating, sleeping, and posture. They include, standalone or in combination, patient-reported data, photo/video/audio-based analysis, smart phone sensing, wearables, Internet of Things

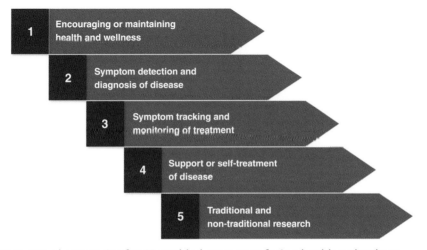

Figure 38.2: Broad categories for AI-enabled consumer-facing health technology.

(IoT) devices, and biomechanical sensors incorporated into clothing or shoes. These data inputs are analysed using AI to provide patients with better awareness of what they are doing as well as increasingly instructions on how to improve. These technologies are fuelling the nascent movements of *quantified self* (the concept of self-discovery via personal analytics) and *biohacking*, also known as human augmentation or human enhancement (self-managed efforts to improve health, well-being, and performance through a strong technology-enabled feedback loop of intervention and results).

- *Related to symptom detection and diagnosis of disease.* AI-based symptom checkers (AISCs) are increasingly used to help manage patient questions and enable self-triage before seeing medical care, both as a replacement for 24/7 health call lines and for triage before in-person or telehealth visits. COVID-19 specific self-assessment websites, apps, and chatbots proliferated in the rapid effort to respond to the pandemic. Natural language processing (NLP) was the starting point for the development of a number of technologies to enable the identification of depression and suicidality in text entered on social media or private devices. Photo-based AI enables self-diagnosis of skin conditions, from acne to cancer to dental caries. Instant AI analysis of audio and video can help provide digital vital signs such as heart rate, respiratory rate, and blood pressure. Tracking of eye movement and vision while using a device or playing games enables diagnosis of eye conditions such as myopia, glaucoma, and retinal disorders. Passive monitoring of typing rhythm and walking rate from smart phones or watches can detect early signs of neuromuscular conditions such as Parkinson's disease. Smart watches and other wearables can detect and monitor arrhythmias, seizures, and frailty.

- *Enabling symptom tracking and monitoring of treatment.* The same technologies listed in the previous two sections can also be applied to symptom tracking. In addition, symptom diaries, usually available online or on mobile device apps, can help with adherence to evidence-proven methods that are otherwise hard to create adherence to without the technological component. Wearables and IoT can make data collection even easier for vital sign collection and for motor symptoms monitoring in conditions like Parkinson's disease, musculoskeletal rehabilitation, arrhythmias, seizures, and frailty. Biomechanical sensors incorporated into clothing or shoes, such as ballistocardiograms, seismocardiograms, and dielectric sensors, can passively and continuously measure variables such as cardiac output, lung fluid volume, and weight, which could be beneficial in managing conditions such as heart failure.

- *Support or self-treatment of disease.* The most frequent conditions that are being targeted with consumer-facing AI-enabled health technology in this subcategory are medication adherence apps; mental health and smoking cessation support using websites, text-based interactions, chatbots, and apps; physical and cognitive exercise support; immersive tools to reduce isolation, distract from pain, or create an immersive environment for rehabilitation; and femtech for digital birth control and fertility support. They are most frequently categorized by regulatory jurisdictions as a subset of DTx and SaMD, so they are often subject to more oversight than the previous two subcategories.

▪ *Powering traditional and non-traditional research.* These new AI-enabled consumer-facing health technologies enable better collection of real-world data (RWD), real-world evidence (RWE), patient-reported outcome measures (PROMs), and patient-reported experience measures (PREMs), as the patient can provide historical data to the research teams that they would not have otherwise been able to access. Data from AI-enabled consumer-facing health technologies and from tools like the Apple ResearchKit now make it possible for non-academic, corporate, and even citizen researchers to access massive datasets, and also to use AI to generate insights in a process that falls outside of regulations and the usual conventions of conducting and disseminating research.

Consumer engagement functionalities are similar to non-AI consumer-facing technology, and include [13]:

▪ Provision of information and reminders.
▪ Gathering, tracking, display, summary, guidance, and alerts using user-entered or user-generated information.
▪ Communication with family, clinician, and peers.
▪ Nudges and rewards for behaviour change.

The AI-enabled component is typically used to simplify insights and to personalize to the end-user.

38.4 Common Issues for Consumer-Facing AI-Enabled Health Technology

Although both public media and a growing body of literature highlight the potential benefit of consumer-facing AI-enabled health technology, it is unclear whether many such solutions are actually available. Most of the published studies conclude that there are many significant, often unintended, issues, and that these solutions are still in the early days of discovering what works and how to proceed while ensuring the protection of the public. The concerns identified range from consumer inconveniences to noticeable consequences without actual harm, to actual or potential adverse events [14].

There is an overlap in both the issues and solutions facing health technology in general, and AI in particular. Other chapters in this book cover issues and solutions for AI-enabled health technologies intended for physicians, most of which also apply to consumer-facing solutions, including, for example, data selection and algorithmic biases. We will not discuss these further here (refer to Chapters 39 and 40).

In regard to both clinician- and consumer-facing solutions, there is an important role for governments, medical, and health organizations to play in raising overall public awareness of these issues, and also in working to eliminate and reduce them through proper consumer protection (using mechanisms such as research, policies, standards, regulations, and quality assurance; see Chapters 36 and 37).

Physicians need to be informed about these issues in order to help protect and educate their patients in the meantime. See [1,13,15] for a deep dive into these issues.

What follows in this section is a quick overview of common issues specifically for consumer-facing AI-enabled health technology, as most issues related to AI for clinicians also apply here and are well covered in other chapters.

38.4.1 Informed Consent Issues

38.4.1.1 Issues Related to Obtaining Informed Consent

There is at present no consensus or recommended approach on how to inform patients about the role of AI in a given health technology used to provide care or in a consumer-facing tool. There are many factors, including societal, cultural, and legislational, that make this a complicated matter [16].

38.4.1.2 Veracity of Description and Claims

Distinguishing between AI-enabled consumer-facing health technology that promotes AI as a marketing strategy and one that actually uses AI (and if so, what type of AI specifically) is important. Currently, outside of a few software and device solutions that have received regulatory approval, there is no verifiable way to understand whether the AI claims of a given health technology are true or not. As most health technology has not received regulatory approval or been subject to peer-reviewed published research, even when there is real AI, there is no ability to verify if it works as promised. Many apps and devices have very narrow functionality that limits their usefulness, or merely provide information about medical conditions, similar to the information that can be read in a pamphlet or on a website. For example, many of the heart rate monitoring devices have wearable sensors that provide a calculation-based average instead of capturing individual heart beats as happens with medical grade devices, but that information is difficult to find or not presented (see Chapter 44 for further discussion of this topic.) There is also another concerning scenario. Many solutions that focus on the dimensions subject to regulation (diagnosis, cure, mitigation, prevention, or treatment of a disease or condition) find ways of describing themselves as information providers only, while they do in fact offer patients recommendations that should be reviewed for safety and quality.

38.4.1.3 Lack of, or Issues with, Terms of Use and Privacy Policy

At least 25% of healthcare apps in the app stores do not have terms of use or a privacy policy [17], and many that do have important omissions or content that is hard to understand for an end-user. This leads to questions over whether the end-user is truly able to provide informed consent to using the technology.

38.4.1.4 Pricing Transparency

Standards for greater pricing transparency do not exist. Many apps are freemium or monetize user data in exchange for being free. Users are often not aware of a pay requirement before the app is downloaded or when purchasing a device, and they invest time and effort in creating data that become potentially inaccessible. They are also not necessarily informed that the use of the app may be free, but that the data are being used for secondary purposes.

38.4.1.5 Technology Stability and Ability to Keep Up to Date

The reality of technology start-ups and companies, as well as groups with limited research or project funding to develop healthcare solutions, is that all too often, creators of such solutions simply have to shut down the offering (either because it was sold and subsumed into another solution or simply as there was no funding to continue to provide it) or change its ownership, terms of use, and pricing. As it is increasingly easy and inexpensive to start a solution, especially a software solution, there is a proliferation of such solutions without the necessary consideration for the sustainability of such solutions. The failure rate of start-ups overall is high, and there is also often very limited funding beyond support for pilots in healthcare. Users can lose all of their data without warning or recourse, which is contrary to the requirement for healthcare retention of medical information in most jurisdictions. In addition, keeping the solution up to date both clinically and from a privacy and security perspective requires continuous investment that is all too often an issue. It is also frequently not clear when a given consumer-facing solution was last updated. Educated consumers can look at the version history section in the app stores, but that information is often not available on websites or while purchasing devices.

38.4.1.6 Unregulated Healthcare Research

AI-enabled consumer-facing health technology has enabled research by new classes of researchers, such as independent researchers, citizen scientists, patient-directed researchers, and self-experimenters. This has provided a wonderful opening for innovative scientific inquiry. However, because these researchers are not recipients of financial assistance or conducting research in anticipation of a submission to the regulators for approval, they are often not covered by the usual research regulations meant to promote the welfare and interests of research participants (to mitigate against unethical collection and use of health data, biases encoded in algorithms, risks to patient safety, and issues with the scientific process) and the public (in terms of making the results of the research available to others) [18].

38.4.2 Privacy and Security Issues

There are many reports of unethical collection and use of health data. For example, as much as 88% of over 18,000 medical health (mHealth) apps studied included code that could potentially collect user data [17] or did not adhere to some of the primary health data privacy principles (limit collection, use, disclosure, and retention). In addition, many of these technologies that are consumer facing present issues relating to security standards, and there are real concerns that data loss or being easy targets for hackers could lead to user data exposure.

38.4.3 Beneficence and Safety Issues

38.4.3.1 Lack of, or Issues with, Clinical Evidence Base

There are numerous analyses demonstrating that many consumer-facing health technologies have critical gaps during their development (including the lack of expert involvement; poor use of evidence base; weak datasets; inadequate process; disparities built into the bias within the data, algorithms, and recommendations; as well as lack of validation). They also have gaps in necessary evidence-based features to correctly address the given health and wellness condition, and issues with quality of the information presented (including incorrect, incomplete, or out-of-date information, and variation in content) [1,13,15,19].

38.4.3.2 Lack of, or Issues with, Clinical Effectiveness and Evidence

There is also widespread lack of evidence of efficacy, especially with performance measures that go beyond patient satisfaction. Although patient experience is a key motivator for adopting consumer technology, better outcomes are a necessary requirement, if there is to be the desired evolution from promise to results.

For example, the proliferation of skin cancer diagnosis apps was heralded as a welcome development to improve the diagnosis of a cancer that has seen both an alarming rise in cases and a high mortality rate unless diagnosed early. However, a 2020 high-quality systematic review of nine studies that evaluated six different identifiable smart phone apps showed that, unfortunately, there is little evidence that current smart phone apps can be useful in self-monitoring and detection of skin cancer [20]. Similarly, reviews of mental health or obesity solutions indicated that, while there is great potential, there is actually little evidence of impact on outcomes [21,22].

38.4.3.3 Risk of Harm

The biggest concern relating to technologies used by users without medical support is the risk of harm, either because the user did something that is harmful as a result of technology-derived information or recommendation (false positive causing an unnecessary or inappropriate action), or because they did not do something that they should have done (a false negative may lead to false reassurance that results in a late or delayed diagnosis) [1].

For example, a systematic review of AI-based symptom checkers showed that there are issues with both false positives and false negatives, and that these lead to negative potential and actual consequences [23]. In another example, this time in mental health, an investigative report by the BBC revealed that some mental health apps failed to identify obvious signs of distress (did not flag self-harm, abuse, or suicidal comments from users, and did not offer escalation paths). This report led to changes in how these technologies are regulated [24].

38.4.4 Usability Issues

38.4.4.1 User-Centred Design Issues

One of the key best practices in technology design is user-centred design (UCD) – the critical importance of designing the solution from the perspective of the end-user so that there is ease of onboarding and ongoing use, ideally without the need for extensive training. In addition, in healthcare there are additional requirements to meet clinical and diversity, equity, and inclusion (DEI) dimensions beyond standard UCD best practices. Many consumer-facing health technologies have extensive issues with usability, identified as one of the key obstacles to their ongoing use [11].

38.4.4.2 Accessibility Gap and Lag

Beyond the UCD issues for all users, people with disabilities or those who experience reduced ability as they age are left behind and unable to use new technologies. There is an 'accessibility gap' or an 'accessibility lag' of at least 12 months, where either the provider of the solution implements the needed changes, or a community of advocates and creators creates a push for the change or adaptive separate solutions that reduce or solve the accessibility issue. While there are a number of suggested standards for accessibility for software and devices, both for health use and non-health use, these are unfortunately voluntary and often not followed, either because of lack of awareness about the guidelines or lack of funding to support the additional costs. All too often, accessibility loses the cost–benefit trade-off, and providers choose to address those issues at a later stage. Increasingly, however, it is relatively easy and inexpensive to resolve accessibility issues because of the availability and reduced costs of new technologies that help with such problems, but many creators are simply not aware of these options or that the accessibility issues exist, as they were not raised in the UCD testing they conducted.

Norms and conventions for both UCD and accessibility are still nascent, and the lack of clear, widely adopted approaches and standards, as well as the absence of regulation on these two dimensions, is contributing to this issue.

38.4.4.3 Health Literacy Issues

In addition to UCD and accessibility, too many consumer-facing solutions are designed by experts who unintentionally contribute to the challenges faced by consumers with low health literacy (defined as the ability for users to understand and act on health information). There is a need to include health literacy strategies throughout the technology development process and in market-use enhancements [25]. Health literacy may also affect the quality of patient-generated data, a factor that needs to be accounted for when using AI to understand and recommend health options that may have been created using a population with greater health literacy than the people using it.

38.4.4.4 Adoption and Ongoing Engagement

Unless there is a dedicated effort to better understand and implement what drives consumers to try and to continue to use health technology, one of the biggest challenges that remains is that consumers do not act on their intent to use software or devices that they have access to, or that they rapidly abandon use of such software or devices. Beyond proving that these new technologies work and are safe to use, it is imperative to ensure that they are actually used in order to fulfil the potential of these new solutions, especially as AI depends on large numbers of users to generate the massive datasets required.

38.4.5 Impact on the Health System

38.4.5.1 Opportunity Cost Compared to Non-AI Solutions

There is a global call to remember that the investment in AI in particular, or technology in general, should not occur at the expense of core investments and strategies required to achieve better healthcare [26]. Similarly, the focus on a consumer-facing solution as a way to bypass hurdles related to regulation, speed to market, and adoption is pulling key resources away from the limited pool of human talent and health tech funding. This reduces those resources' availability to be involved in projects with far greater impact on the health system.

38.4.5.2 Contribution to the Fragmentation of Health Information

These consumer-facing solutions are often created as standalone, and are not easy to integrate into existing and nascent health technologies used in healthcare. This contributes further to the fragmentation of health information. The datasets used need ideally to meet the standards for health data in order to enable the emergence of more comprehensive datasets and AI solutions. This will increase our ability to understand the connections between health, social determinants, and environmental factors.

38.4.5.3 Increased Burden on the Health System and Negative Effects on Diversity, Equity, and Inclusion

Increased awareness through consumer-facing technology often leads to unintended anxiety, unnecessary medical visits, tests for false positives, and harm through complications related to the testing [1,27]. It is also important to consider the DEI perspective on two dimensions: firstly, the increased unnecessary use of the health system by those who have access to technology because of education and/or financial ability creating reduced access for others, and increased costs overall; and, secondly, the ethical dimension of increased awareness without the ability to access the health system for care because of access issues or socioeconomic barriers, and/or consumers taking on additional financial burden to pursue unnecessary care.

38.5 Emerging Standards and Regulation Efforts

Without discouraging enthusiastic innovation, there is a great need for better regulation for market entry and thoughtful post-market surveillance for AI-enabled consumer-facing health technologies that specifically differentiate between systems designed for physicians and those designed for consumer use [1,28]. The current approach, whereby many of these applications focused on health and well-being do not require regulation, is pushing technology creators to choose the consumer-facing path and all too often encouraging them to bypass the need to have oversight. More research is also needed to better understand patients' capabilities and needs in order to explore observations that patients, even when well educated, tend to be limited in their medical and statistical literacy, and are not objective in their decisions to use a given technology or in their understanding of the information presented to them through the technology.

There are emerging regulations for health technologies, including AI and consumer-facing technologies, such as from the US Food and Drug Administration (FDA), the UK's National Health Service (NHS), and Health Canada. In response to incidents, NHS Digital now offers a clinical safety standard, DCB0129: Clinical Risk Management: Its Application in the Manufacture of Health IT Systems, which requires consumer-facing apps to appoint a clinical safety officer and to create 'escalation paths' for people who show signs of self-harm (such as self-harm, abuse, suicidal thoughts, or trauma) [29]. The FDA has created guidance for general wellness apps and 'low-risk devices', and accelerated distribution of these apps during the pandemic in response to the increased need to access services that would otherwise not be available. The FDA and Health Canada now also have regulatory processes for DTx, and plan to increase their oversight in this area.

In addition, app platform owners are acting to some degree as soft regulators, as their business priorities to ensure consumer satisfaction are aligned with the need to offer quality products through their app stores. For example, both Google and Apple have introduced rules on privacy protection and data use limited to the purpose for which the data were collected. App developers have to respect these rules in order to have their apps included in the app stores [28]. Since 2021, both stores have also added mandatory user-facing privacy labels. There have been many calls for a self-regulatory approach for developers of health technology solutions in order to stay ahead of regulatory and public expectations of ethical behaviour, and to avoid a severe backlash through policies and legislation.

38.6 Best Practices for Physician Involvement with the Creation and Validation of Consumer-Facing AI-Enabled Health Technology

Physicians need to become more involved in the creation, validation, and use of AI-enabled consumer-facing health technology in order to ensure that it is created in a way that achieves positive results and integrates well with the tools and workflows of the healthcare system. The alarming lack of professional medical involvement in the development process and design of mobile applications, and a lack of criteria to assess the expert nature or authority of the medical content and workflows [30], has contributed to the many issues described in the previous section, and impedes the fulfilment of the promise of these innovative solutions. The recommendation of the Royal College of Physicians and Surgeons of Canada (RCPSC) 2018 Task Force on Artificial Intelligence and Emerging Digital Technologies is that professional organizations need to work to support more physicians in training and in practice to co-develop, refine, validate, and spread AI-enabled technologies [31].

Physicians can play a significant role in the development of AI-enabled consumer-facing health technologies as founders, advisors, medical consultants, and medical officers to technology companies, remembering that there are guidelines and ethical standards to help avoid conflicts of interest, and uphold the physician's primary duty to patient care when collaborating with industry. Some of the key issues for physicians to address were listed earlier, such as that the solution being developed leverages available evidence and best practices, ensures respect of patient privacy and consent, guides decisions on intervention models to implement, addresses health literacy and DEI, limits the potential for harm through false negatives and false positives, considers the impact on healthcare services and workflows, and includes significant input from end-users during development and optimization [32]. In addition, physicians need to address the requirement for technology sustainability, in terms of availability and keeping it up to date. Physicians can use tools like the mHealth App Trustworthiness (mHAT) checklist. This is useful in the initial stages of creating a consumer-facing technology as well throughout its life cycle [33], and would not be as accessible to, or usable by, traditional technology creators.

The US FDA, the UK Medicines and Healthcare products Regulatory Agency (MHRA), and Health Canada jointly published the Good Machine Learning Practice for Medical Device Development: Guiding Principles, which can be adapted to the creation of AI-enabled consumer-facing health technologies [34]. The document consists of 10 guiding principles (listed in Chapter 36) to help promote safe, effective, and high-quality use of AI/machine learning in medical devices, and these can be adapted to consumer-facing solutions (even though they do not specifically mention them). In addition, physicians can also adapt the 2019 Xcertia guidelines to produce better-quality health technology. The guidelines cover the five key areas of privacy, security, usability, operability, and content. Xcertia is a not-for-profit organization created by the American Medical Association (AMA), the American Heart Association (AHA), and the Healthcare Information and Management Systems Society (HIMSS) in order to provide regularly updated guidelines, with extensive consultation with experts, the public, and technology creators [35]. Similarly, as mentioned earlier, the NHS Digital Clinical Safety team has created clinical risk management standards designed to help creators of health technologies build better and safer products [29].

The validation of innovative technologies is an important step that is often overlooked, especially when developing consumer-facing solutions that do not require regulatory approval, and where there may not be sources of funding. Physicians can lead validation studies as well as demand that such studies are actually done, if asked to start recommending AI-enabled consumer-facing health technology. The evaluation in real-world clinical settings often reveals issues that must be addressed before broader deployment, such as the impact of poor-quality, consumer-captured photos, videos, or audio on the performance of a given technology.

Validation of AI-enabled consumer-facing health technology needs to involve more than metrics such as usability, user satisfaction, growth and patterns in use, and sustainability of use, and should include measures of safety and effectiveness. Randomized trials remain the gold standard. However, single-case designs (systematic provision and removal of an intervention along with continuous assessment in an attempt to identify associated fluctuations in an outcome) and interrupted-time-series designs (which imply causality through showing a disruption in a stable baseline that coincides with the introduction of an intervention) are two other evaluation methods that can be useful [32].

38.7 Best Practices for Recommending and Responding to Patient Queries about AI-Enabled Consumer-Facing Health Technology

Physicians increasingly recommend, or are asked about, AI-enabled consumer-facing health technology. They need to take a similar approach as for other consumer-facing diagnostic, self-management, and self-treatment modalities, in order to be a true medical expert to guide the patient, and to be accountable for these solutions within the healthcare system. Patients are seeking the physician's guidance on or approval of their plans to use AI-enabled consumer-facing health technology, and they are interested in providing the data generated for their direct care and for research. In addition, in some countries such as Germany, the Digital Healthcare Act offers insurance coverage for certain AI-enabled consumer-facing health technologies, but only if prescribed by a physician or granted pre-approval by an insurer [1].

Physicians have always played an important role in mitigating risks for patients, and can help inform patients as to how to better evaluate the consumer health technologies that they are considering. However, there also needs to be greater education of the public about this from governments, health and medical organizations, and social media – this will promote health and technology literacy.

While the majority of physicians are generally willing to engage patients in conversation about specific AI-enabled consumer-facing health technologies relevant to their area of expertise, they face many challenges in doing so. For example, because so many of the AI-enabled consumer-facing health technologies are not subject to regulation as healthcare tools, it is unclear whether health privacy regulations should apply to them. In addition, it is also unclear what a physician's malpractice liability would be if there were a negative outcome for a patient from use of an AI-enabled consumer-facing health technology that the physician recommended. Even when these issues are clarified, physicians will still continue to face a myriad of practical challenges such as lack of time during encounters, difficulty keeping up to date with the increasing volume of options available, lack of information about which options are reliable, and lack of training on how to evaluate the options, as well as concerns about the technologies' privacy, security, quality, safety, and effectiveness.

Only one country has, at the time of writing, created national guidelines for physicians recommending technology to patients. The Canadian Medical Association's Guiding Principles for Physicians Recommending Mobile Health Applications to Patients [36], written in 2015, need to be extrapolated to AI as they do not specifically mention it. The guidelines outline how to do one's own evaluation, and also suggest that the easiest and simplest approach is for physicians to select technologies that are endorsed by a recognized healthcare organization, thus removing from the individual physician the burden of evaluating the given AI-enabled consumer-facing health technology. There are also emerging app libraries subject to rigorous review that are provided by healthcare networks or by groups such as Organisation for the Review of Care and Health Apps (ORCHA).

If a physician is to proceed with their own independent evaluation, there are no specific criteria for AI-enabled consumer-facing health technology, and physicians can adapt one of the 45 emerging evaluation frameworks – all of which, however, have gaps and variation in the quality criteria that are employed [15,21]. These frameworks are based on expert consensus, which can be opaque and difficult to understand, and there is evidence that training on the core concepts is needed to adequately perform the evaluation [37].

These emerging evaluation frameworks are appropriately thorough for emerging technologies, but that also makes them onerous and time-consuming. For example, the six dimensions of quality [38], the 12 guiding principles [39], or the American Psychiatric Association's App Evaluation Model [40] all require an in-depth review of the solution itself, as well as its detailed description, evidence base, terms of use, and privacy policy.

Lack of easy access to information about the technology, including key information such as conflicts of interest, location of data storage, privacy and security, efficacy, undesired effects, and measures taken to avert risks [37], makes such evaluation almost impossible to complete in practice.

38.8 Future Directions for AI-Enabled Consumer-Facing Health Technology

It is key to reiterate that the approach to AI-enabled consumer-facing health technology has great overlaps with AI-enabled health technologies created for clinician-directed use. However, there are unique needs such as the importance of implementing greater consumer protection policies, standards, and mechanisms, similar to other self-directed over-the-counter accessible solutions, in order to ensure quality, usability, safety, privacy, and security without hindering the pace of innovation.

Governments, health organizations, and companies can implement a series of measures that can further improve the quality of, and access to, AI-enabled consumer-facing health technologies, fostering innovation without sacrificing safety and effectiveness. These measures need to include clear standards for technology creators, better consumer education, the establishment of expert curation and post-market surveillance mechanisms, and the encouragement of physicians to recommend these new solutions by providing training and clarifying the liability issues. In addition, the creators of consumer-facing solutions need to consider how they would integrate into, and impact, the clinician-directed healthcare of the person using such solutions in order to first do no harm, and ideally create benefit.

There is no doubt that there is great promise for AI-enabled consumer-facing health technology to provide greater access to health solutions, to empower patients, and to promote further research efforts. Physicians have a key role to play in the creation, validation, and use of these solutions in order to maximize the benefits and minimize the perils. Finally, physicians need to have the same level of knowledge, understanding of development, evaluation processes, and scientific scepticism regarding AI-enabled consumer-facing health technologies as they do for other consumer-facing solutions.

KEY INSIGHTS

- There is an explosive increase in the number and types of AI-enabled consumer-facing health technologies available, and the growth will continue to be fuelled by four main trends: ease of production, private funding support, the increase in consumerization of healthcare, and the growth of patients' unmet needs.
- AI-enabled consumer-facing health technologies can be divided into five categories based on their purpose: (i) encouraging or maintaining health and wellness; (ii) symptom detection and diagnosis of disease; (iii) symptom tracking and monitoring of treatment; (iv) support or self-treatment of disease; and (v) powering traditional and non-traditional research.

- AI-enabled consumer-facing health technologies are similar in many ways to AI-enabled health technologies meant for providers, but have some important unique considerations, including those related to regulation requirements.
- Physicians have not been very involved to date in creating and validating AI-enabled consumer-facing health technologies, and their efforts can make these new modalities much more useful for patient self-management, as well as for clinical care and research.
- Physicians need to be aware of what AI-enabled consumer-facing health technologies their patients may be using or could benefit from. The evaluation by physicians of the quality and safety of AI-enabled consumer-facing health technologies in order to be able to recommend or to respond to patient queries is challenging to complete, due to the lack of a robust established evaluation framework and training on how to use it, as well as the lack of information made available to users by the technology creators.

Conflicts of Interest

Alexandra T. Greenhill is an advisor to a number of technology companies providing healthcare solutions for clinical practice and for consumers, both directly and through accelerators such as New Ventures BC, Founders Institute, FoundersBoost, and The Forum. None of the companies she works with or advises have been mentioned in this chapter.

References

1. Babic B, Gerke S, Evgeniou T, Cohen IG. Direct-to-consumer medical machine learning and artificial intelligence applications. *Nature Machine Intelligence* 2021;3:283–287. https://doi.org/10.1038/s42256-021-00331-0.
2. Cohen AB, Mathews SC, Dorsey ER, Bates DW, Safavi K. Direct-to-consumer digital health. *Lancet Digital Health* 2020;2(4):e163–e165. https://doi.org/10.1016/S2589-7500(20)30057-1.
3. Smith A. Chapter two: usage and attitudes toward smartphones. In: *U.S. Smartphone Use in 2015*. Pew Research Center, 2015. https://www.pewresearch.org/internet/2015/04/01/chapter-two-usage-and-attitudes-toward-smartphones.
4. Owoyemi A, Owoyemi J, Osiyemi A, Boyd A. Artificial intelligence for healthcare in Africa. *Frontiers in Digital Health* 2020;2(6). https://doi.org/10.3389.
5. Yakar D, Ongena YP, Kwee TC, Haan M. Do people favor artificial intelligence over physicians? A survey among the general population and their view on artificial intelligence in medicine. *Value in Health* 2021;25(3):374–381. https://doi.org/10.1016/j.jval.2021.09.004.

6. Young AT, Amara D, Bhattacharya A, Wei ML. Patient and general public attitudes towards clinical artificial intelligence: a mixed methods systematic review. *Lancet Digital Health* 2021;3(9):e599–e611. https://doi.org/10.1016/S2589-7500(21)00132-1.
7. PwC. *What Doctor? Why AI and Robotics Will Define New Health*, 2016. https://www.pwc.com/gx/en/news-room/docs/what-doctor-why-ai-and-robotics-will-define-new-health.pdf.

For additional references and Further Reading please see www.wiley.com/go/byrne/aiinclinicalmedicine.

39

Biases in Machine Learning in Healthcare

Dora Huang[1], Leo Anthony Celi[2,3,4], and Zachary O'Brien[5,6]

[1] Department of Gastroenterology & Hepatology, Beth Israel Deaconess Medical Center, Boston, MA, USA

[2] Department of Medicine, Beth Israel Deaconess Medical Center, Boston, MA, USA

[3] Institute for Medical Engineering and Science, Massachusetts Institute of Technology, Cambridge, MA, USA

[4] Department of Biostatistics, Harvard T.H. Chan School of Public Health, Boston, MA, USA

[5] Australian and New Zealand Intensive Care Research Centre, Department of Epidemiology and Preventive Medicine, Monash University, Melbourne, VIC, Australia

[6] Department of Critical Care, University of Melbourne, Melbourne, VIC, Australia

Learning Objectives

- Recognize biases in existing clinical formulas and algorithms.
- Understand pre-existing biases in healthcare and healthcare providers, and how these influence machine learning in healthcare.
- Appreciate the risks associated with the implementation of machine learning in healthcare in different clinical scenarios and environments
- Consider potential solutions to biases in machine learning in healthcare.

39.1 Introduction

The use of AI and data science in healthcare, together known as machine learning in healthcare (MLHC), has become standard practice. Machine learning works to identify patterns in existing datasets to develop predictive models for future data and outcomes [1]. In healthcare, these models, under the umbrella of clinical informatics, have been used to assess patients' risk of disease, forecast health system burden, and predict clinical results. The models build upon commonly used tools, like traditional scoring systems (e.g. Apgar, Acute Physiology and Chronic Health Evaluation [APACHE]) by combining machine learning and mechanistic models (using theory to predict what might happen in the real world) in their predictions [2,3].

AI in Clinical Medicine: A Practical Guide for Healthcare Professionals, First Edition. Edited by Michael F. Byrne, Nasim Parsa, Alexandra T. Greenhill, Daljeet Chahal, Omer Ahmad, and Ulas Bagci.
© 2023 John Wiley & Sons Ltd. Published 2023 by John Wiley & Sons Ltd.
Companion website: www.wiley.com/go/byrne/aiinclinicalmedicine

The growing use of electronic medical records (EMRs) has provided a unique opportunity to acquire and analyse a large data substrate for MLHC for model training, testing, and validation purposes. Population-level data containing demographic information and variables routinely collected in the process of care can be used to inform MLHC and, subsequently, clinical frameworks and practice. However, while MLHC can potentially inform both providers and patients, it may perpetuate health inequalities due to systematic biases. As healthcare systems continue to digitize their processes and the digital exhaust (excess data collected as a by-product of intentional data collection) of the patient encounters becomes available for analysis, opportunities to include under-represented populations in studies and clinical practice frameworks will become more available. With the ongoing expansion of MLHC, consideration must be given to the risks that arise from its integration into clinical care.

39.1.1 From Biases in Formulas to Algorithmic Biases

Even prior to modern machine learning methods, biases existed in clinical medicine. For example, the formula for estimated glomerular filtration rate (eGFR) has been a commonly used metric for kidney function, based on serum creatinine level [4]. However, the original algorithm made an adjustment for race, under the assumption that Black individuals would have higher serum creatinine levels based on their musculature [5]. This adjustment led to higher estimation of eGFR values for individuals who identify as Black, with potential clinical ramifications including delayed recognition of worsening kidney function, referral to specialist care, or transplantation [6,7]. One study found that removing race adjustments from calculations of eGFR increased the number of chronic kidney disease diagnoses, as well as access to specialist-level care and resources for affected individuals [4].

Other specialties are not immune to such biases. In cardiology and urology, for example, standardized scores such as the American Heart Association Get with the Guidelines-Heart Failure Risk Score and STONE score, used to guide decisions regarding treatment and allocation of resources, assign greater risk to 'non-Black' patients, potentially affecting triaging and therapies offered [8–10]. In obstetrics, the Vaginal Birth after Caesarean (VBAC) algorithm suggests lower success rates for African American or Latina-identifying individuals, which could triage these patients towards caesarean sections over vaginal deliveries (the latter having a much lower risk of harm to both mother and infant) [11].

Advanced MLHC methods have also demonstrated bias. Severity scoring systems used in intensive care medicine have exhibited varying performance across patient ethnicities. The accuracy of these machine learning–derived predictive algorithms has been shown to vary, based on sex and insurance status in intensive care and psychiatry [12,13]. These examples demonstrate how easily implicit biases within datasets can be incorporated into clinical algorithms, and translate into explicit health outcome disparities.

These biases were likely introduced as a result of questionable statistical associations. Many of the algorithmic outputs are based upon associations between race and clinical outcomes found in development datasets. For instance, one study investigated a risk score based on healthcare spending as a surrogate for severity of illness [14]. Such an assumption is flawed, as it is based on observed differences in spending between ethnicities with similar medical histories. When the algorithm was interrogated, it was demonstrated that Black patients were significantly sicker than white patients with the same risk score. This suggested that Black patients received less care, despite a higher illness severity, and that healthcare spending was a biased measure of health [14]. The impact of race and associated biases in algorithms and clinical decision-making cannot be ignored.

39.2 Pre-existing Disparities

Inequities exist throughout the healthcare system. It is of concern that pre-existing biases and disparities embedded within EMRs and treatment guidelines can influence MLHC and perpetuate this imbalance. When these records are used to inform AI technology, ingrained inequalities may be inadvertently integrated into MLHC. This is particularly of concern with the 'black-box' methods in many algorithms, where the relationships between the variables are unclear. Before using EMRs or other population data for MLHC, inherent biases contained in those data must be considered and ultimately addressed.

39.2.1 Social Determinants of Health

Socioeconomic status is tied to health and healthcare outcomes. The individual impact of socioeconomic factors, from health literacy and income to race and ethnicity, is difficult to separate out. Racial and ethnic minorities, as well as individuals with lower socioeconomic status, tend to suffer from poorer health outcomes and have decreased access to healthcare resources [15]. These disparities find their way into medical records and datasets, and unfairly influence models used to predict patient trajectory.

39.2.2 Population-Based Disparities

Health disparities are clearly observed when comparing demographic groups, whether based on race, ethnicity, or gender. These inequities are often reflected in clinical research.

Racial and ethnic minorities are disproportionately affected by major chronic diseases, such as hypertension, obesity, mental illnesses, and certain cancers [16]. The burden of this disease is augmented by unequal insurance coverage, socioeconomic status, and access to health services [17,18]. In solid organ transplant, for example, associations between race and ethnicity and access to transplant and survival after transplant have been observed, though these associations remain difficult to parse from socioeconomic status [19–22].

The disparities seen among racial and ethnic minorities are mirrored when considering gender and sex. Health inequalities, ranging from reproductive health to rates of suicide, were observed within the first two decades of life between females and males [23]. In liver transplant, sex-based disparities in transplant access and pre-transplant mortality are observed, even when adjusted for geography, biological size, or disease aetiology [24–28].

Although racial and ethnic minorities often bear a greater burden of disease, they are not equally represented in clinical datasets or health research [29,30]. The majority of medical research is based on studies of primarily male, white populations, increasing the risk of inaccurate clinical assessments and practices when applied to individuals outside of this population [31–33]. The Framingham Risk Score, widely used to predict cardiovascular risk, was studied primarily on white individuals. One study focusing on racial and ethnic minorities found differences in the associations drawn between risk factors and cardiovascular disease when applied to minority groups [34].

Even 'modern' research, such as in the field of precision medicine, which develops targeted therapies based on individual genomes and lifestyles, suffers from the limited inclusion of non-European participants [35]. Moreover, studies that do include racial and minority populations can inappropriately group individuals to add statistical power to their studies, inadvertently leading to the homogenization of different groups, such as populations classified as 'Asian' or 'Hispanic' [30].

Disparities in research can translate into biases in diagnostic, drug, and device development. For example, one computer model, built to aid in the diagnostic interpretation of X-rays, was found to underperform with under-represented groups, related to gender imbalance in its training datasets [36].

Under-representation in clinical research can occur for a variety of reasons, from language barriers and time constraints to inadequate recruitment or fear of exploitation [30]. When studied, however, racial and ethnic minorities were equally likely to participate in research studies when indications were contextualized and individuals were offered the opportunity [37]. In 1993, the National Institutes of Health (NIH) recognized this problem and mandated greater inclusion of racial and ethnic minorities, as well as study of gender differences, in federally funded research in the USA. Nonetheless, this mandate has been difficult to implement in practice [38]. Ultimately, the health disparities and biases developed by the exclusion of certain population groups from research may be further amplified through MLHC, without active acknowledgement and adjustment [29,30,39]. Moving forward, the lack of racial and gender diversity in research studies needs to be actively prioritized by research and recruitment communities.

39.2.3 Healthcare Provider Bias

Disparities are compounded by unconscious or implicit bias in healthcare providers and can be further perpetuated by inadequate recognition and addressment in medical education [40].

Provider biases impact patients' perceptions of care and the type of treatments offered, as well as patients' outcomes [40]. For example, female patients with acute myocardial infarctions are less likely to survive when treated by a male physician, or similarly, Black newborns have lower survival rates when treated by non-Black physicians [41,42]. Biases can be exacerbated by time constraints, ambiguity in clinical presentations, and increasing clinical and non-clinical demands on providers. In light of this, providers may unconsciously rely on stereotypes for efficient decision-making [40,43].

Historically, medical education has been modelled upon studies that have focused on Caucasian, male populations, often excluding the experiences and perspectives of other social groups, including people of colour and sexual minorities [44,45]. Given this, the standardized illness schemas and patient scenarios that have been taught may unintentionally under-prepare providers for the clinical presentations seen in minority populations [45]. Most medical schools have introduced courses regarding health disparities and prioritize community engagement to address these biases, but there are still issues to address.

39.3 Risks in Implementing Machine Learning in Healthcare

Beyond the development of MLHC algorithms, the implementation of MLHC tools can also generate biases that directly impact patient care. As with any medical intervention, unintended effects may result, and at worst patient harm may occur. Examples of biased implementation may include inequitable access to MLHC technology or the application of MLHC in situations where external factors may affect efficacy.

39.3.1 Resource-Limited and Data-Disadvantaged Communities and Countries

The use of MLHC and AI in low- and middle-income countries (LMICs) is a topic of growing research. To date, such methods have been predominantly applied to the investigation of communicable diseases, health system optimization, and patient outcome prediction models [46]. While the deployment of MLHC in LMICs carries the same challenges as in affluent settings, it also presents its own unique challenges. In addition to the selection and algorithmic biases outlined already, specific concerns regarding accessibility to digital technologies, consent, data protection, and the ethical implications of applying MLHC in LMICs need to be addressed [47].

Patients from LMICs are vastly under-represented in the development of MLHC technology [48]. In much the same way that minority demographics are often excluded from AI training datasets, patients from resource-limited settings are rarely included, despite representing a group that stands to potentially gain the most from these advancements [49]. Consequently, MLHC developed in high-income countries is unlikely to be generalizable to developing countries, due to poor external validity or model misspecifications embedded in its design [47].

The development and implementation of MLHC models in resource-limited settings may also be constrained by existing infrastructure and access to technology [49,50]. However, widespread access to mobile phones and the internet, even in some of the most remote settings, represents a method through which isolated populations can access MLHC [51,52]. Limitations in the use of mobile technologies were seen in previous humanitarian responses, in which concerns regarding data accuracy and completeness were recognized [53–55]. Of particular note was the potential that aid may have been delivered inequitably due to systematic bias, as areas that were the most damaged were more likely to have lost access to telecommunications, and therefore become unable to request aid [55,56]. This may be representative of bias occurring more broadly with the implementation of MLHC in LMICs, as those most in need may lack the technology or digital literacy to utilize such methods, resulting in the further perpetuation of health inequalities [56].

The development of cloud computing may overcome some of these issues by negating the need for resource-limited healthcare providers to purchase and maintain their own computing infrastructure [49,57]. Irrespective of access to technology, the burden of data collection must be considered as an additional barrier to the implementation of MLHC in contexts where resources are already strained. Alternatively, routinely collected data may be utilized, though as already noted, concerns regarding accuracy and completeness may exist [58].

39.3.2 Ethics of Machine Learning in Healthcare in Resource-Limited Settings

Issues regarding informed consent, and other privacy concerns, may arise with mass data collection in LMICs. Few previous studies of AI in LMICs have addressed how informed consent was obtained from individuals included in EMRs or other large datasets [46]. This is particularly true with 'function creep', whereby data are used for purposes other than those for which they were initially collected [47]. Of additional concern is that patients may feel pressured to provide consent if the receipt of care is thought to depend on the provision of their data. Data protection is also of paramount importance given the sensitive nature of health data. Variability in data protection laws, lack of expertise in data governance, the involvement of third-party private entities, and a billion-dollar medical AI industry can all threaten data confidentiality and privacy in developing countries [47,55,59,60].

Finally, the use of MLHC for resource allocation and outcome prognostication raises additional ethical concerns when applied in resource-limited settings or situations, as it may inadvertently cause harm to individual patients. When applied in affluent settings with effectively no resource constraints, MLHC may be used with the aim of identifying high-risk patients, allocating them additional resources, and improving their outcomes without any reduction in the care provided to other patients. However, in a situation where resources are limited, concerns exist that prognostic models may instead be used as a justification to withhold care to the sickest patients to whom the allocation of resources may prove futile [61,62]. By extension, if an AI model is designed with a utilitarian approach, in which the aim is to improve the outcomes of a total population, individual patients may again be 'sacrificed' in pursuit of a net benefit. If a 'black-box' method is used, wherein data inputs are not obvious, then frontline clinicians may be less aware of the value judgements encrypted in the algorithms.

39.3.3 Technologically Advanced Healthcare Systems

In contrast to LMICs and other resource-limited settings, developed countries and healthcare systems with ample resources also carry unique risks resulting from almost ubiquitous access to technology. The popularity of wearable technologies, varying from non-invasive activity trackers to implantable devices such as blood sugar monitors or insulin pumps, has created a source of continuous health information. These increasingly advanced and expensive technologies have the potential to create biases that either positively or negatively affect patients who can afford them [63]. While such devices may improve the quality, efficiency, and timeliness of care, concern exists that they may contribute to 'biosurveillance' and unknowingly provide personal health data to commercial businesses or governments [63,64]. By extension, the use of mobile apps that are marketed as medical or general 'wellness' tools may be unregulated and deter patients from seeking medical care that they falsely believe is being provided by an app [63].

The widespread use of EMRs in affluent countries has created the opportunity for extensive development and publication of MLHC tools of varying quality and usefulness. The exponential creation of healthcare technologies claiming to use MLHC methods risks creating substantial 'noise' in the medical literature, impairing healthcare providers from being able to maintain an understanding of the current evidence at any one time. A 2019 review of MLHC reported that despite more than 10,000 life science publications describing AI and machine learning in healthcare, only 29 US Food and Drug Administration (FDA)-approved medical devices or algorithms existed [65].

The application of AI and MLHC to drug development also creates the potential for inequitable provision of care. With the growing utilization of AI for the analysis of the human genome and drug discovery, concerns exist that ownership and licensing of AI technologies for this purpose may dictate research agendas and control who is able to develop medicines [63]. Furthermore, the legalities of ownership and intellectual property regarding specific medical therapies that were developed using commercial AI tools may be unclear.

39.3.4 Self-Fulfilling Prophecies

Regardless of location, predictive models and decision-support tools using MLHC methods are often considered safe, as clinicians retain control of final decisions regarding patient care – an expert-in-the-loop system. This contrasts with the concept of closed-loop systems, in which AI-determined interventions would be implemented autonomously [66]. Prognostic tools that aim to provide clinicians with insight into a patient's eventual outcome may ultimately cause an innate change in that patient's clinical trajectory – it becomes a self-fulfilling prophecy [67–72].

Self-fulfilling prophecies refer to situations where clinicians make decisions based upon a predictive model, and as a consequence of those decisions the predicted outcome is more likely to occur [67]. If a score that sought to predict in-hospital mortality suggested that a patient was almost certainly going to die, then the treating clinicians may cease curative treatments, because they anticipate further intervention to be futile. As a result, the scoring system becomes correct in its prediction. Conversely, if a score suggests that a patient is very likely to have a good outcome, then additional therapies may be implemented if the patient were to deteriorate because the clinicians expect the patient to do well.

If prediction tools developed using MLHC are inaccurate because of the biases outlined in this chapter, then the resulting care delivered to patients may be systematically altered. As the tendency of such biases is to disadvantage minorities and those already at greater risk of poor outcomes, worsening inequalities may result as prognostic scores influence clinician decisions. This risk may be greatest with the use of 'black-box' methods, which might give clinicians a false sense of impartiality in their decisions, as they presume MLHC tools to be objective and accurate.

39.4 Next Steps and Solutions

MLHC is uniquely positioned to address health disparities and change how individuals and communities interact with the healthcare system. However, conscious and deliberate effort will be required to avoid perpetuating biases [73].

39.4.1 Acknowledging Bias

As highlighted previously, the potential for biases to be conferred from healthcare workers to EMRs and medical notes is a fundamental limitation of the data sources used for training MLHC. Providing tools for self-evaluation and reflection, in both clinical practice and medical education, may reduce the risk of unconscious bias. Explicit acknowledgement of implicit biases and related behaviours through self-assessment, for example, has been shown to change clinician behaviour [40,43]. Instead of judgement-based decisions, physicians are encouraged to engage in 'perspective-taking' of patients' concerns, and to 'individuate' patients, or separate patients' clinical concerns from those of their social group, to reduce implicit biases and differences in treatments offered [40]. The strategies invoked to reduce individual provider biases, such as direct education, reflection, and individuating, can also be applied to MLHC development and analysis.

39.4.2 Advocating for Inclusion

Fundamentally, MLHC has the potential to address biases including the under-representation of certain populations, and factor in the environment in which it is being implemented. Thoughtful questioning of the information included in existing databases, with recognition of (and correction for) under-represented race, gender, socioeconomic status, and other variables, is necessary. New projects and databases should strive to actively involve under-represented populations in original research and development, both in terms of the researchers themselves and the populations they study. This may mean building upon existing policies or mandates (such as ongoing efforts by the NIH to include under-represented populations in research), acknowledging the make-up and potential biases of grant reviewers and funders, or moving primary research sites to more accessible and diverse locations [30].

Existing projects working to engage under-represented populations in research, such as the Heart Health Lenoir Project, found that active community participation led to greater retention of minority groups, likely contributing to the overall applicability of the research [74]. Adaptations such as these may be difficult to apply to groups with unobserved or difficult-to-measure characteristics, such as LGBTQ+ or displaced communities [75]. In these circumstances, it may be appealing to use a proxy measure or a well-intentioned label; however, both options could lead to further bias, as described in the next section [14,76]. Balancing the need for privacy with the desire to explicitly measure characteristics will be a unique challenge for MLHC.

39.4.3 Algorithmic Fairness

Changes to improve the inclusion of previously under-represented populations will require careful, periodical reassessment to determine their impact. In fact, these ongoing efforts, shaped in a field known as 'algorithmic fairness', have helped to advance work in racial and gender biases in particular [75].

Approaches to algorithmic fairness have been divided into 'input-focused' and 'output-focused' strategies [77]. Input-focused refers to determining which variables and labels are considered for inclusion in a MLHC model. However, it should be recognized that black-box methods may unknowingly predict and utilize protected characteristics, such as race, through a combination of other surrogate variables. To avoid such situations, only variables with an established causal relationship with the outcome should be included, though this may reduce model performance and hinder the discovery of new causative relationships [77]. Alternatively, an output-focused strategy relies on an evaluation of the final model, assessing for various indicators of fairness. Such indicators may include measures of anti-classification (protected attributes are not used to make decisions), classification parity (predictive performance is equal across subgroups), and calibration (risk scores are equivalent across subgroups), while recognizing limitations in these metrics [78]. Quantifying objective measures of bias in data and algorithms may allow for the active implementation of methods to reverse such inequalities in the design, implementation, and audit of models [79–82]. Methods may include incorporating 'fairness constraints' or 'affirmative action' rules into MLHC algorithms to proactively target equity with appropriate metrics [77,78,83]. While these actions may reduce the overall performance of a model, ensuring that an MLHC tool does not cause harm to particular populations should be prioritized. Beyond this, the nature of equity being pursued must also be canvassed, as avoiding the provision of disparate treatments versus avoiding disparate outcomes may entail fundamentally different, conflicting processes [83].

39.4.4 Systemic Change

The responsibility for ensuring that MLHC does not prejudice against specific populations extends beyond individual data scientists or clinicians. The need for regulation that mandates minimum requirements for MLHC has been recognized [84,85]. National and international bodies have released regulatory standards to guide the assessment and approval of MLHC before it is implemented into clinical practice, as would occur with any other medical device or drug [65,86,87]. In addition to mandating an assessment of bias in MLHC models, efforts to encourage open-access licensing for MLHC algorithms are slowly gaining steam, so that independent evaluations of their performance and re-calibration can be performed using local data, and clinicians and patients can better understand how MLHC tools produce their outputs. To date, this has been limited by the largely proprietary nature of MLHC, which limits transparency to clinicians, researchers, and patients who may be harmed [88]. Finally, the understanding and 'AI literacy' of clinicians using MLHC will need to be supported, so that they can be involved in creating, overseeing, and monitoring the technology, and, more importantly, recognize its potential limitations when applied at the point of care [89]. This topic is explored more extensively in Chapter 40.

MLHC has the potential to fundamentally transform healthcare by providing tools to individualize tests and treatments, and by expanding the medical knowledge base to learn from populations that were historically excluded in studies. These benefits, among numerous others, are balanced against the significant risk that MLHC may worsen existing health inequalities. By anticipating that biases can arise from the use of health-related data that mirror those of society, and actively working to mitigate the effects, the value of MLHC can be equitably distributed.

KEY INSIGHTS

- ◼ **MLHC is uniquely positioned to address health disparities and to change how individuals and communities interact with the healthcare system.**
- ◼ **Biases and disparities are embedded within EMRs. These ingrained inequalities may be inadvertently integrated into MLHC algorithms.**

- Racial and ethnic minorities often bear a greater burden of disease, yet are not equally represented in clinical datasets or health research.
- Under-represented groups need to be actively prioritized for inclusion in research studies; however, changes to improve the inclusion of previously under-represented populations will require careful, periodic reassessment to determine their impact.
- The use of MLHC for resource allocation and outcome prognostication raises additional ethical concerns when applied in resource-limited settings or situations, as it may cause harm to individual patients.
- Appropriate representation of race and gender in research studies is the best way to ensure that MLHC is a positive addition to the healthcare continuum.

References

1. Callahan A, Shah NH. Machine learning in healthcare. In: Sheikh A, Bates D, Wright A, Cresswell K (eds), *Key Advances in Clinical Informatics: Transforming Health Care through Health Information Technology*. Amsterdam: Elsevier; 2017, 279–291.
2. Apgar V. A proposal for a new method of evaluation of the newborn. *Classic Papers in Critical Care* 1952;32(449):97.
3. Knaus WA, Zimmerman JE, Wagner DP, Draper EA, Lawrence DE. APACHE-acute physiology and chronic health evaluation: a physiologically based classification system. *Critical Care Medicine* 1981;9(8):591–597.
4. Diao JA, Wu GJ, Taylor HA et al. Clinical implications of removing race from estimates of kidney function. *JAMA* 2021;325(2):184–186.
5. Levey AS, Stevens LA, Schmid CH et al. A new equation to estimate glomerular filtration rate. *Annals of Internal Medicine* 2009;150(9):604–612.
6. Eneanya ND, Yang W, Reese PP. Reconsidering the consequences of using race to estimate kidney function. JAMA 2019;322(2):113–114.
7. Levey AS, Tighiouart H, Titan SM, Inker LA. Estimation of glomerular filtration rate with vs without including patient race. *JAMA Internal Medicine* 2020;180(5):793–795.

For additional references and Further Reading please see www.wiley.com/go/byrne/aiinclinicalmedicine.

40

'Designing' Ethics into AI: Ensuring Equality, Equity, and Accessibility

Lisa Murphy

NHS England Centre for Improving Data Collaboration, London, UK

Learning Objectives

- Understand how AI can create or exacerbate health inequalities.
- Identify how inequity and bias can occur at each stage of AI development.
- Appreciate how a collaborative approach is required for identifying and mitigating inequalities from AI use in healthcare.
- Explore how ethical principles can be operationalized.

40.1 Introduction

The numerous benefits of AI are not always realized equitably across health systems or nations. Not only do disparities in access to AI exist, but algorithms and AI-driven technologies can actually introduce, or perpetuate, bias and inequality. These biases and inequalities can be introduced at each point in the AI life cycle – and often there will be interdependencies across each stage. Issues with biases in algorithms can cause a range of harms to individuals, from misdiagnoses to inappropriate treatment to poor patient experience. They can also impact healthcare delivery, inappropriately diverting resources or influencing service design. An ethical approach to AI design, development, and delivery is required to address these potential sources of harm.

In June 2021 the World Health Organization (WHO) released its principles for ethical use of AI in health [1]. One of these states that AI should 'Ensure equity', through addressing data and development choices. The WHO recognized, as a number of research studies have found previously, that there is a particular risk of racial bias being ingrained in algorithms and AI-driven technologies, in both healthcare and beyond. These ethical principles are not the first attempt to address problems of harm and inequity, but add further international consensus to a field that has been working over several decades to develop an ethical practice around the use of AI in healthcare – particularly as bioethical models designed primarily for clinical care do not adequately translate. Ethical principles around the use of AI in healthcare should serve as a starting point for rigorous guidance on determining

AI in Clinical Medicine: A Practical Guide for Healthcare Professionals, First Edition. Edited by Michael F. Byrne, Nasim Parsa, Alexandra T. Greenhill, Daljeet Chahal, Omer Ahmad, and Ulas Bagci.
© 2023 John Wiley & Sons Ltd. Published 2023 by John Wiley & Sons Ltd.
Companion website: www.wiley.com/go/byrne/aiinclinicalmedicine

and integrating ethical practice into design. While implementation through policy, regulatory, and legislative mechanisms is essential, guidance needs to be operational-ized at the appropriate level of abstraction – and considered holistically rather than as a 'tick-box' issue for compliance [2].

Algorithmic bias is often denoted as a 'data problem', but the data reflect the system they were gathered from and the individuals working within it. Any dis-criminatory structures will result in data that have bias embedded within them, as well as within the AI development process. Further, these same systems are those that will be implementing and monitoring algorithms and AI technologies, and thus that may not identify issues arising from their use.

> While many health systems and their organizations have diversity, equity, and inclusion programmes in place, these rarely focus on the use of AI, or digital technologies more broadly.

There is often a general lack of awareness of the bias and inequalities that AI can cause or perpetuate among the healthcare workforce, let alone the tools that could be used to address these.

Looking at each stage of the AI life cycle (Figure 40.1) in turn, there are a number of issues that need to be considered, as well as steps that can be taken to improve equity and accessibility.

40.2 Business and Use Case Development

The potential for inequity in health AI starts with the identification of a problem or need, and a decision to develop an algorithm to address it. The genesis of algo-rithmic development in healthcare can come from a range of sources, and this origin should be included in any ethical evaluation. It is important to consider what issues are being prioritized, whether these are addressing an established healthcare need, and who will be impacted. Ensuring that the problems and pur-poses of desired algorithms are ethical is complex, and this includes assessment of issue prioritization. Research areas that have historically been underfunded, such as diseases that predominantly affect women or minority ethnic groups, are also less likely to receive support for AI development. A lack of diversity in the healthcare and research workforce may confound this, as the sociodemographic composition of those who are determining the research and innovation priorities will impact target issue selection and the associated available funding. Ethnic and gender minority groups will also be impacted by weak incentives to develop prod-ucts for smaller markets.

Setting a clear organizational or even national strategy for AI development, prefer-ably in collaboration with patients and healthcare professionals, is vital for ensuring that innovations are developed in line with the needs of a health system. Diverse repre-sentation at a strategic level in health systems will also be required if decision-making on priorities is to account for all communities within a population. Such strategic

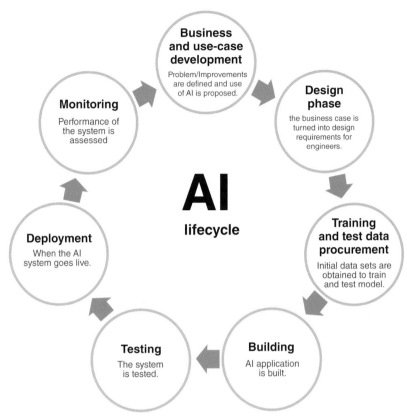

Figure 40.1: The AI lifecycle. UK Information Commissioner's Office algorithmic auditing framework.

Source: AI Lifecycle / ICO / Public domain OGL.

direction would bring numerous benefits, including facilitation of robust research to deployment pipelines that would allow tracking for potential bias and inequity throughout the AI life cycle. Without this coordination, an ad hoc approach to AI development will likely result in a disproportionate focus on areas that are 'high profile' or more prevalent in wealthier populations, leading to further health inequalities.

40.3 Design Phase

Development teams need to identify the modelling approach and associated performance metrics that will drive accuracy while preventing or minimizing disparities. They should consider the needs and social preferences of their context, to determine the ethical principles to which they will adhere. These principles should be utilized as a tool for process review throughout the design and development process, rather than viewed as an end-point to be reached. Documentation of the algorithm should include the ethical principles used, allowing users to understand if and how they align to their own population or practice.

Bias and inequality can be designed into an algorithm or AI-driven technology, particularly if the team involved in its development does not reflect, or engage with, the population it is intended to impact. The power to mitigate this lies with the team developing the algorithm, who make decisions about the critical components of its make-up. For example, using a surrogate loss function (the curve of loss generated by a model's predictions, with minimizing the loss function–enhancing model) can provide computational efficiency, but may not reflect the desired ethical criteria [4].

> Diverse development teams – across sex, gender, race, ethnicity, sexual orientation, and class – are critical to interrogating these components for fairness and providing understanding of the complexities underlying the introduction of discrimination.

Any biases of designers, developers, and researchers might inadvertently be 'designed into' any algorithm or AI-driven technology, such as through the use of label determinations that do not account for patient characteristics. In particular, if a model uses attributes such as race and gender without a clear understanding of their interplay with the outcome of interest, then there is a risk that its performance and interpretation will exacerbate inequities for a wide range of diagnostics and treatments. This has been seen in healthcare delivery more broadly, where 'race corrections' to clinical algorithms have been found to be based on outdated, suspect racial science. When selecting a target variable(s) (what the algorithm is optimizing for), it is essential to measure any potential to introduce bias early in the design process. The choice of target variable or outcome can also obscure underlying issues that are the drivers of bias, such as differences in clinical practice.

Differences in label noise can result in disparities of a model's impact [4], and so development teams have the responsibility to choose, and where possible improve, labels so that these inequalities do not further exacerbate disparities in health. They must consider how labels have been generated, such as diagnostic codes generated by a provider for reimbursement rather than research purposes (and for which incentives to under-report and/or over-report outcomes may exist) [4]. These resulting inequities can lead to unintended and permanent embedding of biases in algorithms used for clinical care.

40.4 Data

Without appropriate data to train and validate an algorithm, it will be unable to perform its intended function safely and successfully. Access to robust, representative, and unbiased data is important throughout development, as even balanced baseline data cannot ameliorate issues of imbalance in downstream tasks. Data issues can arise due to a number of causes, including the following.

40.4.1 Unrepresentative Data

Datasets may not be representative of the population that an algorithm will impact, due to under-sampling, particularly of under-served and marginalized populations. When individuals from these populations do appear in datasets, their data are less likely to be accurately captured due to errors in collection and systemic discrimination. The reasons behind this are complex, and may be due to variations in access to or delivery of healthcare, or even trust in the health system. For example, ethnic minority patients may be less likely to access services even when they have the same levels of medical need and risk as white people; think of the deterrence seen in the UK as a result of so-called hostile environment policies. These issues are compounded by research and engagement programmes designed on available data, driving further bias in datasets.

While some sampling biases can be identified and possibly corrected or adjusted for, others may be more difficult to adjust for, such as rare manifestations of diseases. Communicating to unrepresented communities that their participation in research and/or data-collection activities may lead to increased access to innovation – due to the comparative ubiquity of digital interventions, for instance through integration into electronic health records, or to a 'physical' development such as a medicine that they may need to pay for – is an important step in engendering their engagement.

40.4.2 Missing Data

Access to the right data is paramount to measuring and addressing algorithmic bias. Without data on race, ethnicity, gender, sex, sexual preference, and class, it may be difficult to test and control for fairness. In addition to the population missingness already described, missingness in datasets can be a result of:

- Variations in healthcare service availability, including access to specialist testing or more novel therapeutics. For example, larger genomics datasets often have a disproportionate number of individuals of European descent, producing genetic risk scores that are more accurate in individuals of European ancestry than in others.
- Bias in data collected during clinical trials, which disproportionately include Caucasian participants and thus result in a lack of racial and ethnic diversity.
- The 'digital divide', where disparity in access to the internet and/or digital technology means that datasets generated through use of technology or social media will be biased towards those able to utilize these platforms.
- Variables that are poorly recorded or prone to misclassification. For example, the healthcare needs and experiences of transgender and gender non-conforming individuals are not well documented in datasets because documented sex, not gender identity, is what is usually available. However, documented sex is often discordant with gender identity for transgender and gender non-conforming individuals.

40.4.3 Variations in Data Quality and Availability

Data-collection practices and platforms vary across and between health systems, leading to differences in quality and integrity. These disparities are even more pronounced on a global scale, as low- and middle-income countries have greater variation in coding and digitization of records.

40.4.4 Encoded Bias in Datasets

Data points may carry hidden bias, which can then be perpetuated in any research and innovation in which they are used. Biases among clinical staff can impact what data are recorded and how, as can those from discriminatory practices and policies that affect healthcare delivery. For example, there is evidence that Black patients are under-treated for pain, and so an algorithm developed to determine analgesic provision may under-estimate their need. Biases can also be transcribed into clinical notes, and if these are then used by natural language processing technology to pick up symptom profiles or phenotypic characteristics, those will incorporate real-world biases as well.

40.4.5 Interpretation of Data

How data points are construed and applied can also introduce bias to an algorithm. For example, the use of healthcare spending as a proxy for medical need or healthcare use has resulted in a number of problematic algorithms. As socioeconomic factors affect both access to healthcare and access to financial resources, then models that utilize this measure may yield predictions that exacerbate inequities.

Addressing these issues with the underlying data is not always straightforward, and while some can be addressed with technical interventions (e.g. to improve data quality), others will require policy or programmatic solutions. For example, encouraging health-sector organizations, research bodies, or even nation states to collaborate in AI development could improve the diversity of available data, as well as the expertise for interpreting and incorporating data points. Giving developers access to data from low- and middle-income countries has been cited as an opportunity to support data diversity issues, but there are a number of data protection concerns to be considered. Offers to pay for data may act as a perverse incentive to share, and countries or health-sector organizations may not have the skills and experience to ensure that they are receiving fair-value return for their data assets.

CASE STUDY

Health systems often use clinical prediction tools to support healthcare delivery. A study of one of these commonly used algorithms found that it discriminated against millions of African Americans, whose level of chronic illness was systematically mismeasured due to the label choice of using healthcare costs as a proxy for ill health. As the health system had a higher expenditure, on average, on white patients than on Black patients, the tool returned higher risk scores for white patients than for Black patients. These scores may then have been used to determine care pathways or resource allocation, for example resulting in more referrals for white patients to specialty services, perpetuating both spending discrepancies and race bias in health care [5].

40.5 Building

The build of an algorithm has a number of key decision points where bias and inequity can be introduced. Development teams will need to consider their modelling approach carefully, how it may be vulnerable to bias or influence inequalities, and the interplay with the data available for use. How a team builds 'fairness' into an AI model is not only a technical challenge, but an ideological one. How fairness is determined, quantified, and measured is not straightforward, and often depends on the values of the target population or health system. There may also need to be a determination of how an algorithm's accuracy and achieving fairness are balanced.

Tuning parameter selection, whether a priori or during development, can impact how generalizable a model is. This lack of generalizability is often rooted in the underlying data, with overfitting algorithms to non-representative or biased data having the potential to disproportionately harm already marginalized populations [4].

A model's build will need to adjust for confounders where possible, which can be introduced by individual or societal prejudices. These confounders can result in identification of inequalities as biological in origin, rather than due to socioeconomic or environmental factors, leading to 'automation' of bias into healthcare delivery [6]. For example, an airborne disease might appear to have a higher prevalence in a particular ethnic group, but this may be due to the group being at higher risk of living in damp and overcrowded housing, and thus of disease transmission. Confounders can be controlled by including them as features in classification or regression models. It may not, however, be possible to carry out such adjustment or current techniques may not be sufficient (e.g. as the features have a mediating or moderating effect), and so these need to be incorporated differently into model design and/or accounted for during deployment.

40.6 Testing

Algorithms need to be tested against independent datasets, drawing on real-world data where possible, as well as tested as part of an integrated care pathway and across implementation routes, for example across different imaging machines or electronic health record vendors. Understanding the nuances of the deployment context and evaluating AI performance within it are necessary to identify any potential sources of harm that may emerge, with multi-disciplinary working across technical and clinical staff crucial to share expertise. The target population for an algorithm should also be involved in deployment planning, with engagement strategies exploring how its use will impact their health and healthcare experience. For example, a tool that allocates healthcare appointments may inadvertently adversely impact patients without access to private transport, or may need to be available in multiple languages in order to ensure broad accessibility across the target population.

Commonly used performance metrics, such as area under the receiver operating characteristic curve, only give an indication of global performance. It is therefore key that algorithmic performance is assessed for subgroups within the target population, as while a model may perform well overall, it may not when results are broken down for different groups. Development teams must also test against their fairness metrics during evaluation, to both check for inequity and also validate that these metrics are appropriate for post-deployment monitoring.

While there is work to authenticate more apt and flexible approaches to AI evaluation in healthcare, randomized clinical trials remain the most common way for this to be carried out. The SPIRIT-AI and CONSORT-AI initiative is an international collaborative effort to improve the transparency and completeness of reporting of clinical trials evaluating interventions involving AI [7,8]. This provides guidance on good trial design and reporting, and supports improved transparency, with clear documentation allowing for review into the data-collection and model-development process (see Chapter 42).

CASE STUDY

A research team in Canada developed an AI tool to analyse speech patterns that would allow for identification of early signs of Parkinson's disorder. Despite performing well in evaluation, there were a number of issues with misdiagnoses upon deployment. Investigation by the team discovered that all of the misdiagnoses occurred in individuals for whom English was their second language, as their different patterns of speech were picked up as unusual by the algorithm, which had only been trained on the speech of native speakers.

40.7 Deployment

A development team's post-deployment considerations may not fully account for the impact of deploying a biased model into healthcare settings, particularly if they lack diversity or relevant expertise for the deployment setting. Again, multi-disciplinary working is required to ensure a safe and equitable approach to deployment.

There are a number of human factors that will influence the contribution of an algorithm or AI-driven technology to inequalities. This is more likely to occur in settings where users do not have knowledge or experience of how algorithms or AI-driven technologies work, and thus may not adhere to the developers' instructions for use. For example, clinicians who over-rely on AI to support their decision-making may accept an algorithm's determination even when its models are erroneous, while other clinicians who distrust AI to perform or inform decisions about their patients' care might decide to ignore or adjust its outputs, even if it offers a bias correction.

> **Health-sector organizations must ensure that staff involved in AI deployment have adequate training to understand how to use it safely and equitably – with this understanding also being key for building trust in AI integration into healthcare settings**.

Organizations or health systems deploying AI should ensure that they communicate transparently to their populations on what algorithms are being used, for what purpose, and under what scrutiny [6]. They should also provide avenues for feedback, helping to bring a 'human-centric' approach to algorithmic deployment. This transparency, along with accountability mechanisms for addressing any issues that arise, is important for establishing trust in the use of AI in healthcare. Such an approach has been taken by the city of Amsterdam, which has established an 'Algorithm Register' that provides an overview of the AI systems and algorithms that it uses.

Algorithms and AI-driven technologies cannot necessarily be transferred across deployment settings. For example, even with appropriately diverse training datasets, AI tools developed in high-income nations cannot reliably be rolled out in low-income countries, due to differences in disease profiles. Additionally, AI-driven technologies lauded as answers to global challenges facing health systems, such as algorithms to assess medical images and thus alleviate radiological workforce shortages, will only be available where the technical infrastructure exists for their use.

40.8 Monitoring

Once an algorithm is in use, it is important that there is continuous monitoring of its deployment, such as through regular 'auditing' to assess outcomes for bias or inequity – including a foresight analysis to identify potential future harms. It is possible that any action to adjust the model may increase or decrease its performance for a given subpopulation, and so any change should trigger consideration of an evaluation exercise. Organizations or health systems utilizing these algorithms should perform their own audit activity to identify and mitigate any risk to fairness, security, or human rights. The UK Information Commissioner's Office has developed an AI auditing framework to support organizations in undertaking these activities [3].

> As part of a holistic ethical approach to ongoing evaluation, development teams should openly report their results and algorithmic code for error-checking, and assess for clinical benefit and cost savings rather than algorithmic effectiveness alone.

Where and by whom clinical or cost benefit is being realized should be considered against the demographics of the target population, determining whether these are being distributed as fairly as anticipated.

Importantly, the use of algorithms that introduce or drive inequalities can create a feedback loop whereby they influence the system, its data, and thus further AI development. They should therefore not be viewed in isolation, but as part of the wider digital infrastructure that supports population health and healthcare delivery.

40.9 Conclusion

There are no formulaic or immediate fixes to prevent AI from introducing bias or perpetuating inequalities in healthcare, with a system-wide approach needed to address the complexity of potential sources. Collaboration across sectors, as well as within the international health community, to share knowledge and experience (especially of where harms have been detected) is needed for the development of an evidence base. This community of practice needs to leverage this evidence into establishment of robust standards and validated mitigation approaches for addressing bias in health AI, realizing ethical principles as ethical practice.

KEY INSIGHTS

When developing, assessing, or procuring an algorithm or AI-driven technology, clinical teams should consider:

- The problem that this innovation is trying to address, who selected it, and what the motivation for this was.
- Whether the dataset utilized was representative of the target population, and what biases may have become ingrained within it.
- Whether selection of the algorithm's target outcome and modelling approach took into account the possibility of bias, and if it has appropriately adjusted for confounders.
- How patients and healthcare professionals have been involved in the design, evaluation, and deployment strategy of the algorithm.
- How the evaluation process has assessed for bias and inequalities, including algorithmic impact on clinical outcomes and cost-effectiveness.
- The approach to auditing the algorithms that developers are undertaking, and how findings of this will be made available.

References

1. World Health Organization. *Ethics and Governance of Artificial Intelligence for Health*, June 2021. `https://www.who.int/publications/i/item/9789240029200`.
2. Morley J, Elhalal A, Garcia F. Ethics as a service: a pragmatic operationalisation of AI ethics. *Minds and Machines* 2021;3:239–256.
3. Information Commissioner's Office. An overview of the Auditing Framework for Artificial Intelligence and its core components, 26 March 2019. `https://ico.org.uk/about-the-ico/media-centre/ai-blog-an-overview-of-the-auditing-framework-for-artificial-intelligence-and-its-core-components`.
4. Chen I, Pierson E, Rose S. Ethical machine learning in health care. *Annual Review of Biomedical Data Science* 2021;4:123–144.
5. Obermeyer Z, Powers B, Vogeli C. Dissecting racial bias in an algorithm used to manage the health of populations. *Science* 2019;366(6464):447–453.
6. McCradden M, Joshi S, Mazwi M. Ethical limitations of algorithmic fairness solutions in health care machine learning. *Lancet Digital Health* 2020;2(5):221–223.
7. Rivera SC, The SPIRIT-AI and CONSORT-AI Working Group, Liu X, et al. Guidelines for clinical trial protocols for interventions involving artificial intelligence: the SPIRIT-AI extension. *Nature Medicine* 2020;26:1351–1363.

For additional references please see `www.wiley.com\go\byrne\aiinclinical medicine`.

41

Making AI Work: Designing and Evaluating AI Systems in Healthcare

Niels van Berkel

Department of Computer Science, Aalborg University, Aalborg, Denmark

---

Learning Objectives

- Understand the field of human–computer interaction (HCI), as well as have an overview of relevant work in this area for further reading.
- Understand some of the factors that support the alignment of AI systems with the needs of medical professionals, patients, and other relevant stakeholders.
- Recognize the importance of stakeholder involvement when designing human-AI systems in healthcare.
- Consider the role and importance of a study's ecological validity, longitudinal assessments, validation across diverse datasets, and iterative development when designing human-AI systems in healthcare.
- Discuss recommendations for the development of AI systems in healthcare, with lessons learned from prior deployments.

41.1 Introduction

Promising stories of AI have set sky-high expectations for its ability to transform medical practice. However, living up to even the more modest expectations will require careful consideration of how medical professionals will interact with this technology and how we can successfully embed AI systems within day-to-day clinical practice. Previous attempts at introducing technology into the medical context, such as electronic health records [1], have not been unanimously successful [2]. This is despite what is often initial optimism regarding a technology's ability to transform healthcare. Similarly, in the recent and ongoing battle against COVID-19, many AI systems were developed to support the diagnosis and triaging of patients, the impact of which was ultimately limited [3]. These challenges highlight the difficulties of designing and evaluating digital systems for use in the healthcare context, which may be further exacerbated if the technology does not meet the needs of medical professionals. Yet the potential for AI systems to support medical professionals is

AI in Clinical Medicine: A Practical Guide for Healthcare Professionals, First Edition. Edited by Michael F. Byrne, Nasim Parsa, Alexandra T. Greenhill, Daljeet Chahal, Omer Ahmad, and Ulas Bagci.
© 2023 John Wiley & Sons Ltd. Published 2023 by John Wiley & Sons Ltd.
Companion website: www.wiley.com/go/byrne/aiinclinicalmedicine

vast, covering areas such as diagnosis, prognosis, guided surgery, and assisting in the training of medical personnel. This chapter provides a starting point for developers and clinicians interested in the design and evaluation of AI systems in a healthcare context.

The field of human–computer interaction (HCI) has developed methods and guidelines on how to design and evaluate digital systems so that they align with the needs of the system's users. As a research discipline, HCI has been described as sitting at the intersection of computer science and psychology [4]. Combining these two disciplines and following a mindset in which the user of the system is central in developing new technology, HCI has stressed the importance of understanding user needs and the context in which the technology will be used in order to create successful digital systems. More recently, HCI researchers and practitioners have begun to shift their attention and expertise to the design of AI systems. Following the aforementioned focus on the human stakeholders in any technology, this work has been described as human-AI [5] or human-centred AI [6].

In this chapter, we provide concrete recommendations for the development of AI systems in healthcare. HCI and related disciplines have a long history of contributing to the healthcare technology landscape [7]. While AI has only recently matured to be deployed in real-world applications, experiences obtained in the design and evaluation of non-AI-based systems provide valuable lessons that similarly apply to AI technology design. Through examples from the literature and based on our own experiences in designing and evaluating AI systems, we will illustrate lessons learned from prior deployments. The following section provides a high-level overview of the contributions and history of HCI-driven work in healthcare. This is followed by this chapter's two primary contributions: recommendations for the *design* and *evaluation* of human-AI systems in healthcare.

How do we design systems that medical professionals want to use in their day-to-day activities? Beyond the critical aspect of ensuring the accuracy of these AI systems, the usability and user experience of this technology are vital in ensuring adoption. Failing to meet these aspects will result in the system being abandoned, regardless of its potential in improving healthcare quality or efficiency. The evaluation of human-AI systems is complex, as system behaviour depends heavily on the input received and subsequent assessment of the algorithm. This makes evaluation less predictable. This level of unpredictability, combined with a medical context in which the evaluation of prototype systems on actual patients is often not considered, raises novel challenges for assessing AI systems. However, evaluation is critical, as it can reveal essential shortcomings in a system prior to eventual deployment.

Finally, we outline open research questions that have not been extensively discussed within the literature but require further investigation. These problems deal with embedding AI technology in a team rather than supporting one individual, involving patients in algorithm-driven decision-making, and effectively sharing tasks between the human operator and the AI system.

41.2 Background in Human–Computer Interaction

Prior to the recent increase in AI-driven systems, HCI researchers and practitioners have already gained a wide range of experience in designing interactive systems. Of course, many of the lessons learnt over the past decades will help design useful and effective AI systems. One of the central terminologies used in HCI when designing a digital system is 'usability'. Usability is defined as 'The extent to which a product can be used by specified users to achieve specified goals with effectiveness, efficiency and satisfaction in a specified context of use' [8]. As is clear from the definition, the specification of a system's intended users, goals, and context of use plays a prominent role in determining the usability of a system. Therefore, before developing any system, it is critical to understand the intended users, their goals, and the context in which the system will be used.

The tragic story of Therac-25 is an often-presented case that highlights the potential consequences of a technology that does not sufficiently consider the user or the daily use of the system in its design [9]. Therac-25 was a computerized radiation therapy system used in the USA and Canada to treat patients in the 1980s. After operators of the machine entered the desired radiation dosage, the machine sometimes gave radiation to patients that was hundreds of times greater than the norm. Following several fatal accidents, an investigation revealed that a combination of different factors, including errors in software design, development practices, and user interaction, resulted in massive overdoses of the radiation administered to patients [9]. Considerations for human factors and the design of user interfaces, the layer through which users provide input to a system and subsequently receive output, have since grown substantially. By 1995, James Reason highlighted that 'Human rather than technical failures now represent the greatest threat to complex and potentially hazardous systems' [10]. HCI and related disciplines have since studied human error in a variety of healthcare contexts, for example in the frequently occurring task of numerical entry [11], and in clinical decision-making such as determining correct prescriptions [12]. This increased understanding of human errors has resulted in numerous heuristics to support the design of user interfaces [13,14].

Moving beyond the usability of individual systems, the 1990s saw a shift in thinking towards supporting groups of people working together. Described by Bannon as a transition 'from human factors to human actors' [15], the interaction between users and system was no longer restricted to a one-on-one relationship but allowed for multiple persons to make use of one or even multiple devices collaboratively. Popular platforms like Google Docs and Microsoft Teams highlight the possibilities of this type of multi-device collaboration. Examples within the healthcare context include the early study of working collaboratively and simultaneously with digital and analogue patient records [16], the physical coordination and distribution of work in hospitals [17], and designing technology to support telemedicine [18].

See Fitzpatrick and Ellingsen for a detailed overview of collaboration-focused contributions in the healthcare context [7].

A last major direction within HCI research is a move towards ubiquitous and context-aware computing [19]. Ubiquitous computing describes the notion that computing can appear at any location and is no longer restricted to dedicated desktop-based workplaces [20]. Instead, tablets and smart phones now enable healthcare workers to input and interact with patient data anywhere. These technical possibilities have allowed healthcare technology to leave the hospital and be part of patients' daily lives through smart phone applications and wearable devices [21]. The increasing miniaturization of hardware has furthermore enabled the use of sensors to monitor patients' vital signs or track the flow of patients and equipment in the hospital [22].

Modern digital systems often combine all these focus areas, recognizing the need for usable systems that support real-world collaboration and combine the unique capabilities of multiple devices. As such, prior work in HCI provides the building blocks for AI technology that is usable and aligns with the needs of its end-users. To make AI systems 'work' in the modern healthcare environment, system designers need to provide a clearly understood interface that supports patient safety, enables collaboration between clinical team members, and support data collection, evaluation, and decision-making both inside the hospital and outside in the patients' day-to-day life.

41.3 Designing Human-AI in Healthcare

The design of AI-driven systems introduces novel challenges. In comparison to non-AI-based systems, in which the system's behaviour can be largely pre-defined, the uncertainty of the system's behaviour is much higher [23]. Furthermore, given the novelty of the technology, users are likely uncertain as to what level of support they can expect and, equally important, what type of support the system is unable to provide. Other questions include the long-term effect of the technology on skills development and the possible replacement of human workers. Like the design of non-AI-based systems, however, it is vitally important to involve the envisioned end-users and other relevant stakeholders in the early stages of the design process. In this section, we outline recommendations for the design of human-AI systems in a healthcare context.

41.3.1 Stakeholder Involvement

HCI researchers have long argued for the inclusion of relevant stakeholders early in the design and development process. Within the health domain, these stakeholders typically consist of medical professionals (e.g. nurses, clinicians) and other relevant roles such as patients, family members, and hospital support staff. By involving relevant stakeholders early on in designing a new system, we can grasp the problem domain more clearly, thereby increasing the chance that the eventual outcome will align with real-world problems.

Relevant stakeholders can provide useful information to inform the system's functionality based on their prior experiences and expectations. Techniques for collecting data from these stakeholders include interviews, observations of work-related activities, and focus group discussions. Data collected via these methods are typically converted to concrete user requirements as part of the overall system development process. Different forms of end-user involvement can be considered. For an in-depth discussion of different types of end-user involvement, see Noyes and Baber on user-centred design [24] and Muller and Kuhn on participatory design [25]. Regardless of the exact strategy chosen for end-user involvement, involving relevant stakeholders early on in the development of medical technology is critical to ensure the applicability of the developed system in a real-world context.

> KEY INSIGHT 1: **Collect requirements and expectations from the intended end-users during the initial stages of the project to ensure real-world relevance and fit.**
>
> KEY INSIGHT 2: **Ensure representative end-users of the system are involved in the design and evaluation of your system.**

41.3.2 Explaining AI Decisions

An often-discussed downside of AI systems is the opaque nature of their behaviour, which makes it challenging to determine why certain decisions were made. Moving away from this so-called black-box behaviour, there is an increasing interest in explainable AI. Particularly in the context of healthcare, in which any decision can have far-reaching consequences, relevant stakeholders need to understand why an AI support system would recommend or even autonomously carry out a given action. Providing an insight into the reasoning of these systems can prevent errors, as a medical expert can intervene when incorrect conclusions are drawn.

What makes for a usable explanation differs between stakeholders – for example, clinicians require a different explanation model than patients. As per Key Insights 1 and 2, recognizing user needs is critical to recognizing the type of explanations that might be helpful to specific end-users. For example, prior work highlights that explanations of AI suggestions do not necessarily need to be provided immediately when generated, as such explanations can interrupt physicians during tasks such as surgery, where attention is critical [26].

> KEY INSIGHT 3: **Explanations of an AI system's behaviour align with the needs of the target user group.**

41.3.3 Fit for Context

Existing algorithms typically form the basis of novel AI systems. While this makes for an effective starting point, any new system will need to be designed around the requirements of the context in which it is deployed. This includes both the technical fit of the system, such as whether the data on which the system is trained match the real-world context in which it is deployed, as well as the fit to the user's task. A recent example of poor contextual fit is found in an AI-driven retinal assessment deployment by Google in Thailand. In analysing the system's performance during deployment, Beede et al. highlight how the system often failed when presented with the images provided by the nurses due to poor lighting conditions and the high patient throughput [27]. With more than a fifth of the images rejected, the system subsequently assigned patients to see a specialist on a different day, even when nurses assessed the image they took of a patient as negative. This highlights the potential negative consequences that a poor fit for context can have, resulting in additional work for both patients and medical professionals. When considering the fit of a system to a specific task, the interface between user and system plays a critical role. In designing the visual markers of an AI endoscopy support system, Van Berkel et al. overlaid AI suggestions on patient video footage in a colour very distinct to the colour of the colon wall to ensure that the suggestion would be most visible [26]. This design decision was subsequently evaluated with endoscopists.

> **KEY INSIGHT 4: Align the design of the human-AI system with the specific characteristics of the context in which it is used.**

41.4 Evaluating Human-AI in Healthcare

Before deploying any AI system, it is critical to evaluate its use in a realistic setting. Although lab-based simulations can be used to indicate the accuracy of an AI system, evaluating a system in a clinical environment where people use it outside the development team can highlight previously unconsidered problems. This section outlines the key aspects in evaluating a human-AI system to be used in the healthcare context.

41.4.1 Representing Reality

When considering the evaluation of AI systems, it is critical to consider the day-to-day reality in which the system will be used. The closer the alignment between the evaluation and reality, the more valuable the insights of a conducted evaluation are. This notion is called 'ecological validity', and is defined by Carter et al. as 'the extent to which a study comprises "real-world" use of a system' [28]. Ecological validity is not a straightforward binary state in which a study either achieves or fails to achieve ecological validity. Instead, the concept consists of a wide range of dimensions. The degree to which ecological validity can be achieved is often restricted by practical, ethical, or other limitations. Van Berkel et al. highlight seven primary dimensions of ecological validity as encountered in clinical usability evaluations: user roles, environment, training, scenario, patient involvement, software, and hardware [29]. As stressed in their article, it is impossible to obtain an 'optimal configuration' on each dimension. Instead, it is critical to identify the trade-offs presented in a study to increase ecological validity where possible. For example, while it is often unfeasible to involve actual patients in a medical evaluation, the use of simulated patients has proven effective for training and evaluation purposes [30].

> **KEY INSIGHT 5: Identify and describe the most relevant dimensions of an evaluation's ecological validity prior to evaluation.**
>
> **KEY INSIGHT 6: Maximize a study's ecological validity within the given constraints, and actively consider the effect of these constraints on evaluation outcomes.**

41.4.2 Longitudinal Assessment

Usability evaluations typically focus on questions such as 'Can a user complete the task they set out to do?' and 'Are the instructions and output results clear?' Such usability evaluations are typically of limited duration (i.e. spanning less than one hour), in which the participant is asked to complete a set of typical work-related tasks. Well suited to identifying problems in the design of user interfaces and workflow-related errors, usability evaluations cannot answer all questions in the evaluation of human-AI systems. In particular, understanding the effects of introducing a new AI system into a healthcare organization requires a longitudinal assessment.

Prior work highlights that our interaction with technology changes over time [31,32], with initial interest in a new technological artifact typically waning after a while. Consider, for example, the many activity trackers collecting dust in bedroom drawers after an initial couple of weeks of intense use. This phenomenon is known as the novelty effect. In the medical context, the non-adoption or abandonment of technological solutions is common [33,34] An investigation into this phenomenon by Greenhalgh et al. points to seven aspects that impact technology adoption, including the condition or illness, the technology, and the wider (institutional and societal) context [34]. Greenhalgh et al. furthermore point to the impact of time as a crucial element in an organization's adaptation to introducing a new system. Time allows medical staff and other employees to integrate the technology into their daily workflow or opt to abandon the system altogether. Therefore, it is critical to evaluate systems over an extensive period of deployment to collect insights on the technology's adoption by the intended users.

> **KEY INSIGHT 7: Conduct long-term evaluations to evaluate the adoption and impact of novel systems.**

41.4.3 Validating across Diverse Datasets

AI-driven decision-making relies heavily on the data on which it is trained. A well-known issue in AI systems is the lack of a broad representation in these datasets, most commonly due to limitations in the diversity of race or gender in historical data. Such disparities in the data can result in unexpected and unintended consequences when the system is faced with a person from a group under-represented in the data [35]. This is far from a theoretical problem. Historical data show that, for example, from 2003 to 2009 women were less likely to receive optimal care related to artery diseases in US hospitals compared to men [36]. Such disparities in the rate at which patients received lipid-lowering medications, for instance, will continue with the introduction of algorithmic decision-making if that is trained on biased historical data. Furthermore, and perhaps even more concerning, the opaque nature of the majority of current AI systems essentially hides the underlying reasons for the decision outcome. Given the inherent risk of hidden bias in AI-driven decision-making, it is essential to evaluate an algorithm's performance across a diverse dataset and validate whether the assessments made across the dataset are valid.

> **KEY INSIGHT 8: Validate the decisions made by an AI system across a diverse dataset to identify potential biases and shortcomings in the training data.**

41.4.4 Iterative Development

Lastly, the results of any evaluation should feed back into the system's development to ensure that any identified shortcomings can be resolved. Repeatedly carrying out the process of development and evaluation is known as iterative development [37] and allows for a rapid and agile development process in which the initial requirements of the system are adjusted and refined based on the feedback collected during evaluations. Furthermore, it supports the development and evaluation of individual aspects of a system's software. This is often a necessity, given the many sub-systems that make up the entire system. It is generally recommended to assess the effectiveness of early-stage prototypes with the intended end-users, rather than waiting for a complete system implementation before evaluating the system with users. The early evaluation of prototype implementations ultimately reduces development time, as initial end-user feedback can highlight wrong directions in the development process.

> **KEY INSIGHT 9: Elicit feedback from end-users early on in the development process and iterate development based on user feedback.**

41.5 Open Research Questions

While the development of AI has taken great leaps forward over the past decades in terms of technical capabilities, much work remains to be done to integrate and operationalize AI technology in daily medical practice. This chapter outlines recommendations and best practices for designing and evaluating AI systems in a healthcare context, while acknowledging that the development of best practices is still under development. To inspire and outline future research opportunities in this critical domain, we highlight three open research questions:

- How to support collaborative work in AI-based systems.
- How to involve patients in algorithm-driven decision-making.
- How to design effective task sharing.

41.5.1 Supporting Collaborative Work

Teamwork and collaboration play an essential role in daily healthcare practice and have been described as a necessary element to provide safe, efficient, and patient-centred care [38]. However, most AI systems in healthcare are designed around the notion of a single end-user, providing limited support and tools that allow people to share the input to an AI-support system. In a review of teamwork in dynamic healthcare contexts (e.g. operating rooms, intensive care), Manser identifies patterns of communication, coordination, and leadership that positively affect clinical teamwork [39]. Future AI-driven support systems must incorporate these critical elements not only to support one clinician, but instead to be able to support a team of medical experts.

A promising direction for this is presented in the work by Bardram and Houben on 'collaborative affordances' [40]. Collaborative affordances are defined as 'a relation between a [physical and/or digital] artifact and a set of human actors, that affords the opportunity for these actors to perform a collaborative action within a specific social context' [40]. Within the context of medical records, Bardram and Houben identify four collaborative affordances – 'portability', 'collocated access', 'shared overview', and 'mutual awareness' – which allow for collaboration between medical staff. These affordances, among others, are largely missing from contemporary medical AI systems, prohibiting information sharing and collaboration.

41.5.2 Shared Decision-Making

Effective communication between patients and medical professionals is critical in achieving a successful care trajectory [41]. A widely established concept within the patient–professional relationship is that of shared decision-making [41,42]. Charles et al. define shared decision-making via four criteria: '(1) that at least two participants, physician and patient, be involved; (2) that both parties share information; (3) that both parties take steps to build a consensus about the preferred treatment; and (4) that an agreement is reached on the treatment to implement' [42]. Elwyn et al. highlight that shared decision-making is based on the introduction of choice to the patient, describing different treatment options, and assisting patients in exploring their preferences to arrive at a decision [41]. As seen from these definitions, it is critical for a patient to understand the benefits, trade-offs, and necessity of different treatment options.

The introduction of AI support systems essentially introduces a third party to the shared decision-making process, in which an AI system can support in the identification and selection of suitable treatment options. While the concept of AI explainability has been explored from the perspective of medical professionals (see Cai et al. on dealing with imperfect AI in pathology [43]), the patient perspective in dealing with AI remains under-explored in the current literature. Determining where and how AI support can be integrated into the shared decision-making process is an essential research trajectory given the increased reliance on AI technology by clinical professionals. Failing to ensure that patients can understand and engage with this new technology will ultimately undermine the concept of shared decision-making.

41.5.3 Effective Task Sharing

The ongoing development of AI will increase the types of tasks that AI systems can carry out autonomously. This makes AI support systems more powerful and will require more effective techniques for sharing (sub-)tasks between the human operator and the AI system. For example, even advanced AI systems will encounter scenarios in which their uncertainty exceeds a pre-determined threshold. At this point, a human expert must step in and take over from the AI system to make a decision. This behaviour can already be found in today's autonomous driving systems and will increasingly manifest itself in the healthcare context.

Sujan et al. highlight the various steps required for such task handovers to be successful: the AI system has to recognize its limitations, decide on which elements to hand over, determine how this handover should be accomplished, and decide when it ought to be carried out [44]. Each of these steps requires further investigation of user needs, contextual requirements, and technical capabilities. Prior work has suggested the design of structured communication protocols between the user and AI system, as currently exist in handover protocols between medical professionals [44]. Similarly, a medical professional handing over a task to an AI system requires a pre-defined protocol and interface that outline the expected AI behaviour and provide appropriate mechanisms for the user to intervene if needed.

41.6 Conclusion

Despite the numerous challenges facing the deployment of AI in real medical contexts and applications, AI is likely to transform modern-day healthcare. To maximize its potential, however, we need to ensure that the AI systems we put out into the world align with the needs of medical professionals, patients, and other relevant stakeholders. This chapter outlines the primary steps required to design and evaluate AI systems that bridge computational possibilities and real-world needs and conditions. We highlight the necessity of involving relevant stakeholders early on in the design of human-AI systems. Insights obtained from these stakeholders inform the intended end-users' needs, for example in critical areas such as AI explainability and the unique aspects of the context of use. Subsequently, this chapter provides recommendations for evaluating human-AI systems in a healthcare context, stressing the need for ecologically valid and longitudinal evaluations to obtain the most relevant insights. AI-driven systems provide novel challenges in their evaluation due to the relative unpredictability of their behaviour and concerns about bias introduced into AI decision-making. Furthermore, we highlight open research questions, indicating that while AI technology has made tremendous leaps forward, an extensive amount of work is still required to provide medical professionals with AI systems that can truly be embedded into their everyday tasks. We hope that the recommendations outlined in this work can provide a stepping stone for both medical professionals and system developers who are new to the application of human-AI in healthcare.

References

1. Ratwani RM, Savage E, Will A et al. A usability and safety analysis of electronic health records: a multi-center study. *Journal of the American Medical Informatics Association* 2018;25(9):1197–1201.
2. Kaplan B, Harris-Salamone KD. Health IT success and failure: recommendations from literature and an AMIA workshop. *Journal of the American Medical Informatics Association* 2009;16(3):291–299.
3. The Alan Turing Institute. *Data science and AI in the age of COVID-19 – report*, 2021. https://www.turing.ac.uk/research/publications/data-science-and-ai-age-covid-19-report.
4. Carroll JM. Human-computer interaction: psychology as a science of design. *Annual Review of Psychology* 1997;48:61–83.
5. Amershi A, Weld D, Vorvoreanu M et al. *Guidelines for Human-AI Interaction*. New York: Association for Computing Machinery; 2019, 1–13.
6. Xu W. Toward human-centered AI: a perspective from human-computer interaction. *Interactions* 2019;26(4):42–46.
7. Fitzpatrick G, and Ellingson G. A review of 25 years of CSCW research in healthcare: contributions, challenges and future agendas. *Computer Supported Cooperative Work* 2013;22(4):609–665.

For additional references and Further Reading please see www.wiley.com/go/byrne/aiinclinicalmedicine.

42

Demonstrating Clinical Impact for AI Interventions: Importance of Robust Evaluation and Standardized Reporting

Gagandeep Sachdeva[1], Diana Han[1,2], Pearse A. Keane[3], Alastair K. Denniston[1,2,3,4], and Xiaoxuan Liu[1,2,4]

[1] College of Medical and Dental Sciences, University of Birmingham, Birmingham, UK

[2] Centre for Regulatory Science and Innovation, Birmingham Health Partners, University of Birmingham, Birmingham, UK

[3] National Institute of Health Research Biomedical Research Centre for Ophthalmology, Moorfields Hospital London NHS Foundation Trust and University College London, Institute of Ophthalmology, London, UK

[4] University Hospitals Birmingham NHS Foundation Trust, Birmingham, UK

Learning Objectives

- Clinical evaluation of AI systems is necessary to provide evidence that they are accurate, safe, and effective.
- It is important that clinical evaluation of AI systems is performed iteratively, given the vulnerabilities of AI systems, such as tendency to overfit on training data and poor generalizability to new data examples.
- Robust clinical evidence provides the necessary assurance that the AI system is sufficiently safe and robust to progress to the next evaluation stage and for real-world implementation.
- To ensure the minimum information is included when reporting clinical evidence, a number of AI-specific reporting guidelines (SPIRIT-AI, CONSORT-AI, STARD-AI, TRIPOD-AI and DECIDE-AI) have been, or are being, developed to help authors and readers.

AI in Clinical Medicine: A Practical Guide for Healthcare Professionals, First Edition. Edited by Michael F. Byrne, Nasim Parsa, Alexandra T. Greenhill, Daljeet Chahal, Omer Ahmad, and Ulas Bagci.
© 2023 John Wiley & Sons Ltd. Published 2023 by John Wiley & Sons Ltd.
Companion website: www.wiley.com/go/byrne/aiinclinicalmedicine

42.1 Clinical Evaluation and Study Design for AI in Clinical Medicine

Clinical studies provide evidence as to whether health interventions are effective, and if they will provide the desired outcome for patients and the healthcare system. Clinical evaluation in the context of an AI intervention can be considered an iterative pathway from proof of concept, to in silico evaluation of performance, to real-world evaluation of performance, and to real-world evaluation of outcomes. This stepwise approach allows the necessary safety and performance evidence to be collected, in order to justify proceeding to the next step, which may change the clinical care pathway (thus carrying a higher risk of harm). To be useful, studies should be designed to minimize bias, provide confidence in the results, and therefore provide assurance for decision-makers at each stage to proceed to the next step of evaluation and subsequent real-world implementation.

For AI health interventions, it is even more important that such a stepwise approach is followed, given the known vulnerabilities of AI systems, including the tendency to overfit on training data, learn spurious correlations in data features, and generalize poorly on new data [1–3]. To date, most AI studies in clinical medicine have been retrospective studies, where the patient sample is represented in data rather than patients, and the outcome is the AI system's ability to correctly classify disease status [4–6]. These can be considered proof-of-concept, or early, in silico studies of test performance, but cannot reliably demonstrate how the AI system will perform on new data examples or how it will affect the upstream and downstream clinical pathway. We know the performance of AI systems in silico may not translate into performance in vivo, due to complex technical and human factors [7,8].

As such, AI technologies that demonstrate promising results in retrospective studies should proceed to prospective clinical studies and seek to replicate the results in real-world clinical implementation. Prospective studies allow the downstream and collateral consequences to be measured, and may reveal unintended consequences once implemented [7,9]. Prospective studies may also be observational, where the AI system is evaluated without any change to the clinical pathway. This helps to reduce the risk of harmful consequences if insufficient safety evidence exists. Beyond this, randomized control trials (RCT) remain the benchmark of clinical studies, where key study elements help to minimize bias and increase confidence in the findings. Importantly, RCTs offer the advantage of a counterfactual in the control arm, allowing comparative evidence to be collected [10]. To date, only a handful of prospective comparative trials have been conducted for AI health interventions (Table 42.1).

Where possible, studies should be designed to evaluate impact on the whole clinical pathway, and to understand the outcome for an end-point that is robust and

Table 42.1: Summary of Published Clinical Trials Evaluating Ai Systems.

Publication	Target disease/ outcome	Intervention and control	Summary of results
Diagnosis and AI			
Wang et al. 2019 [11]	Colonic adenoma	AI-assisted real-time polyp detection (n = 522) and routine colonoscopy (n = 536)	Significantly improved adenoma detection rate with AI system (p < 0.001)
Wang et al. 2020 [12]	Colonic adenoma	Deep learning polyp detection system (n = 484) and a sham system (n = 478)	Significantly improved adenoma detection rate with AI (p = 0.030)
Su et al. 2020 [13]	Colonic adenoma	AI polyp detection system (n = 308) and routine colonoscopy (n = 315)	Significantly improved adenoma detection rate (p < 0.001), bowel preparation (p = 0.023) and longer withdrawal time (p < 0.001) with AI system
Gong et al. 2020 [14]	Colonic adenoma	AI adenoma detection system (n = 355) and routine colonoscopy (n = 349)	Significantly improved adenoma detection rate with AI (p = 0.001)
Repici et al. 2020 [15]	Colonic adenoma	AI adenoma detection system (n = 341) and routine colonoscopy (n = 344)	Significantly improved adenoma detection rate with AI (p < 0.001). AI picked up a significantly higher proportion of adenomas smaller than 5 mm (p = 0.038) and between 6 and 9 mm (p = 0.025), regardless of morphology or location
Wang et al. 2020 [16]	Colonic adenoma	AI adenoma detection system (n = 184) and routine colonoscopy (n = 185)	Significantly reduced adenoma (p < 0.0001) and polyp (p < 0.0001) miss rate with AI. Significantly reduced adenoma miss rate in ascending, transverse, and descending colon
Repici et al. 2021 [17]	Colonic adenoma	AI adenoma detection (n = 338) and routine colonoscopy (n = 340) performed by non-expert endoscopists	Significantly improved adenoma detection rate with AI (p = 0.02). Use of the AI system led to a 22% increase in adenoma detection rate and 21% increase in adenoma per colonoscopy detection

(Continued)

Table 42.1: (Continued)

Publication	Target disease/outcome	Intervention and control	Summary of results
Brown et al. 2021 [18]	Colonic adenoma	AI adenoma detection (n = 116) and non AI-assisted high-definition white light colonoscopy (n = 116)	Significantly reduced adenoma missed rate with AI (p = 0.0247) and sessile serrated lesion miss rate (p = 0.0482) with AI. No significant difference in first-pass adenoma detection rate with AI (p = 0.3091)
Lui et al. 2021 [19]	Colonic adenoma	AI adenoma detection system (n = 52)* and routine colonoscopy (n = 52)*	AI detected at least one missed adenoma in 14 patients, and increased adenoma detection by 23.6%
Wu et al. 2019 [20]	Blind spots in oesophagogastro-duodenoscopy (OGD)	AI system for OGD (n = 153) and routine OGD (n = 150)	Significantly reduced blind spot rate (p < 0.001) and longer mean inspection rate (p < 0.001) with AI. No significant difference in completeness of documentation (p = 0.11)
Wu et al. 2021 [21]	Gastric neoplasms	AI system in upper gastrointestinal endoscopy (n = 907) and route endoscopy (n = 905)	Significantly reduced gastric neoplasm miss rate (p = 0.015)
Yao et al. 2021 [22]	Ejection fraction	Electrocardiography (ECG)-based decision support system for early diagnosis of low ejection fraction (n = 11,573) and usual care (n = 11,068)	Significantly improved diagnosis of low ejection fraction with AI system in the overall cohort (p = 0.007) and high-risk cohort (p = 0.01). More echocardiograms obtained in the intervention arm, for patients with AI-positive ECGs (p < 0.001)
Kaura et al. 2019 [23]	Paroxysmal atrial fibrillation (PAF)	Zio® patch (iRhythm Technologies, San Francisco, CA, USA), 14-day continuous ECG monitoring (n = 43) and conventional 24-hour Holter monitoring (n = 47)	Significantly greater rate of PAF detection with Zio patch (p = 0.026). Projected 10.8 avoided strokes annually, medical savings of £113,630, increasing to £162,491 over 5 years

Table 42.1: (Continued)

Publication	Target disease/ outcome	Intervention and control	Summary of results
Lin et al. 2019 [24]	Childhood cataracts	AI platform for cataracts diagnosis and management (n = 175) and routine consultant review (n = 175)	Significantly lower diagnostic and treatment recommendation accuracy, and a shorter mean diagnostic time (p < 0.001) with AI
Disease prediction and AI			
Wijnberge et al. 2020 [25]	Intra-operative hypotension	Machine learning system for intra-operative hypotension (n = 31) and standard monitoring (n = 29)	Significantly reduced intra-operative median time weighted average (p = 0.001) and median time per person (p < 0.001) of intra-operative hypotension with machine learning system
Jaroszewski et al. 2019 [26]	Crisis intervention	Machine learning barrier reduction intervention on mental health support app (n = 325) and standard app access (n = 327)	Participants receiving machine learning barrier reduction intervention were 23% more likely to use crisis services (p = 0.02)
Therapeutic treatment and AI			
Post et al. 2021 [27]	Emergency department visits	Predictive model plus community-based case management plan (n = 486) and usual care (n = 409)	With intention-to-treat effects, no significant difference observed for visits to emergency department (–0.27, 0.55), inpatient (–0.60, 0.18) or outpatient stay (–0.87, 1.12) with case management plan, compared to usual care
Nimrl et al. 2020 [28]	Insulin dose optimization	AI insulin therapy adjustment (n = 54) and physician-guided control (n = 54)	Glycaemic control (time spent within target glucose range) with AI was non-inferior to the physician (p < 0.001)
Labovitz et al. 2017 [29]	Adherence to anticoagulation therapy	AI app, monitoring adherence to anticoagulation therapy (n = 15) and no daily monitoring (n = 12)	Based on plasma drug concentrations, anticoagulation therapy adherence was reported as 100% (15/15) with AiCure and 50% (6/12) with no daily monitoring

* Lui et al. 2021 (non-randomized trial): the same 52 patients received both control and intervention endoscopy. First routine colonoscopy was performed, then during the withdrawal phase the AI system was activated.

meaningful, either clinically or for the health system. Specific elements that should be considered in clinical AI studies include:

- *Study design*: the optimal study design for the intervention that will provide sufficient evidence across key domains (including efficacy, safety, and cost-effectiveness).
- *Population*: ensure that the study population reflects the population in which it is intended to be used, and that it is sufficiently diverse to detect under-performance in population subgroups, such as minority populations.
- *Setting*: ensure that the study setting reflects the setting (or range of settings) where it is intended to be used, to provide sufficient confidence of performance outside of 'tried-and-tested' settings. AI-specific considerations here include the heterogeneity of devices used for data acquisition, data handling and processing procedures, and differences in clinical pathways.
- *Intervention(s):* ensure that the AI component of any intervention is described sufficiently, to guarantee that results are ascribed to a specific AI system (including version identifiers) and would enable replication of the study.
- *Comparator*: the comparator should be a clinically relevant and accepted reference. This reference is commonly 'standard practice' or 'best practice', with a view to informing decision-makers as to whether, and how much, the intervention can bring improvement to the outcome, compared to a reference.
- *Outcomes*: outcomes should include those that are the most important to patients and other key stakeholder groups, and be pre-specified; use of core outcome sets is recommended where they exist for the condition of interest; pre-specification avoids bias through retrospective selection of the most favourable outcome or of a positive result arising through chance and multiple testing.
- *Process measures*: consider relevant impacts on the overall health pathway such as changes in time to diagnosis or treatment, efficiency of service provision, accessibility to care, and cost of healthcare delivery.
- *Balancing measures*: consider relevant consequences of implementing the AI system to the other parts of the healthcare system, including changes in behaviour, changes in resource requirements, and potential ethical implications (such as loss of autonomy).
- *Protocol deviations*: all deviations from study protocol should be recorded and reported. Firstly, such deviations may affect the interpretation of results in relation to pre-specified outcomes. Secondly, such deviations may provide important information regarding the feasibility and safety of deploying the intervention more widely.
- *Analysis*: analysis should be pre-specified. It should include consideration of subgroups to ensure that risks of harm that disadvantage specific groups is detected; errors should be analysed at the individual error level to identify the reasons for failure where possible.

- *Study protocol*: the study should be registered (e.g. on the World Health Organization International Clinical Trials Registry Platform) in advance; additional publication of study protocols may enable helpful independent peer review prior to commencement of the study.
- *Reporting*: open and transparent reporting should align to the registered protocol, including any protocol deviations and full analysis of planned outcomes. Participant flow (including exclusions at participant level, exclusions at input data level, and losses to follow-up) should be reported according to the CONSORT-AI diagram (adapted from the CONSORT 2010 flow diagram, see later). Appropriate reporting guidelines specifically designed for AI are available and discussed later in this chapter.

42.2 Complete and Transparent Reporting of AI Studies

The critical appraisal of clinical evaluation studies is an essential part of evidence-based medicine. Decision-makers such as regulators, commissioners, clinicians, and patients should be able to assess the quality, value, and relevance of a clinical AI study by the way it was designed, conducted, analysed, and reported. This process supports stakeholders when making considered decisions about whether or not an intervention should be approved and commissioned. Critical appraisal is contingent on clear and transparent reporting. Readers cannot assess the validity of study results unless investigators explain exactly what they did, what they found, and how they interpreted the results. A number of reporting guidelines are available, supported by the Enhancing the QUAlity and Transparency Of health Research (EQUATOR) Network, to assist in good reporting of clinical studies.

Reporting guidelines developed should be organized according to study type (i.e. separate guidelines for clinical trials, diagnostic accuracy studies, observational studies, systematic reviews). Specific interventions (e.g. psychological interventions), outcomes (e.g. patient-reported outcomes), and study designs (e.g. n = 1 trials) requiring specific reporting requirements have been extended in addition to previously agreed reporting standards. In the same way, specific considerations for AI interventions have led to the development of AI-specific extensions to existing EQUATOR reporting guidelines.

42.2.1 Reporting Guidelines for Clinical Trial Protocols and Clinical Trial Reports: SPIRIT-AI and CONSORT-AI

RCTs are considered the gold-standard experimental design in the hierarchy of evidence, providing the most rigorous assessment of preventative, diagnostic, and therapeutic interventions. Standard Protocol Items: Recommendations for Interventional Trials (SPIRIT 2013) [30] and Consolidated Standards of Reporting Trials (CONSORT 2010) [31] are the accepted reporting standards for randomized trials, and these guidelines have been widely endorsed by the International Committee of Medical Journal Editors (ICMJE) and medical journals.

Extensions to these two guidelines, SPIRIT-AI and CONSORT-AI, were published in September 2020 [32–37]. These extensions include 14 and 15 new items, respectively, considered as minimum standards of reporting for AI interventions, in addition to reporting core items as outlined by SPIRIT 2013 and CONSORT 2010. AI-specific recommendations include, but are not limited to:

- Description of the type and versions of the AI model and its intended use.
- Access and restrictions to access or re-use of the AI model and/or its code.
- How the AI system was integrated in trial sites.
- Inclusion and exclusion criteria at the level of participants and input data.
- Assessment and handling of poor-quality or unavailable input data.
- Any human–AI interaction elements.
- The output of the AI intervention and its impact on decision-making or other elements of clinical practice.
- Analysis of performance errors of the system.

The full list of recommendations and associated explanatory text can be found in the referenced publications, which include templates for authors to submit alongside their manuscripts. It is highly recommended that each item is read alongside the explanatory information that contextualizes the meaning of each item and provides examples.

42.2.2 Reporting Guidelines for Diagnostic Test Accuracy Studies: STARD-AI

At present, a significant proportion of potential AI healthcare applications are diagnostic systems that classify disease presence/absence, disease subtype, and/or disease severity [38]. Indeed, many areas where AI is expected to have the largest impact are in automated diagnosis of disease for population screening programmes, such as breast cancer screening and diabetic eye disease screening [39,40]. These studies should adhere to STARD 2015 (Standards for Reporting Diagnostic Accuracy Studies) guidelines in the absence of AI-specific reporting guidelines [41]. An AI-specific extension, STARD-AI, is under development (at the time of writing) [42,43].

42.2.3 Reporting Guidelines for AI Prediction or Prognostic Models: TRIPOD-AI

Clinical prediction models estimate the likelihood of an individual having or developing disease using predictor variables (risk factors such as age, sex, and biomarkers). The ability of AI to analyse large and complex datasets of predictor variables has led to the development of several potential AI prediction models, such as AI algorithms for predicting sepsis [44].

The widely accepted EQUATOR reporting guidelines for prediction and prognostic model studies are the TRIPOD 2015 (Transparent Reporting of a Multivariable Prediction Model for Individual Prognosis or Diagnosis) guidelines [45]. An AI-specific extension, TRIPOD-AI, is also under development (at the time of writing) [46].

42.2.4 Reporting Guidelines for AI Usability and Human Factors: DECIDE-AI

Critical to the successful implementation of AI systems is the way in which they are designed to interact with humans, and the learning curve associated with this. Complex decision-support tools such as AI (which are also typically 'black box') may have unpredictable human interaction properties warranting specific investigation. There is an argument that early, small-scale feasibility studies are necessary after initial validation of algorithmic performance, prior to launching into large, expensive prospective trials. To support this stage of evaluation, DECIDE-AI (Developmental and Exploratory Clinical Investigation of DEcision-support systems driven by Artificial Intelligence) makes new recommendations for how such studies should be reported [47]. The DECIDE-AI guidelines are in the last stage of development (at the time of writing).

42.3 Conclusion

This chapter has provided an overview of the principles of clinical evaluation and the specific reporting guidelines that have been, or are being, developed for clinical AI studies. As with all health interventions, clinical evaluation begins with a clear definition of the intended impact and appropriate outcome measures that reflect value to the patient and the health system. Prospective, comparative trials are now beginning to emerge to provide much-needed evidence on safety and effectiveness of AI systems in real clinical environments. This is a pivotal time for evaluating the real-world generalizability of AI algorithms. It is therefore crucial that clinical evaluation studies are of the highest standard, and adhere to appropriate reporting guidelines, to inform on whether the implementation of these systems can bring benefits to patients.

> **KEY INSIGHTS**
>
> - **Robust clinical evaluation of AI systems must be conducted to generate the necessary evidence that AI systems are safe, accurate, and effective.**
> - **Where possible, studies should be designed to evaluate the impact on the whole clinical pathway, and to understand the outcome for an end-point that is robust and meaningful, either clinically or for the health system.**

- Clinical studies in AI should be designed with that intended impact in mind and reported according to the relevant reporting standards.
- AI-specific reporting standards were or are being specifically developed and include SPIRIT-AI, CONSORT-AI, STARD-AI, TRIPOD-AI, and DECIDE-AI.

References

1. Kelly CJ, Karthikesalingam A, Suleyman M et al. Key challenges for delivering clinical impact with artificial intelligence. *BMC Medicine* 2019;17:195.
2. McCradden MD, Stephenson EA, Anderson JA. Clinical research underlies ethical integration of healthcare artificial intelligence. Nature Medicine 2020;26:1325–1326.
3. Futoma J, Simons M, Panch T et al. The myth of generalisability in clinical research and machine learning in health care. *Lancet Digital Health* 2020;2:e489–e492.
4. Liu X, Faes L, Kale AU et al. A comparison of deep learning performance against healthcare professionals in detecting diseases from medical imaging: a systematic review and meta-analysis. *Lancet Digital Health* 2019;1:e271–e297.
5. Nagendran M, Chen Y, Lovejoy CA et al. Artificial intelligence versus clinicians: systematic review of design, reporting standards, and claims of deep learning studies. *BMJ* 2020;368:m689.
6. Aggarwal R, Sounderajah V, Martin G et al. Diagnostic accuracy of deep learning in medical imaging: a systematic review and meta-analysis. *npj Digital Medicine* 2021;4:65.
7. Gaube S, Suresh H, Raue M et al. Do as AI say: susceptibility in deployment of clinical decision-aids. *npj Digital Medicine* 2021;4:1–8.

For additional references and Further Reading please see www.wiley.com/go/byrne/aiinclinicalmedicine

43

The Importance and Benefits of Implementing Modern Data Infrastructure for Video-Based Medicine

Matt Schwartz and Ian Strug

Virgo Surgical Video Solutions, Inc., Carlsbad, CA, USA

Learning Objectives

- Understand the importance of implementing data infrastructure for AI development in video-based medicine.
- Pros and cons of the different methods for video data acquisition and management.
- Optimal process for implementing video data infrastructure in clinical practice.
- Understand ancillary benefits that come from implementing modern video data infrastructure.

43.1 Prevalence of Video in Medicine

Since its use was first documented in 1855 by the French physician Antonin Jean Désourmeaux, endoscopy has gone on to become a critical procedural tool across numerous medical specialties. While early endoscopes were simple hollow tubes with illumination to peer inside organs, modern endoscopy involves the use of miniaturized high-definition digital video cameras. Across procedures such as colonoscopy, upper endoscopy, bronchoscopy, cystoscopy, arthroscopy, and laparoscopic surgery, there are now over 75 million endoscopies performed each year in the USA [1]. Physicians perform these endoscopic procedures for a variety of purposes, ranging from diagnosis to surgery.

Clearly, video now plays a critical role in medicine. To put this in perspective, 1080p video in high-definition quality typically generates about 1–2 gigabytes' worth of data per hour, even using state-of-the-art compression techniques. Assuming the average endoscopy is 30 minutes long, this means each year the USA generates

---

AI in Clinical Medicine: A Practical Guide for Healthcare Professionals, First Edition. Edited by Michael F. Byrne, Nasim Parsa, Alexandra T. Greenhill, Daljeet Chahal, Omer Ahmad, and Ulas Bagci.
© 2023 John Wiley & Sons Ltd. Published 2023 by John Wiley & Sons Ltd.
Companion website: www.wiley.com/go/byrne/aiinclinicalmedicine

approximately 56 *petabytes* worth of endoscopy video data. Again, this is using state-of-the-art data compression. Uncompressed, this data would be measured in *exabytes*.

43.1.1 Why Is Video-Based Medicine So Ripe for Advancement with AI?

Out of all the domains where AI has recently made significant headway, perhaps none has been as substantial as computer vision. In fact, many consider the 2012 ImageNet competition, which was won by a convolutional neural network (CNN) called AlexNet, to be the dawning of the current 'AI Spring' period. After years of stalled progress in computer vision, AlexNet achieved a top-5 error rate in the competition that was a full 10 percentage points lower than previous winners.

Suddenly, the field of computer vision and the broader AI community recognized the massive potential of deep learning. This potential has proven to be particularly potent in fields such as natural language processing, recommendation systems, and computer vision. What makes these fields so ripe for deep learning is that they share a few common traits, such as the ability to generate massive digital datasets and these data often being of high dimensionality. High dimensionality here refers to data in which the number of features for a given sample is significantly larger than the number of samples.

Computer vision in particular deals with highly dimensional digital imaging data. For example, a single frame from a 1080p video consists of 1920 pixels in width by 1080 pixels in height, for a total of 2,073,600 pixels. Each of these pixels contains a red, green, and blue value, and each of those values ranges from 0 to 255. The dimensionality in the pixel values of just a single video frame is immense. Then consider that video frame rates are typically either 30 or 60 frames per second. All of this data dimensionality is very challenging to parse with conventional algorithms; however, deep learning algorithms are well suited to detect patterns within the data.

Video-based medicine generates a significant amount of highly dimensional data and therefore checks the technical boxes for being well suited to AI development. The ways in which video is used clinically also lend themselves to AI playing a significant role in advancing patient care.

Endoscopic medical procedures are generally performed for diagnostic and/or therapeutic applications. In all these modalities, AI has the potential to augment physician performance. In diagnostic endoscopies such as screening colonoscopy and upper endoscopy, real-time AI systems may help physicians detect polyps or identify Barrett's oesophagus that may have otherwise been missed. In therapeutic applications of endoscopy, real-time AI systems may help physicians identify challenging anatomy or assess tumour margins.

In these applications, real-time AI will play a similar role to the perception systems of self-driving cars. The key difference, however, is that the results of the AI perception will help inform the physician's decision-making.

43.1.2 Challenges with Pre-existing Data

When embarking upon the development of new AI applications, the starting point is usually to examine the availability of existing data. However, when it comes to medical video, pre-existing datasets are sparse and of generally poor quality for AI development. Unfortunately, the vast majority of video-based medical procedures are simply not recorded.

In the rare instances where video-based medical procedures are recorded, they are typically captured in low resolution or with distorted compression artifacts. Even more challenging, these videos are often only partial recordings saved in a variety of video formats and poorly archived. It is not uncommon for pre-existing medical video datasets to exist as a hodgepodge of DVDs, thumb drives, and external hard drives. Such datasets can prove useful for developing proofs of concept, but they are ill-suited for production-level AI development.

Another strategy for leveraging pre-existing datasets in AI development for video-based medicine is to focus on development via still imagery, as still images are much more commonly captured to electronic health records in a standardized fashion. For most endoscopic procedures, the performing physician will capture a handful of still images during the procedure, typically representing significant anatomical landmarks or interesting pathology.

AI techniques have been developed for performing still image classification and still image object detection, and these techniques can be extended to perform inference on a sequence of still images, for instance a series of video frames. As such, pre-existing still image datasets have proven useful for developing proofs of concept and even early production-level AI systems in tasks such as colon polyp detection and colon polyp classification. However, pre-existing still image datasets typically continue to be lacking when it comes to standardization, quality, and scale.

As AI techniques for video advance, AI systems trained on high-quality video datasets are likely to outperform those trained on moderate-quality still image datasets.

43.2 The Solution: Thoughtful Video Data Capture

The solution here is to capture medical procedure videos in an organized and standardized fashion. All modern endoscopic video processors known to the authors provide high-definition video outputs. Therefore, it is in theory possible to systematically capture nearly every single endoscopic procedure video in its entirety.

From the perspective of AI development, the optimal solution would in fact be to capture all procedure videos in their entirety. Furthermore, the capture of these procedure videos should take place in high definition and be archived such that they may be easily managed and accessed. It is also very important to consider information security when accumulating such large and sensitive datasets.

43.3 Options for Building Video Data Capture Infrastructure

Several options exist today for video capture. Here we will group these options into local hard media storage, on-premises server storage, and cloud storage. Each of these has its pros and cons.

Local hard media storage systems vary from the use of consumer-grade video capture devices to medical-grade video capture systems manufactured by the endoscopy equipment manufacturers. These systems will often record procedure videos onto DVDs, SD cards, thumb drives, or internal/external hard drives. These systems require limited, or even no, internet connectivity. However, local storage has several drawbacks. DVDs, SD cards, thumb drives, and hard drives are expensive and extremely difficult to manage at scale. It quickly becomes impractical to archive this storage in a way that can be easily searched and accessed for AI development purposes. These systems are often challenging for clinical staff to set up, and require someone from the clinical staff to be responsible for starting and stopping the recording – which detracts from the normal clinical workflow.

Perhaps most importantly, though, it is very difficult to securely manage these hard storage devices. The systems do not properly track utilization, and the media devices themselves require the user to set up proper encryption. Health systems quickly lose the ability to control data security with these systems, and there have been multiple instances where hard media devices containing protected health information (PHI) were lost or stolen, resulting in significant Health Insurance Portability and Accountability Act (HIPAA) fines.

Another option for medical video capture is on-premises server storage. Most healthcare facilities run on-premises server storage in some capacity for electronic health record and imaging data storage. These servers are typically managed directly by the Information technology (IT) staff of the facility.

It is possible to configure endoscopy video processors such that their high-definition video output is routed to these on-premises servers for storage, often with a device in between to handle video compression and data routing. On-premises systems and services may be provided by endoscopy equipment manufacturers, electronic health record system providers, or other companies that specialize in medical video storage solutions.

The third strategy for medical video capture and management is cloud storage. The notion of cloud computing and storage is now a mainstream concept in IT, and involves shifting the location of computer and storage servers from on-premises to a centrally managed data centre. The most popular cloud services providers are Amazon Web Services, Google Cloud Platform, and Microsoft Azure. These providers offer significant economies of scale and state-of-the-art performance and security measures.

When capturing endoscopy video to cloud storage, the video output of the endoscopy video processor is transmitted over a network connection – often intermediated by another device – to the cloud storage host. Authorized users then access their video data using a web-based interface (Figure 43.1). Cloud storage architecture enables nearly

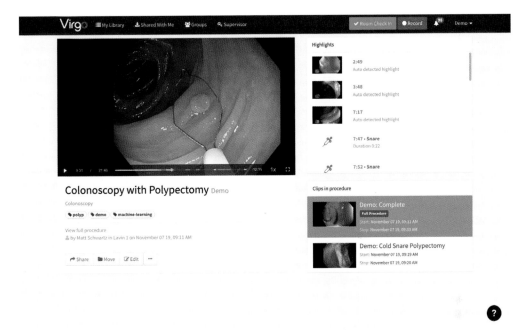

Figure 43.1: Example of a web portal for accessing endoscopy videos in cloud storage with features including video highlights, secure sharing, and annotation.

Source: Matt Schwartz and Ian Strug.

limitless scalability at significantly lower cost than on-premises infrastructure. At the same time, cloud architecture requires unique networking connectivity to ensure robust video uploading. The different options are summarized and compared in Table 43.1.

43.4 How to Leverage Video Infrastructure for AI Development

The optimal video infrastructure for AI development should support highly scalable video capture and programmatic data access. Both on-premises and cloud-based infrastructures are able to meet these requirements; however, cloud-based infrastructure will generally enjoy superior scalability without increased costs.

Ideally, an institution should capture and archive every endoscopic procedure video to maximize data capture, in particular the capture of rare events, which aid in training robust AI models that are capable of handling edge-case scenarios. Certain video capture platforms provide functionality that automatically triggers video capture of a procedure to help ensure all procedures are recorded without disrupting the standard clinical workflow.

With large-scale video capture, it becomes increasingly important to implement supporting infrastructure that aids in video archiving, management, and access. High-volume healthcare providers will commonly perform several thousand video-based medical procedures each month. Procedure videos should be stored with sufficient metadata – such as date, time, location, type, outcomes, and so on – to

Table 43.1: Summary of Capabilities for Different Video Capture Options.

	Local hard media (DVDs, hard drives, USB drives, etc.)	Integrated on-premises servers	Cloud storage solutions
Upfront costs	Ranges from several hundred US dollars for consumer grade to tens of thousands of US dollars for medical grade	Ranges from high tens of thousands of US dollars for servers with limited integration to hundreds of thousands or potentially millions of US dollars for full integration of endoscopy suites	Low installation fees generally ranging from several hundred US dollars to several thousand US dollars
Ongoing costs	Relatively low costs for new storage devices	High costs for additional server capacity and full-time information technology (IT) maintenance staff	Very low-cost plans available for either capped or unlimited data
Security	Very poor security with almost no enforceable controls on data capture or access	Variable, depending on IT capabilities and infrastructure of healthcare provider	Highest possible security leveraging state-of-the-art practices from cloud services providers
Scalability	Extremely low, requiring frequent replacement of storage devices with challenging archiving	Moderate, depending on IT capabilities and infrastructure of healthcare provider	Virtually unlimited scalability available
Data access	Challenging but possible with sufficient work on behalf of clinician and team	May require significant additional infrastructure build on part of IT staff	Generally high accessibility, depending on cloud solution provider

enable targeted video retrieval. Ideally, on-premises and cloud video infrastructure will be integrated with the health system's electronic health records so that each video is specifically linked with a patient and an encounter.

Once a health system deploys video capture infrastructure at scale, it will quickly begin generating substantial volumes of video data for AI development. To leverage this video data for AI development, one must first select and organize videos into specific subsets. Generally, AI development revolves around the use of training data, validation data, and test data. As such, it is critical that AI practitioners have programmatic access to video data, in either on-premises or cloud storage, with the ability to partition data into these subsets.

Video data pose particular challenges around data transfer because of the large file sizes involved. For this reason, it is generally preferable to limit the transfer of video data between infrastructures. With AI training efforts on video data shifting more and more to cloud computing because of the necessary computer resources, it may be advantageous to implement cloud video infrastructure, which will limit the need to make expensive data transfers from on-premises into the cloud.

43.5 IT, Security, and Legal Considerations When Implementing Video Capture Infrastructure

When implementing endoscopic video capture in clinical practice, it is important to consider IT security and legal implications. The authors recommend that clinicians who are interested in endoscopic video capture begin conversations with IT and legal staff at their institutions early in the process.

Endoscopic video data is generally considered de-identified when it consists only of internal video footage without other identifiers; however, it is not uncommon for endoscopy video processors to embed PHI such as a medical record number or patient name directly into the video feed. When video is stored with additional metadata, it almost certainly consists of PHI. In these scenarios, the healthcare provider must consider HIPAA implications related to the storage and management of PHI.

If a healthcare provider is evaluating third-party solutions for endoscopic video capture – regardless of whether they involve the use of local hard media storage devices, on-premises server systems, or cloud-based solutions – it will likely need to perform an appropriate IT security assessment to ensure the solutions are properly secured and implemented in accordance with data security needs. Experienced third-party providers should be capable of efficiently and sufficiently responding to security assessment requests. Clinicians interested in accelerating their timeline for implementing a video capture solution are well served by engaging their IT departments as early as possible and facilitating an introduction to the third-party providers they are evaluating.

Similarly, it is critical that a healthcare provider is obtaining adequate informed consent from patients prior to capturing endoscopic video. While standard informed consent forms for endoscopic procedures typically already include provisions for video capture, healthcare providers should confer with their legal counsel to ensure this is the case. Legal review should also consider whether there are specific provisions surrounding how the video data will be used that require additional informed consent.

43.6 Ancillary Benefits of Implementing Video Capture in Clinical Practice

Beyond creating datasets for AI development, systematic endoscopic video capture provides superior documentation with numerous ancillary benefits. These benefits include, but are not limited to:

- Enablement of video-based research projects.
- Development of video-based training protocols.
- Utilization of video data for clinical trial recruitment.
- Improved defence in malpractice suits.

With the increased utilization of video-based procedures, medical societies are recognizing the need to support video-based research. Creating a library of procedure videos enables researchers to conduct blinded video assessments of technique performance and outcomes. In fact, many video capture and management solutions include built-in analytics and assessment forms to assist with such research. Many clinical specialties provide special research submission opportunities for video-based research projects and case studies. For example, the American Society for Gastrointestinal Endoscopy hosts VideoGIE (`www.videogie.org`), the Society of American Gastrointestinal and Endoscopic Surgeons hosts SAGES TV (`https://www.sages.org/video`), and the Arthroscopy Association of North America hosts Arthroscopy Techniques (`www.arthroscopytechniques.org`), all focused on endoscopy video submissions.

As video-based competency assessments become more standardized and commonplace in endoscopic fields, fellow programmes can adopt video capture and review as a way to enhance their training curricula. Some examples of video-based competency assessments include the Bethesda ERCP Skill Assessment Tool [2], the Cold Snare Polypectomy Assessment Tool [3], and the LAParoscopic Surgery Video Educational GuidelineS [4]. Implementing a video capture and management solution into clinical practice is the easiest way to incorporate such assessment tools into clinical training programmes.

Clinical trials represent another excellent use case for endoscopic video. Many pharmaceutical trials, such as those for inflammatory bowel disease, rely upon endoscopic video assessment for both determination of inclusion eligibility and outcomes measurement. Often, clinical trial sites lacking standardized endoscopic video capture and management infrastructure must deploy ad hoc solutions for trial participation. By deploying scalable video capture and management infrastructure, clinical trial sites can analyse significantly more video data to find trial-eligible patients within their population.

Lastly, standardizing endoscopic video capture provides clinicians with improved documentation, which may help avoid and defend against malpractice lawsuits. Many experts have written about the positive impact that video capture has on procedural quality. For example, in 2013, Makary wrote a viewpoint in *JAMA* highlighting the value of video recording and reviews, as well as the broad patient support for such practices [5]. Simply improving procedural quality in this fashion is likely to reduce the likelihood of adverse events warranting malpractice suits. Additionally, some expert witnesses for malpractice cases, such as Rex [6], believe that video recordings can provide a tremendous advantage to the defence in malpractice suits.

43.7 Conclusion

Video-based medical procedures present innumerable opportunities to improve patient care with AI, and the information-rich, highly dimensional video data generated by these procedures are precisely the type of data coveted by AI practitioners. Unfortunately, standard documentation for video-based medical procedures frequently does not include systematic capture of the procedure video itself, leaving

AI practitioners working with limited still image data that often poorly represent the actual procedures.

Clinicians in endoscopic fields who are interested in furthering AI research and development may open significant research opportunities by implementing systematic video capture infrastructure in their practice. While many solutions are available to achieve such systematic video capture, cloud-based video capture and management solutions offer numerous advantages related to scalability, cost, and data access. In addition to supporting AI research and development, implementing video infrastructure in clinical practice may lead to ancillary benefits related to other research, training initiatives, quality improvement, clinical trials, and generally improved documentation.

KEY INSIGHTS

- **Endoscopy is incredibly prevalent across the healthcare landscape, with over 75 million endoscopic procedures performed in the USA each year.**
- **Endoscopic video data are highly dimensional, making them particularly well suited to many AI techniques related to deep learning.**
- **Solutions are available to today's practitioner that will enable them to systematically capture their endoscopic procedure video at a low cost.**
- **Endoscopic video capture offers additional clinical benefits beyond AI research and development.**

References

1. Dryda L. GI endoscopies make up 68% of all endoscopies in U.S. *Becker's GI & Endoscopy*, 11 April 2019. https://www.beckersasc.com/gastroenterology-and-endoscopy/gi-endoscopies-make-up-68-of-all-endoscopies-in-u-s-5-market-trends.html.
2. Elmunzer BJ, Walsh CM, Guiton G et al. Development and initial validation of an instrument for video-based assessment of technical skill in ERCP. *Gastrointestinal Endoscopy* 2021;93(4):914–923. https://doi.org/10.1016/j.gie.2020.07.055.
3. Patel SG, Duloy A, Kaltenbach T et al. Development and validation of a video-based cold snare polypectomy assessment tool (with videos). *Gastrointestinal Endoscopy* 2019;89(6):1222–1230.e2. https://doi.org/10.1016/j.gie.2019.02.018.
4. Celentano V, Smart N, Cahill RA et al. Development and validation of a recommended checklist for assessment of surgical videos quality: the LAParoscopic surgery Video Educational GuidelineS (LAP-VEGaS) video assessment tool. *Surgical Endoscopy* 2021;35:1362–1369. https://doi.org/10.1007/s00464-020-07517-4.
5. Makary MA. The power of video recording: taking quality to the next level. *JAMA* 2013;309(15):1591–1592.
6. Rex DK. Avoiding and defending malpractice suits for postcolonoscopy cancer: advice from an expert witness. *Clinical Gastroenterology and Hepatology* 2013;11(7):768–773. https://doi.org/10.1016/j.cgh.2013.01.027.

44

AI and the Evolution of the Patient–Physician Relationship

Judy L. Barkal[1], Jack W. Stockert[1], Jesse M. Ehrenfeld[2], and Lawrence K. Cohen[1]

[1] *Health2047, Menlo Park, CA, USA*

[2] *Medical College of Wisconsin, Milwaukee, WI, USA*

Learning Objectives

- Develop appreciation of the current and future impact of AI on the patient–physician relationship.
- Examine positives and pitfalls of consumerization of health and wellness.
- Understand the roles for patient and family participation in the design, co-creation, testing, and deployment of AI.

44.1 Introduction

AI for clinical use is expanding rapidly. AI chatbots, clinical decision-support systems (CDSS), image readers, and diagnostic devices are just a few examples where AI is being developed for clinical use. AI is also showing up in consumer-grade devices, wearables, and smart phone applications for patients to use outside the clinic. Increasingly, both clinicians and consumers expect AI-enabled devices to empower their decision-making. As with any new technology, it is important to consider which AI developments are helpful, which ones might be detrimental, the potential for unintended consequences, and how humans might be impacted.

We begin our discussion by considering key characteristics of patient–physician relationships, and propose questions that can be asked when evaluating potential AI impacts on those relationships. Next, we outline how AI might augment human intelligence in different clinical contexts. We then consider AI impacts on patient–physician relationships, using examples of consumer-grade AI and medical-grade AI. Lastly, we look at opportunities for physicians, patients, families, and caregivers to be involved in the design, development, and deployment of AI.

AI in Clinical Medicine: A Practical Guide for Healthcare Professionals, First Edition. Edited by Michael F. Byrne, Nasim Parsa, Alexandra T. Greenhill, Daljeet Chahal, Omer Ahmad, and Ulas Bagci.
© 2023 John Wiley & Sons Ltd. Published 2023 by John Wiley & Sons Ltd.
Companion website: www.wiley.com/go/byrne/aiinclinicalmedicine

44.2 Patient–Physician Relationship

The patient–physician relationship is the cornerstone of healthcare, on which AI will have many different impacts. We discuss some key characteristics of the patient–physician relationship that will later help us examine potential impacts of AI on that relationship:

- *Trust.* Trust is the foundation of the patient–physician relationship. When AI is augmenting the physician providing medical services to patients, this trust can be impacted. This impact is driven by how AI is integrated into existing workflows, and how AI is experienced by both patients and physicians. Two key questions to consider are: Does AI enhance or diminish patient–physician trust in a given clinical context? Does AI improve the capacity and capability to deliver optimal or better outcomes?
- *Humanization.* Healthcare is a human system. Dr Abraham Verghese, a professor at Stanford University School of Medicine, best captures what AI and humanization of medicine could be:

  > *The way here is not to think technology versus human, but to ask how they come together where the sum can be greater than the parts for an equitable, inclusive, human and humane care and practice in medicine. [1]*

  How does AI support humanized medicine? Does AI potentially dehumanize medical practice? Does AI support equitable practices for all patients regardless of race, ethnicity, gender, or socioeconomic status?
- *Families and caregivers.* Caring for patients may extend to working with family members and patient caregivers. How does AI support the patient's family and caregivers? How does AI present challenges for families and caregivers? How does AI enable physicians to provide an informed view that is understandable and has a context that is appropriate and meaningful for patients?
- *Experience.* AI makers have opportunities to improve the AI user experience by involving physicians, patients, families, and caregivers during development. Involving these key stakeholders helps AI makers build empathy for user needs. AI makers can combine what is technically possible with what users need in order to tailor AI designs for the best user experience. Consider key questions related to experience: How does AI support and enhance patient experience and also the experiences of families and caregivers? How does AI enhance the physician experience?

44.3 AI in the Clinical Context

AI makers might describe AI as a product, a procedure, or a service. If AI makers approach their AI solution using primarily a technology lens, they might miss the importance of the behavioural evolution needed for AI in clinical care delivery.

First, we distinguish between consumer-grade AI and medical-grade AI, and second, we clarify AI use in a clinical context. Further, we consider consumer-grade AI examples and discuss potential impacts on patient–physician relationships, and then move to discussing medical-grade AI.

44.3.1 Consumer-Grade AI

Consumer-grade AI has generally not been clinically validated, which means it has not been certified as generating clinically validated measurements. In some cases, consumer-grade AI may have partial clinical validation for some measurements, but no certification for others. Consumer-grade AI may offer wellness tools for patients. An example might be a smart watch that generates clinically validated blood pressure measurements, but no certification of other measurements that it generates, such as sleep tracking.

Today, individuals can 'hack their health' using consumer-grade AI to help build and maintain healthy habits, such as exercise, diet, or sleep. These individuals who are also patients sometimes want to share their personal wellness information with physicians in a clinical context. If physicians determine that AI is not clinically validated, or is validated but monitoring a lower-priority condition, they may need to discuss further with patients to help them understand the limitations for clinical use or a specific care plan. Physicians may also need to remind patients about the importance of seeking qualified medical care rather than placing trust in AI that is not clinically validated. In this way, AI can generate new conversations that build trust and understanding as well as improve personal care decisions.

The number of consumer-grade AI solutions is growing rapidly, and there are still relatively few that are clinically validated. If patient sharing of consumer-grade AI information with physicians also grows rapidly, the resulting data deluge could possibly hinder or undermine health decisions, and perhaps even erode trust in patient–physician relationships. As consumer-grade AI options become clinically validated, they can offer options that go beyond personal wellness tools, and offer certified information that physicians might use in a clinical context. This situation could help reinforce trust in patient–physician relationships and health decisions.

Patients who are not clinical experts are often unable to place the output of consumer-grade applications into context. For example, in the absence of any prior information about disease prevalence, a consumer is much more likely to incorrectly affirm a false-positive signal from an AI-enabled device. A consumer who thinks they have a disease, as confirmed by a consumer-grade AI tool, may be thought of as base-rate neglect bias, or the human tendency to underweight base rate (prior) relative to individuating information (likelihood) when estimating the probability of uncertain events. Base-rate neglect bias is described as one of the most common fallacies in medical decision-making [2]. Patient–physician conversations can help place the output of consumer-grade applications in an appropriate clinical context.

44.3.2 Medical-Grade AI

Medical-grade AI has been clinically validated and has regulatory approval. Generally, medical-grade AI has an intended clinical use that must be declared and approved by regulatory agencies using evidence provided by AI makers. Regulators assign a category to AI based on intended use and significance of risk to patients [3]. The regulatory approval dictates what work AI can perform in a clinical context. An example might be AI that can analyse a patient's retinal image and generate a diagnosis for a physician to use.

Medical-grade AI can augment human intelligence in different clinical contexts and with different levels of autonomy. To help distinguish different levels of autonomy in medical-grade AI, we adapt some terminology from the American Medical Association taxonomy that provides guidance for classifying various AI (e.g. expert systems, machine learning, algorithm-based services) for medical services and procedures [4]:

- *AI can assist.* Detects clinically relevant data without analysis or generated conclusions. Human interprets and generates reports.
- *AI can augment.* Analyses and/or quantifies data in a clinically meaningful way. Human interprets and generates reports.
- *AI can work autonomously.* Automatically interprets data, and independently generates clinically relevant conclusions without concurrent human involvement.
    - *Level 1*: Interprets and offers results (e.g. a diagnosis). Human can contest. Requires human action.
    - *Level 2*: Draws conclusions and initiates management options, with alerts/opportunities for human override. May require human actions.
    - *Level 3*: Draws conclusions, initiates management options that require human actions to contest.

The adoption of medical-grade AI in clinical use impacts the physician and healthcare organization in many ways. There are other references that go into some detailed considerations of evaluating and adopting AI [5]. We now examine AI impacts on the patient–physician relationship with a particular focus on preserving trust and humanized medicine. We also examine how AI affects patient and physician experiences, and extend our overall AI impact discussion to include patients' families and caregivers.

44.4 AI Impact Scenarios

Each patient–physician relationship is unique. It can be challenging to predict how AI might impact each relationship. Just as with electronic health record adoption, the impact of the technology is often inextricably linked to the specific implementation across different workflows. For this reason, many practices have struggled to implement electronic health records in ways that add support rather than distance to the patient–physician relationship. We describe some example scenarios, and examine what types of AI impacts might be possible.

44.4.1 AI Assisting

AI might assist the physician as a medical scribe, quietly capturing visit notes using natural language processing in the background during physician–patient discussions. The AI assistant might reduce physician time typing at a computer during the visit, and enable more time and attention for patients. A human scribe could do the same, but their presence in the room might also make the patient less comfortable. Conversely, some patients may be reluctant to allow their healthcare encounters to be either recorded or remotely monitored by AI scribing software. Whether there is an AI scribe or human scribe, patients may still have privacy and confidentiality concerns to be addressed. In addition, the physician must have confidence in the AI scribe. If AI transcriptions need many corrections, the experience for physician and patient might be diminished, with time spent correcting AI results, leaving less time and attention for the patient.

An AI assistant might offer other support:

- *Enhancing communication.* AI multilingual capabilities could facilitate patient and family or caregiver communications with physicians.
- *Improving diagnostic capabilities.* AI in a CDSS context can help physicians keep up with the exponential growth of information, and track the most current recommendations.
- *Advancing care adjacency recommendations.* AI's ability to rapidly search and analyse information might enable quick retrieval of recommendations for medical or support services near a patient's home or workplace, potentially reducing delays for patients and lengthy follow-up coordination for physicians and their staff.
- *Ensuring system reliability.* AI can be used to improve the reliability of care processes from a variety of standpoints. Given a low level of process reliability across diverse healthcare settings, there are many opportunities for AI to augment existing systems and enable more equitable and higher-quality patient outcomes.

44.4.2 AI Monitoring

AI monitoring is another area of promise for improving care decisions and outcomes. AI monitoring might be an option if a patient wants help managing a chronic condition at home between physician visits. It can also be particularly helpful for silent diseases such as hypertension, where long-term effects on health and well-being are significant. Family members and caregivers might appreciate the support that AI monitoring can bring to their roles in helping care for patients at home. In these contexts, the key focus areas are:

- *Usability.* The usability of the AI monitor is paramount to a positive experience for patients and caregivers. AI monitors with overly complex operating instructions might lead to less frequent use and diminished benefits for patients. While there is a generation of digital 'natives' who often embrace new technologies, there is also growing awareness of the millions of patients who are digitally 'fragile' and have difficulty adopting and keeping up with updates to new technologies.
- *Function and purpose.* The purpose and functional aspects of AI monitoring should be clear in the discussion between physician and patient. Patients might have trouble understanding the utility and purpose of AI monitoring, or may have concerns about their privacy and confidentiality. These concerns may require further discussion, or they could erode trust.
- *Accessibility.* Some patients may not be able to afford AI monitors if costs are not covered. This can create inequity among patients. Some AI monitors might also have conditional limitations, such as needing a smart phone connection or high-speed internet. It is important to consider when AI might worsen health inequities for patients who cannot use or cannot afford additional devices and services for the AI monitor.

With AI monitoring, preservation of the relationship between physician and patient should be paramount. Successful AI monitoring often requires the use of qualified clinical staff to help patients and caregivers effectively use the AI monitor. Initial patient education is typically needed, as well as regular follow-up discussions with patients. Qualified clinical staff might be from the physician office or might be associated with the AI maker or a third party. In any case, a clinical protocol for escalation of issues to the physician using the physician's specified conditions must be in place for clinical staff to follow, and also be used when the physician must make clinical decisions. The implementation of AI monitoring should be thoughtful and empathetic to patients' and physicians' needs. Implementations that are detached from the care continuum might create unintended consequences where patients perceive that AI monitoring has distanced them from their physician and dehumanized their relationship. Other patients might like having attentive clinical staff checking in with them regularly, and keeping their physician informed of their situation. All interactions with clinical staff should reinforce the trust relationship between individual patient and physician.

Physicians may be hesitant to use outside clinical staff, who may not interact with patients with the same quality and attentiveness that in-house clinical staff do. Physicians want patients to have the same personalized experience with in-house and outside clinical staff, always being attentive to individual patient needs. Likewise, the interactions physicians have with clinical staff supporting patients using AI monitoring is expected to be professional, responsive, and attentive to the physician's protocols and instructions. The addition of the clinical staff with AI monitoring might enhance or diminish both patient and physician experiences, and could further evolve the patient–physician relationship.

44.4.3 AI Performing Clinical Work

AI might perform clinical work that helps a physician with decision-making. One example might be AI that can generate a diagnosis for the physician to consider as part of decision-making. Another example might be AI that helps a physician search for 'patients like this one' to find and consider what other physicians have done in similar cases.

Discussion of AI options with patients should be similar to that for any other type of medical treatment and device options. Physicians discuss the indications, risks, benefits, and alternatives of any intervention. With AI, the augmentation or level of autonomy might become part of the conversation if the patient perceives that AI presents more risk to them. It is important for physicians to understand how AI works so that they can adequately inform their patients. Some other issues may also need to be addressed. Recent research has shown that patients think AI is too standardized and inflexible to deal with their unique needs, and they trust human decision-makers more than AI [6].

The physician's practical experience with AI might help address patient questions and concerns. The AI maker might also offer educational materials for patients, families, and caregivers. Through this discussion of AI, the goal is to preserve the patient–physician relationship and preserve or perhaps enhance trust.

Some patients may alternatively ask why AI is not an option. It is possible that AI does not have the regulatory category certification or lacks real-world evidence for the patient's context. The physician can discuss why AI might not be an option. This discussion is similar to when other medical treatments and devices are not options. Even when AI cannot be used, the discussion can preserve trust between patient and physician.

Some AI limitations might also raise equity concerns with patients. The AI might not have cost coverage and the patient might not be able to afford to pay. AI might not have regulatory certification for the patient's race, gender, or other demographic characteristics. Physicians can raise such equity concerns with AI makers on behalf of patients, and help reinforce the patient–physician relationship based on ethical, equitable, and evidence-based medical practice.

There are examples of equitable AI that improve patient access to care. One example is AI that can reliably detect diabetic retinopathy [7]. This AI may assist a primary care physician in a rural community by providing the option of screening patients before referring them to an eye specialist, whose practice may be many hours away. This type of AI use may create a positive experience for patients and physicians, and potentially strengthen the patient–physician relationship. In addition, patients who get earlier treatment from an eye specialist might show an improved outcome of keeping their eyesight.

We have discussed how different levels of autonomous AI might impact patient–physician relationships. We have presented the importance of the work that AI performs and also the experiences of patients, families, and caregivers in addition to physicians. We now move to our discussion of why and how AI makers might engage physicians, patients, families, and caregivers in the development of AI.

44.5 AI Development with Humans

AI makers must do technical development of AI and provide sufficient evidence to regulators for approval. This is a big task, and takes significant time and resources. We suggest that AI makers proceed with development work involving key stakeholders who will potentially adopt and benefit from AI: physicians, patients, families, and caregivers. Their involvement in empathetic design will help expedite adoption and shape AI usability by real-world users. This is a critical component to ensure that AI technical innovation can truly impact health and care.

There are clear advantages in building human–computer interfaces that human stakeholders have helped define, test, and validate as early as possible. Changes and additional work late in development can cost great amounts of time and resources that were not in the development plan and budget. Next, we suggest some ways to involve physicians and patients earlier in the development process.

44.5.1 Physician Advisory Groups

AI makers should work with existing physician advisory groups or help bring together physicians interested in helping them develop AI [8]. Some of these physicians might help train AI, validate AI, or participate in clinical research (see later discussion). Initial engagement can lead to having an ongoing advisory group for the AI maker and other physicians wanting to adopt and improve AI. Further, it is important to seek diversity in the physician group to ensure that the development process does not introduce bias into AI.

44.5.2 Patient Advocacy Groups

AI makers can reach out to existing patient advocacy groups for feedback, or form a patient advisory group made of diverse patients, families, and caregivers. These groups provide feedback to AI makers on the AI experience, and communicate patient preferences for use and sharing of their data by the AI maker. Patient families and caregivers can offer feedback on how well AI supports their role in providing care at home, or in advocating for patients who may be unable to advocate for themselves. Patient advocacy groups can also help AI makers develop educational content about AI.

44.5.3 Clinical Research

Throughout this chapter we have excluded discussion of experimental AI. Here we recognize that AI is developed using the regulatory guidelines of clinical research, which regulate the involvement of physicians and patients. There are still many important opportunities to learn from the experiences of physicians and patients beyond whether AI works or not. The clinical research phase is an opportunity to include patients from diverse racial, ethnic, and socioeconomic backgrounds so that the certified AI is more equitable and accessible to broader populations. By including diverse physicians, AI makers can also help reduce bias in AI users.

If regulations permit, observed physician and patient experiences during clinical research can inform further development of AI to achieve greater usability. Using this development time to collect learning can sometimes help AI makers develop plans for AI features or products for future development.

44.6 Conclusion

Many AI options will continue to emerge in consumer-grade and medical-grade AI. We can envision AI assisting and augmenting physicians and performing increasingly autonomous work as new decision-making capabilities are developed. How AI might affect the patient–physician relationship can be learnt by involving physicians, patients, their families, and caregivers in AI design, adoption, experience, education, and evaluation. Patient and physician will continue to discuss healthcare options in the context of patient circumstances and potential risks, as well as preferences for privacy and confidentiality, including use and sharing of their data. We look forward to a future where AI is highly usable, accessible, and equitable for all patients. Further, we hope AI and physicians working together can help patients achieve improved outcomes.

We have seen technology transform other industries outside of healthcare by embracing the key stakeholders – the primary users and beneficiaries of the technology. The technology systems had to fit into existing workflows and implement human interfaces that enhanced user experiences and improved safety and business outcomes. Airlines and aviation have been transformed by integrating systems with pilots, airports, maintenance, and airline staff, to name a few key stakeholders.

It is critical that AI be designed, developed, and adopted with shared perspectives around capabilities and diverse stakeholder needs. Otherwise, AI will not contribute to transforming healthcare as we all hope. Physicians and patients as well as regulators and payers want AI to be safe, usable in a clinical context, and effective as a tool for improving outcomes. As AI makers partner with healthcare stakeholders, we are encouraged by the progress that can and will be made for AI to transform health and care.

KEY INSIGHTS

■ **The impact that AI has on the patient–physician relationship will be influenced by trust, humanization, families, and caregivers, as well as experience.**

■ **AI in the clinical context needs to be distinguished as either consumer-grade AI, which is not clinically validated, or medical-grade AI, which is clinically validated and has regulatory approval. The risks and applications of these two types differ.**

■ **Likely scenarios for AI in clinical contexts include AI as a medical assistant, AI as a patient monitor, and AI conducting clinical work.**

■ **It is crucial for AI makers to engage physicians, patients, families, and caregivers in the development of AI to ensure that AI be designed, developed, and adopted with shared perspectives around capabilities and diverse stakeholder needs.**

References

1. Hansen AJ. Stanford Presence Center symposium grapples with balancing human and artificial intelligence in medicine. *Scope*, 6 March 2018. https://scopeblog.stanford.edu/2018/03/06/stanford-presence-center-symposium-grapples-with-balancing-human-and-artificial-intelligence-in-medicine.
2. Babic B, Gerke S, Evgeniou T, Cohen IG. Direct-to-consumer medical machine learning and artificial intelligence applications. *Nature Machine Intelligence* 2021;3:283–287.
3. IMDRF. Software as a Medical Device (SaMD): Clinical Evaluation. International Medical Device Regulators Forum; 2017. https://www.imdrf.org/sites/default/files/docs/imdrf/final/technical/imdrf-tech-170921-samd-n41-clinical-evaluation_1.pdf.
4. American Medical Association. CPT® Appendix S: Artificial Intelligence Taxonomy for Medical Services and Procedures, 2021. https://www.ama-assn.org/system/files/cpt-appendix-s.pdf.
5. American Medical Association. Advancing Health Care AI through Ethics, Evidence and Equity, 2022. https://www.ama-assn.org/practice-management/digital/advancing-health-care-ai-through-ethics-evidence-and-equity.
6. Cadario R, Longoni C, Morewedge C. Understanding, explaining, and utilizing medical artificial intelligence. *Nature Human Behaviour* 2021;5L1636–1642. https://doi.org/10.1038/s41562-021-01146-0.
7. Digital Diagnostics. IDx-DR, 2022. https://www.digitaldiagnostics.com/products/eye-disease/idx-dr.

For additional references please see www.wiley.com/go/byrne/aiinclinicalmedicine

45

Virtual Care and AI: The Whole Is Greater Than the Sum of Its Parts

Junaid Kalia

NeuroCare.AI, Prosper, TX, USA

Learning Objectives

- ▤ Understand digital transformation.
- ▤ Appreciate the vision of virtual care and AI in synergy.
- ▤ Understand the Virtual Care as a Service (VCaaS) model.
- ▤ Understand Artificial Intelligence as a Service (AIaaS) model.
- ▤ See the convergence and synergy between VCaaS and AIaaS.
- ▤ Review the evolution of legal and regulatory frameworks.
- ▤ Recognize the Food and Drug Administration's encouragement of the use of AI in virtual care.
- ▤ See examples of the evolution of stroke care and also VCaaS and AIaaS in practice.

45.1 Understanding Digital Transformation

Digital transformation in any field should be understood as an ongoing process or a journey, and not a static destination. Let us take the example of maps and mapping technology. The simple digitization of maps did not bring about the radical change that enabled new core competencies (e.g. Lyft, Uber, DoorDash, etc.) but rather a digital transformation of mapping technology itself. This transformation continues to this day as these companies strive to improve upon their current mapping systems – the journey continues. The enablers in these radical changes depend on two technologies: (i) systems for the continuous user-generated collection of quality data; and (ii) the ability of AI to interpret and learn from these data. The systems enable the continued collection of high-quality data while simultaneously improving underlying AI models. More importantly, these applications are packaged and distributed as a *Software as a Service* (SaaS) model [1]. SaaS enables and incorporates user-generated data to be used to create value. It is cloud-based, decentralized, democratized, and, most importantly, scalable.

AI in Clinical Medicine: A Practical Guide for Healthcare Professionals, First Edition. Edited by Michael F. Byrne, Nasim Parsa, Alexandra T. Greenhill, Daljeet Chahal, Omer Ahmad, and Ulas Bagci.
© 2023 John Wiley & Sons Ltd. Published 2023 by John Wiley & Sons Ltd.
Companion website: www.wiley.com/go/byrne/aiinclinicalmedicine

Virtual care (VC) is the digitization of the front door of healthcare, the first step of which is getting comprehensive care online for both the patient and provider. It is a paradigm shift in care delivery, drastically transforming how we expect to receive care. VC is the first step to bridging the chasm in the adoption of digital health for the masses; the only silver lining of the COVID-19 pandemic is the spotlight that it cast on the need for VC. In April 2020, overall telehealth utilization for office visits and outpatient care was 78 times higher than in February 2020, and remained 38 times higher than pre-pandemic [2]. Digital transformation also assists in collecting high-quality, relevant data at source by enabling and integrating new forms of data, as discussed in the next section. The growing acceptance of, and access to, VC will enable a further digital transformation of healthcare with AI at the heart of it.

45.2 Vision of Virtual Care and AI Synergy

Before we dive into the details of the models of VC and AI synergy, let us understand how these models will integrate into real-life situations. VC enables new forms of data, and with the power of AI these data can be turned into actionable intelligence. The digitized patient will create more data in various forms. Some highlighted examples include:

- Automated digital video analysis can be applied to facial asymmetry detection in stroke [3], smile detection in autism [4], tremor detection in movement disorders [5], event detection in seizure [6] and falls [7], and gait analysis in orthopaedics, rehabilitation, and multiple sclerosis [8].
- Automated digital audio analysis can be applied to dysarthria in Parkinson's [9], tonality and sentiment analysis in psychiatric disorders [10], and cough frequency in pulmonology [11].
- Automated Health Internet of Things (HealthIoT) will bring various forms of data in terms of identification, communication, location, and sensors. These are already used for atrial fibrillation, diabetes, pneumonia, and hypertension [12], but these examples barely scratch the surface of the potential.

VC is the first step in digitization. However, data alone will not improve patient outcomes – they need to be analysed in context. AI is critical in this area and needs to be deployed contextually according to a patient-driven as a service model that we will discuss later. We will also see increased digitization of in-person visits to incorporate these new data points, moving us closer to a true digital health vision with ambient intelligence [13].

45.3 Understanding the Virtual Care as a Service (VCaaS) Model

The future healthcare model is forecast to be virtual first, augmented by in-person visits (if required), rather than the other way around. This digital transformation will first and foremost make high-quality data collection at the source a priority. This fact

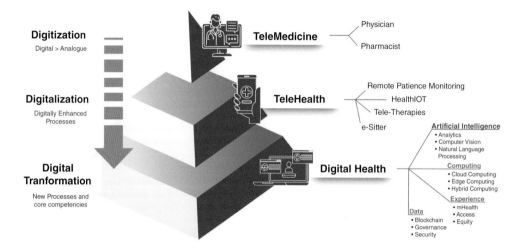

Virtual care Continuum

Convergence of Technologies | Enabling Core Competencies

Figure 45.1: Digital transformation of healthcare in the context of the virtual care (VC) continuum. The increasing digitalization of the patient journey is exemplified by the VC continuum from telemedicine to telehealth to true digital health. VC is the digitalization of the front door of healthcare, the first step of which is getting comprehensive care online (telemedicine) for both patient and provider. This is enabling heath data to move from analogue to digital formats. Digitalization is the next step in the process and includes telehealth enabled by digitally enhanced processes. Necessary steps are required to ensure that new processes and core competencies – inclusive of AI – are included as we move forward towards a full digital transformation of healthcare.

will act as fertile soil for the fruits of AI to blossom, enabling new core technologies that will parse through multi dimensional multi-modal data. This increasing digitization of patient journeys is exemplified in the VC continuum from telemedicine to telehealth to true digital health, as shown in Figure 45.1.

The very essence and expectations of care will change once the VC model is fully adopted. The patient experience is being transformed, and care delivery expectations are radically changing. VC allows for more robust communication between patient and clinician, receiving and sending important data electronically, and opens avenues to new therapy and patient monitoring formats, as discussed in the earlier examples. These avenues are, in themselves, great sources of new kinds of high-quality data, and also allow AI to learn patterns and develop new tools for disease detection, prevention, and management.

VC is already being delivered exactly like a SaaS. It is cloud-based, on-demand, and, in most cases, web based. It has also enabled choice for patients and hospitals, as geographical boundaries are no longer constraints [14]. Hospitals choose which services they want to augment, replace, or create. As examples, Tele-ICU was rapidly adopted during the pandemic to improve staff safety. Tele-stroke has been part and parcel of many hospital systems due to a shortage of neurologists.

The ultimate expression of the VC continuum is the 'Virtual Hospital at Home', shown in Figure 45.2 [15,16]. These initiatives are being delivered on the same as

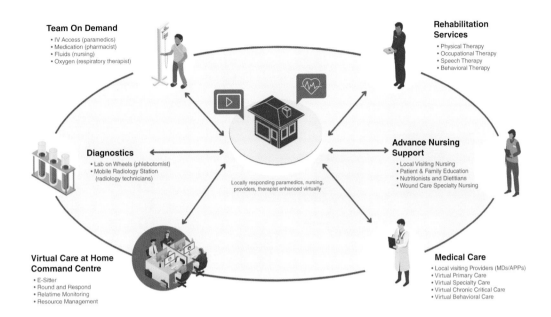

Team On Demand
• IV Access (paramedics)
• Medication (pharmacist)
• Fluids (nursing)
• Oxygen (respiratory therapist)

Rehabilitation Services
• Physical Therapy
• Occupational Therapy
• Speech Therapy
• Behavioral Therapy

Diagnostics
• Lab on Wheels (phlebotomist)
• Mobile Radiology Station (radiology technicians)

Advance Nursing Support
• Local Visiting Nursing
• Patient & Family Education
• Nutritionists and Dietitians
• Wound Care Specialty Nursing

Locally responding paramedics, nursing, providers, therapist enhanced virtually

Virtual Care at Home Command Centre
• E-Sitter
• Round and Respond
• Realtime Monitoring
• Resource Management

Medical Care
• Local visiting Providers (MDs/APPs)
• Virtual Primary Care
• Virtual Specialty Care
• Virtual Chronic Critical Care
• Virtual Behavioral Care

Virtual Hospital at Home
Your home is your care site

Figure 45.2: Virtual Hospital at Home. This is the ultimate expression of the virtual care continuum, where different healthcare initiatives are delivered on an as a service model, including laboratory services, mobile radiology, diagnostics, and tele-rehabilitation services. Patients will be able to select providers and services based on cost, convenience, and urgency in their own homes, making home their 'care site'.

a service model, where patients will choose providers and services based on cost, convenience, and urgency. We have already seen the development, and implementation, of laboratory-on-wheels [17], HealthIoT devices [18], mobile radiology stations [19], and tele-rehabilitation services [20]. These services will be integrated according to patients' needs, creating value and improving outcomes along the way. Hospitals will need to develop a new use case as the care environment shifts [21].

45.4 Understanding the AI as a Service (AIaaS) Model

AI in healthcare has been developed as marketplaces by IBM [22] and Nuance [23], which will follow the SaaS model, similar to an app store model as shown in Figure 45.3. However, given the high-stakes nature of medicine, sweeping changes cannot suddenly be implemented. To mitigate some of these risks, AI in healthcare will initially be developed and deployed in smaller modules and integrated (see Chapter 2).

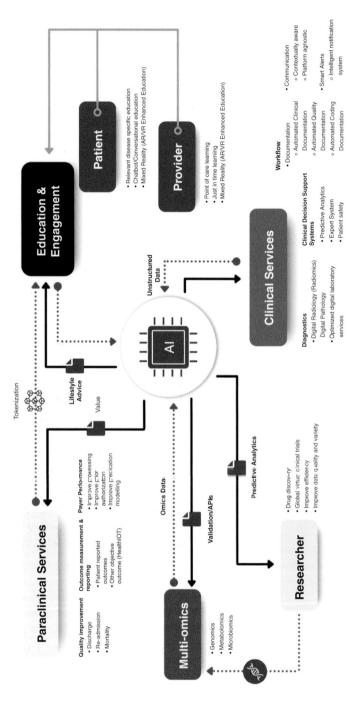

Artificial intelligence as Service (AIaas)

Plug-n-play modular services to enhance and enable new competencies

Figure 45.3: AI as a Service (AIaaS) in healthcare can be provided as a modular strategy, bridging the gap from proof of concept to production. The modular approach enhances the chances of adoption, expanding upon usage where needed and tweaking processes along the way. Hospitals and clinicians can choose the modules that will have the greatest impact on their population, saving cost and time in the process.

The advantage of a modular strategy is that it ensures privacy, reduces risk, and improves value measurement. It bridges the gap from proof of concept to production. The best examples are Viz.ai and RapidAI [24,25]. These use AI to synchronize stroke care, reducing systemic delays that stand between patients and life-saving treatments through care coordination and automated detection of (i) brain haemorrhage, (ii) large vessel occlusion, and (iii) salvageable brain tissue. Both companies developed one module and then added other modules to their ever-evolving AI product suite. This is the true evolution of AIaaS in action. The modular approach enhances the chances of adoption, expanding upon usage where needed, and tweaking processes along the way. Hospitals and clinicians can choose the modules that will have the greatest impact on their population, saving cost and time in the process. For example, a dermatologist will choose a different module that a cardiologist or a neurologist serving their respective patient populations.

45.5 Convergence and Synergy between VCaaS and AIaaS and Other Technologies

As both technology and societal acceptance evolve, VC and AI will continue to converge. As VC expands and creates more quality data, it will require algorithms, specifically AI, to make sense of that data and develop decision-support tools. With AI becoming increasingly indispensable, both VCaaS and AIaaS services will complement and synergistically move digital health forward. This synergy will create an exponential expansion, especially with other emerging technologies like 5G, Wifi6, edge and node computing, and mixed reality [26].

This convergence will also usher in a new era of quality improvements, as precise patient-level data will become available to ensure the accurate quantification of outcomes [27]. This will have major ramifications, as one of the key deterrents to 'value-based care' has been accurately capturing outcomes. With enhanced objectivity and patient-reported outcome data, we can finally create policies that reimburse outcomes compared to activity (fee for service), realizing the dream of value-based care.

45.6 Evolution of Legal and Regulatory Frameworks

The expansion of VC during the pandemic arose from the need for contactless care. However, realizing the great potential for faster and improved care, numerous societies and agencies are now arguing to make these benefits permanent [28,29]. Similarly, in AI the US Food and Drug Administration's (FDA) Software as a Medical Device (SaMD) approach inherently creates an environment where specific modules are approved, which opens the potential for a holistic suite of AI. Combining both, we now see a regulatory framework where VCaaS and AIaaS approaches are encouraged.

One of the biggest hurdles to health information exchange was removed with the Cures Act, ensuring interoperability [30]. Interoperability is expected by default, and information blocking is penalized. As an example, the Centers for Medicare & Medicaid Services (CMS) set up a Trusted Exchange Framework to enhance the sharing of medical data [31]. CMS also ensures that interoperability falls at the level of the Health Maintenance Organization (HMO) rather than electronic health record (EHR) vendors [32]. There are clear certification requirements for vendors, but moving the responsibility from EHR vendors to the HMOs creates an opportunity to untether VCaaS and AIaaS from EHR vendors. EHR vendors are required to enable application programming interfaces (APIs) within 24 hours to ensure continued data services without delay. This will empower HMOs and clinicians to deliver cost-effective care to their respective patients, as they can now choose which services are to be enabled or disabled, based on a patient's demands.

45.7 FDA Encourages the Use of AI in Virtual Care

The FDA's SaMD model [33] is in evolution, and rightly so. Technologies evolve at a breakneck speed, and the accompanying regulatory framework continues to lag and evolve slowly, but the FDA has now approved multiple AI algorithms through various pathways [34]. Although not explicitly documented but communicated through public meetings, the FDA's current thinking has grown to encourage the use of VC to improve data quality, volume, variety, and velocity [35]. This will enable continuous learning models [36] and account for data shifts [37]. To date, there are no FDA-approved continuous learning algorithms. The expansion of VC has become a requirement. It is essential to collect clinically validated data and develop models that can be improved while preserving patient safety and privacy, which points to a symbiotic, synergistic relationship between VC and AI (see Chapter 36).

45.8 Value and Reimbursement

Reimbursement is a core issue in healthcare. Unlike other economies, the drive for innovation in healthcare is severely restricted by heavily regulated financial or business models. The VC business was initially driven by the lack of physicians for essential medical services, for example tele-stroke and tele-psychiatry. The spread of the COVID-19 pandemic then made contactless care a necessity. Now payments for VC are becoming mainstream.

Compensation related to AI services is still in its early stages. CMS created a programme, New Technology Add-On Payment (NTAP) [38], as a bridge effort to promote new technologies in healthcare for Medicare patients until the diagnosis-related group (DRG) reimbursement system is calibrated. Viz.ai and RapidAI are the only AI-based platforms awarded additional reimbursement modes [39,40]. The requirements for reimbursement are stringent, and demonstrating cost benefits for new technology can be challenging. In the future, as we see AI evolving from proof of concept to delivering real value to patients, more payers will initiate programmes to reimburse AI companies, with payers and patients both saving money.

Integrating VC and AI is a colossal opportunity waiting to be seized. The USA wastes about $1 trillion annually in healthcare [32]: 1% of $1 trillion is $10 billion. If we can design systems that can save 1% of waste, we are looking at significant value for society, patients, providers, and entrepreneurs. This value creation is, and will be, the reimbursement pathway for new technological advancements in healthcare.

45.9 Evolution of Stroke Care in the Digital Era

Stroke care serves as a prime example of the significance of AI and VC in clinical care, in both acute and chronic settings. Stroke is a perfect storm; in an acute care setting 'time is brain', where latency and accurate information can have a transformative impact on the patient's life. Hence, tele-stroke was one of the first services approved for reimbursement regardless of location requirements [41]. Tele-stroke enables the rapid, virtual (via video) examination of a suspected stroke patient, including a review of imaging, and recommendation for or against the administration of a clot-busting drug. Advice is also given on whether the patient should receive endovascular treatment.

Even before the reimbursement programme, many hospitals were paying themselves to enable stroke services at their hospitals. Reimbursement led to an explosion in the use of alteplase (a thrombolytic medication) for selected stroke patients [42]. Patient selection for alteplase became increasingly complex with new forms of imaging like computed tomography angiography and perfusion. Manual imaging performance wastes precious time; thus, automated processing is crucial to decrease latency in care for stroke patients [43,44]. From this need grew the availability of commercial software for rapid detection and patient selection, such as RapidAI, AIDoc [25], Viz.ai, and Brainomix (www.brainomix.com). VC necessitates AI in healthcare with new imaging data and decision support.

Given that the cost of disability from a stroke is huge, for both the patient and society, technologies that can decrease latency in care such as Viz.ai or RapidAI were the first ones to be recognized by the CMS NTAP program. The upfront cost of such technologies also becomes more attractive and affordable when compared to the value they bring.

In the chronic care setting, we have seen increasing use of telehealth to remove barriers to care, providing access, equity, and convenience. As disability decreases mobility, care now comes to the patient rather than the other way around. The use of new HealthIoT devices like blood pressure monitoring, pulse oximetry, and fall detection is already commercially available, for instance with Biointellisence™ (https://biointellisense.com). Increasingly these new HealthIoT devices are being incorporated into telehealth platforms [45]. Moreover, services like tele-rehabilitation can enhance in-person rehabilitation and decrease time to institutionalized rehabilitation, saving costs while increasing safety and convenience [46].

Other benefits, like getting therapy in one's native language, can now be realized as telehealth opens the opportunity to provide care without geographical limitations [47]. New forms of objective monitoring are emerging for rehabilitation via wearables and will need AI to parse through data that these new devices will generate [48,49]. Digital health platforms will also improve medication adherence to empower patients and family members, thus improving care and decreasing complications [50,51].

45.10 Full-Stack Digital Clinician

'Full-stack' is a term used to describe software engineers that can handle complete end-to-end processes from data to a server to clients. The exponential change and shift towards digital health will come with its challenges. Clinicians will need to relearn the new paradigm of medicine, which will result in a shift from population-based (evidence-based) medicine to personalized (precision) medicine. This will require the re-education of clinicians, as they will be bombarded with multi-dimensional, multi-modal data and analysis. There will be a need to retrain current clinicians to use AI responsibly and ethically [52,53]. Medical school curricula and continued medical education (CME) also need to incorporate AI in healthcare as mandatory learning [54,55]. We will soon see the birth of Clinician 4.0, a full-stack digital clinician.

45.11 Conclusion

VC and AI services will continue to evolve and converge with additional technologies, realizing the goal of value-based, personalized, precision care. VC, enhanced with AI, will lead to true digital transformation, and give birth to full-stack digital clinicians. Eventually, we will see systems developed from the ground up to use VC and AI first rather than following or add-on services. Until then, we need to keep moving the needle towards digital transformation by creating and adopting VC and AI as services.

KEY INSIGHTS

- Virtual care is the first step in the digital transformation of healthcare.
- Virtual care as a service model will continue to evolve the virtual care continuum, enabling new core competencies with the convergence of technologies.
- This continuum will provide high-quality and new forms of data to create clinically validated data for AI services.

- ■ **Inter-operability and information-blocking rules will tear down data silos and democratize healthcare data.**
- ■ **AI in healthcare needs to fill the production gap, which is possible with the AIaaS model.**
- ■ **As services model thinking will create minimal viable products that can be scaled and deployed and then further integrated**
- ■ **As these services converge and evolve, a marketplace and eventually platforms will emerge to create a value chain of VCaaS and AIaaS in synergy.**
- ■ **There will be a need for the re-education of the clinical workforce in the new digital healthcare era enhanced by AI.**

References

1. Software as a service. *Wikipedia*, 2022. `https://en.wikipedia.org/wiki/Software_as_a_service`.
2. Torous J, Myrick KJ, Rauseo-Ricupero N, Firth J. Digital mental health and COVID-19: using technology today to accelerate the curve on access and quality tomorrow. *JMIR Mental Health* 2020;7(3):e18848.
3. Chang C-Y, Cheng M-J, Ma MH-M. Application of machine learning for facial stroke detection. In: *2018 IEEE 23rd International Conference on Digital Signal Processing (DSP)*. New York: IEEE; 2018, 1–5.
4. Wu C, Liakat S, Helvaci H et al. Machine learning based autism spectrum disorder detection from videos. In: *2020 IEEE International Conference on E-health Networking, Application & Services (HEALTHCOM)*. New York: IEEE; 2021, 1–6.
5. Kovalenko E, Aleksandr T, Anikina A et al. Distinguishing between Parkinson's disease and essential tremor through video analytics using machine learning: a pilot study. *IEEE Sensors Journal* 2020;21(10):11916–11925.
6. Tian J, Yu W, Chen J et al. Automated analysis of seizure behavior in video: methods and challenges. In: *2020 2nd World Symposium on Artificial Intelligence (WSAI)*. New York: IEEE; 2020, 34–37.
7. De Miguel K, Brunete A, Hernando M, Gambao E. Home camera-based fall detection system for the elderly. *Sensors* 2017;17(12):2864.

For additional references and Further Reading please see `www.wiley.com/go/byrne/aiinclinicalmedicine`

46

Summing It All Up: Evaluation, Integration, and Future Directions for AI in Clinical Medicine

Mark A. Shapiro[1] and Marty Tenenbaum[2]

[1] *xCures, Inc., Oakland, CA, USA*

[2] *Cancer Commons, Mountain View, CA, USA*

Learning Objectives

- Recall AI foundations and key definitions.
- Discover a framework for assessment and evaluation of AI systems in clinical medicine.
- Review ethical and regulatory issues associated with AI in clinical medicine.
- Be aware of future directions for AI in clinical medicine.

46.1 Introduction

Clinicians are increasingly presented with 'AI-enabled' software, systems, and other technology. With more than 340 software or medical devices already approved by the US Food and Drug Administration (FDA) [1], medical practitioners can expect these systems to become ubiquitous in their clinical practice. AI-enabled systems are or soon will be involved in all parts of the clinical workflow, from scheduling of patient encounters and retrieval of relevant medical history, to diagnosis, treatment planning, and surveillance. The aim of this chapter is to recap the key ideas within this textbook and leave clinicians with a solid understanding of how AI systems work. This will prepare them both to critically evaluate if an AI medical system is operating correctly, and to participate in the development and refinement of such systems. Finally, we present a vision for the future of AI in clinical medicine.

46.2 Foundations of AI and Machine Learning

A useful working definition of *AI* is:

> *Computer algorithms or systems that can perform complex tasks typically requiring human intelligence or expertise.*

AI in Clinical Medicine: A Practical Guide for Healthcare Professionals, First Edition. Edited by Michael F. Byrne, Nasim Parsa, Alexandra T. Greenhill, Daljeet Chahal, Omer Ahmad, and Ulas Bagci.
© 2023 John Wiley & Sons Ltd. Published 2023 by John Wiley & Sons Ltd.
Companion website: www.wiley.com/go/byrne/aiinclinicalmedicine

This definition is more aspirational than technical. As Mat Velloso, the technical advisor to the CEO of Microsoft, observed, 'If it is written in Python, it is probably machine learning. If it is written in PowerPoint, it's probably AI.'

Until the term AI has a more precise definition, we urge clinicians to ask clarifying questions when confronted with systems that claim to deliver AI in clinical medicine. As the many examples in this book can attest, AI can provide substantial benefits to clinicians and patients, but in order to understand whether the outputs of a system are relevant in a specific clinical situation or for a specific patient, more information about the AI model is required. As developers of AI systems and software, we encourage the field to learn from the experience of pharmaceutical, biological, and medical device developers, in order to avoid repeating mistakes that led to a backlash for their industries from patients or clinicians.

Machine learning has a more widely understood and technical meaning. We definite it as:

> *The subfield of computer science that is focused on developing or implementing algorithms that apply statistics, linear algebra, calculus, and other mathematical methods for prediction, recommendation, and classification tasks.*

The key difference between machine learning and traditional statistical modeling methods is the derivation, tuning, or selection of model parameters from the data. Data Scientist Juan Lavista Ferres observed, 'When we raise money it's AI, when we hire it's machine learning, and when we do the work it's logistic regression.' So, when presented with software or systems that employ machine learning, a clinician should reasonably expect answers to specific questions about the algorithm(s) being used, and what metrics were used to evaluate and validate the model, among other specifics.

Because machine learning models typically *learn aspects of the model from the data*, the developer must make several choices that an end-user should be mindful of. The first is the choice of model itself. It is quite common to try several models for a given task and simply select the model with the top score on some chosen performance metric. It should be obvious that because the model is somewhat reliant on the data, the selection of data used to develop a model is critical. It is at this stage where it is possible for the developer to introduce *hidden biases* in the model.

Some examples of hidden biases are bias in how the data were selected, whether those data were representative (e.g. the patients used to train the model do not generalize to the setting where it is being used), and biases inherent in the data themselves (such as might arise from bias in the medical system, access to care, geography, patient demographics, etc.). Consider the critique of the IBM Watson for Oncology system, which was trained on data from a top cancer centre in the USA, but which did not always generalize for patients in other countries, both due to demographics, but also to the differences in local practice patterns and treatment options [2–4].

Both developers and users of AI-enabled systems must consider the sources of the data and take great effort to ensure that those data are fit for the intended purpose.

Many machine learning models may be thought of as extensions to traditional statistical methods. For example, when fitting a normal regression equation by minimizing the sum of squared errors, a machine learning model might add an additional penalty to account for model complexity. The concept of a *penalty function* was a key insight necessary for modern machine learning methods. In addition to a sum of square error terms, a penalty can be introduced to shrink the number of model parameters, hence the description of machine learning as selecting a model using the data. This contrasts with a standard statistical approach where the statistician chooses which independent variables are thought to contribute to the dependent variable. It should be noted that several authors have shown that *complex models do not necessarily outperform simpler statistical models* [5] on out-of-sample data [6], and that machine learning approaches primarily outperform statistical methods only when the dimensionality of the data grows large [7].

Within machine learning, the two main tasks are *prediction* and *classification*. Prediction normally involves a real-valued objective, which can be a probability (expressed as a percentage or number between zero and one), a time to event (in days, months, years, or other units), or any other numerical objective. In contrast, classification is concerned with assigning a label. This is also called a 'categorical' output and could be a binary classification (e.g. is the patient expected to be alive or dead at 30 days?), or a multi-class classification (e.g. is a magnetic resonance image [MRI] worsening, improving, stable, or equivocal?).

Prediction and classification methods can be 'fuzzy', meaning that they may have probabilities associated with multiple outputs. The outputs (or dependent variables) are not limited to a single scalar value, and in fact could be a vector, matrix, or tensor. They may also include point estimates with a variance or even a full probability distribution. In clinical medicine, this means that the AI outputs could range from very complex things like a suspected lesion boundary on a serial MRI scan (which may be presented visually, but is computed as a tensor) to a simple risk score.

Natural language processing (NLP) is:

> *The application of machine learning and other computational methods to the analysis of language.*

The most important insight catalysing progress in language modelling for AI was the development of vector representations of words and sentences (see Figure 46.1) [8,9].

GloVe was a 300-dimensional model, and the developers showed no enhancement from a larger, 1000-dimensional model. This means that in a dictionary of tens of thousands of words, each word can be represented as a combination of those 300 features. More recent developments, for example GPT-3, BERT, and ELMO, include very large embedding models based on transformer architectures that can represent language as high-dimensional vectors (typically 768-dimensional) with embeddings that depend on context from surrounding words and sentences, providing more

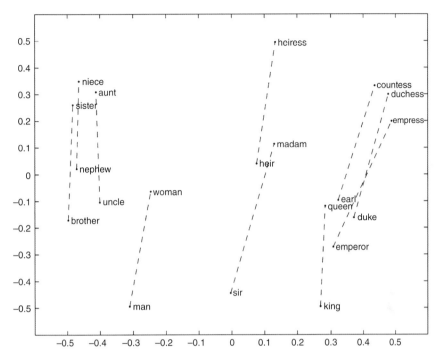

Figure 46.1: Linear relationships between words denoting male and female relationships.

Source: Adapted from Jeffrey Pennington et al. [8].

nuance than GloVe since they can handle words having different meanings depending on context. While these models can perform exceptionally well on general tasks such as language translation, domain-specific tasks, particularly in biomedicine, can be challenging. These models can struggle to contextualize jargon, patterns of speech, abbreviations, and terms of art that were rarely encountered during model training, such as rare symptoms or conditions. It can be difficult, though not impossible, for these models to handle words that were never seen in the training data. Moreover, these models are *generative*, meaning that they can be trained to generate text from different inputs. The generated text sounds credible even when it is untrue. These systems require large amounts of text for training, and there is a lot of untrue text out in the world. Learning relationships from text that includes biases and falsehoods, while accurately reflecting human language, can lead to a model that incorporates those biases and untruths. It is the text analogue to deep fake images.

The limitations of transformer language models can sometimes be resolved by 'unlocking' a deep layer in the model and training on domain-specific text, such as radiology reports or clinical notes. This is an example of *transfer learning*, where a highly trained language model is tuned on a smaller amount of domain-specific information. Large amounts of text may still be required.

More generally, the goal of transfer learning is to develop a model that correctly learns to recognize distinguishing features in one domain that can be applied to another. Transfer learning has great potential in any medical AI application requiring large-scale data collection and labelling, especially when clinically important but rare subgroups are involved. A non-textual example of transfer learning is training a neural network model to recognize pancreatic tumors, and then retraining it on a smaller set of data to identify liver tumours. Of course, this is potentially risky and requires careful validation, but it can be highly cost-effective.

46.3 Types of Learning

In practice, most AI methods involve one of two approaches, and it is important to understand the differences when considering the applicability of an AI system to a patient or clinical setting. *Supervised learning* requires labelled data to train the AI algorithm. This is an approach that is well suited to situations where there are a lot of data available ('Big Data') and there is broad consensus on the correct labelling of those data (see Figure 46.2). Such might be the case when training an AI to identify areas of clinical interest in radiographic images or pathology slides. However, getting access to large volumes of high-quality, labelled medical data for AI model development is often a major challenge. It is costly to have physicians manually label data, and the task cannot easily be delegated to untrained personnel. Thus, supervised learning in medicine is heavily dependent on situations where labels are created during routine practice, such as coded data in an electronic health record. For clinicians, it is important to be mindful of the fact that coding systems developed for billing (e.g. ICD-9 and ICD-10) may not translate to accurate labels for training a clinical model.

Many of the clinical AI systems in this book involve supervised learning on labelled training data, where there is high inter-rater agreement among clinicians. For example, systems designed to classify electrocardiogram (ECG) abnormalities have remarkably high accuracy that is comparable to that of cardiology residents

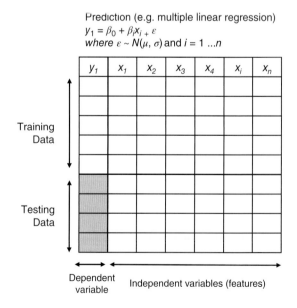

Figure 46.2: Schematic depiction of supervised learning set up as a prediction problem. In this example the training data are used to create a model that can predict the shaded testing data (dependent variable) using the unshaded testing data (independent variables) as input.

Source: Image created by Mark A. Shapiro and Marty Tenenbaum.

[10]. These systems have been trained on tens of thousands or millions of normal and abnormal ECGs, labelled using a reproducible process, such as having two independent readers provide a label with a referee process to produce a 'reference standard' or 'gold standard'. Unfortunately, not all of medicine is as well characterized and in many applications human experts do not agree. Although this issue is not insurmountable, developing AI in areas where there is an imperfect reference standard creates practical limits to supervised learning.

Overfitting can be an issue with supervised learning AI models. This is especially true in medicine, where there may be more predictor (independent) variables than there are examples. The definition of overfitting is creating a model that is more complex than can be justified by the data. Taken to the extreme, this would simply be a lookup table that takes each input and returns the labelled output. Such a model would be unable to generalize to unseen data but would still fit the training data perfectly. The major risk of an overfitted model is that, while displaying very high performance on the training data, it will generalize poorly to new data, a situation that creates unacceptable clinical risks.

To mitigate the risk of overfitting, AI models should be developed by separating the data used for training from those used for testing and validation. This may be accomplished through n-fold *cross-validation*, in which the data are randomly partitioned into test data that are held out for validation and training data that are themselves randomly portioned into 'folds' (see Figure 46.3). For example, in a dataset of 100 examples, 20 may be randomly selected for validation, the other 80 are then randomly split into five groups (called folds) each of 16 examples. Note the use of randomization in this process. Unlike prospective experiments, like clinical trials, machine learning often relies on retrospective analysis of data. Random splitting of the retrospective data helps to guard against bias in a manner similar to randomization in a prospective clinical trial.

To avoid 'leaking' information from validation data (and thus overfitting) into the AI model, *hyperparameters* should be fitted during the cross-validation stage. Hyperparameters are inputs into the model that must be specified by the developer. Both supervised and unsupervised learning techniques have hyperparameters. Because the model itself is a choice of the developer, it too may be considered an example of a hyperparameter. Thinking critically at this level, a clinician might ask 'why a support vector machine instead of a random forest?' Does the model really make sense given the data and task? It has become relatively easy to train many different models at the push of a button. Often different models have comparable performance, meaning that they are all using most of the available information within the training data. However, situations where one model dramatically outperforms other models should be treated with caution unless there is a clear, explainable reason. For example, a risk-scoring algorithm might more logically flow from a rules-based approach or a decision tree and would be expected to perform better than a linear regression for that task.

Expert systems and rule-based methods are a traditional approach for AI dating to the 1970s, and are based on learning rules that encode or infer the knowledge of

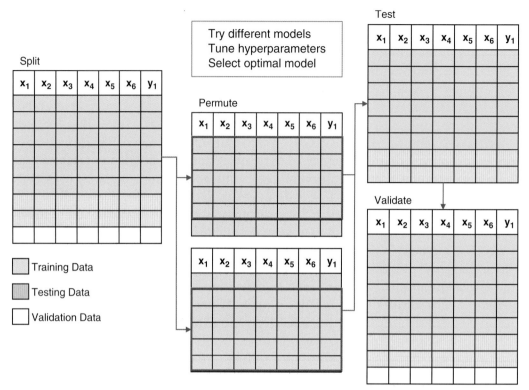

Figure 46.3: Schematic depiction of cross-validation. A set of labelled data is randomly split into three groups, training, testing, and validation data. The training data are then randomly split again into five groups, where each of four of the five groups is used to train a model against the held-out fold, which is used to evaluate the model. In this step, the training data are not independent, but by repeating the process and averaging the models, a good model is advanced to testing on the held-out test data.

Source: Image created by Mark A. Shapiro and Marty Tenenbaum.

domain experts [11]. These approaches are closely related to tree-based, supervised learning models and to non-parametric statistical models. Modern implementations incorporate many elements of more recent AI and machine learning techniques to generate rules. Whereas early systems relied on rules that were manually entered by 'knowledge engineers', today's systems can learn rules as features from data through stepwise analysis processes.

It is complex and potentially costly to elicit rules from clinical experts or to produce datasets from which these rules can be inferred, but the benefits include high accuracy, agreement with human experts, and a straightforward way to explain model reasoning and decisions – by citing the relevant rules. Often rule-based methods are a useful tool to augment biomedical and clinical NLP tasks: a simply formulated rule by an expert could eliminate the need for hundreds of labelled examples from which that rule would otherwise have to be learned.

Unsupervised learning, as the name implies, does not rely on external labels for the data. Instead, unsupervised learning methods look for patterns in data to form groups of similar or dissimilar items. These approaches can be useful where there is not an expert consensus on how to label items, or where the number of measured features is too large for human experts to identify what is relevant for a task. Examples include NLP, where each word represents a unique dimension. Patterns of words can quickly convey information such that a few words or sentences can convey the theme of a book, article, or patient history. A digital image has millions of pixels or voxels, each of which can take on a wide range of values. Just as a radiologist does not interpret a scan by evaluating each pixel, unsupervised learning methods discover boundaries where shapes and textures change. These are both examples of *dimensionality reduction*. The resulting features may be different and more discriminating than those used by clinicians.

In AI, unsupervised learning is often synonymous with *clustering* techniques, which attempt to find groups or classes of similar items within a dataset. Most clustering methods use the entire dataset, looking for structure without known labels, leading to a lower-dimensional representation of the data. However, supervised learning methods may benefit from clustering before machine learning or by performing dimensionality reduction by penalizing model complexity during the fitting process. An example would be least absolute shrinkage and selection operator or *LASSO regression* [12], which creates a penalty for the number of parameters retained in the model in addition to the normal objective of minimizing the mean squared error.

Another way to think about unsupervised learning is as an attempt to discover a hidden data-generating process. This concept comes from *Bayesian statistics*, in which an AI model is measured against how well it can reproduce observed data. These types of unsupervised learning models are called *generative models* and are closely related to simulation. In medicine, generative models have the potential to learn how to create convincing synthetic cases, which can enable privacy-preserving research or create synthetic data for human reviewers to label; a powerful technique for dealing with conditions where there may be extremely limited data available. Examples of generative models include variational autoencoders and generative adversarial networks. Both are types of *deep-learning neural network*.

Deep learning is another very important term that is often associated with medical AI systems. Most commonly, the term is applied to a neural network with multiple hidden layers between the 'input' layer and the 'output' layer. A classic example is a convolutional neural network, which is currently the most widely used architecture for computer vision applications. Here, the hidden layers are learning different aspects of the image, such as the edges between different objects or the difference between the foreground or background of the image. This *dimensionality reduction* can be accomplished using different AI techniques, such as unsupervised learning algorithms.

However, the term deep learning can also apply to systems that are not neural networks. In those cases, the AI pipeline would typically include sequential models, such as a dimensionality reduction step followed by a prediction or classification step.

Other types of learning commonly employed by AI systems include semi-supervised learning and weakly supervised learning, transfer learning, and reinforcement learning. These hybrid methods are useful when there are limited or low-quality labelled data from which models attempt to generalize by first learning how to label and then how to predict or classify. *Semi-supervised learning* has proven effective and popular in a wide variety of medical image analysis applications [13]. In other cases, a model trained for one task on a large amount of data may be re-trained on a new but similar task with fewer training data. That is called *transfer learning*.

46.4 AI Model Review

Supervised learning machine learning models include kernel methods, such as support vector machines; k-nearest neighbours; decision trees; penalized regression models; naïve Bayes; and neural networks. Unsupervised learning includes common dimensionality reduction or clustering methods, such as principal components analysis (which has long been used in the development of psychiatric and psychological ratings scales), and newer methods such as latent Dirichlet analysis (LDA) [14], a method based on non-parametric Bayesian statistics; T-distributed stochastic neighbour embeddings (t-SNE) [15], a nearest neighbour method based on robust regression; density-based agglomeration methods; and uniform manifold approximation and projection (UMAP) [16], a non-linear technique based on topology theory. The latter two methods are effective for visualizing high-dimensional data in two dimensions.

Common to unsupervised learning methods is the notion of *distance* (see Figure 46.4). The choice of the distance metric for unsupervised learning algorithms is an important one. Distance is typically normalized to a range from zero to one. In medicine, often we are more interested in *similarity*, which in machine learning is one minus the normalized distance. Depending on the clustering algorithm, distance or similarity might be an expected input.

Euclidean distance, based on the Pythagorean theorem, is a standard and conceptually simple choice but, depending on the application, there are dozens of distance metrics that might be suitable. Euclidean distance is poorly suited to

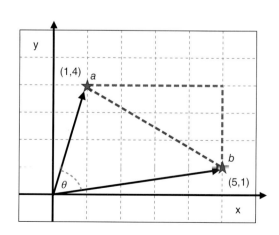

Figure 46.4: Three types of distance measures between points *a* and *b*. Euclidean distance is shown in red (5 units), Manhattan distance in blue (7 units), and cosine distance (θ) shown in green. Cosine distance is measured from zero to pi in radians, which can be normalized by converting to a scale from zero to one. In this example the normalized cosine distance is 0.25.

Source: Image created by Mark A. Shapiro and Marty Tenenbaum.

high-dimensional data, such as language data, due to the *curse of dimensionality*. To understand this concept, consider two randomly selected points on a one-dimensional line segment of length one. The average distance of points on this segment is one-half. Moving to two dimensions, on a circle of diameter one, the average distance between any two points is pi/2, about 0.63. As the number of dimensions increases, the average distance between points increases, such that in high-dimensional space, meaning problems with many variables, all points will, on average, be equidistant from one another. A similar situation arises when distance is measured on categorical features, which are commonly captured by *one-hot encoding* (each feature is present or absent, coded as zero or one in the dataset): the number of dimensions increases as the number of features does, and with many binary features there is inevitably a high combinatorial distance between any points. It is for these reasons that dimensionality-reduction methods become important in AI and machine learning. In NLP, one common solution is to use cosine distance rather than Euclidean distance, which is the angle from the origin between points. Examples are shown in Figure 46.4. For a clinician evaluating an AI system, the relevant question is whether the distance metric makes sense relative to the structure or type of data and the method being used for clustering.

An important but less widely used model for AI systems in clinical medicine is a *recommender system*. These types of AI are designed for information retrieval. They are ubiquitous in modern internet technology, helping to identify and retrieve personally relevant information from the ocean of information available. Among the best-known examples are the old Google PageRank [17] search and the Netflix movie recommendation algorithms. Almost all websites use these systems to retrieve information that is relevant to the user. Recommender systems typically have aspects of both supervised and unsupervised learning methods.

Recommender systems were originally based on algebraic techniques that represented users (e.g. patients) and items (e.g. treatments), each as a set of features. They rely on observed favourable or unfavourable interactions to provide a real, definite basis for recommendations using observation. The system will suggest items to a new user that similar previous users interacted with. This user–user approach is called a collaborative filter (see Figure 46.5). Likewise, items can be recommended based on a previous user interacting with similar items, which is called a content filter.

A challenge with recommender systems is the need for many user–item observations before the system can reliably make recommendations. This is termed the *cold start problem*. There is the potential for each user and each item to have many features, making the problem very complex. Current systems involve the use of mixed content and collaborative filters, with user and item metadata (information about the users or items), latent and hierarchical features (features can belong to groups, such as 'glioblastoma' belonging to the class 'brain tumours'), and temporal features (the time order of features matters). These involve complex computational challenges that are not tractable with matrix algebra alone.

An important tool for producing better information retrieval in recommender systems has been the use of what is called 'side information', which can help with

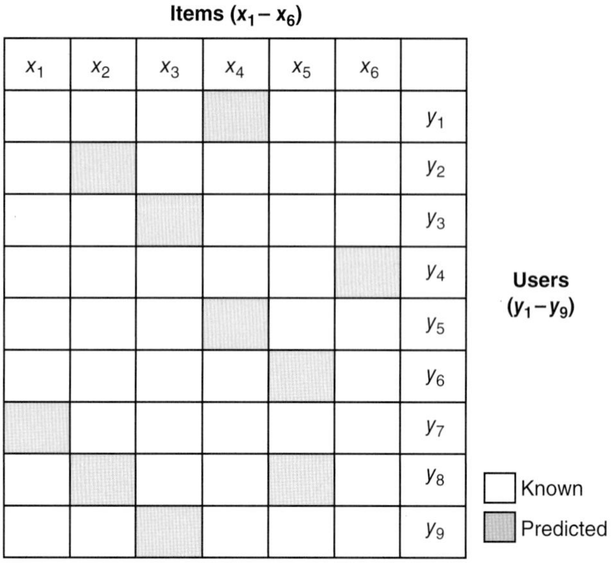

Items ($x_1 - x_6$)

Figure 46.5: A schematic of a collaborative filter recommender system.

Source: Image created by Mark A. Shapiro and Marty Tenenbaum.

the cold start problem. Side information could be things like treatment guidelines or clinical trial results. This information reduces sparsity and improves the connectedness of the user–item relationships. Recommender systems are also an example of an *active learning* AI system. These systems learn from each observation to sequentially improve recommendations, and are not typically 'static' algorithms, as are trained and validated AI prediction models.

Active and reinforcement learning AI is dynamic the system evolves by trying to balance exploration (try new things) with exploitation (try things that seem to work). This involves a trade-off between providing 'good' outputs and testing for 'better' outputs. This type of pre-planned A/B testing is common in e-commerce. In medicine, the best example of active learning would be adaptive clinical trials that use a *multi-armed bandit* allocation. However, active learning systems introduce an increased level of complexity, and raise important clinical and ethical questions that must be addressed prior to their application in practice.

46.5 Data Quality and Data Standards

With any scientific endeavour, the quality of the data collected for research matters. Computer scientists have long used the phrase '*Garbage in, garbage out*' to describe this situation. With AI algorithm development, the data should be '*fit for use*', meaning that they are reliable for and relevant to the intended analysis. However, it is helpful to think about the volume of data. In a small research study, great care must be taken to ensure that all the data are accurate and complete. In a large data-mining exercise, the analyst may rely more on the fact that missing or erroneous data will be a small fraction of the total. With AI applications, putting time and effort into more and better-quality labelled data is much more valuable than building complex models.

Clinical medicine is full of *data standards* and *coding systems*. Examples of coding systems include ICD-10 codes for diagnosis [18], LOINC codes for procedures [19], RxNORM codes for drug names, SNOMED for standardizing clinical terms [20], plus many others. Coding systems and *data models* vary by application. While the pharmaceutical industry relies on the CDISC standards [21] for study data models, real-world data have recently coalesced around the OMOP clinical data model [22]. Together these standardization efforts help to define common, inter-operable frameworks that can be fit for specific uses.

Most, if not all, AI algorithms will require some transformation of the input data as a *pre-processing* step. Data transformations are an essential part of creating quality data that are fit for use, but they can also introduce subtle biases. In addition to transforms that encode data, algorithms typically require treatment of missing data through imputations (i.e. replacing a missing value with the average value across that variable, creating a 'dummy' variable or code for missing values) to prevent the observation from being lost. Treatment of missing data in clinical trials and AI algorithms is extremely important. Were data *missing at random* or were they informative? Correctly censoring missing observations is critical for predictive models to avoid introducing *immortal time bias*, a situation where the event being predicted cannot occur due to missing observations. There is an extensive literature on this topic from traditional statistics, but a rigorous and light-hearted review can be found in 'Do Oscar winners live longer than less successful peers? A reanalysis of the evidence' by Sylvestre and colleagues [23].

46.6 Measures of AI Model Performance

The objective of this section is to review how AI system performance is typically measured or reported. Many approaches to performance assessment of AI are quite similar or even identical to those used to evaluate diagnostic tests.

For about 20 years, the field of AI has been dominated by papers that report new model architectures with slight improvements on existing models when measured against common open-source benchmark datasets. While the availability of open datasets as standards for performance comparison has undoubtedly advanced the field, reports of AI model or system performance should be considered critically in the clinical setting. While a clinical trial may report an apparently highly significant result of, for example, $p < 0.001$, the associated effect size may be clinically insignificant, or the measured effect may be completely clinically irrelevant.

Performance metrics fall into different categories depending on the type of task that the AI system is performing. For binary classification tasks, clinicians should be familiar with sensitivity and specificity from diagnostic tests. The measured performance of AI and machine learning systems is often reported using these same measures. Performance metrics are typically defined on a scale from zero to one, but depending on the nature of what is being measured and the context of the measurement, the scores can be misleading. Clinicians should adopt a Bayesian approach to interpreting many of these metrics based on their clinical 'prior' information.

With diagnostic tests, when the prevalence of positive cases is low in a population, an abnormal test result might constitute a false positive. In such cases, the clinical action is typically a retest, where the probability of a true positive is very high when a repeat test confirms the first finding. With AI-based systems, it is often not possible to perform an independent 'retest'.

46.6.1 Sensitivity and Specificity

Sensitivity is the ability to correctly detect a condition. This is commonly given as the number of true-positive (TP) results reported by the test or algorithm divided by the actual number of positive cases (P) in the sample. When there is a 'gold standard' or 'reference standard' to measure against, sensitivity is an appropriate choice for reporting performance. A *confusion matrix* is a helpful tool to understand and report the results of a classifier; an example is shown in Figure 46.6. These tables are used for diagnostic devices and AI alike.

Specificity is the ability to correctly report a negative result in cases where the true result is negative (TN). For example, in a diagnostic test, high specificity implies that the test correctly identifies patients who *do not* have the condition being tested. High specificity implies a low type I error rate, meaning few false-positive (FP) results. However, *high specificity should be interpreted with caution*. A test that *only* reports negative results will have a high specificity but no practical value, since it will have poor sensitivity. Thus, these two measures are typically reported together. This is also why *accuracy should typically be avoided* when reporting classification results: it is highly sensitive to *class imbalances*. Class imbalance is a very common challenge in AI. When training an AI system, great care must be taken to consider and manage imbalances between classes in the training data.

It is important to note that if the comparison is between an AI model (or diagnostic test) and a non-reference standard, agreement that an item is a TP or TN does not mean that either the model or non-reference standard is correct, merely that they agree. In such cases, differences in the prevalence of positive and negative examples in the training and reference datasets can have a large effect on the

Total population = P + N	Predicted Positive PP = TP + FP	Predicted Negative PN = FN + TN	
Actual Positive (P)	True Positive (TP)	False negative (FN)	**Sensitivity/ Recall** = TP / P
Actual Negative (N)	False positive (FP)	True negative (TN)	**Specificity** = TN / N
Prevalence = P / (P + N)	**Precision** = TP / (TP + FP)	**F₁ Score** = 2 TP / (2 TP + FP + FN)	Accuracy = (TP + TN) / (P + N)

Figure 46.6: A confusion matrix with several classification metrics listed.
Source: Image created by Mark A. Shapiro and Marty Tenenbaum.

measured sensitivity and specificity [24]. Where there is a very low prevalence of actual positive cases in the intended use population, even a 0.99 sensitivity is subject to wide confidence intervals that are rarely reported. In medicine, the quality of the labelled data is thus of paramount importance if the reported performance of an AI system is to be accurate.

46.6.2 Precision, Recall, and F_1 score

In AI applications, it is more common to see precision and recall reported. While the terms come from the field of information retrieval, they are other names for performance metrics found in diagnostic testing. *Recall* is the same as sensitivity defined earlier. *Precision* is defined as the number of TP results divided by the sum of TP and FP results, which is called *positive predictive value* in diagnostic testing. From a statistician's perspective, precision is one minus the type II error rate.

Because there is a potential trade-off between type I and type II errors in the development of AI algorithms (and clinical trials or diagnostic tests), it Is considered good practice to report the F_1 score, which is the harmonic mean of precision and recall. This measure provides a more balanced perspective on the overall performance of a classification algorithm. However, depending on the clinical situation, an algorithm might be developed to optimize a particular metric. If the clinical setting calls for accurate screening, for example to avoid missing early detection of cancer, the algorithm might be optimized for recall/sensitivity. However, if the harms from over-treatment are significant, precision or a balanced approach based on the F_1 score is more logical.

46.6.3 Area Under the Receiver Operating Characteristic Curve

Because the sensitivity and specificity of a classification algorithm are subject to trade-offs such that the developer could gain sensitivity at the expense of specificity or vice versa, it is common to include a plot of the receiver operating characteristic showing how these trade-offs occur over the range of possible values. In this way, it is easy to visualize how a classifier performs relative to *random guessing*. As seen in Figure 46.7, the area under the receiver operating characteristic curve (AUROC) for random guessing is one-half, while for a perfect oracle the AUROC would be 1.0. For a multi-class problem, the chance of randomly picking the correct class declines as the number of classes increases. In such cases, the performance of random guessing will decline towards the x-axis of Figure 46.7. Just as imbalanced examples of class data can pose problems with a supervised learning classifier, the presence of small but clinically important subgroups in training data can lead to high-validation performance that hides errors for these rare subgroups. Examples of this issue in computer vision applications are discussed in the work of Oakden-Rayner and colleagues [25].

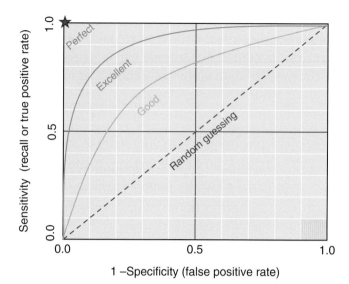

Figure 46.7: Understanding an ROC diagram for a binary classifier.

Source: Image created by Mark A. Shapiro and Marty Tenenbaum.

46.7 Validation of AI Systems

Medical interventions have long been subject to various standards for conducting and reporting the results of evaluations (Consort, ICH E6, ICH E9) [26,27]. This area is highly developed in regulated medical products, including pharmaceuticals, medical devices, and diagnostic tests. The lessons learned from the development of those other medical interventions and the principles that underpin those standards should inform the development and evaluation of AI systems in clinical medicine.

More recently, suggestions and principles for developing and validating AI systems in clinical medicine have been proposed [28]. The FDA, Medicines and Healthcare products Regulatory Agency (MHRA), and Health Canada, which oversee medical product regulation in the USA, UK, and Canada, respectively, put forth proposed guidelines for *Good Machine Learning Practices* (GMLP) [29], which are analogous to but much less developed than existing Good Clinical Practice (GCP), Good Laboratory Practice (GLP), and Good Manufacturing Practice (GMP) standards for other medical products. They recognize 10 guiding principles, which are included and discussed in more detail in Chapter 36.

We believe that these provide a compass for developers of AI systems for clinical medicine, and are the basis for what a clinician should expect to see in the product label or product information from an AI system deployed into clinical practice.

Like clinical trials, AI and machine learning algorithms are the product of complex scientific investigations. It is important that they have enough transparency for physicians, allied health professionals, and patients to understand their inner workings and performance. Just as the clinical trials that form the basis for the approval of medical products are published and disclosed, the investigation and validation of AI systems should be available at a level of detail that people knowledgeable in the field may scrutinize to evaluate the results.

We recommend that when machine learning models are deployed into production, having completed validation, a label (sometimes called a model card in the AI and machine learning community) should be produced. This is analogous to a clinical study report or publication of a clinical trial with methods. It should include:

- A general description of the model, including why and how it was developed.
- An overview of how the model works, including the software used to develop it.
- The intended use population.
- A description of the expected inputs and the form and format of the expect output.
- What hyperparameters are required for the model and how they were chosen.
- A description of the source of the training, testing, and validation data.
- A description of how the data were generated, collected, selected, and/or processed.
- An overview of the quality control plan used to ensure the quality of data in the model.
- The performance metrics used to train the model.
- An explanation of why the chosen metrics were selected over alternatives.
- Factors affecting model performance.
- How the model was validated.
- A sensitivity analysis of the model over ranges of inputs.
- A discussion of the possibility of biases in the model.

We believe that AI/machine learning models deployed in, or as, medical devices should generally adhere to existing frameworks for protecting health and ensuring that the product is safe and effective when used as directed. Some additional questions that must be considered in order to have confidence in a clinical AI model include:

- What is the gold standard against which the model is trained or measured?
- How was the gold standard defined or evaluated?
- Was the model tested on data from a single or multiple centres?
- Was an out-of-sample replication test performed?
- Was the evaluation retrospective, prospective, or both?
- How sensitive is the model to changed estimates of population information or hyperparameters?

In summary, as with medical products approved and used based on analysis from classical statistical models, clinicians presented with AI systems should be prepared to ask critical questions about how the data used to develop the model were collected. They should insist on systems that were developed and implemented in accordance with good software development practices. As we have seen with pharmaceuticals, there is a move to encourage information sharing during the peer review or regulatory review process. Clinicians should be prepared to ask questions. To what extent were the training data used for the model made available to independent researchers? If the datasets are proprietary, were they available to regulatory reviewers and did those expert reviewers make public a summary of their findings? Because AI systems can be opaque in both development and description, we encourage transparency as a guiding principle to ensure that these systems are safe and effective when used in clinical medicine.

46.8 Review of AI Applications in Clinical Medicine

As shown throughout this textbook, AI systems are already widely deployed in clinical medicine. They assist with the diagnosis of patients, the transcription of medical records, the scoring of prognostic risk, and even the recommendation of treatments or clinical trials. We can summarize the many distinct applications of AI in medicine under three main use types.

46.8.1 Big Data Applications

The most common AI applications apply pattern recognition to Big Data. These point solutions work well in applications such as ECG and MRI interpretation, where data are plentiful and there is general consensus on what constitutes a normal versus abnormal result.

Given adequate quantities of labelled data, supervised, semi-supervised, and deep learning algorithms can all quickly learn simple classification tasks. We caution that as the number of classes of output increases, the performance of such algorithms can degrade quickly. For complex tasks involving many distinct features of interest and many output classes, an ensemble of AI models may be a better choice. Breaking problems down into clearly defined – and manageable – parts can improve the quality of the resulting model(s). Breaking the problem down into separate sub-models will also make the interpretation clearer. This strategy is widely used in non-medical AI applications.

In clinical workflows, Big Data systems can help clinicians sift through large numbers of images or high volumes of telemetry data, by alerting them to abnormalities that need their attention. Learning when not to alert is just as important. With AI, a clinician can manage multiple data feeds from many patients across many types of sensors – both inpatient and from at-home devices. Using AI to identify important signals can improve utilization of expert clinical resources, reduce clinician decision fatigue, improve patients' clinical experience, and ideally lead to better patient outcomes.

Today's clinical AI systems tend to use static algorithms. In the near future, AI algorithms will be able to adapt to the local clinical environment, for example adjusting prior probabilities to take account of differences in patient demographics between centres. We can also expect to see tighter integration across algorithms. Predictions from diagnostic scans will inform treatment recommendations. In-patient tests will set the alert parameters of at-home monitoring devices. Intelligent radiology platforms will track lesion volumes from scan to scan, calling out very subtle changes, even when the patient is assessed using different equipment.

Another area where AI systems can improve clinical practice is through real-time feedback and continuous learning. Enabling a clinician to confirm or correct an AI system's diagnostic prediction or therapy recommendation provides an immediate learning opportunity for both human and computer. These learnings can then be validated and reinforced by tracking longitudinal outcomes. In the reverse scenario, an AI system can periodically insert test cases into a clinical review workflow in order to gauge performance quality and identify opportunities for retraining. During residency, gamification (turning the interface into a 'game-like' experience) using AI can increase engagement, help trainees identify areas of competence, and integrate targeted retraining if necessary.

There are challenges to realizing these advances, first and foremost the need to integrate data across health systems. Data sharing has been a longstanding challenge in healthcare, due to issues around patient *and* clinician privacy. Consider the story of Henrietta Lacks, whose cancer cells became one of the most widely used tools of biomedical research. Her cells have contributed to innumerable discoveries and commercial products. These cells were taken, modified, and used without her consent and the entire story was virtually unknown until 50 years after her death [30]. In developing AI systems, we urge that care is taken to avoid a similar situation where patient or clinician data are incorporated into AI systems without their knowledge or consent.

46.8.2 Prognostic and Diagnostic AI Applications

In addition to Big Data applications that rely on pattern recognition, this book has reviewed AI applications for the diagnosis or prognosis of medical conditions. In the diagnostic setting, AI can sift through large amounts of external data, such as publications and guidelines, to suggest potential conditions. Information retrieval from text sources has been an area where AI has proven highly successful outside of medicine. Even within medicine, the objective of practising 'evidence-based medicine' often necessitates quick searches to confirm the latest guideline or researching a treatment when a clear guideline does not exist. Studies have shown that both clinicians and patients rely on search engines to find relevant information [31]. The quality and provenance of the sourced information can vary based on how effective the searcher is and their choice of search tool. Proactive retrieval of high-quality information that is directly relevant to a patient case is an area where AI systems should be able to help. This can include both curated literature and guidelines search, as well as cross-institutional 'federated' searches of electronic health record systems seeking similar cases.

The evidence level for information-retrieval tasks can be quite different than that needed for Big Data tasks. In contrast to an ECG classification task, diagnostic and treatment decisions can involve substantial clinical ambiguity. Clinicians and patients both benefit when a comprehensive set of possible decisions and actions has been considered. Busy human beings may recall the top two or three options but struggle to recollect less common possibilities, especially under time pressure. In areas of medicine where practice is changing (such as oncology), or where a large amount of data must be cross-indexed (e.g. pharmacy drug–drug interaction systems), AI provides another layer of quality control and thus can improve patient safety.

AI systems used for prognosis are typically extensions of statistical models used for prognostic prediction and risk scoring or stratification. AI models can utilize more information (i.e. higher-dimensional data) than hand-built statistical models. They can also select features and feature–feature interactions to focus attention on the most relevant information. However, users of these risk-scoring and prognostic algorithms should take care to ensure that the models were properly validated. For example, in a train–test–validate paradigm, the model is selected and optimized in the training phase and accepted in the test phase, based on its performance on held-out data. At this stage, it should be explainable to a domain expert. Finally, the model can be considered clinically validated when replicable performance on another out-of-sample dataset has been completed. While complicated, this paradigm is not dissimilar from the approach the FDA uses to approve new drugs (two adequately powered, well-controlled studies that include pre-specified analysis plans). AI systems, which may be classified as medical devices, should – like other devices – have valid scientific evidence that they are safe, effective, and reliable when used as intended.

46.8.3 Learning in the Absence of Big Data

There are many important applications where Big Data are not available, where there are no data at all, and where the correct answer is unknown. Take oncology as an example. Back in the 1970s, at the start of Nixon's War on Cancer, there were 10 types of cancer, defined principally by organ of origin, and about 10 commonly used cancer chemotherapies. If we arrayed these cancer types and treatments on a 10×10 grid (cancer types on the horizontal axis, therapies on the vertical), we would have 100 boxes representing a therapy applied to a cancer type. With approximately a million patients a year diagnosed in the USA, one could in principle allocate 10,000 patients per box and run clinical trials testing all treatments against all cancer types.

Fast forward 50 years. Today, there are tens of thousands of cancer subtypes, defined by morphology, histopathology, and genetics. There are also tens of thousands of plausible multi-drug anti-cancer regimens. (The authors of this chapter maintain a treatment library of more than 10,000 current regimens compiled from published literature, online databases, and a large cancer patient registry [32].) The 10×10 grid is now a $10,000 \times 10,000$ grid representing 100 million potential clinical trials. Fortunately, there are still only about a million patients per year in the USA available for trials, so most of these cells are empty; there are likely *no data* on whether a given regimen would be effective on a given patient, because that regimen has never been tried for that subtype of cancer. It is a safe bet that no one knows the optimal way to treat any cancer with currently available drugs.

This is truly the challenge of precision medicine. It is a challenge that can only be met with a new generation of AI systems that can (i) prospectively plan individualized treatment regimens to optimize individual outcomes; (ii) continuously learn from each patient's results; and (iii) coordinate treatments across all patients to maximize collective (system-wide) learning. Such systems will need to integrate vast amounts of data and knowledge from many sources, enable distributed expert hypothesis generation and testing, and assist with information retrieval, outcomes assessment, and data analysis. This 'Learning Health System' framework was dubbed 'Precision Oncology 3.0' by Schrager and Tenenbaum [33]. It has been nearly a decade since this problem and suggested AI-based solution were proposed. An early implementation is being piloted in the form of an Institutional Review Board–approved observational registry trial called XCELSIOR [32].

Going forward, systems that are capable of continuously learning from medical practice will require the full complement of AI learning approaches, from transfer learning and few-shot learning models to active learning and causal inference. We expect ensembles of learning and information-collection techniques will be required. At many steps, the system will need to fall back on human expertise and human–machine cooperative problem solving. Such systems will require an openness to innovation in medicine, a willingness to prioritize transparency, and no small amount of legal and regulatory innovation. In return, they can drive transformational changes in healthcare. By continuously learning from every patient, learning health systems will eliminate the barriers between clinical research and clinical care, thereby both improving outcomes and accelerating the development of promising therapies. By codifying the collective knowledge of experts and tumour boards, and making it available at the point of care through decision-support apps, these systems will help eliminate the gaping disparities in knowledge and outcomes that exist among academic medical centres and community hospitals and physicians, especially those in rural, disadvantaged, and developing-country communities.

46.9 Future Directions

46.9.1 Implications for Clinical Medicine

The pace of change in AI outside of medicine has been extraordinary. In many cases this has been invisible to consumers, but AI is infused into almost every electronic device or software with which we interact. AI will become deeply integrated into medicine for two main reasons. The first is that medicine is a field that is heavily dependent on electronic technology, and AI can improve software and systems in well-established ways. The second, perhaps less obvious driver is that medicine is highly subject to what economists call Baumol's disease. The example that Baumol gave was that it still takes the same number of people and the same amount of time to play a Beethoven string quartet as it did 200 years ago, but it costs a great deal more money.

In reflecting on the state of medicine, outcomes have improved but costs have increased dramatically. Physicians continue to see an average of about 20 patients per day, a number that has not changed much in decades. Instead, medicine has seen a growth in mid-level practitioners and technical personnel. Despite productivity gains in some areas, technology has not led to more medicine at a lower cost. AI systems could help reduce the 20 hours per week that physicians spend on non-patient-facing activities, from scheduling and chart review to researching treatment options.

We envision AI-based intelligent agents that can extend the physician in ways that nurses and medical technicians have in the past: aggregating records and creating a crisp case summary, assembling relevant diagnostic test results and scheduling additional tests if required, flagging issues in the test results, researching prospective treatment options, and monitoring the patient's progress. By supporting such activities, AI agents will help maximize the 15 minutes that each patient has with their physician, and allow good medicine to happen continuously behind the scenes, even when the patient is away from the clinic.

As healthcare moves to precision medicine, the possibilities for AI expand far beyond these basic support services. Imagine basing treatment decisions on outcomes data from every similar patient; predicting therapy response based on deep patient-level simulations (so-called digital twins and in silico clinical trials); or, in equipoise situations, globally coordinating treatment decisions across similar patients to maximize information gain. None of these would be possible without AI. Arguably, precision medicine itself would not be possible without AI.

Such is the potential of AI in the coming decade. AI-powered learning healthcare systems can deliver better outcomes for patients and clinicians, better value for insurers and health plans, and far faster and cheaper clinical studies. However, these potential benefits must be balanced against the potential harms. Algorithms that are hastily developed and deployed can increase disparities in care and, more importantly, cost lives. Everyone involved in healthcare has a responsibility to become knowledgeable about what AI can and cannot achieve.

46.9.2 Concluding Thoughts

We wish to leave the reader armed with a newfound understanding of how AI will be deployed in their clinical practice, as well as the tools and perspectives needed to be a critical evaluator and effective user of those systems. Building safe and effective clinical AI systems is challenging, as we have tried to outline in Figure 46.8. However, the recent speed of innovation in this field has been staggering, even for those pioneers who have been working on AI for more than 50 years. It is the rapid advances against problems thought to be nearly intractable that have been possible with more and better data and computing power, the theoretical and applied improvements in AI algorithms, and the ease of deploying those solutions with accessible software.

Chess or Go	Self-driving cars	Medicine
Closed world	Relatively open world	Open world
Static rules	Mostly static rules	Dynamic rules
Perfect information	Most information available	Partial information
Simulation is trivial	Model-based simulation is possible	Simulation is less reliable with partial information
Experiments are free	Experiments are affordable, but errors can kill	Experiments are expensive, and errors can kill
Feedback is instant	Feedback is instantaneous	Feedback takes years
Data are nearly unlimited	Data are massive	Data are limited and costly

Figure 46.8: Relative comparison of different tasks in which AI solutions have been or are under development. While AI systems have proven superior to human intelligence in perfect information games for 20 years, most medical applications are harder. It is only recently that AI is starting to prove that it is up to handling medical tasks.

Source: Image created by Mark A. Shapiro and Marty Tenenbaum.

We also wish to leave the reader with a sense of the incredible promise of AI in medicine, and the expectation that this technology will be transformative on the practice of medicine during the next decade. Perhaps the most apt parting quote is from Jim Keller, the former head of Tesla's self-driving AI programme, who said, 'Progress disappoints in the short run, [but] surprises in the long run' [34].

Conflicts of Interest

Mark Shapiro is an employee of xCures, Inc., a developer of AI-enabled clinical decision-support software and systems. Marty Tenenbaum is a co-founder of xCures, Inc. The authors have an equity interest in xCures, Inc.

References

1. US Food and Drug Administration. Artificial intelligence and machine learning (AI/ML)-enabled medical devices, 2021. https://www.fda.gov/medical-devices/software-medical-device-samd/artificial-intelligence-and-machine-learning-aiml-enabled-medical-devices.
2. Tupasela A, Di Nucci E. Concordance as evidence in the Watson for Oncology decision-support system. *AI & Society* 2020;35:811–818.
3. Jic Z, Zhiying Z, Li L. A meta-analysis of Watson for Oncology in clinical application. *Scientific Reports* 2021;11(1):5792.
4. Cavallo J. Confronting the criticisms facing Watson for Oncology: a conversation with Nathan Levitan, MD, MBA. *The ASCO Post*, 10 September 2019. https://ascopost.com/issues/september-10-2019/confronting-the-criticisms-facing-watson-for-oncology.

5. Christodoulou E, Ma J, Collins GS et al. A systematic review shows no performance benefit of machine learning over logistic regression for clinical prediction models. *Journal of Clinical Epidemiology* 2019;110:12–22.

6. Makridakis S, Spiliotis E, Assimakopoulos V. Statistical and machine learning forecasting methods: concerns and ways forward. *PLoS One* 2018;13(3):e0194889.

7. Austin PC, Harrell FE, Steyerberg EW. Predictive performance of machine and statistical learning methods: impact of data-generating processes on external validity in the 'large N, small p' setting. *Statistical Methods in Medical Research* 2021;30(6):1465–1483.

For additional references please see `www.wiley.com/go/byrne/aiinclinical medicine`

47

A Glimpse into the Future: AI, Digital Humans, and the Metaverse – Opportunities and Challenges for Life Sciences in Immersive Ecologies

Siddharthan Surveswaran[1] and Lakshmi Deshpande[2]

[1] *Department of Life Sciences, CHRIST (Deemed to be University), Bangalore, India*

[2] *XR Labs, Tata Consultancy Services, Mumbai, India*

47.1 Introduction to the Metaverse

The Metaverse is a three-dimensional (3D), immersive, persistent, and virtual space, featuring digital assets and cryptocurrencies in virtual lands where social collaborations and businesses will flourish. The Metaverse is predominantly extended reality (XR). It is an immersive spectrum encompassing burgeoning technologies – virtual, augmented, and mixed reality (VR, AR, MR); spatial sound and haptics; digital humans; and cryptocurrency using blockchain technology. The co-mingling of physical and virtual interactions is aided by AI and 5G connectivity.

The Metaverse is poised to grow at a rate of over 40% to reach a net revenue of about $1600 billion by 2030 [1]. It will significantly impact every sector: retail and media; banking, financial services, and insurance (BFSI); and healthcare. Cryptocurrencies, non-fungible tokens (NFTs), and virtual lands will be the newer ways in which people will have digital lives. This is very evident when we see that retail giants like Walmart, Nike, Gap, Verizon, and others have invested in virtual land, and have started selling virtual goods in the Metaverse [2]. In addition to social media, virtual properties, and cryptocurrencies, the Metaverse is poised to have a

AI in Clinical Medicine: A Practical Guide for Healthcare Professionals, First Edition. Edited by Michael F. Byrne, Nasim Parsa, Alexandra T. Greenhill, Daljeet Chahal, Omer Ahmad, and Ulas Bagci.

significant impact in life sciences, especially in the healthcare sector. In this chapter, we examine aspects of XR and AI that will play important roles in various areas of life sciences, and discuss the future of life sciences in the Metaverse.

47.2 Digital Humans and Genomic Information

Digital humans are 3D virtual beings that look almost like physical human beings, mimicking human traits such as physical movements, facial expressions, non-verbal cues, and conversational exchange. They are visually rich entities, ready to converse in virtual worlds, a leap ahead of the conversational bots of today. They require:

- AI to process human input and provide responses.
- Natural language processing to comprehend voice commands.
- Natural language generation so that the digital human can respond via voice.
- High-fidelity 3D modelling to accurately imitate facial expressions displaying empathy.

A fascinating progression of a digital human is a digital twin of a human for interactions in the virtual world. XR companies are designing algorithms to generate realistic 3D models, employing deep learning techniques and neural networks [3]. Life science advances, particularly genomics, could provide additional valuable data to generate realistic 3D avatars, though this concept is in its infancy at present.

A genome is defined as a complete set of genes or DNA sequence information of a haploid set of chromosomes of an organism. Genome-wide association studies (GWAS) focus on identifying genomic variants that are statistically associated with the occurrence of a particular trait. A GWAS analyses the genome sequence information of several thousand individuals to look for single-nucleotide polymorphisms (SNPs) that frequently occur in relation to a disease or trait. This analysis uses Big Data analytics involving the entire genome sequence of many individuals to look for millions of genetic variants that manifest as disease outcomes. GWAS have a huge application in the healthcare sector, aiding in the prediction of the susceptibility of an individual to an array of diseases, and predicting the response of individuals to drugs [4]. They show the correlation between a trait and its underlying SNPs, such as height, skin colour, hair colour, eye colour, and some behavioural and personality traits [5]. Thanks to high-throughput parallel sequencing technologies – also known as next-generation sequencing (NGS) – the cost of human genome sequencing can be as low as $1000 per individual genome.

In the Metaverse, digital humans are designed using several data points and genome sequences, which are important data to create lifelike avatars. Personal genomics services, such as 23andMe, generate personal genome sequences for genetic testing and ancestry determination. Recently, a South Korean AR company, in collaboration with Eone Diagnomics (a personalized genome-sequencing company), used genome information from models featured in its VR Asian model festival event [6]. This is a novel application in the virtual world to make realistic avatars by leveraging genetic information.

Combining genomics with AI would potentially permit the creation of a 'true-to-life' virtual being. In the near future, an individual's digital human would be so real that his or her ticking 'genomic clock' would determine the time when they would manifest a genetic disorder in the Metaverse. Potentially, it would then be possible to virtually repair DNA and thus to live longer in the Metaverse. In other words, it would be possible to transcend our mortal life in the Metaverse. Since only genome sequence Big Data along with AI can predict the future using this information, we would need to amend genetic data privacy laws for digital humans to organically thrive in the Metaverse. The implications of this are beyond the reach of this book.

47.2.1 Genomic Data in the Metaverse

Data in the Metaverse are basically decentralized, so that users would carry their digital assets as well as their profile information from one Metaverse to the next. The same will hold true for genomic information, so that a finite amount of vital genetic sequence information in encrypted form will be associated with an individual's digital avatar. This information could be passed on along with the avatar across different Metaverses, where it could be used by that platform's Metaverse requisites based on user permissions. Once in the new Metaverse, the avatar could be tweaked according to the application programming interface (API) of the new Metaverse. Similarly, the genomic information could be upgraded to the avatar based on new genomic sequence paradigms.

47.2.2 Use and Monetization of Genomic Data in the Metaverse

The encrypted genomic information associated with an avatar has numerous use cases. For example, we could consider the concept of 'virtual hospitals'. The avatars of accomplished physicians could treat multiple patients at once in the Metaverse, using the genomic information associated with patient avatars. When a patient's avatar walks into a virtual clinic carrying genomic information, treatment could be provided by AI physicians, and this could help in the treatment of diseases of patients in the real world. In this way, treatment could be given to an infinite number of patients in the virtual world. Digital human physicians are scalable and omnipresent, with no language barriers. Virtual avatars could participate in medical research, providing their encrypted genomic information on a voluntary basis. Users participating in such research could be incentivized to share their genomic identities for research purposes through NFTs or other cryptocurrencies.

Currently, medical research in hospitals is carried out at a local scale with a local demographic, so the results obtained are often biased to a particular race or ethnicity. However, research using virtual avatars that can participate across the globe would yield better and more robust results, as they would represent a wide range of demographics. A wide range of participants who come with their genomic information would be indispensable to the pharmaceutical industry. This would be very helpful, for example, to enable pharmaceutical companies to develop efficient drugs at a much reduced cost. Similarly, drug adverse reactions, drug dosage, and drug responses could be studied on digital twins of real-life patients in the Metaverse – the realm of pharmacogenomics.

47.3 Immortality in the Metaverse

Genome information stored in avatars could be carried on for generations to come, and AI digital avatars could outlive our real selves in the Metaverse. Imagining how your baby will look and behave based on a combination of your genomic identities could be possible with digital avatars. A digital human of a future baby would be possible using AI tools that would take the Metaverse to the next level.

47.4 AI and VR in Drug Discovery

The analysis of the 3D molecular structures of drug candidates is already a powerful drug discovery tool. Target structure analysis including detecting possible binding sites, generating candidate molecules, anticipating interaction sites between the generated molecules with a target, ranking candidate molecules according to their biomolecular affinities, and optimizing molecules for further refinement are all areas where AI-based drug discovery is already employed. Combining technologies like AI, automation, and high-throughput screening will result in much faster drug discovery than is currently achieved.

VR technology is now being used to visualize molecular structures in 3D and at real-life size, to evaluate and refine the interaction of drug candidates and their targets. This permits scientists to understand the binding-pocket interactions where the drug–target interaction takes place, and revise the molecules to modulate the interaction as necessary. All this can be interactive, with different scientists in different physical locations working together in the virtual world. Such technologies are already on the horizon, and a California-based company, Nanome.ai, is a pioneer in this space [7].

47.5 Immersive Environments in Life Sciences

Immersive environments in digital health serve educational, assistive, and therapeutic purposes. On the education front, some start-ups provide digital medical libraries with VR content and surgical training platforms. Health Scholars immerses clinicians in emergency situations to practise rapid responses where caregivers empathize with the patient's condition [8]. Metaverse experiences can also be used by patients to receive or amplify treatments. One value-add of these immersive environments is that they can heighten the intensity of patients' therapeutic experiences. Heightened experiences draw consumers to meditation Metaverses such as DehaVR and Tripp, and highlight AppliedVR's and XRHealth's treatments for chronic pain.

Therapeutic Metaverse environments can scale access to the specialized settings required for certain types of healthcare interventions. For example, Metaverse start-up *OxfordVR* allows patients to try exposure therapy in virtual spaces to address phobias and post-traumatic stress disorder (PTSD). Floreo VR lets children with autism practise behavioural skills in different social contexts, and Luminopia generates digital scenes to treat neuro-visual disorders like amblyopia. We expect to see more Metaverse innovation in clinical areas that rely heavily on interaction with one's environment: developmental disorder support, neurological rehabilitation, and musculoskeletal care, to name a few.

47.6 Digital Twins

Other digital health Metaverse start-ups are creating digital twins: representations of real-world entities (e.g. organs, individuals, patient populations) that exist in virtual worlds and can be manipulated to obtain insights for healthcare decision-making. Digital twins are a form of synthetic data, the broad class of artificially generated information used in place of real-world data. However, unlike other forms of synthetic data, digital twins are modelled on real entities, and are often connected in an ongoing manner to their real-world counterparts. This hybrid connection places digital twins squarely in the Metaverse.

One type of healthcare digital twin is that of organs and muscle groups. Siemens Healthineers is pioneering cardiac digital twins, complex digital simulations that reflect the molecular structure and biological function of the hearts of individual patients. Using cardiac digital twins, doctors can simulate how a patient's heart would respond to medications, surgery, or catheter interventions, before making any real-world decisions. Similarly, Virtonomy builds digital twins of bone and muscle groups to simulate how medical devices or implants might degrade within a patient's body over time [9]. On a larger scale, digital twins can also simulate how populations might respond to disease outbreaks or new drugs, paving the way for clinical trials in the Metaverse. For example, Unlearn incorporates prognostic information from multiple patients' digital twins into randomized controlled studies. As this would reduce the need for intrusive and onsite monitoring, the promise that digital twins hold for longitudinal studies on chronic conditions such as long COVID is intriguing.

Robotics have been used in surgery for some time now. Going forward, complicated surgeries are all set to use augmented realities. Whether it be removal of cancerous tumours or performing a complicated spinal surgery, doctors are looking forward to new ways of performing these surgeries with precision.

47.7 Gamification to Connect and Bring Healthcare Providers and Consumers Together

As platforms like Roblox have changed the way gamification is perceived, more and more users are finding ways to collaborate and connect with other users. Now anyone can imagine, create, or have fun with friends through such platforms.

When it comes to healthcare, gamification is restricted largely to wellness and fitness apps. Augmented reality has been seen in smarter workouts through virtual instructors [10].

47.8 Telemedicine

The use of telemedicine has increased dramatically since the start of the COVID-19 pandemic. The Metaverse will supplement telemedicine visits with a virtual office, where patients and physicians can meet in a 3D clinic or any other location. This is projected to improve the user experience for teleconsultation services significantly. Using VR, the Metaverse in healthcare can enable next-level immersion, by providing a considerably higher sense of 'being there' than other virtual environments like websites, messaging applications, or social media.

47.9 Facilitating Collaboration Among Healthcare Professionals

The ability to immediately share information between healthcare professionals would allow for quicker identification of the underlying causes of illness. Monitoring patient activity in the Metaverse also allows for easier tracking of variables like compliance, which will aid in the diagnosis and treatment of illnesses. Healthcare companies will need to develop a new business model that is connected with patient health insurance and reimbursement bodies, all in this new virtual space. Any limitations will be offset by an essentially boundless user experience, breaking down geographical constraints and creating limitless possibilities for patients all over the world.

47.10 Conclusions

XR, along with AI, will power the new Web 3.0, or its buzzword 'the Metaverse'. The potential applications of XR in the life sciences are immense, and the futuristic ideas in this chapter will soon become a reality. There is huge opportunity in using genomic data along with AI and XR. This will need to be done carefully, thoughtfully, and ethically, but if done in that way, the positive ramifications are very exciting.

References

1. Emergen Research. *Metaverse Market, by Component (Hardware, Software), by Platform (Desktop, Mobile), by Offering (Virtual Platforms, Asset Marketplace, Avatars, and Financial Services), by Technology, by Application, by End-Use, and by Region Forecast to 2030*, April 2022. https://www.emergenresearch.com/industry-report/Metaverse-market.

2. J.P. Morgan. *Opportunities in the Metaverse: How Businesses Can Explore the Metaverse and Navigate the Hype vs. Reality*, 2022. https://www.jpmorgan.com/content/dam/jpm/treasury-services/documents/opportunities-in-the-metaverse.pdf.

3. Chen X, Jiang T, Song J et al. gDNA: towards generative detailed neural avatars. *arXiv*, 13 April 2022. https://doi.org/10.48550/arXiv.2201.04123.

4. Cano-Gamez E, Trynka G. From GWAS to function: using functional genomics to identify the mechanisms underlying complex diseases. *Frontiers in Genetics* 13 May 2020. https://doi.org/10.3389/fgene.2020.00424.

5. Mick E, McGough J, Deutsch CK et al. Genome-wide association study of proneness to anger. *PLoS One* 2014;9(1):e87257. https://doi.org/10.1371/journal.pone.0087257.

6. Choi J-W. Asian models' genes to be used to create metaverse characters. *Korea Times*, 11 January 2022. https://www.koreatimes.co.kr/www/art/2022/04/398_322088.html.

7. Nanome. https://nanome.ai.

For additional references please see www.wiley.com/go/byrne/aiinclinicalmedicine

Index

AI in Clinical Medicine: A Practical Guide for Healthcare Professionals, First Edition. Edited by Michael F. Byrne, Nasim Parsa, Alexandra T. Greenhill, Daljeet Chahal, Omer Ahmad, and Ulas Bagci.
© 2023 John Wiley & Sons Ltd. Published 2023 by John Wiley & Sons Ltd.
Companion website: www.wiley.com/go/byrne/aiinclinicalmedicine